CARE PLANS LISTED ACCORDING TO BEHAVIORAL CONCERNS

D1515545

KEY TO ESSENTIAL TERMINOLOGY

CLIENT ASSESSMENT DATA BASE:

Provides an overview of the more commonly occurring etiology and co-existing factors associated with a specific psychiatric diagnosis as well as the corresponding abnormal diagnostic findings and signs/symptoms.

NURSING PRIORITIES:

Establishes a general ranking of needs/concerns upon which the Nursing Diagnoses are ordered. In actual care plan construction, this ranking would be altered according to the individual client situation.

DISCHARGE CRITERIA

Identifies generalized statements which could be developed into short-term and intermediate goals to be achieved by the client before being "discharged" from nursing care. They may also provide guidance for creating long-term goals for the client to work on after discharge.

NURSING DIAGNOSES:

The general problem/concern (Diagnosis) is stated without the distinct etiology and signs/symptoms which would be added to create a client problem statement when specific client information is available. For example: when a client develops increased tension, apprehension, quivering voice, focus on self, the nursing diagnosis of Anxiety could be stated "Anxiety, Severe, related to unconscious conflict, threat to self-concept as evidenced by statements of increased tension, apprehension, observation of quivering voice, focus on self." In addition, diagnoses which have been identified within these care plan guides as actual or potential may be changed/deleted or diagnoses may be added, dependent on specific client information.

MAY BE RELATED TO/POSSIBLY EVIDENCED BY:

Lists the usual/common reasons (etiology) why a particular problem may occur and the probable signs/symptoms which would be used to create the "related to" and "evidenced by" portions of the client problem statement when the specific client situation is known.

CLIENT OUTCOMES/EVALUATION CRITERIA:

These give direction to client care as they identify what the client/nurse hope to achieve. They are stated in general terms in this book to permit the practitioner to modify/individualize them by adding time lines and individual client criteria so they become "measurable," e.g., "Client appears relaxed and reports anxiety is reduced to a manageable level within 24 hours."

INTERVENTIONS:

Divided into independent and collaborative, interventions are ranked only by most to least common. When creating the individual care plan, these interventions would normally be reordered to reflect the client's specific needs/situation. In addition, the division of independent/collaborative is arbitrary and is actually dependent on the individual nurse's capabilities and hospital/community standards.

RATIONALE:

Although not commonly appearing in client care plans, rationale has been included here to provide a psychiatric and pathophysiological basis to assist the nurse in deciding about the relevance of a specific intervention for an individual client situation.

PSYCHIATRIC CARE PLANS
Guidelines for Client Care

Marilynn E. Doenges, M.A., R.N., C.S.

Clinical Specialist
Adult Psychiatric/Mental Health Nursing
Private Practice
Colorado Springs, Colorado

Mary C. Townsend, R.N., M.N.

Nurse Specialist and Clinical Instructor
Psychiatric/Mental Health Nursing
Wichita, Kansas

Mary Frances Moorhouse, R.N., C.C.P., CCRN

Consultant and Contract Practitioner
Critical Care
Colorado Springs, Colorado

 F. A. DAVIS COMPANY • PHILADELPHIA

Library of Congress Cataloging-in-Publication Data

Doenges, Marilynn E., 1922-
   Psychiatric care plans.

   Bibliography: p.
   Includes index.
   1. Psychiatric nursing—Handbooks, manuals, etc.
I. Moorhouse, Mary Frances, 1947-   .   II. Townsend, Mary C., 1941-   III. Title.   [DNLM:
1. Nursing Assessment—handbooks.   2. Patient Care Planning—handbooks.   3. Psychiatric Nursing
—handbooks.
WY 39 D651p]
RC440.D64   1988   610.73′68   88-11825
ISBN 0-8036-2672-X

DEDICATION

We dedicate this book to ourselves: our own intestinal fortitude, our unfailing optimism, our dogged perseverance, and our own increasing conviction in the value of Nursing Diagnosis and the future of the profession of nursing.

Special thanks to:

our families, the Doenges' and Daigle's, the Moorhouse's, and the Townsend's, who have continued to support our dreams, fantasies, and obsessions;

our colleagues, who continue to provide a sounding board and feedback for our professional beliefs and expectations.

Kudos to the F. A. Davis staff, Robert Martone, Ruth DeGeorge, who have shown great patience and helped maintain our sanity (or contributed to our insanity), and to Herb Powell who facilitated the review process to get this project completed in a timely fashion.

Lastly, to the nurses who have patiently awaited this book, we hope it will help in applying theory to practice and enhance the delivery and effectiveness of your care.

PREFACE

This book is primarily designed to meet the needs of nurses in the psychiatric setting (hospital, clinic, private practice) who are using the nursing process to identify client needs. A holistic/humanistic focus is presented in which the nurse serves as advocate for the client. Care Plans are formulated using nursing diagnoses with interventions and rationale based on current scientific premises. They encompass psychosocial/psychodynamic concepts and have been organized according to psychiatric diagnoses as listed in the Diagnostic and Statistical Manual of Mental Disorders, Third Edition-Revised (DSM III-R). ANA standards are used as a basis for the nursing process and development of care plans which serve as a guide to the therapeutic nurse/client relationship.

Chapter 1 examines current issues and their implications for the nurse caring for the client and family who are experiencing emotional difficulties. An overview of cultural, community, sociological, and ethical concepts impacting on the nurse in a variety of health care settings is included. The need for cooperation and coordination with other health care professionals is an important concept which is highlighted.

Chapter 2 reviews the use of nursing process as it applies to therapeutic interventions for all nurses in whatever setting they may encounter individuals with psychiatric diagnoses and/or experiencing emotional stresses/disorders. Nursing Diagnosis, as proposed by the North American Nursing Diagnosis Association (NANDA), is discussed to provide the nurse with an understanding of its application in the psychiatric setting. The use and adaptation of the care plan guides presented in this book are discussed. An assessment tool to assist the nurse to identify appropriate nursing diagnoses and a sample care plan based on a client situation are also included.

Chapters 3 through 15 apply the nursing process in developing care plans for specific psychiatric diagnoses using nursing diagnoses to identify individual client needs in acute care as well as community settings. Psychodynamic concepts are identified in the rationale as it relates to nursing actions appropriate to the nursing diagnosis.

The client data base for each care plan includes information gathered from the nursing history, physical findings, and laboratory data from which nursing priorities are established. A decision-making model is used to organize and prioritize nursing interventions based on the nurse acting independently or collaboratively within the health team. Discharge criteria guidelines are included for each care plan to assist in determining what might be appropriate for the individual client and the setting.

This book is designed to be a ready reference for the practicing nurse as a catalyst for thought in planning and evaluating care of the client experiencing emotional turmoil. Students will find the care plans helpful as they learn and develop skills for using nursing process and nursing diagnosis in the psychiatric setting.

M.E.D.
M.C.T.
M.F.M.

CONTRIBUTORS

ANDERSON, ALICE Y, CAPTAIN (P), AN, BSN, MSN
Head Nurse, Inpatient Psychiatry
Tripler Army Medical Center
Tripler AMC, Hawaii

BEAM, IDA MARLENE, BSN
Retired, Army Nurse Corps
Private Home Respite Care
Colorado Springs, Colorado

BOTKIN, PAULETTE, RN
Institute of Forensic Psychiatry
Colorado State Hospital
Pueblo, Colorado

BUFFUM, MARTI DAVIS, RN, MS
Nursing Faculty/Lecturer, San Francisco State
  University
Staff Nurse III, Inpatient Psychiatry, Marin General
  Hospital
Greenbrae, California
Private Practice, Clinical Specialist
San Anselmo, California

CANTIN, WM G., Lt, NC, USN
Consultant/Liaison Nurse
Alcohol Rehabilitation Facility
Tripler Army Medical Center, Hawaii

CARSON, VERNA, RN, MS, DOCTORAL CANDIDATE
Assistant Professor in Psychiatric/Community
  Health Nursing
University of Maryland School of Nursing
Baltimore, Maryland

DUNCANSON, KATHLEEN K, BSN, CRRN, CRC
Senior Rehabilitation Specialist
Intracorp
Woodland Park, Colorado

GEISER, ROSEMARIE, RN, MSN, CS
Clinical Nurse Specialist, Adult Psychiatry
Palo Alto Veterans Administration Medical Center
Menlo Park Division
Palo Alto, California

HUGHES, MARYANNIE LEWIS, MSN, BSN, RN, CS
Captain, U.S. Army Nurse Corps
Clinical Head Nurse
Clinical Specialist at Tri-Services Alcoholism Recovery
  Facility (TRI-SARF)
Tripler Army Medical Center, Hawaii
Nurse Recruiter-Counselor
Ft. Sheridan, Illinois

LANGE, NOLA, BSN, MA
Contract Practitioner
Colorado Springs, Colorado

McCOMB, MARGARET D, RN, MN, CS
Clinical Specialist for Nursing Process
Nursing Quality Assurance Coordinator
Veterans Administration Medical Center
Portland, Oregon

MEIDER, JILL G, MS, RN, CS
Clinical Specialist Child/Adolescent Psychiatric Nurse
N.E.E.D. Foundation Day Treatment Program and
  Mental Health Clinic
Colorado Springs, Colorado

MULLANEY, JOANNE BARNES, RN, PhD
Associate Professor
Salve Regina College
Newport, Rhode Island

PETERSON, EARLENE, RNC, BSN
Ob/Gyn Nurse Practitioner
Academy Women's Clinic
Colorado Springs, Colorado

RYNIER, LEANN G, RN, BSN Ed, M.Ed
Patient Care Education Specialist
Philhaven Hospital
Mount Gretna, Pennsylvania

LEDERACH, NAOMI K, RN, BSN, MN
Director of Education
Philhaven Hospital
Mount Gretna, Pennsylvania

REVIEWER/RESEARCHER

LANGE, NOLA, BSN, MA
Contract Practitioner
Colorado Springs, Colorado

REVIEWERS

BRICKER, PAM, RNC
Unit Coordinator
Cedar Springs Psychiatric Hospital
Colorado Springs, Colorado

CARTER, NANCY LEA, RN, BSN, MA
Hospital Nursing & Management
Counseling of Children
Child Care Provider
Albuquerque, New Mexico

DANNEWITZ, KAREN, RN, MS, CS
Private Practice, Consultant
Colorado Springs, Colorado

JIMERSON, SUZANNE SAYLE, RN, MS, CS
Clinical Specialist in Adult/Family Psychiatric Nursing
Dover, Massachusetts

THOMAS, BARBARA E, RN, BSN, C.
Coordinator of Partial Hospitalization and
   Specialty Groups
Cedar Springs Psychiatric Hospital
Colorado Springs, Colorado

SPECIAL THANKS TO

DAVID U. CASTER, M.D., F.A.P.A.
Psychiatrist
Colorado Springs, Colorado

CONTENTS

xiv

ISSUES AND TRENDS IN PSYCHIATRIC NURSING

Within the past century, psychiatry has begun to emerge from behind the veil of mystery and superstition. The two most significant factors in bringing psychiatric care to the arena of scientific study and therapeutic modalities are the work of Sigmund Freud and the advent of psychotropic drugs. Although there now are many theories and techniques of communication therapies, Freud was most responsible for establishing communication as therapy and for studying mental and emotional dysfunction in a scientific manner.

Psychotropic drugs, many of which have only been available since 1955, have made it possible to control symptoms of psychiatric illnesses. The major tranquilizers (phenothiazines) are used as therapy by themselves and as a means of enabling the client to benefit from other therapies and live as normal a life as possible.

Current Treatment

In spite of these advances, much of psychiatry is still veiled in mystery. True scientific study of the relationship between therapy and change in human behavior is difficult at best. However, the etiology of many disorders is still unknown or only partly understood. Biomedical research has greatly increased in recent years with ongoing research into the biologic and psychologic bases for mental illness. Intervention is still based on theory and on the personality and "style" of the therapist. Although theoretical approaches are many and varied, e.g., psychoanalytic, family systems, and behavioral, there are three basic forms of treatment in use today. These are (1) the use of drugs (neuropsychopharmacology), (2) conditioning or behavior modification and (3) communication therapies.

Today there are many economic and social factors that influence the care given psychiatric clients. Psychiatric nursing has also been changing in many ways. Nurses no longer give only long-term custodial care. They are qualified and expected to participate in therapy, including group therapy. The role of the nurse in administration of medications has expanded to include discussions of side effects and expected therapeutic results to assist clients in making informed choices about their care.

Financial Considerations

The need to provide an economic base for long-term, treatment-oriented psychiatric care remains a challenge for the health care system. Medical costs are skyrocketing, and there is a strong push to economize in all areas. A major step in cost-cutting was the passage by Congress of prospective payment by DRGs (diagnostic related groups), in which Medicare reimburses a predetermined amount for hospitalization for each admission diagnosis. While DRGs are an option in psychiatry at this time, there are strong indications that this will one day be the method of reimbursement for all health care. Already, other third-party payers are using these criteria for establishing payment.

This trend tells us, as health care providers, that psychiatric nurses need to develop new methods of providing effective client care. Goal-oriented, time-limited interventions are necessary if we are to continue to provide quality mental health care to our clients. The nursing process as a model for problem-solving can be used to achieve this goal. Development of nursing diagnoses has provided impetus to more effective care-planning and documentation, providing a framework for systematic nursing care based on scientific knowledge.

Historical Factors

Within the last 20 to 30 years, there has been a movement to release chronically ill clients from state hospitals and other mental health institutions. The reason for this was partially economic. It is expensive to keep people institutionalized and unproductive in large hospital settings. Another reason was a growing awareness of the civil rights of the individual and a belief that the rights of the chronic psychiatric client were being violated. Changes in treatment made it possible to begin to look at what could be done to help this population become more self-sufficient, contributing members of society. Clinics, day treatment programs, and other alternate facilities have been established in an attempt to meet these goals. A major concern, however, is that these community facilities have not been sufficient to meet the increasing need for mental health treatment and care.

Cultural Impact

The result of these changes has been a dramatic reduction in the number of long-term clients in institutions. However, new problems have been created and the system has failed to care adequately for the clients who have been returned to their community. The decrease in cost of care is dubious since many nonfunctional or borderline individuals have been released only to become dependent on other community agencies and/or wander the streets.

Care providers find themselves working with persons who have difficulty or cannot adapt to society as self-sufficient members, either because of chronic illness or because of long-term institutionalization. Nurses are challenged to assist these clients to reach realistic goals with a minimum of dependency on community resources.

Concern for civil rights has also had an impact on involuntary commitment. It must be demonstrated that a person poses a danger to self/others and/or the community before legal commitment to an institution can be accomplished. While this protects the individual against unjust confinement, there seems to be little recourse for families of disturbed persons who will not voluntarily seek treatment. Inevitably, some people who would greatly benefit receive no treatment and, without adequate care, join the chronically psychotic or nonfunctional clients in board-and-care facilities or other community agencies. Others fade into the anonymity of "street" or "bag" people subsisting by whatever means possible. Occasionally much publicity is given to the infrequent client who commits violent acts after having been discharged from the psychiatric system, creating fear and anger among the general populace with an accompanying demand for tighter controls.

Ours is an aging society. More and more people are reaching middle and late years. An increasing awareness of midlife crises and the emotional impact that it has on the individual has encouraged more people to seek help with the problems which may be created at this time. More individuals are willing to disrupt their lives to seek "happiness" and "find themselves." As a person ages, many losses occur, e.g., job, loved ones, health, and ability fo function (sexually and otherwise), and often the individual's self-image suffers. Chronic depression and substance abuse are increasing problems in the older population. There is also an increase of suicide in this neglected segment of our society, as depression may go unnoticed simply because no one pays attention. Nurses are in an excellent position to detect these problems and initiate goal-setting and treatment referrals with the elderly. In the past, goals for the elderly were not given much consideration because of limited life expectancy. Obviously, this view is quite short-sighted and clearly discriminating. With this awareness comes a need for more programs to meet these needs.

On the other end of the spectrum, children's and adolescents' psychiatric needs are growing and requiring expansion of facilities and programs. More recognition is being given to the reality that delinquent youngsters are very often troubled and may in fact be mentally ill. While facilities and programs specifically designed for children and/or adolescents are becoming more available, there is still a reluctance to acknowledge the reality of mental illness, substance abuse, and suicide in young people.

Substance Abuse

Substance abuse has come full force to national and worldwide attention. Society's awareness of this problem has brought both legal and therapeutic means of solving it to the forefront. Very specific modalities have been developed to work with the addicted client. Psychiatric nurses need awareness of the specific concerns of the substance abuser related to chemical imbalances, as well as the unique problems and needs of the individual. Although recognition of the effect on the family, as well as issues of co-dependence, is resulting in more effective methods of treatment, many of the needs related to therapy for addicted individuals remain unfulfilled.

Suicide

As noted, suicide is on the increase. The statistical rise may be due in part to the identification of some deaths as suicide that formerly may have been labeled accidental. With an alarming rise in the incidence of suicide among children, adolescents and the elderly, specific interventions are necessary in determining what kinds of preventive actions can be helpful. The nurse is often in a position to recognize the potential for suicide in the client and take effective action.

Stress

An increased awareness of the effects of stress on our lives is emerging. Of special interest is the influence of stress in the development of many psychologic problems. Manifestations of stress, e.g., ulcers, asthma, and perhaps any or all of the physical illnesses humans experience, have also been acknowledged. While many psychiatric treatment modalities, e.g., biofeedback, relaxation skills, and guided imagery, are directed at stress reduction/management, it is often a neglected area for the client with physical illness.

In psychiatry, the phenomenon of delayed stress reactions (the belated response of victims to violence or chronic deprivation) is being given more attention. This is now recognized as a significant cause of many disorders which may appear years after the occurrence of the stressor.

Societal changes, such as increased divorce rates resulting in stepfamilies and single-parent homes, create problems which demand new and creative approaches to treatment. Fathers are taking on more child-rearing responsibilities, and mothers are combining careers with homemaking. Increased mobility of individuals often results in the lack of extended family available for role-modeling and assistance, leaving nuclear families vulnerable to added stress. With the wide use of television, rapid travel, and the opening of third world countries to the West, our world is shrinking, and what happens in one area affects and influences all other areas. At the same time, space travel with its concomitant scientific discoveries has expanded our knowledge base and influenced the medical care system.

Nursing

New developments and changes in the nursing profession are impacting the psychiatric nursing field. One of these changes is the development and implementation of nursing diagnoses, which is making the use of care plans for documentation more efficient. Identification of specific problems and determination of individual interventions necessary for reaching timely goals have enhanced the care-planning process. Independent roles for the nurse, such as private practice and liaison/consultant positions in institutions/community settings, are impacting how health (psychiatric) care is delivered. Nursing involvement in the interdisciplinary team approach to psychiatric care is more frequently acknowledged. The nurse requires greater clinical expertise, maturity, critical thinking ability, assertiveness, and client management skills to meet these needs. More recognition is being given to the need for the client to be an active participant in the therapeutic process. Nurses enter into therapeutic relationships with clients, which become the cornerstone of quality care. Assessments are made, nursing diagnoses identified, and nursing care is implemented and evaluated with the active involvement of the client.

Psychiatric nursing is a specialized area of nursing which uses theories of human behavior as its science and the purposeful use of self as its art. Nursing organizations, such as the American Nurses Association (ANA), have established programs to credential nurses, e.g., Clinical Specialist in Psychiatric/Mental Health Nursing. These specialty certification programs share common goals: to provide consumer protection, to enhance nursing knowledge and competency, to increase nursing autonomy, and to strengthen collaboration. Specialty certification will take on more importance in this cost-conscious era as managers seek to hire competent professionals.

As health care delivery becomes more complex and more economically centered, the need for communication and collaboration among health care professionals is intensified. Collaboration between the medical professionals of different departments/services/facilities enhances efficient and comprehensive care. The therapeutic relationship with the client provides a milieu in which the art of nursing can be practiced. The nurse, as the primary coordinator of overall client care, strives to assure that the client receives quality but cost-effective care. The care plan serves as the vehicle for/and documentation of this ongoing communication among nurses and other disciplines. Client care conferences provide a forum for communication and collaboration with other disciplines.

Care-planning provides a means to increase nursing knowledge and enhance practice. Standardized care plans establish priorities of care and define minimum standards of safe practice. They also serve as "memory joggers" to nurses caring for clients not usually seen in their area of clinical practice by providing information and promoting safe, effective care. Conversely, standardized care plans are not intended to be all-inclusive. Nursing judgment is required to individualize the care plan for each specific client. Care plans also provide an outline for documentation of the care which has been given and how the client responded to that care.

Computerization

Many nurses believe that their limited time can be better spent with the client, giving care, rather than generating written care plans. Institutions using computerized care-planning report increased numbers of care plans being generated and maintained than occurred previous to computerization (Lombard and Light, 1983). Computerization can decrease time spent in generating and maintaining care plans and may improve the quality of record-keeping, as nurses may quickly enter, display, evaluate, update, and print a care plan.

Most computerized systems use standardized client care plans, with many using the nursing diagnoses accepted for testing by the North American Nursing Diagnosis Association (NANDA). These basic care plans reflect standards of care for particular client problems and are designed to meet specific needs. Since the plans reflect a wealth of varied nursing experience, they allow even novice practitioners to formulate effective care strategies. These computerized care plans can provide psychiatric nurses with an efficient means to develop comprehensive, continuous, individualized, and legible care plans for each client.

Conclusion

With these rapid changes affecting the health care system, nurses need resources to help them stay current and provide quality care for their clients. Efficient and effective use of the client care plan helps ensure that the psychiatric client receives individualized quality care in the midst of cost containment. It also provides documentation of the impact of nursing on client care. This book is designed to assist the psychiatric nurse in planning and delivering this care to the client in the hospital and/or community setting. The care plans provide a means of identifying nursing diagnosis for many of the most common psychiatric conditions the nurse/student deals with in daily practice.

CHAPTER 2

NURSING PROCESS: PLANNING CARE WITH NURSING DIAGNOSIS

There is a growing awareness that nursing care is a key factor in client survival and in the maintenance, rehabilitative, and preventive aspects of health care. Publication of the American Nurses Association Social Policy Statement (1980), defining nursing as the diagnosis and treatment of human responses to actual and potential health problems, in combination with the ANA Standards of Practice, have provided impetus and support for the use of nursing diagnosis in the practice setting. Prospective payment plans, movement from acute care (hospital) to community settings (mental health centers, group homes/foster care), and other changes in the health care system are highlighting the need for a common framework of communication and documentation. This can promote continuity of care for the client who moves from one area of the health care system to another. Evaluation and documentation of care are an important part of this process.

Nurses have visionary ideas for delivery of quality care to all clients. Often, turning those ideas into action becomes a frustrating exercise in futility, as what appears easy to do in theory becomes difficult in practice. In a hectic schedule, many nurses believe that time spent in writing care plans is time taken away from client care. In reality, the delivery of quality care involves planning and coordination. It is our belief that, as the nurse works with nursing diagnosis, learning the etiology and defining characteristics, goals become apparent and interventions for attaining these goals become clear. Care plans, properly written and utilized, provide tools for client care assessment, guidelines for documentation, and direction for continuity of care among nurses and other caregivers.

Nursing Process

The term Nursing Process was introduced in the 1950s, but it has taken many years to develop national acceptance of the process as an integral part of nursing care. It is adapted from the scientific approach to problem-solving and requires the skills of: (1) assessment (systematic collection of data relating to clients and their problems), (2) problem identification (analysis/interpretation of data), (3) planning (choice of solutions), (4) implementation (putting the plan into action), and (5) evaluation (assessing the effectiveness of the plan and changing the plan as indicated by the current needs). While nurses use these terms separately, in reality they are interrelated and form a continuous circle of thought and action, providing an efficient method of organizing thought processes for clinical decision-making. Nursing process is now included in the conceptual framework of most nursing curricula and accepted in the legal definition of nursing in most nurse practice acts.

To use this process, the nurse must demonstrate fundamental abilities of knowledge, intelligence, and creativity, as well as expertise in interpersonal and technical skills. Some *critical assumptions* for the nurse to consider in the decision-making process are that:
- the client is a human being with worth and dignity;
- there are basic human needs which must be met. When they are not, problems arise requiring interventions by another person until the individual can resume responsibility for self;

- the client has a right to quality health and nursing care delivered with concern, compassion, and competence; focusing on wellness, prevention, and restoration;
- the therapeutic nurse-client relationship is a critical element in this process.

Nursing Diagnosis

Nurses have struggled for years to define nursing by identifying its parameters with a goal of attaining/verifying professional status. To this end, nurses have been meeting and conducting research to develop nursing diagnosis. While there are differing definitions of nursing diagnosis, we have chosen to use Shoemaker's, taken from the *Classification of Nursing Diagnosis, Proceedings of the Fifth National Conference* (Kim, et al, 1984): "Nursing diagnosis is a clinical judgment about an individual, family, or community which is derived through a deliberate, systematic process of data collection and analysis. It provides the basis for prescriptions for definitive therapy for which the nurse is accountable. It is expressed concisely and it includes the etiology of the condition when known."

Nursing diagnosis provides a framework for using the nursing process and is the crux of the nursing care plan, focusing attention on client needs/responses and serving as the prime determinant of the style of nursing care to be delivered. Nursing actions have often been based on variables, such as signs and symptoms, tests, and medical diagnosis. Accurate diagnosis of a client problem can become a standard for nursing practice, understood by all who are using the plan of care, and thus can lead to improved delivery of care. The nursing diagnosis is as precise as the data will allow. It communicates the client's situation at the present time and reflects changes as they occur. It is necessary to seek, incorporate, and synthesize all the relevant data and make the statement meaningful so as to provide direction for nursing care.

The affective tone of the nursing diagnosis can shape expectations of the client's response and influence the nurse's behavior toward the client. For instance, if the nurse sees the client as noncompliant, the nurse's attitudes and behavior may reflect anger and mistrust, and judgmental decisions may be made which do not accurately treat the client's problem. In addition, the nurse needs to be aware of biases which may interfere with reaching an accurate diagnosis. Keeping an open mind to numerous possibilities and not getting stuck on a single symptom/thought will facilitate this process. For example, as cues are identified, e.g., restlessness, an inference may be made by the nurse that the client is anxious. If the nurse assumes that this is only psychological, the possibility that it may be physiologically based may be overlooked.

Nursing diagnosis provides a common language for identifying client problems, nursing interventions, and evaluation tools. This common language is important for several reasons. It promotes communication between nurses, shifts, units, alternate care settings, and other health care professionals. It provides a base for clinicians, educators, and researchers to document, validate, and/or alter the nursing process.

Care Planning

Medicine, nursing, and other health disciplines are interrelated with implications for each other. This interrelationship should include the exchange of data, sharing of ideas or thoughts, and development of plans of care which include all data pertinent to the individual client/family.

The written care plan communicates the past and present status and needs of the client to all members of the health care team. It identifies problems solved and those yet to be solved, approaches that have been successful, and patterns of client responses. It provides a mechanism to help assure continuity of care. It can document client care in areas of accountability, quality assurance, and liability.

The care plan should contain more than actions initiated by medical orders. The use of care plans reflecting only functional divisions of tasks/duties perpetuates the notion that care plans are "busy work," unrelated to caregiving. It needs to contain the written coordination of care given by all disciplines. The nurse becomes the person responsible for coordinating these different activities into a functional plan necessary to provide holistic care for the client. Independent nursing actions are an integral part of this process. Interdependent/collaborative actions are based on the medical regimen, as well as suggestions and orders from other disciplines involved with the care of the client. Restructuring care plans using "nursing models" can increase usage and provide succinct documentation/relevance, demonstrating the relationship between planning and documentation.

In the past, nurses believed that since no two clients are identical, no two care plans could be alike. Therefore, care plans were formulated from the beginning for each client. An awareness evolved that this approach was not practical or cost-effective, as the information and interventions documented were frequently repeated from one care plan to the next. Nurses recognized that although clients are, in fact, individual and have many differences, they also have many common characteristics, needs, and problems. Therefore, today's approach to the use of the nursing process is to consider similarities as well as differences among clients.

Standardized care plans or care plan guides are a method of responding to these similar problems and needs, which can then be modified to meet individual differences.

Care Plan Components

The format for each care plan presented consists of the **Client Assessment Data Base** constructed from information obtained from the **History, Physical Examination,** and **Diagnostic Studies. Nursing Priorities** are then determined/ranked and **Discharge Criteria** identified. The priorities in this book are a general ranking system for the nursing diagnoses in the care plan and, along with the discharge criteria, can be reorganized with time lines according to the individual client/situation to create short/long-term goals. The choice of a **Nursing Diagnosis** is supported by criteria that identify possible cause ("related to") and defining characteristics ("evidenced by"). **Client Outcomes/Evaluation Criteria** for each problem area/diagnosis are identified. Appropriate independent and collaborative interventions with accompanying rationales follow.

Care plan construction begins with the collection of data (assessment). The **History** consists of subjective and objective information encompassing the various concerns reflected in the 1986 list of Nursing Diagnoses (NANDA). Subjective data are those which are reported by the client and significant other(s). This information includes the client's perceptions—what the client wants to share. It is important to accept what is reported, as the client is the "expert" in this area, but the nurse needs to note incongruencies/dissonances which may indicate the presence of other factors, such as lack of knowledge, myths/misconceptions, and/or fear.

Objective data are those which are observed or described (quantitatively or qualitatively) and are verified by others. They include results of the **Physical Examination** and **Diagnostic Testing** (including psychological findings). Evaluation of both subjective and objective data leads to the identification of problems or areas of concern/need. These problems/needs are expressed as nursing diagnoses (Table 2-1).

The key to accurate nursing diagnosis is problem identification which focuses attention on a current/potential physical or behavioral response that interferes with the client's accustomed or desired quality of life. It deals with concerns of the client, significant other(s), and/or nurse, which require nursing intervention and management. In this text the choice of individual nursing diagnosis is validated by the **Related to/Evidenced by** statements which reflect the etiology and defining characteristics most consistent with a specific psychiatric situation.

Nurses may feel at risk in committing themselves to documenting a nursing diagnosis. However, many references are currently available to aid in identifying and formulating the problem statement. In addition, unlike medical diagnoses, nursing diagnoses change as the client progresses through various stages of illness/maladaptation to problem resolution. From the specific information obtained in the **Client Assessment Data Base,** the etiology and signs/symptoms can be identified and an individualized client problem/diagnostic statement formulated. For example, a client may complain of "feelings of worthlessness and inability to make decisions," leading to a choice of the nursing diagnosis: Self-concept, disturbance in: Self-esteem related to the client's belief that the decisions the client makes are not satisfactory and evidenced by client questioning of others "Do you think that's right?"

Goal statements/outcomes are then formulated to give direction to nursing care. These **Client Outcomes/Evaluation Criteria** emerge from the diagnostic statement and are what the client/nurse hopes to achieve. They have been stated in general terms in this book to permit the practitioner to modify/individualize them by adding time lines, considerations of client circumstances and needs, and other specifics. When identified, the terminology needs to be concise, realistic, measurable, and stated in words the client/reader can understand. Beginning the goal statement with an action verb (for example, "verbalizes an increased sense of self-worth") provides direction that is measurable. It is important that multidisciplinary goals do not conflict.

Interventions communicate actions to be taken to achieve desired client outcomes. Again using an action verb, e.g., "assess," provides direction for the nurse. The rationale for interventions needs to be sound and feasible with the intention of providing individualized care. Actions may be independent or collaborative and encompass orders from nursing, medicine, and other disciplines. In this book, collaborative actions in conjunction with other disciplines are identified to assist the nurse in choosing appropriate interventions for the individual/ setting. The educational background/expertise of the nurse, standing protocols, and areas of practice (rural/urban, acute/community care settings) can influence whether an individual intervention is actually an independent nursing function or requires collaboration.

The nurse should plan care with the client when possible, as both are accountable for that care and for achieving the desired goals. The written interventions which guide client care need to be dated and signed to identify the person who is initiating and coordinating the care.

This book is intended to facilitate the application of the nursing process for the psychiatric client and family/ significant other(s). Each care plan is intended to be an informational guide so that the individual practitioner will need to modify/extract only that information that is pertinent to the specific client situation. In addition, a psychiatric assessment tool with data collection organized according to Diagnostic Divisions (Table 2-2) has been included to assist the nurse in identification of nursing diagnoses. A client situation and sample care plan to illustrate this process are also provided at the end of this chapter.

In summary, the authors believe that any nursing diagnosis can be actual or potential, and although this issue has not been resolved by NANDA, it has been used in this manner in this book. Recognizing that the current NANDA list of diagnoses is not comprehensive, nurses need to use the accepted diagnoses on a daily basis to become familiar with their parameters and validate their usefulness, identifying strengths and deficiencies. As noted, with few exceptions, we have presented NANDA's recommendations as formulated by the Conferences. Brackets indicate additions/changes the authors have made to clarify/enhance the accepted nursing diagnoses, e.g., [Learning Need]. Some diagnoses have been combined for convenience, indicating that two or more factors may be involved, e.g., Coping, Family: Potential for Growth/Ineffective Family: Compromised. It is anticipated that the nurse will choose what is appropriate. Nurses can be creative in working with the standardized format, redefining and sharing interventions as they are used with individual clients. We appreciate that not all diagnoses presented in these care plans may be appropriate for your client/locale, and alternatives should be chosen to meet individual client needs. We support the belief that practicing nurses and researchers need to study, use, and evaluate the diagnoses as presented. As new nursing diagnoses are developed, it is important that the information they encompass is reflected in the data base. The nurse is encouraged to share insights and ideas with the North American Nursing Diagnosis Association (NANDA), St. Louis University School of Nursing, 3525 Caroline Avenue, St. Louis, Missouri 63104.

Psychiatric Assessment/Data Base

The client assessment is the foundation upon which identification of individual needs, responses, and problems are based. To facilitate assessment and diagnosis in the nursing process, a Psychiatric Client Assessment Tool has been constructed using a nursing focus instead of the familiar medical approach of "review of systems."

To achieve this nursing focus, we have grouped the 72 NANDA nursing diagnoses (Table 2-1) into related categories titled **Diagnostic Divisions** (Table 2-2), which reflect a blending of Maslow's Hierarchy of Needs and a self-care philosophy. These divisions serve as the framework or outline for collection of data. The nurse is directed to the appropriate corresponding nursing diagnosis as the client information is recorded.

Since these divisions are based on human responses and needs and not specific "systems," information gathered may occasionally be recorded in more than one area. For this reason, the nurse is encouraged to keep an open mind, pursue leads, and collect as much of the data as is available before choosing the nursing diagnosis that best reflects the client's situation. Once the appropriate nursing diagnosis is identified, appropriate goals and interventions can be established.

Recognizing and reflecting on current changes in the delivery and utilization of health care, and realizing that many people may not be seen in the health care system except when their illness has exacerbated, we have not restricted this assessment tool to psychiatric data but have included general health information. In addition, physiologic well-being may affect or be affected by the individual's psychologic state, and base-line information is necessary to assist in recognition of changes which may occur in relation to subsequent therapies or state of wellness.

PSYCHIATRIC CLIENT ASSESSMENT TOOL

This is a suggested guide/tool for development by an individual/institution to create a data base reflecting Diagnostic Divisions of Nursing Diagnoses. Although the divisions are alphabetized for ease of presentation, they can be prioritized or rearranged to meet individual needs.

Name: _____
Age: _____ DOB: _____ Sex: _____ Race: _____
Admission Date: _____ Time: _____ From: _____
Source of Information: _____ Reliability (1–4): _____
Family member/Significant other(s): _____

ACTIVITY/REST

Subjective

Occupation: _____ Usual activities/Hobbies: _____
Leisure time activities: _____
Limitations imposed by condition: _____
Sleep: Hours: _____ Naps: _____ Aids: _____
　　Insomnia: _____ Related to: _____
　　Rested upon awakening: _____

Objective

Observed response to activity: Cardiovascular: _____
　　　　　　　　　　　　　　Respiratory: _____
Mental status (e.g., withdrawn/lethargic): _____
Neuro/muscular assessment:
　　Muscle mass/tone: _____
　　Posture: _____ Tremors: _____
　　ROM: _____ Strength: _____
　　Deformity: _____ Other: _____

CIRCULATION

Subjective

History of: Hypertension: _____ Heart Trouble: _____
　　　　　Rheumatic Fever: _____ Ankle/leg edema: _____
　　　　　Phlebitis: _____ Slow healing: _____
　　　　　Claudication: _____
Extremities: Numbness: _____ Tingling: _____
Cough/hemoptysis: _____
Change in frequency/amount of urine: _____

Objective

B/P: R: Stand: _____ Sit: _____ Lying: _____
　　L: Stand: _____ Sit: _____ Lying: _____
Pulse (palpation): Carotid: _____ Radial: _____
　　Femoral: _____ Popliteal: _____
　　Post Tibial: _____ Dorsalis pedis: _____
Heart sounds: _____ Rate: _____
　　Rhythm: _____ Quality: _____ Murmur: _____
Breath sounds: _____
Jugular vein distention: _____
Extremities: Temperature: _____ Color: _____
　　Capillary refill: _____
　　Homan's sign: _____ Varicosities: _____

Color/cyanosis: Overall: _____ Mucous membranes: _____ Lips: _____
Nail beds: _____ Conjunctiva: _____ Sclera: _____

ELIMINATION

Subjective

Usual bowel pattern: _____ Laxative use: _____
Character of stool: _____ Last BM: _____
 History of Bleeding: _____ Hemorrhoids: _____
 Constipation: _____ Diarrhea: _____
Usual voiding pattern: _____ Incontinence: _____
 Urgency: _____ Frequency: _____ Retention: _____
Character of urine: _____
Pain/burning/difficulty voiding: _____
History of kidney/bladder disease: _____

Objective

Abdomen tender: _____ Soft/firm: _____
 Palpable mass: _____ Size/girth: _____
 Bowel sounds: _____
Bladder palpable: _____ Overflow voiding: _____

EMOTIONAL REACTIONS

Subjective

What kind of person are you (positive/negative, etc.)? _____
What do you think of your body? _____
How would you rate your self-esteem (1–10)? _____
What are your moods?: depressed: _____ guilty: _____
 unreal: _____ ups/downs: _____ apathetic: _____
 separated from world: _____ detached: _____
Are you a nervous person? _____
Are your feelings easily hurt? _____
Report of stress factors: _____
Previous patterns of coping with stress: _____
Defense mechanisms:
 Projection: _____ Denial: _____ Undoing: _____
 Rationalization: _____ Passive-aggressive: _____ Repression: _____
 Intellectualization: _____ Somatization: _____ Regression: _____
 Identification: _____ Introjection: _____ Reaction formation: _____
 Isolation: _____ Displacement: _____ Substitution: _____
 Sublimation: _____
Financial concerns: _____
Relationship status: _____
Cultural factors: _____
Lifestyle: _____
Significant losses/changes (date): _____
Stage of grief/manifestations of loss: _____
Religion: _____ Practicing: _____

Objective

Emotional status (check those that apply):
 Calm _____ Friendly _____ Cooperative _____ Evasive _____
 Fearful _____ Anxious _____ Irritable _____ Withdrawn _____
 Restive _____ Passive _____ Dependent _____ Euphoric _____
 Angry/hostile _____ Other (specify) _____

Consistency of behavior: _____
    Verbal: _____
    Nonverbal: _____
    Characteristics of speech: _____
    Motor behaviors: _____ Posturing: _____
    Under/overactive: _____ Stereotypic: _____
Observed physiological response(s): _____
Other: _____

FOOD/FLUID

Subjective

Usual diet (type): _____ # meals daily: _____
Last meal/intake: _____
Loss of appetite: _____ Nausea/vomiting: _____
Heartburn/Indigestion: _____ Related to: _____ Relieved by: _____
Allergy/Food Intolerance: _____
Mastication/swallowing problems: _____
    Dentures: upper _____ lower: _____
Usual weight: _____ Changes in weight: _____
Use of diuretics: _____
Known thyroid problems: _____

Objective

Current weight: _____ Height: _____ Body Build: _____
Skin turgor: _____ Mucous membranes, moist/dry: _____
Edema: General: _____ Dependent: _____
Condition of teeth/gums: _____ Halitosis: _____
Appearance of tongue: _____
    mucous membranes: _____
Bowel sounds (previously assessed): _____
Breath sounds (previously assessed): _____
Urine S/A or Chemstix: _____

HYGIENE

Subjective

Activities of daily living: Independent: _____
    Dependent (specify): Mobility: _____ Feeding: _____
        Hygiene: _____ Dressing: _____
        Toileting: _____ Other: _____
    Assistance provided by: _____

Objective

General appearance: _____
Manner of dress: _____ Personal habits: _____
Body odor: _____ Condition of scalp: _____
Presence of vermin: _____

NEUROLOGIC

Subjective

Dreamlike states: _____ Walking in sleep: _____
Automatic writing: _____
Believe/feel you are another person: _____
Reports perception different than others: _____

Fainting spells/dizziness: _____

Headaches: Location: _____ Frequency: _____

Tingling/Numbness/Weakness (location): _____

Stroke (residual effects): _____

Seizures: _____ Aura: _____ How controlled: _____

Eyes: Vision loss: R _____ L _____

Ears: Hearing loss: R _____ L _____

Objective

Mental status:

   Oriented/disoriented: Time: _____ Place: _____ Person: _____

   Level of consciousness: _____

   Cooperative: _____ Combative: _____

Memory: Immediate: _____ Recent: _____ Remote: _____

Intellectual function: _____

Judgment: _____

Comprehension: _____

Thought processes (assessed through speech): _____

   Patterns of speech: _____

   Content: _____

      Delusions: _____ Hallucinations: _____ Illusions: _____

   Rate or flow: _____

   Clear, logical progression: _____

   Expression: _____

Speech: Clear: _____ Slurred: _____

   Unintelligible: _____ Aphasic: _____

   Unusual speech pattern/impairment: _____

Mood: _____

Affect: _____ Appropriateness: _____ Intensity: _____

   Range: _____

Insight: _____

Pupil size/reaction: R: _____ L: _____

Handgrasp: R: _____ L: _____

Paralysis: _____

Glasses: _____ Contacts: _____ Hearing Aids: _____

PAIN

Subjective

Location: _____ Intensity (1–10): _____ Quality: _____

   Duration: _____ Radiation: _____

Precipitating factors: _____

How relieved: _____

Objective

Emotional response: _____ Narrowed focus: _____

RELATIONSHIP ALTERATIONS

Subjective

Memory of early years: _____

Marital status: _____ Years in relationship: _____

   Living with: _____

Genogram: _____

Family dynamics: _____

Extended family: _____

Other support person(s): _____
Role within family structure: _____
Report of problems: _____
Coping behaviors: _____
Frequency of social contacts (other than work): _____

Objective

Verbal/nonverbal communication with family/S.O.(s): _____
_____

Family interaction (behavioral) pattern: _____

SAFETY

Subjective

Allergies/Sensitivity: _____ Reaction: _____
History of sexually transmitted disease (date/type): _____
Blood transfusion: _____ When: _____
History of accidental injuries: _____
Fractures/Dislocations: _____
Arthritis/Unstable joints: _____
Back problems: _____
Impaired: Vision _____ Hearing _____
Prosthesis: _____ Ambulatory Devices: _____
Expressions of ideation of violence (self/others): _____

Objective

Temperature: _____ Skin integrity: _____
Scars: _____ Rashes: _____
Lacerations: _____ Ulcerations: _____
Ecchymosis: _____ Blisters: _____
Burns, degree/percent: _____
General strength: _____
Muscle tone: _____
Gait: _____ ROM: _____
Paresthesia/Paralysis: _____

SEXUALITY

Sexual orientation/variant preferences: _____
Sexual concerns: _____

Female

Subjective

Age at Menarche: _____ Length of Cycle: _____ Duration: _____
Last menstrual period: _____ Menopause: _____
Method of birth control: _____
Complaints: _____

Objective

Vaginal warts/lesions: _____ Other: _____

Male

Subjective

Penile discharge: _____ Prostate disorder: _____
Vasectomy: _____ Use of condoms: _____
Concerns/Complaints: _____

Objective

Warts/lesions: _____ Other: _____

TEACHING/LEARNING

Subjective

Dominant language (specify): _____
Education level: _____
Learning disabilities (specify): _____
Cognitive limitations (specify): _____
Health beliefs/practices: _____
Special health care practices: _____
Familial risk factors (indicate relationship):

    Diabetes: _____ Tuberculosis: _____
    Heart Disease: _____ Strokes: _____
    High B/P: _____ Epilepsy: _____
    Kidney disease: _____ Cancer: _____
    Mental illness: _____ Other (specify): _____

Prescribed medications: (circle last dose)

Drug	Dose	Times	Take regularly	Purpose
_____	_____	_____	_____	_____
_____	_____	_____	_____	_____

Nonprescription drugs: OTC: _____
           Street drugs: _____
Use of alcohol (amount/frequency): _____
Admitting diagnosis (physician): _____
Reason for hospitalization (client): _____
History of current complaint: _____
Client expectations of this hospitalization: _____
Previous illnesses and/or hospitalizations/surgeries: _____
_____
Evidence of failure to improve: Physical: _____
    Mental: _____
Last complete physical exam: _____ By: _____

Discharge Considerations

Date data obtained: _____
1. Anticipated date of discharge: _____
2. Resources available: Persons: _____
   Financial: _____
3. Do you anticipate changes in your living situation after discharge? _____
   specify: _____
4. Living facility other than home (specify): _____
     5. Community supports: _____
        Groups: _____ Socialization: _____

VENTILATION

Subjective

Dyspnea (related to): _____
Cough/sputum: _____
History of Bronchitis: _____ Asthma: _____
        Tuberculosis: _____ Emphysema: _____
Smoker: _____ Pk/day: _____ # of years: _____

Objective

Respiratory: Rate: _____ Depth: _____ Symmetry: _____

Cyanosis: _____ Clubbing of fingers: _____

Mentation/restlessness: _____

Use of respiratory aids: _____

TABLE 2-1. Nursing Diagnoses (through 7th NANDA Conference)

Activity intolerance
Activity intolerance, potential
Adjustment, impaired
Airway Clearance, ineffective
Anxiety

Body Temperature, potential, alteration in
Bowel Elimination, alteration in: Constipation
Bowel Elimination, alteration in: Diarrhea
Bowel Elimination, alteration in: Incontinence
Breathing Pattern, ineffective

Cardiac Output, alteration in: decreased
Comfort, alteration in: Pain, acute
Comfort, alteration in: Pain, chronic
Communication, impaired: Verbal
Coping, Family: potential for growth
Coping, ineffective Family: Compromised
Coping, ineffective Family: Disabled
Coping, ineffective Individual

Diversional Activity, deficit

Family Process, alteration in
Fear
Fluid Volume, alteration in: excess
Fluid Volume, deficit, actual (1)
Fluid Volume, deficit, actual (2)
Fluid Volume, deficit, potential

Gas Exchange, impaired
Grieving, anticipatory
Grieving, dysfunctional
Growth and Development, altered

Health Maintenance, alteration in
Home Maintenance Management, impaired
Hopelessness
Hyperthermia
Hypothermia

Incontinence: Functional
Incontinence: Reflex
Incontinence: Stress
Incontinence: Total
Incontinence: Urge
Infection, potential for
Injury: potential for: Poisoning; Suffocation; Trauma

Knowledge deficit (specify) *[Learning Need]

Mobility, impaired, physical

Neglect, unilateral
Noncompliance, specify *[Compliance, alteration in]
Nutrition, alteration in: Less than body requirements
Nutrition, alteration in: More than body requirements
Nutrition, alteration in: potential for more than body requirements

Oral Mucous Membrane, alteration in

Parenting, alteration in: actual or potential
Post-trauma Response
Powerlessness

Rape Trauma Syndrome

Self-Care Deficit: Feeding; Bathing/Hygiene; Dressing/Grooming; Toileting
Self-Concept, disturbance in: Body image; Self-esteem; Role performance, Personal identity
Sensory-Perceptual alteration: Visual; Auditory; Kinesthetic; Gustatory; Tactile; Olfactory
Sexual Dysfunction
Sexuality Patterns, altered
Skin Integrity, impairment of: actual
Skin Integrity, impairment of: potential
Sleep Pattern disturbance
Social Interaction, impaired
Social Isolation
Spiritual Distress (distress of the human spirit)
Swallowing, impaired

Thermoregulation, ineffective
Thought Processes, alteration in
Tissue Integrity, impaired
Tissue Perfusion, alteration in: Cerebral; Cardiopulmonary; Renal; Gastrointestinal; Peripheral

Urinary Elimination, alteration in patterns
Urinary Retention *[acute/chronic]

Violence, potential for: Self-directed or Directed at others

---

*Brackets indicate authors recommendations

TABLE 2-2. Diagnostic Divisions

After data have been collected and areas of concern/need have been identified, the nurse is directed to the Diagnostic Divisions to review the list of nursing diagnoses that fall within the individual categories. This will assist the nurse in choosing the specific diagnostic label to describe the data accurately. Then with the addition of etiology (when known) and signs and symptoms, the client problem statement emerges.

ACTIVITY/REST
Activity intolerance
Activity intolerance, potential
Diversional Activity, deficit
Sleep Pattern disturbance

CIRCULATION
Cardiac Output, altered: decreased
Tissue Perfusion, altered: (specify)

ELIMINATION
Bowel Elimination, altered: Constipation
Bowel Elimination, altered: Diarrhea
Bowel Elimination, altered: Incontinence
Incontinence: Functional
Incontinence: Reflex
Incontinence: Stress
Incontinence: Total
Incontinence: Urge
Urinary Elimination, altered patterns
Urinary Retention [acute/chronic]

EMOTIONAL REACTIONS
Adjustment, impaired
Anxiety
Coping, ineffective Individual
Fear
Grieving, anticipatory
Grieving, dysfunctional
Hopelessness
Post-trauma Response
Powerlessness
Rape Trauma Syndrome
Self-concept, disturbance in: Body image; Self-esteem; Personal identity
Spiritual Distress (distress of the human spirit)

FOOD/FLUID
Fluid Volume, altered: excess
Fluid Volume deficit, actual 1 [failure of regulatory mechanisms]
Fluid Volume deficit, actual 2 [active loss]
Fluid Volume deficit, potential
Nutrition, altered: Less than body requirements
Nutrition, altered: More than body requirements
Nutrition, altered: potential for more than body requirements
Oral Mucous Membranes, altered
Swallowing, impaired

HYGIENE
Self-care deficit: Feeding; Bathing/Hygiene; Dressing/Grooming; Toileting

NEUROSENSORY
Communication, impaired: Verbal
Neglect, unilateral
Sensory-Perceptual alteration
Thought Processes, altered

PAIN/COMFORT
Comfort, altered: Pain, acute
Comfort, altered: Pain, chronic

RELATIONSHIP ALTERATIONS
Coping, Family: potential for growth
Coping, ineffective Family: Compromised
Coping, ineffective Family: Disabling
Family Process, altered
Parenting, altered: actual or potential
Self-concept, disturbance in: Role performance
Social Interaction, impaired
Social Isolation

SAFETY
Body Temperature, potential alteration in
Health Maintenance, altered
Home Maintenance Management, impaired
Hyperthermia
Hypothermia
Infection, potential for
Injury, potential for: Poisoning, Suffocation, Trauma
Mobility, impaired physical
Skin Integrity, impairment of: actual
Skin Integrity, impairment of: potential
Thermoregulation, ineffective
Tissue Integrity, impaired
Violence, potential for

SEXUALITY
Sexual Dysfunction
Sexuality Patterns, altered

TEACHING/LEARNING
Growth and Development, altered
Knowledge deficit (specify) [Learning need (specify)]
Noncompliance (specify) [Compliance, altered (specify)]

VENTILATION
Airway Clearance, ineffective
Breathing Pattern, ineffective
Gas Exchange, impaired

Client Situation: Anorexia Nervosa/Bulimia

The following reflects an individual client situation to guide the nurse through the activities of data collection, problem identification, goal setting, and the choosing of interventions for a specific client:

M.J.B., a 33-year-old female, presented at Dr's office with complaints of light-headedness, fatigue, weakness, and history of eating disorders. Admitted to the Eating Disorders program on referral by her family physician for controlled environment and monitoring of physiologic well-being.

ADMITTING PHYSICIAN'S ORDERS

CBC, electrolytes, blood sugar on adm.
ECG in A.M.
Endocrine studies, Dexamethasone suppression test (DST) in A.M.
Urinalysis in A.M.
Regular diet with selective menu; schedule dietary consult
Weigh on adm and according to protocol
Trilafon 8 mg/t.i.d.

NURSING HISTORY AND ASSESSMENT

Name: Mary Jane B.
Age: 33   DOB: Feb. 13, 1954   Sex: F   Race: C
Admission Date: 6/23/87   Time: 3:30 P.M.   From: Home
Source of information: Self   Reliability: 2 to 3
Family member/Significant other(s): Family not in area, no contact
Friend: Mrs. C. P.

ACTIVITY/REST

Subjective

Occupation: Receptionist, city government office.
Usual activities/Hobbies: Volunteers for church, says has "lots of projects, but can't get them completed," "would like to learn new vocation."
Leisure time activities: "Not much. I don't like to get out with people and I just don't seem to have the energy."
Limitations imposed by condition: "Afraid people will know about my problem."
Sleep: "Not enough, maybe 4–5 hours."
Insomnia: "I have some problem, usually because I don't get to bed."
    Says this is her "binge time," finds things to do to avoid going to bed.
    Not rested on awakening, "tired all the time."

Objective

Observed response to activity: Respiratory: tachypnea/28
                                    Cardiovascular: elevated pulse/120
Mental status: withdrawn
Posture: sits hunched over, not looking up

CIRCULATION

Subjective

History of: occasional ankle/leg edema

Objective

B/P: 106/68 lying   90/63 sitting   Pulse: 104 at rest

Heart sounds/Breath sounds: deferred
Color: skin, pale   Conjunctiva/mucous membranes/lips: pale

ELIMINATION

Subjective

Usual bowel pattern: irregular, constipation an ongoing problem. Uses an herbal laxative once or twice a week.
    Last BM: 2 days ago.
        Character: dry, light-colored.
Usual voiding pattern: no problem but voiding less frequently (once/twice a day).
Character of urine: dark yellow.

Objective

Deferred

EMOTIONAL REACTIONS

Subjective

What kind of person are you? "I'm a nothing, a zero."
What do you think of your body? "I don't like my body, it's too fat." Doesn't do anything where she has to expose her body. Would like to learn massage but doesn't want to have a man touch her body (a requirement of the class is that students practice on one another).
How would you rate your self-esteem (1–10)? "Zero."
What are your moods? "depressed, lonely."
Are you a nervous person? "Yes."
Are your feelings easily hurt? "Yes. I'm afraid I'm a bother to other people. They think I'm not doing a good job."
Report of stress factors: worries about "everything," binge eating, having to deal with people in her job, limited income, no savings/health insurance.
Previous patterns of coping with stress: Previously anorectic, avoided eating, running (frequently 10 miles a day); withdrawal (ran away from the hospital last time she was hospitalized).
Financial concerns: is in a low-paying job, no resources.
Relationship status: Single, has never been married nor had a relationship. Says "I don't like men, can't trust them."
Cultural factors: white, middle class.
Lifestyle: Has no home of her own, house-sits for people who are gone, stays with church friends between house-sitting jobs ("helps with the money"). Is alone a lot in this situation.
Significant losses/changes (Date): Left home and moved to another state ten years ago. Does not have contact with family. Father died four years ago; did not see him or return for funeral.
Stage of grief/manifestations of loss: Stated matter-of-factly, "I don't want to have any contact with family. I was glad to get away from them and really don't want to have any contact with them now."
Religion: Catholic   Practicing: Yes

Objective

Emotional status: Calm, cooperative, fearful, anxious, dependent.
Behavior: Consistent. Verbal responses are congruent. Speech is modulated, congruent; voice low.
Defense mechanisms: Uses rationalization—"I ate lunch, some lettuce and sunflower seeds"; denial—"I'm not a worthwhile person"; and projection—"I don't like the way people act. They lie, cheat, and steal."
Body language: Sitting quietly with head down; looks up occasionally and maintains eye contact when she does; "playing" with a tissue.

FOOD/FLUID

Subjective

Usual diet: Vegetarian, does not eat eggs or chicken. Eats one meal a day; no breakfast; snacks on lettuce, nuts, may have tuna for lunch. "Afraid to eat for fear she can't stop." Binges on whatever is available, usually carbohydrates (candy bars, cookies). Drinks occ. glass of water, diet colas (2–3/day).

Usual weight: 130, no recent weight changes. Weighed 85 lb when she was hospitalized for anorexia the first time, 12 years ago.

Vomiting: "Usually once a day, sometimes only two or three times a week."

Swallowing problem: Sore mouth and throat frequently.

Objective

Current weight: 128 #   Height: 5 ft 4 inches   Body build: slight
Skin turgor: tight   Mucous membranes/lips: dry
Edema: none   Halitosis: sour breath
Condition of teeth/gums: tooth decay/erosion evident, gums inflamed, salivary glands slightly swollen.

HYGIENE

Subjective

Independent in self-care.

Objective

General appearance: Neatly dressed in boxy style blue suit; oxford type shoes, in good condition; dark, short hair curled around face; eye makeup lightly applied; nails well kept, no nail polish; no jewelry noted.

NEUROLOGIC

Subjective

Reports sees self as "fat," even though others don't.

Reports fainting spells/dizziness several times a week, recurrent headaches. Says tires easily but works hard.

Eyes: No complaints of eye strain or change in acuity. Does not wear glasses.

No report of hearing loss.

Says concerned because she is not remembering things, "being forgetful."

States she is "depressed, feels tense and anxious, empty."

Objective

Mental status: Alert and oriented to time, place, and person. Memory intact.

Intellectual functioning: States has a problem concentrating, difficulty making decisions.

Thought processes: Speech pattern is normal. Thinking seems fairly rational and logical with organized, coherent flow of ideas. Occ. evidence of distorted thinking, e.g., "I'm afraid my electrolytes are out of balance, but I take vitamins every day." Speaks in a quiet voice. Defensive thinking is apparent with occ. ideas of reference; "people will say I'm weird if they find out about me."

Mood: Depressed, fearful, consistent, verbalizes feelings appropriate to the situation.

Affect: Behavior is consistent with expression of feelings.

Insight: Demonstrates some awareness of extent of condition. Says "I think my electrolytes are out of balance." Verbalizes awareness of not being sure she wants to give up behavior. "What will I have if I don't binge/purge anymore?" States "it makes her feel, knows she is alive."

PAIN

Subjective

No complaints of pain at present.

Headaches occasionally "all over head," 2–3 times/wk last 3 mo. Says did not have headaches until recently when vomiting became more frequent.

RELATIONSHIP ALTERATIONS

Subjective

Memory of early years: F. alcoholic, Mo. rejecting person who often told the children she wished she had not gotten married or had children. Physical abuse common in the family. Reports "F. occasionally belted Mo.," children were frequently "beaten" when they had displeased parents/done something wrong.

Marital status: Single. Living with church friends, house-sitting.

Genogram: Deferred.

Family dynamics: "Mo. was angry with F. most of the time." Sister and brother are two and five years younger, says "felt responsible for them when they were little, grew apart as I became older." Has not had contact with them in past ten years.

Extended family: None.

Other support persons: Employer; church friends, including Mr. and Mrs. S., an older couple she describes as surrogate parents.

Role within family structure: Oldest child with younger sister and brother.

Report of problems: Says feels lonely, doesn't have friends, knows she has to stop the binging/vomiting cycle. Doesn't trust people. Does have limited relationship with church friends, doesn't want them to know about her problem.

Coping behaviors: Preoccupation with food and compulsive need to binge/purge, withdrawal from interaction with others.

Frequency of social contacts (other than work): none other than church, attends mass once or twice a week.

Objective

Has not been observed with family/significant other(s).

SAFETY

Subjective

Temperature: 99.4 po

No history of accidents/injuries

No known allergies

States has frequent colds "every few months"'

Expressions of ideation of violence (self/others): has suicidal thoughts occasionally, recognizes behavior as suicidal

Objective

No physical evidence of self-harm.

SEXUALITY

Subjective

Age at menarche: 12 yr   Length of cycle: irregular   Duration: 2 days

Last menstrual period: 2 months ago

Is not sexually involved with anyone and does not use birth control

Objective

Deferred

TEACHING/LEARNING

Subjective

Dominant language: English

Education Level: HS, graduated from business program, secretarial

Learning disabilities/Cognitive limitations: not aware of any

Health beliefs/practices: Vegetarian. Believes if she eats something, "cannot" stop. Believes if she eats sugar, her body craves it and she will just keep on eating.

Familial risk factors: F. died of stroke, age 67, maternal gmo had a "bad" heart. Not aware of any other significant family history, although mother was "not well."

Prescribed medications: none

Nonprescription drugs: does not take any OTC or illicit drugs. Takes an herbal laxative once or twice a week. Takes vitamins "because I know I don't eat right."

Use of alcohol: None

Admitting diagnosis (physician): Anorexia/Bulimia

Reason for hospitalization (client): "To get my electrolytes under control."

History of current complaint: Long-standing eating problems (20 yr), anorectic as an adolescent, binging and purging for last ten years.

Client expectations of this hospitalization: "I want to begin to feel good about myself and my work, spiritually, mentally, and physically."

Previous hospitalization: Hospitalized twice 10 and 12 years ago. Ran away from the hospital the last time and moved to another state.

Evidence of failure to improve: Physical: having blackouts, fainting spells, says "electrolytes are out of balance."
Mental: States has difficulty thinking, relaxing, complains of inferiority feelings.

Date of last physical exam: 1983

Discharge Considerations

Date data obtained: 6/23

Anticipated date of discharge: 7/14 (21 days)

Resources available: Persons: Employer and church friends.
Financial: has job "not doing what she was trained to do," which employer will hold for her.

Anticipated changes in living after discharge: None, at the moment. Would like to get own place as soon as feasible.
Living facility other than home: would like to continue to house-sit, "helps with the money."

Community supports: Church   Socialization: no social activities

VENTILATION

Subjective

Respiratory rate: 28 with activity/22 at rest

Dyspnea related to: exertion

Does not smoke. Says does not cough except with colds

Care Plan: Anorexia Nervosa/Bulimia

NURSING DIAGNOSIS:	NUTRITION, ALTERED: LESS THAN BODY REQUIREMENTS related to inadequate food intake and self-induced vomiting evidenced by pale conjunctiva and mucous membranes, poor skin turgor, inflamed gums, tooth decay/erosion, slightly swollen salivary glands, complaints of sore mouth/throat.
CLIENT OUTCOMES/EVALUATION CRITERIA:	Verbalizes understanding of nutritional needs within 72 hours. Establishes a dietary pattern with caloric intake adequate to maintain appropriate weight within 72 hours.

INTERVENTIONS

Independent

Establish a minimum weight goal to be maintained, 125–130#.

Maintain a regular weighing schedule, M-W-F, before breakfast in same attire and graph results.

Make selective menu available and allow client to control choices, as much as possible.

Be alert to choices of low-calorie foods; hoarding food; disposing of food in various places such as pockets or wastebaskets.

Use a consistent approach. Present and remove food without persuasion and/or comment. Sit with client while eating, also without comment.

Provide one-to-one supervision. Have client remain in the room with no bathroom privileges for 1/2 hour following eating.

Avoid room checks and control devices.

RATIONALE

When this is agreed upon, psychological work can begin. Malnutrition is a mood-altering condition leading to depression and agitation so that adequate nutrition is important for psychologic well-being.

Provides accurate ongoing record of weight loss and/or gain. Also diminishes obsession about gains and/or losses.

Client needs to gain confidence in self and feel in control of environment. More likely to eat preferred foods.

Client may try to avoid taking in what she views as excessive calories.

Client detects urgency and reacts to pressure. When staff responds in a consistent manner, client can begin to trust her responses. Avoids manipulative games. Any comment which might be seen as coercion provides focus on food. Client may experience guilt if forced to eat. The one area in which she has exercised power and control is food/eating. Structuring meals and decreasing discussions about food will decrease power struggles with client.

Prevents vomiting during/after eating. Note: sometimes clients desire food and use a binge-purge syndrome to maintain weight. Purging may occur for the first time in a client as a response to establishment of weight program.

Reinforces feelings of powerlessness and are usually not helpful.

INTERVENTIONS

Independent

Establish exercise program with the client, discussing likes and dislikes, e.g., walking, aerobics, swimming.

Monitor exercise program and set limits on physical activities. Chart activity/level of work (pacing, etc.).

Provide regular diet and snacks with substitutes and preferred foods available.

Carry out program of behavior modification. Involve client in setting up program. Provide reward for maintaining weight, ignore gain/loss.

Avoid giving laxatives.

Schedule dietary consultation.

Administer drug therapy, as indicated:
    perphenazine (Trilafon) 8 mg. t.i.d. (8 A.M., 2 & 10 P.M.)

Review laboratory studies, e.g., blood sugar, CBC, endocrine studies

RATIONALE

A gradually increasing exercise program can help client begin to improve muscle tone and control weight in a more satisfactory manner.

Client may exercise excessively to burn calories.

Having a variety of foods available will enable client to have a choice of potentially enjoyable foods/may enhance intake.

Provides structured eating situation while allowing client some control in choices. Note: Behavior modification may be effective only in mild cases or for short-term weight maintenance.

Use is counterproductive as they may be used by client to rid body of food/calories.

Helpful in establishing individual dietary needs/program and provides educational opportunity.

Antipsychotic drug which blocks postsynaptic dopamine receptors in the brain. Given to manage underlying pathology, e.g., depression/anxiety.

Provides information about dietary status/needs/effectiveness of therapy.

NURSING DIAGNOSIS:	**FLUID VOLUME, DEFICIT, ACTUAL #2, related to inadequate intake of food and liquids, consistent self-induced vomiting evidenced by dry skin/mucous membranes, decreased skin turgor, increased pulse rate (104), body temperature (99.4° F), orthostatic hypotension (90/63), concentrated urine/decreased urine output, change in mental state, states she is "flaky, forgets things she ought to remember," observed reports of client being forgetful and "out of it."**
CLIENT OUTCOMES/EVALUATION CRITERIA:	**Reports fluid intake of 2000 cc/day with increased urine output within 36 hours. Verbalizes understanding of causative factors and behaviors necessary to correct fluid deficit within one week. Demonstrates improvement in**

vital signs, skin turgor, and moisture of mucous membranes within three days.

INTERVENTIONS	RATIONALE
Independent	
Discuss strategies to stop vomiting, e.g., saying positive affirmation of "I can stop vomiting," talking to friend/therapist, use of imagery/relaxation.	Helping the client to deal with anxiety feelings which lead to vomiting and decision to stop will prevent continued fluid loss.
Have client measure urine output accurately.	Reduced urinary output may be a direct result of reduced food/fluid intake and continued vomiting.
Monitor amount and types of fluid intake. Be aware of diet soft drink intake.	Increased intake of diet pop results in adequate output, even though there is no protein/calorie intake.
Monitor vital signs, capillary refill, and dizziness. Recommend rising slowly, sitting, then standing.	Orthostatic hypotension can occur with fluid deficit.
Note complaints of muscle pain/cramps, generalized weakness, paresthesia, nausea.	Signs of potassium deficit and may reflect inadequate intake, starvation state, deficit from self-induced vomiting.
Discuss actions necessary to regain optimal fluid balance, e.g., drinking a glass of fluid every two hours. Encourage use of calorie containing beverages as well as water.	Involving client in plan to correct fluid imbalances may enhance success and provides sense of control over what is happening to her.
Review laboratory studies, e.g., electrolytes, CBC, urinalysis.	Syndrome may result in electrolyte imbalances, hemoconcentration.

NURSING DIAGNOSIS:	**THOUGHT PROCESSES, ALTERED related to severe malnutrition, psychologic conflicts, e.g., sense of low self-worth, perceived lack of control evidenced by impaired ability to make decisions, problem-solve, non-reality-based verbalizations ("I need to lose 30 lb"; "I ate a lot of food today, sesame seeds and lettuce"); ideas of reference (says people think she isn't doing a good job); altered sleep patterns (goes to bed after midnight, often 2 A.M., gets up early); altered attention span, distractibility.**
CLIENT OUTCOMES/EVALUATION CRITERIA:	**Verbalizes awareness and understanding of relationship of lack of food intake to problems of concentration and decision-making within 48 hours. Demonstrates improved ability**

CLIENT OUTCOMES/EVALUATION CRITERIA—*continued*	to make decisions, problem-solve, and memory of daily/recent events within three weeks.

INTERVENTIONS	RATIONALE

Independent

Be aware of client's distorted thinking ability.	Allows the caregiver to lower expectations and provide information and support.
Listen to and do not challenge irrational, illogical thinking. Present reality concisely and briefly.	It is not possible to respond logically when thinking ability is physiologically impaired. The client needs to hear reality, but challenging leads to distrust and frustration.
Encourage strict adherence to nutrition regime.	Improved nutrition is essential to improved brain functioning. (Refer to ND: Nutrition, alteration in, less than body requirements.)

NURSING DIAGNOSIS:	**SELF-CONCEPT, DISTURBANCE IN: BODY IMAGE/SELF-ESTEEM related to morbid fear of obesity; perceived loss of control in some aspect of life, (e.g., ability to interact satisfactorily with others, eating); unmet dependency needs; dysfunctional family system evidenced by distorted body image, view of self as fat, even in the presence of normal body weight (states "need to lose 30#"); expresses concern, uses denial as a defense mechanism and feels "powerless to prevent binge/purging and make changes in my life"; perceptual disturbances with failure to recognize hunger; fatigue, anxiety, and depression.**
CLIENT OUTCOMES/EVALUATION CRITERIA:	**Identifies physical assets/strengths, accepts compliments and verbalizes a more realistic body image within three weeks. Acknowledges self as an individual who has responsibility for own actions and voluntarily stops binging and purging by the end of the program (3 weeks).**

INTERVENTIONS	RATIONALE

Independent

| Establish a therapeutic nurse/client relationship. | Within a helping relationship, the client can begin to |

INTERVENTIONS	RATIONALE
Independent	
	trust and try out new thinking and behaviors.
Promote self-concept without moral judgment.	Individual sees self as weak-willed, even though a part of the person may feel a sense of power and control.
State rules re: weighing schedule, remaining in sight during medication and eating times, and consequences of not following the rules. Be consistent in carrying out rules without undue comment.	Client is obsessed with fear of weight gain. Regular monitoring of client's weight is important to nutritional status. Consistency is important in establishing trust. As part of the behavior modification program, the client knows the risks involved in not following established rules (e.g., decrease in privileges). Failure to do so is viewed as the client's choice and accepted by the staff in matter-of-fact manner so as not to provide reinforcement for the undesirable behavior.
Respond (confront) with reality when client makes unrealistic statements, such as, "I've stopped vomiting so there's nothing really wrong with me."	Provides constructive feedback about how improving nutrition will give her energy to look at other aspects of her life so that food will not be so all-consuming. Individual needs to be confronted because she denies the psychological aspects of her situation, and often expresses a sense of inadequacy and depression.
Be aware of own reaction to the client's behavior. Avoid arguing.	Feelings of disgust, hostility, and infuriation are not uncommon when caring for these clients. Prognosis remains poor even with stabilization of weight, as other problems may remain. Many continue to see themselves as fat, and there is also a high incidence of affective disorders, social phobias, obsessive-compulsive symptoms, substance abuse, and psychosexual dysfunction. The nurse needs to deal with own response/feelings so they do not interfere with care of the client.
Encourage client to recognize positive characteristics related to self.	Discussion of positive aspects of the self system, such as social skills, work abilities, education, talents, and appearance can reinforce client's feelings of being a worthwhile/competent person.
Assist the client to assume control in areas other than dieting/weight loss, e.g., management of own daily activities, work/leisure choices.	Feelings of personal ineffectiveness, low self-esteem, and perfectionism are often part of the problem. Client feels helpless to change and requires assistance to problem-solve methods of control in life situations.
Help the client formulate goals for self not related to eating, e.g., choice of a satisfying vocation/avocation, and formulate a manageable plan to reach those goals, one at a time on a short-/long-term basis.	Client needs to recognize ability to control other areas in life and may need to learn problem-solving skills in order to achieve this control. Client may not know how to set realistic goals and choices may be influenced by altered thought processes.
Assist client to confront sexual fears. Provide sex education as necessary.	Major physical/psychologic changes in adolescence can contribute to development of this problem. Feelings of powerlessness and loss of control of feelings, in particular sexual, sensations, and physical development lead to an unconscious desire to desexualize self. Client often believes that these fears can be overcome by taking control of bodily appearance/development/function.

INTERVENTIONS	RATIONALE

Independent

Encourage client to take charge of own life in a more healthful way by making own decisions and accepting self as is. Encourage acceptance of inadequacies as well as strengths. Let client know that it is acceptable to be different from family, particularly mother.	Client often doesn't know what she may want for self. Parents (mother) made decisions for her. Client also believes she has to be the best in everything and holds self responsible for being perfect. She needs to develop a sense of control in other ways, besides dieting and weight loss.
Involve in personal development program.	Learning about proper application of makeup, methods of enhancing personal appearance may be helpful to long-range sense of self-esteem.
Use interpersonal psychotherapy rather than interpretive therapy.	More helpful for the client to discover feelings/impulses/needs from within own self. Client has not learned this internal control as a child.
Encourage client to express anger and acknowledge when it is verbalized.	Important to know that anger is part of self and as such is acceptable. Expressing anger may need to be taught to client, as anger is generally considered unacceptable in the family and therefore client does not express it.
Assist client to learn strategies other than eating for dealing with feelings. Have client keep a diary of feelings, particularly when thinking about food.	Feelings are the underlying issue and clients often use food instead of dealing with feelings appropriately. May need to learn to recognize feelings and how to express them.
Assess feelings of helplessness/hopelessness.	54% of clients with anorexia have a history of major affective disorder; 33% have a history of minor affective disorder.
Be alert to suicidal ideation/behavior.	Intensity of anxiety/panic about weight gain, depression, hopeless feelings may lead to suicidal attempts, particularly if client is impulsive.
Involve in group therapy.	Provides an opportunity to talk about feelings and try out new behaviors.

NURSING DIAGNOSIS:	**KNOWLEDGE DEFICIT [Learning Need] related to learned maladaptive coping skills; lack of exposure to/ unfamiliarity with information about condition evidenced by verbalization of misconception of relationship of behaviors (preoccupation with extreme fear of obesity and distortion of own body image; refusal to eat, binging, and purging; and current hospitalization), need for new information, and expressions of desire to learn more adaptive ways of coping with stressors.**

CLIENT OUTCOMES/EVALUATION CRITERIA:	**Verbalizes awareness of and plans for lifestyle changes to maintain normal weight without aberrant eating pattern within two weeks. Identifies relationship of signs/symptoms (weight loss, tooth decay, skin problems) to behaviors of not eating or binge-purging within three days. Assumes responsibility for own learning within two weeks.**

INTERVENTIONS	RATIONALE

Independent

Determine level of knowledge and readiness to learn.	Learning is easier when it begins where the learner is.
Note blocks to learning, e.g., physical/intellectual/emotional.	Malnutrition, family problems, affective disorders, and obsessive-compulsive symptoms can be blocks to learning.
Review dietary needs, answering questions as indicated.	May need assistance with planning for new way of eating.
Provide information about and encourage the use of relaxation and other stress management techniques.	New ways of coping with feelings of anxiety and fear will help client to manage these feelings in more effective ways, assisting in giving up maladaptive behaviors of not eating/binging-purging.
Assist with establishing a sensible exercise program. Caution regarding overexercise.	Exercise can assist with developing a positive body image and combat depression.
Review appropriate skin care needs. Encourage bathing every other day. Use skin cream twice a day and after bathing; massage skin, especially over bony prominences. Observe for reddened/blanched areas.	Frequent baths contribute to dryness of the skin. Supplemental lubrication of the skin decreases itching/flaking and reduces potential for breakdown. Massage improves circulation to the skin and skin tone. Involves client in monitoring and intervening in own therapy.
Stress importance of adequate nutrition/fluid intake. (Refer to ND: Nutrition, altered: Less than body requirements.)	Improved nutrition will improve skin condition.
Provide written information for client.	Helpful as reminder of and reinforcement for learning.
Encourage client to ask friends and coworkers to provide support for necessary changes.	Can serve as a support system to help client make necessary lifestyle changes.
Refer for dental consult/care.	Purging behavior (stomach acids) has damaged gum tissues and tooth enamel.
Refer to National Association of Anorexia Nervosa and Associated Disorders.	May be helpful source of support and information for client and significant other(s).

31

CHAPTER 3

CHILDHOOD AND ADOLESCENT DISORDERS

Pervasive Developmental Disorder: Autistic Disorder

DSM III-R: 299.00 Autistic disorder (specify if childhood onset)
299.80 Pervasive developmental disorder NOS

ETIOLOGIC THEORIES

PSYCHODYNAMICS

The autistic child is described as fixed in the presymbiotic stage of development. These children do not achieve a symbiotic attachment, nor do they differentiate self from mother. They do not communicate or form relationships with others.

BIOLOGIC THEORIES

It has been hypothesized that this severe psychiatric disorder of childhood is the result of a disturbance in central nervous system integration and in the biologic process of maturation. Predisposing organic factors which have been associated with this disorder are maternal rubella, phenylketonuria, encephalitis, meningitis and tuberous sclerosis.

FAMILY DYNAMICS

This disorder has been viewed in the past as a result of a severe disturbance in parent-child interaction. Lack of bonding and stimulation as well as maternal deprivation have been listed as causative factors. More recently, dysfunctional parenting has been seen less as contributing to the disorder and more as a response to the disturbed behavior.

CLIENT ASSESSMENT DATA BASE

HISTORY

Onset during infancy or early childhood
Abnormalities may be noted in almost every sphere of development; e.g., disturbed patterns are reported in eating, sleeping, and elimination and motor, perceptual, cognitive, and language development, as well as severely disturbed social relationships (characteristic of this disorder).
Displays poor eye contact, responsiveness/communication when interacting with others.

PHYSICAL EXAMINATION

Determine physical causes for disturbances in age-appropriate functions and behaviors, e.g., toileting problems.
Neurologic examination to determine presence and/or extent of organic impairment. "Soft" neurologic signs are often seen.
Varied responses to the environment; alterations in mood, language development, or self-mutilative behaviors, e.g., head-banging, hair-pulling may be noted.

DIAGNOSTIC STUDIES

EEG: May be abnormal, reflecting presence/extent of organic impairment.
Psychologic testing/IQ: Provides information about cognitive and personality functioning; IQ below 70 may be noted.
Biochemical studies: Abnormalities have not been consistently noted.
Laboratory tests: As indicated by antipsychotic drug therapy.
Hearing testing: To rule out deafness as a cause of speech problems.
Vision testing: To differentiate responses to auditory and visual stimuli as abnormal reactions versus distorted perceptions.
Developmental testing, e.g., Denver Developmental: may reveal delays.

NURSING PRIORITIES

1. Facilitate control/decrease of behavioral symptoms.
2. Enhance communication skills and social interaction.
3. Promote family involvement in treatment process and acceptance of child's disability.

DISCHARGE CRITERIA

1. Current behavior problems or troublesome symptoms for which treatment is being sought are alleviated.
2. Maintains treatment within the community, avoiding institutionalization when possible.
3. Family verbalizes knowledge about resources to meet the need for a long-term structured therapeutic program.

NURSING DIAGNOSIS:	SOCIAL INTERACTION, IMPAIRED
MAY BE RELATED TO:	Disturbance in self-concept
	Lack of bonding and development of trust
	Inadequate sensory stimulation or abnormal response to sensory input
	Organic brain dysfunction
POSSIBLY EVIDENCED BY:	Lack of responsiveness to others, lack of eye contact or facial responsiveness
	Treating persons as objects, lack of awareness of feelings in others
	Indifference or aversion to comfort, affection or physical contact

CLIENT OUTCOMES/EVALUATION CRITERIA:	Failure to develop cooperative social play and peer friendships in childhood
	Increases periods of eye contact
	Tolerates short periods of physical contact with another person
	Initiates interactions between self and others

INTERVENTIONS

Independent

Assign limited number of caregivers to child.

Convey manner of warmth, acceptance, and availability.

Reinforce eye contact with something acceptable to the child (food, object). Eventually replace with social reinforcement.

Gradually increase proximity and planned intrusion into child's isolation.

Be available as support during child's attempts to interact with others.

Collaborative

Work with others who are involved, e.g., teachers, to maintain a structured environment.

Maintain contact with social services caseworker and involve in team conferences.

RATIONALE

Consistent approach by familiar persons increases chances for establishing trust.

These characteristics encourage nonthreatening interaction.

Establishing eye contact is essential to interventions for other symptoms.

Caregivers need to initiate interaction as avenue toward social response.

Presence of a trusted person provides a feeling of security.

Coordinated, consistent efforts are more effective for helping the child to learn new behaviors.

Provides continuity of care when child/family are involved with social services system.

NURSING DIAGNOSIS:	COMMUNICATION, IMPAIRED VERBAL
MAY BE RELATED TO:	Inability to trust others
	Withdrawal into self
	Organic brain dysfunction
	Inadequate sensory stimulation
	Maternal deprivation
POSSIBLY EVIDENCED BY:	Lack of interactive communication mode; does not use gestures or spoken language

35

POSSIBLY EVIDENCED BY— *continued*	Absent or abnormal nonverbal communication; lack of eye contact or facial expression
	If speech is present, peculiar patterns exist in form, content, or speech production.
	Impaired ability to initiate or sustain conversation despite adequate speech
CLIENT OUTCOMES/EVALUATION CRITERIA:	Uses sounds, words, or gestures in an interactive way with others
	Communicates needs/desires to significant others/caregivers
	Initiates verbal or nonverbal interaction with others

INTERVENTIONS	RATIONALE
Independent	
Maintain consistency in caregivers assigned to child.	Familiarity helps child to develop trust and caregivers to learn ways child attempts to communicate.
Anticipate and fulfill needs until communication can be established.	Reduces frustration while child is learning communication skills. Some therapists believe this process should be limited in order to force verbal requests for wants beyond basic needs.
Assess previously used words or sounds. Seek validation and clarification in order to decode communication attempts.	Facilitates recognition of speech efforts. These techniques are useful in determining accuracy of messages received.
Reinforce eye contact with something acceptable to the child, e.g., food, object.	Eye contact is essential to capture child's attention to successfully initiate conversation.
Repeat and reinforce approximations of sounds or words whenever used (shaping).	Response gives child information about the caregiver's expectations and may encourage attempts to communicate.
Teach deaf sign language as alternate communication tool for children with minimal language development.	Signing may produce less anxiety than verbal expression for some children.
Collaborative	
Refer for assessment and testing in cooperation with special education teachers and speech pathologists.	Provides for treatment planning with appropriate specialized interventions/techniques.

NURSING DIAGNOSIS:	VIOLENCE, POTENTIAL FOR, SELF-DIRECTED
MAY BE RELATED TO:	Organic brain dysfunction

POSSIBLE INDICATORS:	Inability to trust others
	Disturbance in self-concept
	Inadequate sensory stimulation or abnormal response to sensory input
	Maternal deprivation
	Response to demands of therapy
	Head-banging
	Biting, scratching, or pinching self
	Pulling out own hair
	History of self-mutilation as response to anxiety
	Indifference to environment or marked distress over changes in environment
CLIENT OUTCOMES/EVALUATION CRITERIA:	Diminishes violent responses and does not engage in self-mutilating behavior

INTERVENTIONS

Independent

Note prior history of violent behaviors and relationship to anxiety or stressful events. Identify events or stimuli that precipitate self-mutilating behavior and intervene before these occur.

Reinforce acceptable behavior; provide other satisfying activities (rocking, swinging).

Apply protective devices (e.g., helmet, padded arm covers, bandages over sores or scabs).

Avoid physical restraint if possible, but holding a child until agitation subsides may be necessary.

Collaborative

Administer antipsychotic medications as indicated.

RATIONALE

Useful in determining patterns and predicting and controlling violent behavior. Self-mutilation may be prevented if causes can be determined and averted. Note: May be first priority if this behavior is a prominent symptom.

Diversion or replacement activities may become substitutes for self-mutilation.

Provides protection when potential for self-harm is present.

Restriction of movement may increase anxiety. Protection from self-harm is essential for safety. (Note: Some therapists advocate use of aversive conditioning to eliminate life-threatening behaviors.)

May exert symptomatic control of agitated behaviors.

NURSING DIAGNOSIS:	SELF-CONCEPT, DISTURBANCE IN: PERSONAL IDENTITY
MAY BE RELATED TO:	Organic brain dysfunction
	Lack of development of trust
	Maternal deprivation
	Fixation at presymbiotic phase of development
POSSIBLY EVIDENCED BY:	Lack of awareness of the feelings or existence of others
	Increased anxiety resulting from physical contact with others
	Absent or impaired imitation of others; repeats what others say
	Persistent preoccupation with parts of objects; obsessive attachment to objects
	Marked distress over changes in environment
	Severe panic reactions to everyday events
	Autoerotic, ritualistic behaviors, self-touching, rocking, swaying
CLIENT OUTCOMES/EVALUATION CRITERIA:	Shows signs of developing awareness of self as separate from others and environment (e.g., discontinuing echolalia, knows body boundaries). Tolerates separations and environmental changes without undue anxiety.

INTERVENTIONS	RATIONALE
Independent	
Use positive reinforcement to encourage eye contact.	Eye contact focuses child on the recognition of another person.

INTERVENTIONS	RATIONALE

Independent

Assist child in learning to name own body parts. Provide mirrors and pictures for self-identification.

This activity may increase awareness of self as separate from others.

Encourage appropriate exploratory touching of others and touching by caregivers.

If done gradually, child can feel the differences between self and others without excessive anxiety.

Encourage self-care activities which differentiate child from environment (self-feeding, washing, dressing, etc.).

Activities may help child to identify body boundaries.

NURSING DIAGNOSIS:	**COPING, INEFFECTIVE FAMILY: COMPROMISED/DISABLING**
MAY BE RELATED TO:	**Family members unable to express feelings related to having a severely disturbed child**
	Excessive guilt, anger, or blaming among family members regarding child's condition
	Ambivalent or dissonant family relationships; disagreements regarding treatment, coping strategies.
	Prolonged coping with problem exhausts supportive ability of family members
POSSIBLY EVIDENCED BY:	**Denial of existence or severity of disturbed behaviors**
	Describes preoccupation with personal emotional reaction to situation (anger, guilt)
	Show persistent lack of acceptance of chronic nature of child's disorder; rationalization that problem is developmental and will eventually be outgrown
	Attempts to intervene with child are achieving increasingly ineffective results

POSSIBLY EVIDENCED BY— *continued*	Withdraws from/becomes overly protective of child
FAMILY OUTCOMES/EVALUATION CRITERIA:	Verbalizes knowledge and appropriate understanding of child's disorder
	Expresses feelings appropriately with decreased defensive behavior (denial, projection, rationalization)
	Demonstrates more consistent, effective methods of coping with child's behavior
	Seeks outside therapeutic support as needed

INTERVENTIONS	RATIONALE
Independent	
Meet regularly with family members in order to discuss feelings and attitudes.	Supportive counseling can help family members express feelings, explore own reactions to child's disorder.
Assess underlying circumstances which may be contributing to ineffective family coping (e.g., financial problems, health of other members, needs of other children).	Identification of stressors may help parents sort out feelings related to child and other issues.
Assist family to develop new methods for dealing with the child's behaviors. Reinforce effective parenting methods. (Refer to CP: Parenting.)	Effective intervention skills can assist family to regain self-esteem and control of their environment.
Collaborative	
Refer to other resources as necessary, e.g., psychotherapy, financial aid, respite care, clergy.	Developing a support system can sustain family coping skills.

Disruptive Behavior Disorders of Childhood

DSM III-R: 314.01 Attention-Deficit Hyperactivity Disorder

ETIOLOGIC THEORIES

PSYCHODYNAMICS

The child with this disorder has impaired ego development. Behavior manifested represents id impulses unchecked, as in severe temper tantrums.

GENETIC/BIOLOGIC THEORIES

This disorder may be sex-linked, since the incidence is much higher in boys than in girls. There is some evidence that fathers of hyperactive children are more likely to be alcoholic or to have antisocial personality disorders. Hyperactivity is sometimes associated with other disorders involving brain damage or dysfunction, such as mental retardation, seizure disorders, and brain lesions. Studies have shown the presence of subtle chromosomal changes and mild neurologic deficits among some hyperactive children. Other physical conditions considered as possible causative factors are: birth injury or anoxia, central nervous system infection, and food/other allergies.

FAMILY DYNAMICS

This theory suggests that disruptive behavior is learned as a means for a child to gain adult attention. It is likely that whether or not the impulsive irritability seen in attention-deficit hyperactivity disorder was present from birth, some parental reactions tend to reinforce and thus maintain or increase its intensity. Anxiety generated by a dysfunctional family system, marital problems, etc., could also contribute to symptoms of this disorder.

CLIENT ASSESSMENT DATA BASE

HISTORY

Onset usually noted before age 7.
Reports from parents and teachers of:
　　Being easily distracted, unable to sustain attention in order to remain on task or complete projects.
　　Having difficulty sitting still, are sometimes physically over-active, and may engage in disruptive behavior or dangerous activities without considering the consequences.
May have difficulty following instructions and appear not to listen or to hear what is said to them.
Family may report emotional lability.

PHYSICAL EXAMINATION

Note presence of physical symptoms which might indicate the existence of physical illness, e.g., rashes, upper respiratory illness, or other allergic symptoms, CNS infection (cerebritis).

DIAGNOSTIC STUDIES

Thyroid studies: May reveal hyper/hypothyroid conditions contributing to problems.
Neurologic testing, e.g., EEG, CT scan: To determine presence of organic brain disorders.
Psychologic testing as indicated: To rule out anxiety disorders; identify gifted, borderline retarded, or learning disabled child; and to assess social responsiveness and language development.

NURSING PRIORITIES

1. Facilitate child's achievement of more consistent behavioral self-control and improvement in self-esteem.
2. Promote parents' development of effective means of coping with and interventions for their child's behavioral symptoms.

3. Participate in the development of a comprehensive, ongoing treatment approach using family and community resources.

DISCHARGE CRITERIA

1. Extremely disruptive and/or dangerous behavior is minimized or eliminated.
2. Child is able to function in a structured learning environment.
3. Parents have gained or regained the ability to cope with internal feelings and to intervene effectively with their child's behavioral problems.

NURSING DIAGNOSIS:	**COPING, INEFFECTIVE, INDIVIDUAL**
MAY BE RELATED TO:	**Situational or maturational crisis**
	Mild neurological deficits
	Retarded ego development
	Low self-esteem
	Dysfunctional family system
POSSIBLY EVIDENCED BY:	**Easily distracted by extraneous stimuli**
	Unable to meet age-appropriate role expectations
	Excessive motor activity; cannot sit still
	Unable to delay gratification
	Shifts from one uncompleted activity to another
CLIENT OUTCOMES/EVALUATION CRITERIA:	**Demonstrates a decrease in disruptive behaviors. Shows improvements in attention span, concentration, and appropriate activity level.**

INTERVENTIONS	RATIONALE
Independent	
Provide quiet atmosphere; decrease amount of external stimuli.	Reduction in environmental stimulation may decrease distractibility.
Provide area and activities for gross motor movement, e.g., gym and/or outdoor area for running, large balls, climbing equipment.	Appropriate outlets are necessary to discharge motor activity.

INTERVENTIONS

Independent

Reinforce attending, concentrating, and completing tasks.

Set limits on disruptive behaviors (e.g., talking incessantly); suggest alternative competing behaviors such as playing quietly.

Collaborative

Administer medication as indicated, e.g., methylphenidate, imipramine.

Investigate alternative treatments, e.g., diet, allergy.

RATIONALE

Desired behaviors will increase with positive reinforcement.

Child needs to know expectations and to learn competing acceptable behaviors, e.g., shouting out vs. raising hand, pushing others vs. keeping hands to self.

Amphetamines and antidepressants have been shown to improve attention and reduce impulsiveness in hyperactive children.

Some children respond favorably to control of refined sugar, food dyes, and allergins.

NURSING DIAGNOSIS:	SOCIAL INTERACTION, IMPAIRED
MAY BE RELATED TO:	Retarded ego development
	Low self-esteem
	Dysfunctional family system
	Neurological impairment
POSSIBLY EVIDENCED BY:	Difficulty waiting turn in games or group situations
	Doesn't seem to listen to what is being said
	Difficulty playing quietly, maintaining attention to task or play activity
	Often shifts from one activity to another
	Interrupts or intrudes on others
CLIENT OUTCOMES/EVALUATION CRITERIA:	Participates appropriately in interactive play with another child or group of children. Develops a mutual relationship with another child or adult.

INTERVENTIONS	RATIONALE
Independent	
Develop trust relationship with child, show acceptance of child separate from unacceptable behavior.	Acceptance and trust encourage feelings of self-worth.
Offer positive reinforcement for appropriate social interaction. Ignore ineffective methods of relating to others; teach competing behaviors.	Behavior modification can be an effective method of reducing disruptive behaviors in children.
Provide opportunities for group interaction and encourage a positive and negative peer feedback system.	Appropriate social behavior is often learned from age-mates.
Collaborative	
Arrange staffings with other professionals, e.g., social workers, teachers. Include parents and child when possible.	Cooperation and coordination among those working with these children will enhance the treatment program. Including the child and parents provides them with understanding of the total problem and proposed treatment program.

NURSING DIAGNOSIS:	**SELF-CONCEPT, DISTURBANCE IN: SELF-ESTEEM**
MAY BE RELATED TO:	**Retarded ego development**
	Lack of positive feedback with repeated negative feedback
	Dysfunctional family system
	Mild neurological deficits
POSSIBLY EVIDENCED BY:	**Derogatory remarks about self**
	Engagement in physically dangerous activity
	Lack of self-confidence
	Hesitance to try new tasks
	Distracts others to cover up own deficits or failures, e.g., acts the clown
CLIENT OUTCOMES/EVALUATION CRITERIA:	**Verbalizes increasingly positive self-regard. Demonstrates beginning awareness and control of own behavior.**

INTERVENTIONS

Independent

Convey acceptance and unconditional positive regard.

Assist child to identify positive aspects of self; give immediate feedback for acceptable behavior.

Provide opportunities for success; plan activities with short time span and appropriate ability level.

Collaborative

Provide learning opportunities, structured learning environment, e.g., self-contained classroom; individually planned educational program.

RATIONALE

May help child to increase own self-esteem.

Positive reinforcement enhances self-esteem and increases desired behavior.

Repeated successes can help to improve self-esteem.

Successful school performance is essential to preserve a child's positive self-image.

NURSING DIAGNOSIS:	COPING, INEFFECTIVE FAMILY: COMPROMISED/DISABLING
MAY BE RELATED TO:	**Excessive guilt, anger or blaming among family members regarding child's behavior**
	Parental inconsistencies; disagreements regarding discipline, limit-setting, and approaches
	Exhaustion of parental resources due to prolonged coping with disruptive child
POSSIBLY EVIDENCED BY:	**Unrealistic parental expectations**
	Rejection or over-protection of child
	Exaggerated expressions of anger, disappointment, or despair regarding child's behavior or ability to improve or change
PARENT OUTCOMES/EVALUATION CRITERIA:	**Demonstrates more consistent, effective intervention methods in response to child's behavior. Expresses and resolves negative attitudes toward child. Identifies and uses support systems as needed.**

INTERVENTIONS	RATIONALE

Independent

Provide information and materials related to child's disorder and effective parenting techniques.

Appropriate knowledge and skills may increase parental effectiveness.

Encourage parents to verbalize feelings and explore alternative methods of dealing with child.

Supportive counseling can assist parents in developing coping strategies.

Provide feedback and reinforce effective parenting methods. (Refer to CP: Parenting.)

Positive reinforcement can increase self-esteem.

Involve siblings in family discussions and planning for more effective family interactions.

Family problems affect all members, and treatment is more effective when everyone is involved in therapy.

Collaborative

Refer to community resources as indicated, e.g., psychotherapy, parent support groups, parenting classes (Parent Effectiveness).

Developing a support system can increase parental confidence and effectiveness.

Disruptive Behavior Disorders of Adolescence

DSM III-R: 309.40 Adjustment Disorder with mixed disturbance of emotions and conduct (formerly Adolescent Adjustment Disorder)

309.90 Conduct Disorder

312.90 Conduct Disorder

ETIOLOGIC THEORIES

PSYCHODYNAMICS

According to psychoanalytic therapy, these children are fixed in the separation-individuation phase of development. Ego development is retarded and id behavior is prominent.

BIOLOGIC THEORIES

Differences in temperament of infants at birth have been observed in relation to attention span, excitability, and adaptability. Correlation between these findings and the development of behavioral disorders in adolescence remain uncertain.

FAMILY DYNAMICS

Certain family patterns contribute to the disruptive behavior. They include parental rejection; inconsistent or rigid, harsh discipline; unstable spousal relationship; and lack of feeling of security within the family system.

CLIENT ASSESSMENT DATA BASE

HISTORY

Symptoms most often appear during prepubertal-to-pubertal period and may predispose the child to conduct or adjustment disorders in adolescence.

Note family constellation/stability, presence/absence of parents/extended family, and other factors which may affect situation.

May be involved with juvenile court, have record of antisocial behavior.

May have had frequent/recurrent life changes, e.g., multiple moves, schools, lifestyle changes.

Parents may report client isolates self, plays stereo loudly, does not participate in family activities, skips meals, eats excessive amounts of "junk" foods.

May have history of poor school/work performance, if applicable.

Blames others for what happens to self.

May complain of nausea, nervousness, worry, and jitteriness. May be depressed, angry, or react with ambivalence or hostility.

May report recent weight gain.

Style of dress may reflect fashion trends or be atypical.

May be involved in drug use/abuse, including cigarettes/chewing tobacco.

May/may not participate in social activities.

May have had previous psychiatric hospitalization for same or other problems.

PHYSICAL EXAMINATION

Affect may be labile.

Physical characteristics/development may not be normal for age range.

Weight may be excessive for height.

DIAGNOSTIC STUDIES

Drug screen: To identify substance use/abuse.

NURSING PRIORITIES

1. Provide a safe environment and protect client from self-harm.
2. Promote development of strategies which regulate impulse control, regain sense of self-worth and security.
3. Facilitate learning of appropriate and satisfying methods of dealing with stressors/feelings.
4. Promote client's ability to engage in satisfying relationships with family members, peer group.

DISCHARGE CRITERIA

1. Exhibits effective coping skills in dealing with problems.
2. Understands need and strategies for controlling negative impulses/acting-out behaviors.
3. Anger expressed in appropriate/nonviolent ways.
4. Family is involved in group therapy/participating in treatment program.

NURSING DIAGNOSIS:	**COPING, INEFFECTIVE, INDIVIDUAL**
MAY BE RELATED TO:	**Inadequate coping strategies**
	Maturational crisis
	Multiple life changes
	Lack of control of impulsive actions
	Personal vulnerability
POSSIBLY EVIDENCED BY:	**Inappropriate use of defense mechanisms**
	Inability to meet role expectations
	Poor self-esteem
	Stealing and other acting-out behaviors.
	Failure to assume responsibility for own actions
	Verbalization of inability to cope
	Excessive smoking/drinking
CLIENT OUTCOMES/EVALUATION CRITERIA:	**Expresses realistic view of the consequences of impulsive behavior. Verbalizes understanding of the relationship between emotional needs and acting-**

out behaviors. Identifies and demonstrates ways to meet own needs.

INTERVENTIONS	RATIONALE
Independent	
Encourage client to express fears and concerns. Offer support and confront when appropriate.	Self-understanding and further exploration are enhanced when verbalizations of concern and anxiety are received in a nonjudgmental manner.
Assist client to recognize the reality and nonproductivity of maladaptive behaviors (failing grades, in trouble with the law, running away).	Old patterns of behavior tend to recur under stress. Continuous monitoring of behavior is necessary to avoid old, unproductive methods of coping and problem-solving.
Focus on specific behaviors, e.g., poor academic performance, antisocial behavior, which are amenable to change.	Energy is best used when focus is on those areas which can be altered.
Reinforce client positively when change in behaviors indicate effective coping through behavior modification system. Anticipate and accept occasional regressive behavior.	Adolescence is a time of stress and vulnerability because of a lack of well-developed coping skills. Positive reinforcement encourages continuing personal growth. Hospitalization may precipitate periodic regression.
Assess religious beliefs/affiliations. Encourage client to draw again on spiritual resources which had been useful in the past.	When these ties have been previously established, they may be helpful in providing resources for the adolescent to enhance inner controls.
Explore possible ways to rekindle relationships with former peers, influential adults, organizations/church youth group, if appropriate.	Attaining peer acceptance is of primary importance during adolescence. Peer groups that share common values promote the formation of belonging and identity.

NURSING DIAGNOSIS:	**VIOLENCE, POTENTIAL FOR, SELF-DIRECTED OR DIRECTED TOWARD OTHERS**
MAY BE RELATED TO:	**Dysfunctional family system and loss of significant relationships**
	Retarded ego development
POSSIBLE INDICATORS:	**Behavior changes, e.g., absenteeism, poor grades, hostility toward authority figures and stealing**
	Poor impulse control
	Feelings of rejection
	Powerlessness; loss of self-esteem

POSSIBLE INDICATORS— continued	Overt aggressive acts directed at the environment
	Self-destructive behavior and/or active suicidal threats/gestures
CLIENT OUTCOMES/EVALUATION CRITERIA:	Verbalizes understanding of behavior and factors which precipitate violent behavior. Expresses anger in appropriate ways and does not make hostile or suicidal gestures/statements or harm self or others. Identifies and uses resources and support systems in an effective manner.

INTERVENTIONS	RATIONALE
Independent	
Assess stresses and warning signals such as behavior changes, anger, anxiety, and recently disrupted family.	Impulsive reactions to stressful situations may be a cry for help and directed toward harm to self or others.
Assess seriousness of suicidal tendency, gestures, threats, or previous attempts. (Use scale of 1–10 and prioritize according to severity of threat, availability of means.)	Knowledge of past and present behavior in reference to suicidal ideation will assist in assessing client's tolerance for stress, degree of concern. Note: May be #1 priority if suicide scale is 8–10.
Maintain a therapeutic milieu which includes a safe environment ("suicide precautions").	Internal controls may be inadequate, requiring some external controls and interventions until internal control is learned.
Establish trusting relationship with client in order to allow exploration and verbalization of feelings related to suicide.	Client's expression of internal conflicts in words, rather than action, will more likely be made to knowledgeable and accepting staff.
Observe client unobtrusively for signs of potential violence toward others.	Intervention before the onset of violence could prevent injury to the client and others.
Have sufficient staff available to indicate a show of strength to client if it becomes necessary.	This conveys to client evidence of control over the situation and provides some sense of security for the client and staff.
Explore and offer more satisfying alternatives to aggressive behavior, e.g., physical outlets for redirection of angry feelings; use of quiet room, e.g., "Soft Spot" with soft balls, pillows to pound. Have staff member stay with client. Encourage client to choose own "Time out," go to room for "alone time."	Increased ability to discover satisfying alternatives in coping with stresses will decrease need for aggressive behavior. Physical outlets help to relieve pent-up tension and anxiety. Staff member can help client to express feelings and begin to recognize value of appropriate handling of anger. Adolescent may see "Time out" as punishment if staff imposes, but begins to take responsibility for own self by recognizing and choosing own quiet/alone time.
Encourage client to ask for time with staff, give permission to express angry feelings.	Recognizing feelings and taking responsibility by asking for time to discuss them helps adolescent learn more effective ways of dealing with problems which lead to anger and acting-out behaviors.

INTERVENTIONS	RATIONALE
Independent	
Include significant other(s) in discussion to educate regarding suicidal ideation/warnings.	May be unaware of/ignorant of meaning of warning signals when suicidal ideation exists.
Assess how unit functioning affects adolescent behaviors.	Milieu stresses, such as vacations, personnel changes, staff conflict, can affect client's own issues, e.g., abandonment. It is important to look at the psychodynamics as well as the unique meaning of individual behavior.
Collaborative	
Place in seclusion or apply restraints as necessary.	May need external restraints until client regains control of own behavior.

NURSING DIAGNOSIS:	ANXIETY [SPECIFY LEVEL]
MAY BE RELATED TO:	**Situational or maturational crises**
	Threat to physical integrity or self-concept
	Dysfunctional family system
POSSIBLY EVIDENCED BY:	**Somatic complaints**
	Excessive psychomotor activity
	Poor attention to task
	Poor impulse control
CLIENT OUTCOMES/EVALUATION CRITERIA:	**Verbalizes awareness of propensity toward increased psychomotor activity, poor attention to task, and poor impulse control. Demonstrates self-initiated intervention strategies which facilitate more effective coping skills. Reports absence of/demonstrates relief from somatic manifestations of anxiety.**

INTERVENTIONS	RATIONALE
Independent	
Assign primary nurse to foster a trusting relationship.	Continuity of care for client builds trust and clarifies expectation.

INTERVENTIONS	RATIONALE

Independent

Observe/assist client to recognize manifestations of anxiety (e.g., nausea, compulsive eating).

Signs and symptoms of anxiety need to be identified before client can make constructive changes.

Identify factors that precede symptoms of anxiety.

Correct assessment and interpretation of premonitory conditions provide for timely intervention.

Support client's exploration to identify those behaviors or interventions which offer relief.

Connecting feelings of anxiety with behaviors that afford relief will encourage the development of more productive behaviors.

Channel excessive energy into physical activity such as exercises, noncompetitive games, jogging in gym, etc.

Discharge of physical energy tends to decrease built-up tensions which lead to manifestations of anxiety. Note: Competitive games may increase anxiety.

NURSING DIAGNOSIS:	**ADJUSTMENT, IMPAIRED**
MAY BE RELATED TO:	**Nonexistent or unsuccessful ability to be involved in problem-solving or goal-setting**
	Losses connected with current/past occurrences in individual situation, e.g., loss of self-esteem, family member/friends; poor school performance; relocation
	Lack of movement toward independence
	Difficulty limiting expectations of self
POSSIBLY EVIDENCED BY:	**Ambivalence toward parent(s)**
	Anxiety
	Self-blame, anger, and feelings of rejection
	Inadequate support systems
	Assault to self-esteem, altered locus of control
	Incomplete grieving (severe emotional loss, physical and/or learning disability)

CLIENT OUTCOMES/EVALUATION CRITERIA:	Verbalizes and recognizes significance of losses in life. Expresses feelings and grieves appropriately. Evaluates realistic potential for forming relationships. Develops a sense of autonomy in current life situation.

INTERVENTIONS

Independent

Promote a trust relationship which is reliable, supportive, and reassuring.

Review previous life situations and role changes determining coping skills already developed. (Refer to ND: Coping, ineffective, Family, Compromised/Disabling.)

Listen to client's perception of inability to adapt to situations presently occurring.

Identify significant support systems past and present.

Develop with the client a plan of action to meet immediate needs, e.g., physical safety, hygiene, emotional support.

Provide opportunities for client to make short-term attainable goals, e.g., crafts, activities.

Encourage client to recognize significance of losses and express feelings regarding these.

Encourage exploration of the relationship of behavior, anxiety, and somatic symptoms to the grief process.

Discuss appropriateness and desirability of the grief process as it relates to the loss(es). Discuss stages of the grief process and behaviors associated with each stage.

Encourage the development of a positive relationship with an adult.

RATIONALE

Communication, growth, and insight flourish in an atmosphere of acceptance and trust.

Provides information about availability of skills for current use.

Provides clues to reality of these perceptions and avenues to assist in dealing with them.

Reinforces availability of resources to aid the client to develop new coping skills.

Provides opportunity for client to learn sense of control and fosters self-esteem.

Promotes feelings of self-worth which can lead to increased risk-taking and the development of more elaborate future-oriented goals.

Grief work cannot begin until losses are acknowledged.

Knowledge regarding possible psychologic and physiologic manifestations of the grief process aids in identifying etiology of existing symptoms and helps in the alleviation of denial.

Grief work is necessary and a natural reaction to loss. A period of time is required (6–12 months) to work through grief. The process gives the client permission to grieve and offers hope for eventual acclimation to the loss.

A quality relationship with an adult (preferably a parent) reinforces the strength and supportive function of the relationship (family) and is a positive factor when setting limits with the adolescent.

NURSING DIAGNOSIS:	SELF-CONCEPT, DISTURBANCE IN: BODY IMAGE; SELF-ESTEEM; ROLE PERFORMANCE; PERSONAL IDENTITY
MAY BE RELATED TO:	Failure at life events (adolescence)

MAY BE RELATED TO— *continued*	Situational/developmental crisis, slow physical maturation
	Disruption of family by divorce/death/ absence of parent or other factors
POSSIBLY EVIDENCED BY:	Behavioral signs, e.g., poor academic performance, stealing, loss of job, bragging about alleged sexual exploits
	Rebellion against generally accepted fashion styles
	Alteration in weight
	Poor hygiene/personal habits
	Difficulty accepting positive reinforcement
	Not taking responsibility for self
	Self-destructive behavior
	Failure to assume role
	Confusion about sense of self
CLIENT OUTCOMES/EVALUATION CRITERIA:	Verbalizes a sense of a more positive self-concept. Realistically identifies and appraises what can be actively influenced by own actions. Develops ego strength sufficient to cope with inner impulses.

INTERVENTIONS	RATIONALE
Independent	
Explore and discuss feelings of rejection and anger related to individual situation.	Recognition and expression of feelings eliminate need for displacement and denial. This directs focus of energy to problems and alternative solutions.
Point out past academic success in order to assist in preserving self-esteem.	Past performance is a more accurate portrayal of ability than that indicated by recent grades.
Assist client in understanding transient nature of poor academic performance related to current stresses.	High anxiety levels affect motivation, attention to task, and performance.
Provide activities in areas of client's interest, tasks which can be completed successfully, and reinforce when these are accomplished.	Success in accomplishing goals builds self-esteem and diminishes need for disruptive acting-out behaviors.

INTERVENTIONS

Independent

Encourage participation in activities with peer group, e.g., outings, hikes, swimming.

Schedule time for one-to-one client/nurse interaction and communication.

Schedule regular exercise activities.

Involve in activities to improve personal appearance, e.g., makeup, hair-styling, how to dress.

Collaborative

Consult with resident educational therapist (teacher) regarding academic pursuits while hospitalized.

Schedule staffings with "home" school counselors, social worker, teachers, and client/parents as possible.

RATIONALE

Social interaction and peer acceptance is one of the tasks of this developmental stage. Participation helps to develop social skills.

Individual attention conveys the importance of the individual. Communication skills are refined with frequent interaction.

Can enhance physical appearance and strength, aids in weight loss, lessens anxiety and stress, and builds positive self-esteem.

How an individual looks affects feelings about inner self and can improve self-esteem.

Continuation of educational process while hospitalized will decrease further loss of self-concept. Can be an opportunity to form a positive relationship with teacher.

Maintains contact with own school setting, fosters continuity for return and sense of importance for the student.

NURSING DIAGNOSIS:	**COPING, INEFFECTIVE FAMILY: COMPROMISED/DISABLING**
MAY BE RELATED TO:	**Loss of significant relationship (parent/child)**
	Highly ambivalent family relationships
	Family disorganization/role changes
	Presence of other situational/developmental crises affecting family members
POSSIBLY EVIDENCED BY:	**Client statement of feelings of abandonment, rejection, and guilt about parent's response to adolescent's problems**
	Client expresses sense of powerlessness and lack of control.
	Parents describe preoccupation with own reactions, e.g., fear, guilt, anxiety.

POSSIBLY EVIDENCED BY— *continued*	Parents withdraw or have limited communication with adolescent or display protective behavior disproportionate (too little or too much) to client's abilities or need for autonomy.
FAMILY OUTCOMES/EVALUATION CRITERIA:	Reestablishes relationship with one another. Expresses feelings openly and honestly. Evaluates individual role in family problems. Identifies factors and decisions which can be made and controlled. Explores possibility of positive changes in the family in the future. Identifies need for/seeks outside support as appropriate.

INTERVENTIONS	RATIONALE
Independent	
Foster trust through one-to-one family/nurse relationship.	Basic trust and stability can be established through continuity and consistency of care.
Encourage client to identify and appropriately verbalize feelings of rejection, abandonment, and ambivalence related to individual situation.	Verbalizing feelings tends to alleviate tensions which may be internalized or somatized, e.g., complaints of nausea.
Focus on specific behaviors which are amenable to change.	Changing of some behaviors can enhance feelings of self-esteem and encourage willingness to make other changes.
Identify underlying family dynamics and determine how they are operating in the present.	Established family patterns affect how the current situation has arisen as well as how the problems need to be resolved and changed now.
Guide client/family in correlating anger and feelings which are centered around lack of influence in family behavior.	Understanding internal dynamics of anger leads to acceptance of locus of control.
Encourage client and family to make as many decisions as are possible within the milieu. Example: client decision to participate in choice of evening activity.	An increase in autonomy and decision-making enhance feelings of self-esteem and competency.
Explore feelings of self-blame and guilt related to problems/changes in the family system. Assist individual in realistic appraisal and verbalization of own role in situation.	Change or disruption in the family system affects all other parts of the system. Children may incorrectly assume that they were instrumental in family problems/marital disruption.
Encourage open communication between client and family when they visit.	Communication patterns affect the functional level of each family member.
Explore ways client and family can be mutually supportive without fostering overdependence on each other.	Security and trust provide a climate for growth and risk-taking.
Give immediate, consistent, and positive reinforcement when desired behaviors are observed. Converse reinforcement/ignore negative behaviors.	Consistent reinforcement of appropriate behaviors fosters continuation of those behaviors. Consequences for inappropriate behaviors and no reinforcement (ignoring) tends to extinguish these behaviors.

INTERVENTIONS

Independent

Discuss reasons for adolescent behaviors.

Collaborative

Explore potential sources of assistance available to meet needs. Refer to social services, other agencies as indicated.

Encourage family to participate in family therapy.

(Refer to CP: Parenting.)

RATIONALE

Understanding of adolescent tasks, ambivalent feelings, etc., can help individual(s) accept and deal more appropriately with difficult behaviors.

Knowledge of resources available in the event they are needed tends to decrease fears of the unknown.

Enables family to work on issues which affect all of the system.

NURSING DIAGNOSIS:	NUTRITION, ALTERED: LESS THAN/ MORE THAN BODY REQUIREMENTS.
MAY BE RELATED TO:	Inadequate intake of balanced, nutritional meals
POSSIBLY EVIDENCED BY:	Reported/observed inadequate food intake and lack of weight gain
	Excessive intake in relation to metabolic need
	Satisfaction of hunger through consumption of excessive amounts of "junk food" with subsequent weight gain
CLIENT OUTCOMES/EVALUATION CRITERIA:	Verbalizes understanding of the relationship of food intake, exercise, and metabolism. Demonstrates positive eating habits with appropriate nutritional intake. Achieves desired weight level.

INTERVENTIONS

Independent

Encourage client to eat well-balanced meals on a regular basis.

Provide information regarding nutritional intake and selection of appropriate foods which will encourage weight loss/gain as indicated.

RATIONALE

Hunger can be satisfied with food intake eliminating "empty calories."

The correlation of food intake and weight gain/loss, if understood, can lead to food choices which result in achieving appropriate weight. Foods which are self-selected are more likely to be eaten and enjoyed.

Assist client in developing insight into eating habits as they relate to feelings of anxiety. Encourage keeping a diary of food intake and related feeling(s).

Increased anxiety may lead to anorexia or frequent snacking as a response to feelings of tension.

Collaborative

Refer to dietician as needed.

May require additional help with determination of caloric needs and intake.

NURSING DIAGNOSIS:	SOCIAL INTERACTION, IMPAIRED
MAY BE RELATED TO:	**Lack of social skills**
	Developmental state (adolescence)
POSSIBLY EVIDENCED BY:	**Verbalized or observed discomfort in social situations and use of unsuccessful social interaction behaviors**
	Dysfunctional interactions with peers, family, and/or others
	Family report of change of style or pattern of interaction
	Self-concept disturbance
CLIENT OUTCOMES/EVALUATION CRITERIA:	**Verbalizes awareness of factors and identifies feelings related to impaired social interactions. Involved in achieving positive changes in social behaviors and interpersonal relationships. Develops effective social support systems.**

INTERVENTIONS

RATIONALE

Independent

Assess individual causes and contributing factors, e.g., disruption of the family, frequent moves during adolescent's life, individual's poor coping, and adjustment to developmental stage.

While learning social skills is one of the adolescent tasks, many factors can interfere with the client's ability to interact satisfactorily with others in social situations.

Review medical history.

Long-term illness/accident may have interfered with development of social skills at earlier stages.

Observe family patterns of relating and social behaviors. Explore possible family scripting of expectations of the adolescent. Note prevalent patterns.

Family may not have effective patterns of relating to others and the child learns these skills in this setting. Often child is reflecting family expectations rather than own desires. Identification of patterns will help with plan for change.

INTERVENTIONS

Independent

Encourage client to verbalize feelings about discomfort, noting recurring factors or precipitating patterns.

Active listen verbalizations indicating hopelessness, powerlessness, fear and anxiety, grief, anger, feeling unloved or unlovable, problems with sexual identity and/or hate (directed or not).

Assess client's coping skills and defense mechanisms.

Have client identify behaviors that cause discomfort and review negative behaviors others have identified.

Explore with client and role-play new ways of handling identified behaviors/situations.

Provide positive reinforcement for positive social behaviors and interactions.

Work with client to correct basic negative self-concept. (Refer to ND: Self Concept, disturbance in: Body Image, Self-esteem, Role Performance, Personal Identity.)

Help client to identify responsibility for own behavior. Encourage the keeping of a daily journal of social interactions and feelings.

Collaborative

Involve in group therapy as indicated.

Encourage reading, attendance at classes (e.g., Positive Image, Self-help, Assertiveness), and community support groups.

RATIONALE

Identifies areas of concern and suggests ways to learn new skills.

Client may have belief that nothing can be done to change the way things are and that own actions do not make a difference.

May be effective for dealing with individual situation and/or provide a base for learning new skills.

Listing specific behaviors will help the client know where change is possible. Knowing what others see can assist the client to accept and effect change.

Active involvement is the most effective way to create change.

Promotes feelings of self-worth and helps to reinforce desired behaviors.

Negative self-concepts may be a major factor impeding positive social interactions.

Enhances self-esteem and provides feedback to improve skills. Journal-keeping can provide an ongoing record to note improvement and/or areas of need for change.

Helpful arena to practice new social skills, receive feedback with support for efforts to improve.

Assists in alleviating negative self-concepts that lead to impaired social interactions.

Eating Disorders

DSM III-R: 307.10 Anorexia Nervosa
Anorexia nervosa is an illness of starvation, brought on by severe disturbance of body image and a morbid fear of obesity. Presently, there is no strong evidence of heredity.

DSM III-R: 307.51 Bulimia Nervosa
This eating disorder (binge-purge syndrome) is characterized by extreme overeating, followed by self-induced vomiting, and may include abuse of laxatives and diuretics.

ETIOLOGIC THEORIES

PSYCHODYNAMICS

The individual reflects a developmental arrest in the very early childhood years. The tasks of trust, autonomy, and separation-individuation are unfulfilled, and the individual remains in the dependent position. Ego development is retarded. Symptoms are often associated with a perceived loss of control in some aspect of life.

BIOLOGIC THEORIES

It is suggested that the cause of these disorders may arise out of neuroendocrine abnormalities within the hypothalamus. Symptoms are linked to various chemical disturbances normally regulated by the hypothalamus.

FAMILY DYNAMICS

The issue of control becomes the overriding factor in the family of the patient with an eating disorder. These families often consist of a passive father, a domineering mother, and an overly dependent child. There is a high value placed on perfectionism in this family, and the child believes he or she must satisfy these standards.

CLIENT ASSESSMENT DATA BASE

HISTORY

Anorexia Nervosa

The onset of the illness is between the ages of 10 and 18.
Distorted (unrealistic) body image. Reports self as fat regardless of weight; sees thin body as fat.
Expresses intense fear of gaining weight.
No medical illness evident to account for weight loss.
Refusal to maintain body weight over minimal norm for age/height.
Exhibits irrational thinking about eating, food, and weight.
May be hungry all the time, but deny hunger; appetite may be normal or exaggerated and rarely vanishes until late in the disorder. May talk about/do gourmet cooking, exhibit preoccupation with food by hiding it, cutting food into small pieces, rearranging food on plate.
Displays an unrealistic pleasure in weight loss, while denying self pleasure in other areas.
Exhibits sense of helplessness.
May have a hysterical or obsessive personality style.
May have depressive affect; be depressed; have family history of higher than normal incidence of depression.
Displays appropriate affect, except in regard to body and eating.
Usually intelligent and a good student. Often from middle- or upper-class family.
History of being a quiet, cooperative child.
May be evidence of an emotional crisis of some sort, such as the onset of puberty or a family move.
May be an avid exerciser. While anorectics are predominantly female (94%), there is evidence that male "obligatory" runners and wrestlers, etc., share common characteristics with female anorectics, e.g., high self-expectations, depressive tendencies, hold back on expression of anger.
Disturbed sleep patterns, commonly early morning insomnia.

May have frequent infections indicative of depressed immune system.

Denial/loss of sexual interest.

May complain of fatigue, feeling "hyper" and/or anxious, and of feeling cold even when room is warm.

Often presents with no other psychiatric illness and with no evidence of the presence of a psychiatric thought disorder.

Bulimia Nervosa

In addition to above history:

Recurrent episodes of binge eating (rapid consumption of a large amount of food in a discrete period of time).

A feeling of lack of control over eating behavior during the eating binges.

Regularly engages in either self-induced vomiting, use of laxatives or diuretics, strict dieting or fasting, or vigorous exercise in order to prevent weight gain. Bloody vomitus may indicate esophageal tearing (Mallory-Weiss).

A minimum average of two binge eating episodes a week for at least three months.

Complains of diarrhea/constipation; vague abdominal pain and distress, bloating.

May complain of continuous sore throat.

Persistent overconcern with body shape and weight.

PHYSICAL EXAMINATION

Presence of weight loss leading to maintenance of body weight 15% or more below that expected. In bulimia, weight may be normal or slightly below.

Cachectic appearing. Skin may be dry, yellowish/pale.

Absence of at least 3 consecutive menstrual cycles (amenorrhea).

May exhibit periods of hyperactivity.

Hair growth may be increased on body (lanugo), but may have hair loss.

May have low B/P, bradycardia, decreased body temperature.

Vomiting may occur; may have binge-purge syndrome (bulimia) independently or as a complication of anorexia.

Dehydration may be evident.

Peripheral edema may be noted.

May have swollen salivary glands; sore, inflamed buccal cavity.

Mental status exam may reveal mental changes (apathy, confusion) brought on by malnutrition/starvation.

DIAGNOSTIC STUDIES

Electrolytes: often imbalanced with decreased potassium, sodium, and chloride.

Endocrine studies:

    Thyroid function:

        Thyroxine levels: usually normal; however, circulating triiodothyronine (T3) levels may be low.

    Pituitary function:

        TSH (thyroid stimulating hormone) response to TRF (thyrotropin releasing factor) is abnormal in anorexia nervosa.

        Propranolol-glucagon stimulation test: studies the response of human growth hormone (GH) which is depressed in anorexia nervosa.

        Gonadotropic hypofunction.

    Hypothalamic function: Abnormality may be a cause of anorexia (rare).

        Cortisol: metabolism may be elevated.

        Dexamethasone suppression test (DST): evaluates hypothalamic-pituitary function; dexamethasone resistance, indicating cortisol suppression, suggests malnutrition/depression.

        Luteinizing hormone secretions test: pattern like those of prepubertal girls.

Leukopenia, elevated SGOT, hypercarotenemia, anemia.

    Blood platelets show significantly less than normal activity by the enzyme monoamine oxidase, which is thought to be a marker for depression.

MHP 6 levels: decreased, suggestive of malnutrition/depression.

Urinalysis and renal function: BUN may be elevated, ketones present, reflecting starvation.

Blood sugar and basal metabolism: may be low.

EKG: abnormal with low voltage, T-wave inversion.

NURSING PRIORITIES

1. Reestablish adequate nutritional intake.
2. Correct fluid and electrolyte imbalance.
3. Assist client to develop realistic body image/improve self-esteem.
4. Provide support/involve family, if available, in treatment program.
5. Coordinate total treatment program with other disciplines.

DISCHARGE CRITERIA

1. Verbalizes importance of adequate nutrition and consequences of fluid loss resulting from self-induced vomiting, laxative/diuretic use.
2. Recognizes maladaptive coping behaviors and stressors that precipitate anxiety.
3. Identifies adaptive coping strategies and techniques for anxiety reduction and maintaining self-control.
4. Verbalizes an increased sense of self-esteem.
5. Achieves and maintains at least 90% of expected body weight with vital signs and laboratory serum studies within normal limits.

NURSING DIAGNOSIS:	**NUTRITION, ALTERED: LESS THAN BODY REQUIREMENTS.**
MAY BE RELATED TO:	**Inadequate food intake**
	Self-induced vomiting
	Laxative use
POSSIBLY EVIDENCED BY:	**Body weight 15% (or more) below expected but may be within normal range (bulimia)**
	Pale conjunctiva and mucous membranes
	Poor muscle tone
	Excessive loss of hair; increased growth of hair on body (lanugo)
	Amenorrhea
	Poor skin turgor
	Electrolyte imbalances
	Hypothermia
	Bradycardia; cardiac irregularities
	Hypotension

Edema

CLIENT OUTCOMES/EVALUATION CRITERIA:

Demonstrates adequate nutritional intake with weight gain to within expected range. Verbalizes understanding of nutritional needs and establishes a dietary pattern with caloric intake adequate to regain/maintain appropriate weight.

INTERVENTIONS	RATIONALE
Independent	
Establish a minimum weight goal.	When this is agreed upon, psychological work can begin. Malnutrition is a mood-altering condition leading to depression and agitation so that adequate nutrition is important for psychologic well-being.
Maintain a regular weighing schedule, such as M-W-F before breakfast in same attire and graph results.	Provides accurate ongoing record of weight loss and/or gain. Also diminishes obsessing about gains and/or losses.
May weigh with back to scale (dependent on program protocols)	Forces issue of trust in client who usually does not trust others.
Make selective menu available and allow client to control choices, as much as possible.	Client needs to gain confidence in self and feel in control of environment. More likely to eat preferred foods.
Be alert to choices of low-calorie foods/beverages; hoarding food; disposing of food in various places such as pockets or wastebaskets.	Client will try to avoid taking in what is viewed as excessive calories.
Use a consistent approach. Present and remove food without persuasion and/or comment. Sit with client while eating, also without comment.	Client detects urgency and reacts to pressure. When staff responds in a consistent manner, client can begin to trust their responses. The one area in which the client has exercised power and control is food/eating. Client may experience guilt if forced to eat. Any comment which might be seen as coercion provides focus on food. Structuring meals and decreasing discussions about food will decrease power struggles with client and avoid manipulative games.
Provide one-to-one supervision. Have the client remain in the room with no bathroom privileges for a specified period (½ hour) following eating.	Prevents vomiting during/after eating. Sometimes clients desire food and use a binge-purge syndrome to maintain weight. Note: Purging may occur for the first time in a client as a response to establishment of weight gain program.
Avoid room checks and control devices.	Reinforces feelings of powerlessness and are usually not helpful.
Monitor exercise program and set limits on physical activities. Chart activity/level of work (pacing, etc.).	Moderate exercise helps in maintaining muscle tone/weight and combating depression. Client may exercise excessively to burn calories.
Maintain matter-of-fact, nonjudgmental attitude if giving tube feedings, hyperalimentation, etc.	Perception of punishment may be counterproductive to promoting self-confidence and faith in own ability to control destiny.

INTERVENTIONS	RATIONALE

Independent

Be alert to possibility of patient disconnecting tube and emptying hyperalimentation if used. Check measurements and tape tubing snugly.

Sabotage behavior is common in attempt to prevent weight gain.

Collaborative

Hospitalize for nutritional therapy, as indicated.

Provides a controlled environment in which food intake, output, medication, and activities can be monitored. Separates client from family (which may be contributing factor) and provides exposure to others with the same problem, creating an atmosphere for sharing. Note: Cure of the underlying problem cannot happen without improved nutritional status.

Provide regular diet and snacks with substitutes and preferred foods available.

Having a variety of foods available will enable the client to have a choice of potentially enjoyable foods.

Carry out program of behavior modification, involving client in setting up program. Provide reward for weight gain; ignore loss.

Provides structured eating situation while allowing client some control in choices. Behavior modification may be effective only in mild cases or for short-term weight gain.

Avoid giving laxatives.

Use is counterproductive, as they may be used by client to rid body of food/calories.

Administer liquid diet and/or tube feedings/hyperalimentation.

When caloric intake is insufficient to sustain metabolic needs, nutritional support can be used to prevent malnutrition/death while therapy is continuing.

Blend and tube feed anything left on the tray after a given period of time, if indicated.

May be used as part of behavior modification program to provide total intake of needed calories.

Provide high-caloric liquid feedings.

May be given as medication, at preset times separate from meals, as an alternate means of increasing caloric intake.

Administer medications as necessary: e.g.,
    cyproheptadine (Periactin);

A serotonin and histamine antagonist used in high doses to stimulate the appetite, decrease preoccupation with food, and combat depression. Does not appear to have serious side effects.

    tricyclic antidepressants, e.g., amitriptyline (Elavil);

Lifts depression and stimulates appetite.

    major tranquilizers, e.g., chlorpromazine (Thorazine)

Promotes weight gain and cooperation with psychotherapeutic program. Major tranquilizers are used only when absolutely necessary due to extrapyramidal side effects.

Assist with electroconvulsive therapy. Help client understand this is not punishment.

In difficult cases where malnutrition is severe and may be life-threatening, a short-term ECT series may enable the client to begin eating and become accessible to psychotherapy.

NURSING DIAGNOSIS:	**FLUID VOLUME DEFICIT, POTENTIAL/ ACTUAL 2**

MAY BE RELATED TO:	Inadequate intake of food and liquids
	Consistent self-induced vomiting
	Laxative/diuretic use
POSSIBLY EVIDENCED BY:	Dry skin and mucous membranes, decreased skin turgor
	Increased pulse rate, body temperature
	Output greater than input (diuretic use)
	Concentrated urine/decreased urine output
	Hemoconcentration
	Hypotension
	Weakness
	Change in mental state
	Altered electrolyte balance
CLIENT OUTCOMES/EVALUATION CRITERIA:	Demonstrates improved fluid balance as evidenced by adequate urine output, stable vital signs, moist mucous membranes, good skin turgor. Verbalizes understanding of causative factors and behaviors necessary to correct fluid deficit.

INTERVENTIONS	RATIONALE
Independent	
Discuss strategies to stop vomiting and laxative/diuretic use.	Helping the client to deal with anxiety feelings which lead to vomiting and decision to stop using laxatives/diuretics will prevent continued fluid loss.
Monitor amount and types of fluid intake. Measure urine output accurately.	Client may abstain from all intake or substitute fluids for caloric intake impacting fluid balance/renal function. Note: Reduced urinary output may be a direct result of reduced food intake.
Monitor vital signs, capillary refill.	Orthostatic hypotension may occur.

INTERVENTIONS	RATIONALE

Independent

Discuss actions necessary to regain optimal fluid balance.

Involving client in plan to correct fluid imbalances provides more option for success.

Collaborative

Review results of electrolyte/renal function (e.g., BUN, creatinine).

Fluid/electrolyte shifts, decreased renal function can adversely affect client's recovery/prognosis and may require additional intervention.

Administer/monitor I.V., hyperalimentation;

Used as an emergency measure to correct fluid/electrolyte imbalance

   potassium supplements, oral or I.V., as indicated.

Restores electrolyte balance. Low potassium levels can lead to cardiac arrhythmias.

NURSING DIAGNOSIS:	**THOUGHT PROCESSES, ALTERED**
MAY BE RELATED TO:	**Severe malnutrition/electrolyte imbalance**
	Psychologic conflicts, e.g., sense of low self-worth, perceived lack of control
POSSIBLY EVIDENCED BY:	**Impaired ability to make decisions, problem-solve**
	Non-reality-based verbalizations
	Ideas of reference
	Altered sleep patterns (may go to bed late and get up early)
	Altered attention span/distractibility
	Perceptual disturbances with failure to recognize hunger; fatigue, anxiety, and depression
CLIENT OUTCOMES/EVALUATION CRITERIA:	**Verbalizes understanding of causative factors and awareness of impairment. Demonstrates behaviors to change/prevent malnutrition and improved ability to make decisions, problem-solve.**

INTERVENTIONS	RATIONALE
Independent	
Be aware of client's distorted thinking ability.	Allows the caregiver to lower expectations and provide information and support
Listen to and do not challenge irrational, illogical thinking. Present reality concisely and briefly.	It is not possible to respond logically when thinking ability is physiologically impaired. The client needs to hear reality, but challenging leads to distrust and frustration.
Adhere strictly to nutrition regime.	Improved nutrition is essential to improved brain functioning. (Refer to ND: Nutrition, altered, Less than body requirements.)
Collaborative	
Review electrolyte/renal function tests.	Imbalances negatively affect cerebral functioning.

NURSING DIAGNOSIS:	**SELF-CONCEPT, DISTURBANCE IN: BODY IMAGE/SELF-ESTEEM**
MAY BE RELATED TO:	**Morbid fear of obesity**
	Perceived loss of control in some aspect of life
	Unmet dependency needs
	Dysfunctional family system
POSSIBLY EVIDENCED BY:	**Distorted body image, views self as fat, even in the presence of normal body weight or severe emaciation**
	Expresses little concern, uses denial as a defense mechanism and feels powerless to prevent/make changes
CLIENT OUTCOMES/EVALUATION CRITERIA:	**Establishes a more realistic body image. Acknowledges self as an individual who has responsibility for own actions.**

INTERVENTIONS	RATIONALE
Independent	
Establish a therapeutic nurse/client relationship.	Within a helping relationship, the individual can begin to trust and try out new thinking and behaviors.
Promote self-concept without moral judgment.	Individual sees self as weak-willed, even though a part of the person may feel a sense of power and control.

INTERVENTIONS	RATIONALE

Independent

State rules re: weighing schedule, remaining in sight during medication and eating times, and consequences of not following the rules. Be consistent in carrying out rules without undue comment.

Client is obsessed with fear of weight gain. Regular monitoring of client's weight is important to nutritional status. Consistency is important in establishing trust. As part of the behavior modification program, the client knows the risks involved in not following established rules (e.g., decrease in privileges). Failure to do so is viewed as the client's choice and accepted by the staff in matter-of-fact manner so as not to provide reinforcement for the undesirable behavior.

Respond (confront) with reality when client makes unrealistic statements such as "I'm gaining weight, so there's nothing really wrong with me."

Provides constructive feedback about how the weight gain will give the client energy to look at other aspects of their lives so that weight concerns will not be so all-consuming. Individuals need to be confronted because they deny the psychologic aspects of their situation and are often expressing their sense of inadequacy and depression.

Be aware of own reaction to the client's behavior. Avoid arguing.

Feelings of disgust, hostility, and infuriation are not uncommon when caring for these clients. Prognosis remains poor even with a gain in weight, as other problems may remain. Many continue to see themselves as fat, and there is also a high incidence of affective disorders, social phobias, obsessive-compulsive symptoms, drug abuse, and psychosexual dysfunction. The nurse needs to deal with own response/feelings so they do not interfere with care of the client.

Assist the client to assume control in areas other than dieting/weight loss, e.g., management of own daily activities, work/leisure choices.

Feelings of personal ineffectiveness, low self-esteem, and perfectionism are often part of the problem. Client feels helpless to change and requires assistance to problem-solve methods of control in life situations.

Help the client formulate goals for self not related to eating and formulate a manageable plan to reach those goals, one at a time.

Client needs to recognize ability to control other areas in life and may need to learn problem-solving skills in order to achieve this control. Client may need help in setting realistic goals.

Assist client to confront sexual fears. Provide sex education as necessary.

Major physical/psychologic changes in adolescence can contribute to development of this problem. Feelings of powerlessness and loss of control of feelings (in particular sexual), sensations, and physical development lead to an unconscious desire to desexualize themselves. Client often believes that these fears can be overcome by taking control of bodily appearance/development/function.

Encourage client to take charge of own life in a more healthful way by making own decisions and accepting self as is. Encourage acceptance of inadequacies as well as strengths. Let client know that it is acceptable to be different from family, particularly mother.

Client often doesn't know what s/he may want for self. Parents (mother) usually make decisions for them. Client may also believe s/he has to be the best in everything and hold self responsible for being perfect. Needs to develop a sense of identity as separate from family and maintain sense of control in other ways, besides dieting and weight loss.

INTERVENTIONS	RATIONALE
Independent	
Involve in personal development program.	Learning about proper application of makeup, methods of enhancing personal appearance may be helpful to long range sense of self-esteem.
Use interpersonal psychotherapy rather than interpretive therapy.	More helpful for the client to discover feelings/impulses/needs from within own self. Client has not learned this internal control as a child.
Encourage client to express anger and acknowledge when it is verbalized.	Important to know that anger is part of self and as such is acceptable. Expressing anger may need to be taught to client, as anger is generally considered unacceptable in the family and therefore client does not express it.
Assist client to learn strategies other than eating for dealing with feelings. Have client keep a diary of feelings, particularly when thinking about food.	Feelings are the underlying issue, and clients often use food instead of dealing with feelings appropriately. May need to learn to recognize feelings and how to express them.
Assess feelings of helplessness/hopelessness.	54% of clients with anorexia have a history of major affective disorder, and 33% have a history of minor affective disorder.
Be alert to suicidal ideation/behavior.	Intensity of anxiety/panic about weight gain, depression, hopeless feelings may lead to suicidal attempts, particularly if client is impulsive.
Collaborative	
Involve in group therapy.	Provides an opportunity to talk about feelings and try out new behaviors.

NURSING DIAGNOSIS:	**FAMILY PROCESS, ALTERED**
MAY BE RELATED TO:	**Issues of control in family**
	Situational/maturational crises
	History of inadequate coping methods
POSSIBLY EVIDENCED BY:	**Dissonance among family members**
	Family developmental tasks not being met
	Focus on "identified patient" IP
	Family needs not being met
	Family member(s) acting as "enablers" for IP

POSSIBLY EVIDENCED BY—
continued

**FAMILY OUTCOMES/EVALUATION
CRITERIA:**

Ill-defined family rules, function, and roles

Demonstrates individual involvement in problem-solving processes directed at encouraging client toward independence. Expresses feelings freely and appropriately. Demonstrates more autonomous coping behaviors with individual family boundaries more clearly defined. Recognizes and resolves conflict appropriately with the individuals involved.

INTERVENTIONS	RATIONALE
Independent	
Identify patterns of interaction. Encourage each family member to speak for self. Don't allow two members to discuss a third without that member's participation.	Helpful information for planning interventions. The enmeshed, over-involved family members often speak for each other and need to learn to be responsible for their own words and actions.
Discourage members from asking for approval from each other. Be alert to verbal or nonverbal checking with others for approval. Acknowledge competent actions of client.	Each individual needs to develop own internal sense of self-esteem. Individual often is living up to others' (family's) expectations rather than making own choices. Provides recognition of self in positive ways.
Listen with regard when the client speaks.	Sets an example and provides a sense of competence and self-worth in that the client has been heard and attended to.
Encourage individuals not to answer to everything.	Reinforces individualization and return to privacy.
Communicate message of separation, that it is acceptable for family members to be different from one another.	Individuation needs reinforcement. Such a message confronts rigidity and opens options for different behaviors.
Encourage and allow expression of feelings (e.g., crying, anger) by individuals.	Often these families have not allowed free expression of feelings and will need help and permission to learn and accept this.
Prevent intrusion in dyads by other members of family.	Inappropriate interventions in family subsystems prevent individuals from working out problems successfully.
Reinforce importance of parents as a couple who have rights of their own.	The focus on the child with anorexia is very intense and often is the only area around which the couple interact. The couple needs to explore their own relationship and restore the balance within it in order to prevent its disintegration.
Prevent client from intervening in conflicts between parents. Assist parents in identifying and solving their marital differences.	Triangulation occurs in which a parent-child coalition exists. Sometimes the child is openly pressed to ally with one parent against the other. The symptom (anorexia) is the regulator in the family system, and the parents deny their own conflicts.

INTERVENTIONS

Independent

Be aware and confront sabotage behavior on the part of family members.

Collaborative

Refer to community resources, such as family group therapy, parents' groups, as indicated.

RATIONALE

Feelings of blame, shame, and helplessness may lead to unconscious behavior designed to maintain the status quo.

May help reduce overprotectiveness, support/facilitate the process of dealing with unresolved conflicts and change.

NURSING DIAGNOSIS:	SKIN INTEGRITY, IMPAIRMENT OF, POTENTIAL/ACTUAL
MAY BE RELATED TO:	Altered nutritional state
	Edema
	Dehydration/cachectic changes (skeletal prominence)
POSSIBLY EVIDENCED BY:	Dry/scaly skin
	Dry rash
	Pressure areas/decubitus
	Dermal abrasions (from scratching)
CLIENT OUTCOMES/EVALUATION CRITERIA:	Verbalizes understanding of causative factors and relief of itching. Identifies and demonstrates behaviors to maintain soft, supple, intact skin.

INTERVENTIONS

Independent

Encourage bathing every other day.

Use skin cream twice a day and after bathing.

Massage skin, especially over bony prominences.

Observe for reddened/blanched areas.

Discuss activity needs, importance of frequent change of position.

RATIONALE

Frequent baths contribute to dryness of the skin.

Contributes to lubrication of the skin. Decreases itching.

Improves circulation to the skin and skin tone.

Indicators of increasing risk of breakdown requiring more intense treatment.

Altered circulation affects perfusion to skin.

INTERVENTIONS	RATIONALE

Independent

Stress importance of adequate nutrition/fluid intake. (Refer to ND: Nutrition, altered: Less than body requirements.)

Improved nutrition will improve skin condition.

NURSING DIAGNOSIS:	KNOWLEDGE DEFICIT [LEARNING NEED] (SPECIFY)
MAY BE RELATED TO:	Lack of exposure to/unfamiliarity with information about condition
	Learned maladaptive coping skills
POSSIBLY EVIDENCED BY:	Verbalization of misconception of relationship of current situation and behaviors (preoccupation with extreme fear of obesity and distortion of own body image, refusal to eat, binging and purging, abuse of laxatives and diuretics, excessive exercising)
	Verbalization of need for new information
	Expressions of desire to learn more adaptive ways of coping with stressors
CLIENT OUTCOMES/EVALUATION CRITERIA:	Verbalizes awareness of and plans for lifestyle changes to maintain normal weight. Identifies relationship of signs/symptoms (e.g., weight loss, tooth decay) to behaviors of not eating/binge-purging. Assumes responsibility for own learning. Seeks out sources/resources to assist with making identified changes.

INTERVENTIONS	RATIONALE

Independent

Determine level of knowledge and readiness to learn.

Learning is easier when it begins where the learner is.

Note blocks to learning, e.g., malnutrition, family problems, drug abuse, affective disorders, obsessive-compulsive symptoms.

Physical/intellectual/emotional factors can interfere with learning.

INTERVENTIONS	RATIONALE

Independent

Review dietary needs, answering questions as indicated. (Refer to ND: Nutrition, altered, Less than body requirements.)

Client/family may need assistance with planning for new way of eating.

Provide information and encourage the use of relaxation and other stress management techniques.

New ways of coping with feelings of anxiety and fear will help client to manage these feelings in more effective ways, assisting in giving up maladaptive behaviors of not eating/binging-purging.

Assist with establishing a sensible exercise program. Caution regarding overexercise.

Exercise can assist with developing a positive body image and combats depression. Client may use excessive exercise as a way of controlling weight.

Provide written information for client/significant other(s).

Helpful as reminder of and reinforcement for learning.

Discuss need for information about sex and sexuality.

Since avoidance of own sexuality is an issue for this client, realistic information can be helpful in beginning to deal with self as a sexual being.

Collaborative

Refer to therapist trained in dealing with sexuality.

May need professional assistance to accept self as a sexual adult.

Refer to National Association of Anorexia Nervosa and Associated Disorders.

May be a helpful source of support and information for client and significant other(s).

Eating Disorders: Obesity

DSM III-R: Although considered to be a type of eating disorder, simple obesity is listed as a physical disorder, but may be considered under the category 316.00 Psychological Factors Affecting Physical Condition.

ETIOLOGIC THEORIES

PSYCHODYNAMICS

Food is substituted by the parent for affection and love. The child harbors repressed feelings of hostility toward the parent, which may be expressed inward on the self. Because of a poor self-concept, the person has difficulty with other relationships. Eating is associated with a feeling of satisfaction and becomes the primary defense.

BIOLOGIC THEORIES

It is suggested that the cause of these disorders may arise out of neuroendocrine abnormalities within the hypothalamus, which result in various chemical disturbances. Familial tendencies have been identified, but obesity is not clearly identified as being hereditary. People who are overweight have more fat cells than thin people and are known to be less active.

FAMILY DYNAMICS

Parents act as role models for the child. Maladaptive coping patterns (overeating) are learned within the family system and are supported through positive reinforcement.

CLIENT ASSESSMENT DATA BASE

HISTORY

Problem may be lifetime or related to life event.
Higher incidence with family history of obesity.
May/may not perceive weight as a problem.
Cultural factors may affect value for thinness/weight.
Client may perceive body image as undesirable.
May have history of recurrent weight loss and gain.
Often has tried numerous types of diets (yo-yo dieting) with varied/short-lived results.
Less likely to be active or engage in regular exercise.
Note presence of associated diseases, cardiovascular, hypertension, diabetes, and endocrine disturbance, as well as pertinent psychologic factors.
Family/significant other(s) may be supportive or resistant to weight loss (sabotage client's efforts).

PHYSICAL EXAMINATION

Weight disproportionate to height.
Body measurements, including skinfold, to estimate fat/muscle mass.
Concomitant health problems may be present, e.g., hypertension, diabetes, cardiovascular.

DIAGNOSTIC STUDIES

May be "normal" or reflect concomitant problems.
Endocrine studies: Thyroid series and pituitary function may reveal abnormalities.

NURSING PRIORITIES

1. Assist client to identify a pattern of weight control containing needed nutrients.
2. Promote improved self-concept, including body image, self-esteem.
3. Encourage health practices to provide for weight control throughout life.

DISCHARGE CRITERIA

1. Identifies healthy pattern for nutrition and weight control.
2. Establishes weight loss pattern of 1 pound/week to desired weight.
3. Verbalizes positive perception of self in relation to change in body image.

NURSING DIAGNOSIS:	**NUTRITION, ALTERED: MORE THAN BODY REQUIREMENTS**
MAY BE RELATED TO:	**Food intake which exceeds body needs** **Psychosocial factors**
POSSIBLY EVIDENCED BY:	**Weight of 20% or more over optimum body weight** **Reported or observed dysfunctional eating patterns** **Denial of excessive food intake**
CLIENT OUTCOMES/EVALUATION CRITERIA:	**Verbalizes a more realistic self-concept/body image, mental and physical. Identifies inappropriate behaviors associated with weight gain or overeating. Demonstrates change in eating patterns and involvement in individual exercise program. Attains desirable body size and composition with optimal maintenance of health.**

INTERVENTIONS	RATIONALE
Independent	
Identify daily caloric intake, types of food, and eating habits via 24-hour recall or diary.	Provides realistic record of amount of food ingested and corresponding eating habits.
Review emotions/events associated with eating.	Helps to identify when client is eating to satisfy an emotional need rather than hunger.
Determine the diet in consultation with the client, avoiding fad diets. Use knowledge of height, body build, age, gender, and individual patterns of eating. Stress the importance of a balanced diet.	A diet which has been developed and agreed to by the client is more apt to be followed. While there is no basis for recommending one diet over another, it needs to provide nutrients with fewer calories than energy expenditure. Standard tables are subject to error when applied to individual situations as circadian rhythms and lifestyle patterns need to be considered. Elimination of carbohydrates from the diet can lead to metabolic acidosis (ketosis) and fatigue, headache, instability, and weakness.

INTERVENTIONS	RATIONALE

Independent

Discuss realistic goals for weekly weight loss. May be increment goals.

One/two pounds per week is reasonable and achieves a more lasting loss. Too rapid a loss may result in fatigue and irritability, which may lead to failure in meeting goals and losing weight. Motivation is more easily maintained by meeting stair-step goals instead of one large goal of the total desired weight loss.

Reassess caloric requirements q 2–4 weeks to determine need for adjustment. Be aware of plateaus when weight remains stable for periods of time. May need emotional support at this time.

Changes in weight and exercise will necessitate changes in diet. As weight is lost, changes in metabolism occur. Distrust and accusations of "cheating" on caloric intake are not helpful.

Determine current activity levels and plan increasing exercise program tailored to individual goals and choice.

Added activity increases energy output and tones the muscles. Commitment on the part of the client enables the setting of more realistic goals and adherence to the plan. No evidence exists that spot reducing or mechanical devices aid in weight loss in specific areas. Loss occurs on a generalized overall basis. Exercise further aids in weight loss by reducing appetite and enhancing sense of well-being and accomplishment.

Develop an appetite reeducation plan with the client.

Signals of hunger and fullness often have become distorted, ignored, and are not recognized without reeducation.

Stress the importance of avoiding tension at mealtimes as well as not eating too fast. Encourage client to eat only at a table or designated eating place and to avoid standing while eating. (Behavior modification techniques may be helpful.)

Reducing stress provides an opportunity for a more relaxed eating atmosphere and more leisurely eating patterns. A period of time is required for the appestat mechanism to know the stomach is full. A designated place is helpful in avoiding snacking.

Collaborative

Consult with dietician to determine caloric requirements for individual weight loss. (Actual weight minus 15# should be used for very obese clients.)

Individual intake can be calculated by several different formulas but is based on the basal caloric requirement for 24 hours.

Administer medications as indicated, e.g.,

appetite-suppressant drugs;

Used with caution at the beginning of a weight loss program. They are effective for only a few weeks and may cause problems of addiction in some people.

hormonal therapy, such as thyroid;

May be necessary when hypothyroidism is present. Replacement when no deficiency is present is not helpful and may actually be harmful. Other hormonal treatments, such as human chorionic gonadotropin (HCG), although widely publicized, have no documented evidence of value.

vitamin, mineral supplementation.

While obese individuals have large fuel reserves, this does not hold true for vitamins and minerals.

Discuss restriction of salt intake and diuretic drug use.

Water retention may be a problem because of increased fluid intake, as well as the result of fat metabolism.

Hospitalize for fasting regime and/or stabilization of medical problems.

Aggressive therapy/support may be necessary to initiate weight loss. Program can be monitored and controlled more effectively in a structured setting. Rapid

INTERVENTIONS	RATIONALE
Collaborative	
	weight loss may encourage adherence to long-term program. Fasting is not generally treatment of choice as success rates have been low and complications such as postural hypotension, anemia, cardiac irregularities, and decreased uric acid excretion with hyperuricemia may occur.
Refer for surgical interventions, e.g., gastric bypass, stapling, if indicated.	Occasionally, these interventions assist the client to lose weight when obesity is life-threatening.

NURSING DIAGNOSIS:	SELF-CONCEPT, DISTURBANCE IN: BODY IMAGE; SELF-ESTEEM
MAY BE RELATED TO:	Client's view of self
	Psychosocial factors: Slimness is valued in this society, and mixed messages are received when advertising stresses thinness.
	Family/subculture encouragement of overeating.
	Control/sex and love issues
POSSIBLY EVIDENCED BY:	Negative feelings about body (mental image often does not match physical reality)
	Preoccupation with change (attempts to lose weight)
	Lack of follow-through with diet plan
	Verbalization of powerlessness to change habits of overeating
CLIENT OUTCOMES/EVALUATION CRITERIA:	Verbalizes a more realistic self-image. Demonstrates acceptance of self as is rather than an idealized image. Acknowledges self as an individual who has responsibility for own self. Seeks information and actively pursues appropriate weight loss.

INTERVENTIONS	RATIONALE
Independent	
Discuss with the client view of being fat and what it does for the individual.	Mental image includes our ideal and is usually not up to date. Fat and compulsive eating behaviors may have deep-rooted psychologic implications, e.g., compensating for love and nurturing, as well as a defense against intimacy. People often eat because of depression, anger, and guilt.
Determine the client's motivation for weight loss and set goals.	A client losing weight for someone else is less likely to be successful/maintain weight loss.
Be alert to myths the client and significant other(s) may have about weight and weight loss.	Beliefs about what an ideal body looks like and unconscious motivations such as the feminine thought of "if I become thin, men will follow me, throw me on the ground, and rape me" and the masculine counterpart "I don't trust myself to stay in control of my feelings," as well as issues of strength, power, and "good cook," can lead to frustration, fear, and sabotage behavior.
Assist client to identify feelings which lead to compulsive eating. Keeping a diary can be helpful. Develop strategies for doing something other than eating for dealing with these feelings.	Awareness of emotions which leads to overeating can be the first step in behavior change.
Graph weight on a weekly basis.	Provides ongoing visual evidence of weight changes which are reality oriented.
Be alert to binge-eating, and develop strategies for dealing with these episodes.	The client has a considerable amount of guilt related to binging, and this is counterproductive to success.
Outline responsibilities of client and nurse being sure they are clearly stated.	It is helpful for each individual to understand area of own responsibility so misunderstandings do not arise.
Provide for privacy as care is given.	May experience sense of shame due to stigma of being fat.
Encourage client to use imagery to visualize self at desired weight. Imagery may also be used to practice handling of new behaviors.	Mental rehearsal is very useful to help the client to plan for and deal with anticipated change in self-image and occasions which may arise, such as family gatherings, special dinners, or other confrontations with food temptations.
Discuss the use of makeup, hairstyles, and ways of dressing to maximize figure assets.	Enhances feelings of self-esteem, promotes improved body image.
Encourage buying clothes as a reward for weight loss instead of food treats.	Properly fitting clothes are comfortable and enhance the body image as small losses are made and the individual feels more positive. Waiting until the desired weight loss is reached can become discouraging.
Suggest the client dispose of "fat clothes."	Removes the "safety valve" of having clothes available "in case" the weight is regained. Also carries the message that the weight loss will not occur.
Staff needs to be aware of and deal with own feelings when taking care of these clients.	Judgmental attitudes, feelings of disgust, anger, weariness, and despair can interfere with care.
Collaborative	
Refer to support and/or therapy group.	Group therapy can be helpful in dealing with underly-

INTERVENTIONS	RATIONALE
Collaborative	
	ing psychologic concerns. Support groups can provide companionship, increase motivation, decrease loneliness and social ostracism, and give practical solutions to common problems.

NURSING DIAGNOSIS:	SOCIAL INTERACTION, IMPAIRED
MAY BE RELATED TO:	**Verbalized or observed discomfort in social situations**
	Self-concept disturbance
POSSIBLY EVIDENCED BY:	**Reluctance to participate in social gatherings**
	Verbalization of a sense of discomfort with others
CLIENT OUTCOMES/EVALUATION CRITERIA:	**Verbalizes awareness of feelings that lead to poor social interactions. Involved in achieving positive changes in social behaviors and improving interpersonal relationships.**

INTERVENTIONS	RATIONALE
Independent	
Review family patterns of relating and social behaviors.	Social interaction is primarily learned within the family of origin and when inadequate patterns are identified, actions for change can be instituted.
Encourage client to express feelings and perceptions of problems.	Helps to identify and clarify reasons for difficulties in interacting with others. May feel unloved/unlovable, or insecure about sexuality.
Assess client's use of coping skills and defense mechanisms.	May have developed coping skills in some areas of life which can be transferred to social settings. Defense mechanisms are used to protect the individual but may be used to contribute to isolation.
Have client list behaviors that cause discomfort.	Identifies specific actions that can be taken to effect change.
Involve in role-playing new ways to deal with identified behaviors/situations.	Practicing these new behaviors enables the individual to become comfortable with them in a safe situation.
Discuss negative self-concepts which may be impeding positive social interactions.	Client may be doing negative self-talk, e.g., ''no one wants to be with a fat person''; ''who would be interested in talking to me?''

79

INTERVENTIONS

Collaborative

Encourage ongoing family or individual therapy as indicated.

RATIONALE

Client benefits from involvement of family/significant other(s) to provide support and encouragement.

NURSING DIAGNOSIS:	KNOWLEDGE DEFICIT [LEARNING NEED], SPECIFY
MAY BE RELATED TO:	**Lack of information**
	Misinterpretation of information
	Lack of interest in learning
	Inaccurate/incomplete information presented
POSSIBLY EVIDENCED BY:	**Statements of lack of and request for information about obesity and nutritional requirements**
	Verbalization of problem with weight reduction
	Inadequate follow-through with previous diet and exercise instruction
CLIENT OUTCOMES/EVALUATION CRITERIA:	**Assumes responsibility for own learning and begins to look for information about nutrition and ways to control weight. Verbalizes understanding of need for lifestyle changes to maintain/ control weight.**

INTERVENTIONS

Independent

Determine level of nutritional knowledge and what client believes is most urgent need.

Provide information about ways to maintain satisfactory food intake in settings away from home.

Provide information about books and other learning tools, e.g., tapes. Encourage attendance at classes, groups.

RATIONALE

Necessary to know what additional information to provide. When client's views are listened to, trust is enhanced.

"Smart" eating when dining out or when traveling helps to maintain weight at desired level while still enjoying social outlets.

Using different avenues of accessing information will further client's learning. Involvement with others who are also losing weight can provide support.

Parenting

DSM III-R: No listing

ETIOLOGIC THEORIES

PSYCHODYNAMICS

Effective parenting is a learned skill and is not a set of instinctive behaviors. Parental roles are derived from many factors, e.g., the family of origin, family myths and scripts, parental skills, knowledge and level of differentiation, socioeconomic and cultural factors, and the marital relationship.

BIOLOGICAL THEORIES

There is a genetic plan for the growth and development of the physical body. In the same way there is a biologic plan for intelligence which is genetically encoded within the individual and drives the child from within. At the same time, parents provide an anxiety-conditioned view of the world which is at conflict with the child's nature. Many of the problems of parenting are man-made, caused by ignoring this plan of nature.

FAMILY DYNAMIC THEORIES

A family is seen as a natural social system, with their own set of rules, definition of roles, power structure, and methods of communication, negotiating, and problem-solving that provide a means of dealing with the process of daily living. These family patterns are largely unconscious and set the emotional tone. These systems are multigenerational, with underlying family dynamics affecting all members in some way. These patterns may be functional or dysfunctional.

CLIENT ASSESSMENT DATA BASE

HISTORY

Family structure may be traditional two-parent, single-parent (mother or father as head), or blended (stepfamily).
Describe family genogram, noting patterns between members and generations. Note presence/geographic distance of extended family.
Varied socioeconomic/cultural factors may impact on parenting, e.g., financial status, structure of family, family myths and beliefs.
Higher risk for families suffering loss, e.g., death, divorce, other separations.
History of period of family disorganization often present.
Child-rearing practices may be ineffective.
Note history of child abuse/sexual abuse.
Family may be in crisis, e.g., situational/maturational.
Broad range of feelings (e.g., calm to hysterical) may be noted.
May display increasing tension and disorganization, e.g., crying, exhaustion, depression, complaints of difficulty sleeping/eating, may repeat the same question over and over. (Note family member(s) who do not appear to be experiencing symptoms of stress or those who may have changed their usual patterns.)

PHYSICAL EXAMINATION

General appearance of family members (neat or disheveled; clean or odious) may be indicators of coping ability, state of denial, presence of crisis.
Behavior: upset, anxious, rapid speech or quiet and withdrawn; appropriate or inappropriate.

NURSING PRIORITIES

1. Promote positive feelings about parenting abilities.
2. Involve parents in problem-solving solutions for current situation.

3. Provide assistance to enable family to develop skills to deal with present situation.
4. Facilitate learning of new parenting skills.

DISCHARGE CRITERIA

1. Understands parenting role, expectations, and responsibilities.
2. Aware of own strengths, individual needs, and methods/resources to meet them.
3. Appropriate attachment/parenting behaviors demonstrated.
4. Involved in activities directed at family growth.

NURSING DIAGNOSIS:	**PARENTING, ALTERED: ACTUAL OR POTENTIAL**
MAY BE RELATED TO:	**Lack of role model**
	Lack of support between or from significant other(s)
	Interruption in bonding process
	Lack of knowledge
	Unrealistic expectations for self, child, partner
	Presence of stress: crisis, financial or legal, cultural move (from one area/country to another, etc.)
	Lack of appropriate response of child to parent/parent to child
POSSIBLY EVIDENCED BY:	**Frequent verbalization of disappointment in child; resentment toward child; inability to care for/discipline child**
	Lack of parental attachment behaviors, e.g., negative characterizations of child; lack of touching; inattention to child's needs
	Inappropriate or inconsistent discipline practices and/or caretaking behaviors
	Growth and/or development lag in child

CLIENT(S) OUTCOMES/EVALUATION CRITERIA:	Presence of child abuse or abandonment **Verbalizes realistic information and expectations of parenting role and acceptance of situation. Identifies own needs, strengths and methods/resources to meet them. Demonstrates appropriate attachment or parenting behaviors.**

INTERVENTIONS

Independent

Determine existing situation and parent(s)'s perception of the problems, noting presence of specific factors such as psychiatric/physical illness; disabilities of child or parent.

Determine developmental stage of the family, e.g., first child/new infant; schoolage/adolescent children; step-family.

Assess parenting skill level, considering intellectual, emotional, and physical strengths and limitations.

Note attachment behaviors between parent and child(ren). Encourage the parent(s) to hold and spend time with the child, particularly the newborn/infants.

Note interactions between parent(s) and child(ren).

Note presence/effectiveness of extended family/support systems.

Stress the positive aspects of the situation, maintaining a positive attitude toward the parents' capabilities and potential for improving.

Involve all members of the family in learning activities.

Provide specific information about limit-setting, time management, and conflict resolution.

Encourage parent(s) to identify positive outlets for meeting own needs, e.g., going to a movie, out to dinner. (Refer to ND: Self-concept, disturbance in: Self-esteem/Role performance.)

RATIONALE

Identification of the individual factors will aid in establishing the plan of care.

These factors affect how family members view current problems and how they will solve them.

Identifies areas of need for further information, skill training, and factors which might interfere with ability to assimilate new information.

Lack of eye contact, touching may be indicative of problems of bonding. Behaviors such as eye-to-eye contact, use of en face position, talking to the infant in a high-pitched voice are indicative of attachment behaviors in American culture. Failure to bond effectively is thought to affect subsequent parent-child interaction.

Identifies relationships, communication skills, feelings about one another.

Provides role models for parent(s) to help them develop own style of parenting.

Helping the parent(s) to feel positive about self and individual capabilities will promote growth.

Learning new skills is enhanced when everyone is interacting.

Helpful in managing parenting responsibilities.

Parent often believes it is "selfish" to do things for own self, that children are primary. However, parents are important, children are important, and the family is important. When parents take care of themselves, they are better parents.

NURSING DIAGNOSIS:	SELF-CONCEPT, DISTURBANCE IN: SELF-ESTEEM/ROLE PERFORMANCE
MAY BE RELATED TO:	View of self as "poor," ineffective parent(s)
	Problems of child(ren), psychiatric/physical illness of the child
	Belief that seeking help is an admission of defeat/failure
POSSIBLY EVIDENCED BY:	Change in usual patterns/responsibility
	Expressions of lack of information about parenting skills
	Lack of follow-through of therapy
	Not keeping appointments
	Nonparticipation in therapy
CLIENT(S) OUTCOMES/EVALUATION CRITERIA:	Verbalize acceptance of selves as parents who are not perfect. Verbalize understanding of role expectations/obligations. Demonstrate personal growth by seeking information, setting of realistic goals, and active participation in improving parent/child relationship.

INTERVENTIONS	RATIONALE
Independent	
Assess level of parent's anxiety, and determine the parent's perception and reality of the situation.	Identification of how family members view the situation and their role in what is happening is essential to the development of the plan of care. The difference between what is actually happening and individual perception can provide helpful clues to family problems and defense mechanisms.
Discuss parental perceptions of their skills and roles as parents. Give information as need is identified.	Parent may see self as a "bad parent" when children have problems and do not live up to expectations of either the parents or society. Information can be given and accepted in casual learning environment.
Listen to expressions of concern about others' reac-	Parent(s) may allow themselves to be influenced by

INTERVENTIONS	**RATIONALE**
Independent	
tions to child's behavior/problems, sense of control over self/situations.	"what others think" rather than establishing their own actions, beliefs, and control.
Note previous and current level of adaptive behaviors/defense mechanisms.	Identifies positive/negative skills and establishes baseline for assisting parents to identify things they already do well and to learn new ways of parenting.
Encourage open discussion of situation/expression of feelings.	Assists individuals to identify areas of concern, hear own ideas, and share with other members of the family.
Acknowledge and accept feelings of anger and hostility.	May believe that expression of negative feelings is not acceptable.
Set limits on maladaptive behaviors and suggest alternative actions, such as hitting pillows, pounding mattress.	Anger may be expressed by unacceptable actions such as hitting/breaking objects in the environment or in violence toward themselves or others.
Have parent(s) identify positive behaviors present, such as the use of positive I-messages, hugging one another.	Improves feelings of self-worth and increases sense of self-esteem when parents recognize that they do have strengths on which to build/establish more positive family interactions.
Encourage individuals to become aware of own responsibility for dealing with what is happening.	Each person has control over own self only and cannot control or make another do anything.
Assist parent(s) to look at own role(s) as actor/reactor to what has been happening in the family.	May limit options to reacting to situations rather than taking action to make things better.
Help parent(s) to avoid comparisons with others.	Each family and the individuals involved have unique ways of dealing with own problems, and comparisons are usually used in a negative way to prove own lack of self-worth.
Assist parents to learn therapeutic communication skills, e.g., I-messages, active listening. Discuss the use of positive I-messages instead of praise.	Improving skills for talking to others offers the opportunity to improve relationships. Positive I-messages help the individual to develop own internal sense of self-worth, enhancing self-esteem.
Provide empathy, not sympathy.	Empathy is objective and communicates an understanding of the other's problems as viewed by that individual, promoting the "I-Thou" relationship. Sympathy is subjective and expresses concern for the nurse's own feelings.
Use positive words of encouragement for improvements noted.	Assists in developing positive coping behaviors.
Discuss inaccuracies in perception as they become apparent.	Helps parents to identify areas of needed action.
Collaborative	
Encourage attendance at group therapy (family and multifamily), assertiveness training, and positive self-esteem classes.	Learning new skills helps individuals develop an improved sense of self-esteem.

NURSING DIAGNOSIS:	FAMILY PROCESS, ALTERED
MAY BE RELATED TO:	**Situational crisis of child/adolescent, e.g., illness/hospitalization, delinquency**
	Maturational crisis, e.g., adolescence, midlife
POSSIBLY EVIDENCED BY:	**Expressions of confusion and difficulty coping with situation**
	Family system not meeting physical emotional/security needs of members
	Having difficulty accepting help, not dealing with traumatic experiences constructively
	Parents don't respect each other's parenting practices
FAMILY OUTCOMES/EVALUATION CRITERIA:	**Expressing feelings appropriately. Demonstrating individual involvement in problem-solving. Verbalizing understanding of child/family problems.**

INTERVENTIONS

Independent

INTERVENTIONS	RATIONALE
Assess family components, roles, dynamics, developmental stage (e.g., young/adolescent children, divorced with step-parents, children leaving home), and cultural influences	Information essential to development of plan of care.
Identify patterns of communication within family.	Helps to establish areas of positive and negative patterns.
Determine boundaries within the family system.	Boundaries need to be clear so individual family members are free to be responsible for themselves.
Assess use of addictive substances by members of the family.	Alcoholism and other drug use may be a critical issue in the interacting of the family as well as in developing a treatment plan. (Note: Individuals may be reluctant to share this information until they feel safe within the therapeutic relationship.)
Identify patterns of communication between individual members and the family as a whole.	May be ineffective to accomplish family tasks. These patterns may be maintaining the maladaptive behaviors/relationships.

INTERVENTIONS	RATIONALE
Independent	
Identify and encourage previously successful coping mechanisms.	Using these behaviors will be comfortable for the individual and a sense of competence and assurance will be gained.
Acknowledge differences among family members with open dialogue about how these differences have been derived.	Conveys an acceptance for these differences among individuals and helps to look at how the differences can be used to facilitate the family process.
Identify effective parenting skills already being used and suggest new ways of handling difficult behaviors.	Allows the individual to realize that some of what has been done already has been helpful and assists in learning new skills to manage the situation in a more effective manner.
Encourage participation in role-reversal activities.	Helps to gain insight and understanding of the other person's feelings and point of view.

NURSING DIAGNOSIS:	**COPING, INEFFECTIVE FAMILY: COMPROMISED/DISABLING**
MAY BE RELATED TO:	**Individual preoccupation with own emotional conflicts and personal suffering/anxiety about the crisis**
	Temporary family disorganization
	Situational crisis
	Exhausted supportive capacities of family members
	Chronically unexpressed feelings of guilt, anger, etc.
	Highly ambivalent family relationships
	Arbitrary handling of a family's resistance which solidifies defensiveness
POSSIBLY EVIDENCED BY:	**Expressions of concern**
	Complaints about S.O.(s) response to problem
	Withdrawal and/or display of protective behavior

POSSIBLY EVIDENCED BY— *continued*	Expressions of despair about family reactions
	Intolerance, agitation, depression, hostility, aggression
	Neglecting relationships
	Distortion of reality about problems; denial
	Decisions/actions which are detrimental
FAMILY OUTCOMES/EVALUATION CRITERIA:	Express more realistic expectations of themselves and situation. Identify internal and external resources. Interact with each other realistically and with understanding. Participate in activities to promote coping.

INTERVENTIONS

Independent

Identify premorbid behaviors and interactions. Note current behaviors.

Note readiness of family to be involved in treatment.

Establish rapport with family members.

Encourage communication, free expression of feelings without judgment.

Note other stressors impacting the family, e.g., financial, physical illness.

Encourage questions, provide accurate information, involving family in treatment planning. (Refer to ND: Knowledge deficit.)

Reframe individual's negative statements when possible.

Encourage dealing with the problems in small increments.

Collaborative

Refer to social services, support group, marriage counselor, community/spiritual resources as indicated.

RATIONALE

Necessary baseline to establish treatment goals. May be withdrawn, angry, hostile, and ignoring other family members (or one specific member).

Readiness is necessary for the success of therapy.

Helps the family to feel comfortable and talk freely about the problems they are experiencing.

Promotes understanding of how others are feeling, perceiving what is happening.

May need assistance with these factors before the family can begin to deal with the issues at hand.

Personal involvement by client and family enhances learning and promotes cooperation with/success of therapy.

Provides a different way of looking at the problem/situation.

One moment at a time can seem more manageable than looking at the whole picture.

Family may need additional help and support at this time.

NURSING DIAGNOSIS:	COPING, FAMILY: POTENTIAL FOR GROWTH
MAY BE RELATED TO:	Surfacing of self-actualization goals
FAMILY OUTCOMES/EVALUATION CRITERIA:	Expresses willingness to look at own role in the problem. Verbalizes desire to change, feelings of self-confidence, satisfaction with progress.

INTERVENTIONS	RATIONALE
Independent	
Determine situation and stage of growth family is experiencing. Note verbalizations of awareness of the growth, impact of the crisis, and expressed interest in learning opportunity.	Baseline data required to establish plan of assistance.
Listen to expressions of hope, planning, etc.	Acknowledgment by the nurse provides reinforcement of hopes and desires for positive change for the future.
Note expression of change of values, discussion of value beliefs.	Willingness to look at own values, discuss meanings, and make decisions about own beliefs is helpful to growth of family members.
Provide role model for parent(s) to be involved with and observe.	Role model provides opportunity for individual members to learn new ways of behaving.
Involve with others who have had similar experiences, e.g., multifamily group therapy, support groups.	Sharing of experiences provides opportunities to develop empathy and understanding of parenting roles.
Provide opportunities for role-play.	Role-play allows client and family to "practice" how they will respond in stressful situations, in an effort to prevent future crises.
Provide experiences to assist family to learn new ways of interacting, group therapy, parenting classes, etc.	Involvement with others helps individuals to see how they and others solve problems, effectively or ineffectively, and provides opportunities to learn new skills.
Encourage open communication within the family (no "family secrets") and use of effective communication skills, e.g., I-messages, active listening.	Open acceptance of a variety of feelings and attitudes is necessary for growth within the family system.
Assist individuals to learn new effective ways of dealing with feelings.	Learning to identify and express feelings provides opportunity to act in different ways.

NURSING DIAGNOSIS:	KNOWLEDGE DEFICIT [LEARNING NEED] SPECIFY
MAY BE RELATED TO:	Lack of information about child growth and development
	Ineffective parenting skills

POSSIBLY EVIDENCED BY:	Angry expressions about parenting role
	Verbalization of problems in dealing with child(ren)
	Statements of misconceptions about how to parent
	Inappropriate or exaggerated behaviors, e.g., hostile, agitated, apathetic
CLIENT(S) OUTCOMES/EVALUATION CRITERIA:	Participates in learning process. Assumes responsibility for learning new parenting skills. Identifies stressors and actions to deal effectively with them. Initiates necessary lifestyle changes and participates in learning activities.

INTERVENTIONS	RATIONALE
Independent	
Determine level of knowledge of parenting skills and beliefs.	Individual needs are based on current information and/or beliefs and misconceptions.
Note level of anxiety and signs of avoidance; cultural beliefs about parents and children; feelings about self as a parent.	Moderate to severe anxiety, level of self-esteem, cultural beliefs can interfere with desire/ability to learn new information.
Provide information and help parent(s) learn new communication skills of active-listening, declarative, responsive, preventive, and positive I-messages.	Learning new methods of interaction promotes improved relationships among family members and helps to resolve current situation.
Discuss conflict-resolution concepts of "Who owns the problem?" problem-solving and resolving of value collisions.	Conflict is inevitable in relationships with others, and learning to understand the other person's point of view and effective ways to deal with differences can strengthen and enhance the relationship between family members.
Be aware of "teachable moments" that occur during interaction with the family and/or individual members.	Taking advantage of opportunities as they present themselves can enhance the learning situation.
Promote active participation in learning by the use of role-play, participant discussion, and other activities.	Learning is enhanced when the individual is actively engaged in the process.
Provide positive reinforcement for attempts to learn new behaviors/communication skills.	Parent frequently feels guilty and critical of self when a child has difficulties, and positive feedback can help individual to be more realistic about own self, the child, and the situation.
Provide information about additional resources, e.g., books on related topics, tapes.	Bibliotherapy can be a helpful adjunct to information given by other means as well as providing a continuation of learning in informal/home setting.

INTERVENTIONS	RATIONALE
Collaborative	
Refer to social workers, clergy, psychotherapy, and/or classes such as Parent Effectiveness, assertiveness training.	Additional resources may help with resolution of other, deeper problems/concerns.

CHAPTER 4

ORGANIC MENTAL DISORDERS (Non-Substance-Induced)

Dementias Arising in the Presenium and Senium (Alzheimer's Disease)

DSM III-R: 290.1 x Primary degenerative dementia
290.4 x Multi-infarct dementia
Organic mental syndromes associated with other
Physical disorders (see DSM III-R for specific code listing)

ETIOLOGIC THEORIES

PSYCHODYNAMICS

A chronic organic mental disorder that has an insidious onset and runs a uniform, gradual, progressive course. Presenile onset occurs before age 65 (e.g., Alzheimer's, Pick's). Symptoms of senile onset appear after age 65 (e.g., senile dementia of the Alzheimer's type [SDAT]); however, the pathophysiologic process is the same.

BIOLOGIC THEORIES

Multi-infarct dementia reflects a pattern of intermittent deterioration in the brain. Symptoms fluctuate and are determined by the area of the brain that is affected. Deterioration is thought to occur in response to repeated infarcts of the brain. Predisposing factors include cerebral and systemic vascular disease, hypertension, cerebral hypoxia, hypoglycemia, and cerebral embolism. Genetics may also be a factor. Studies reveal a familial pattern of transmission that is four times greater than in the general population. Down syndrome may have some relationship to Alzheimer's Disease. At autopsy, both have many of the same pathophysiologic changes. Down patients who survive to adulthood eventually develop Alzheimer's lesions, which has led researchers to theorize that the extra chromosome of Down might be related to the cause of Alzheimer's.
Serious head injury may be a predisposing factor.
Abnormally high levels of antibodies have been found, leading to the theory of an immunologic defect.

CLIENT ASSESSMENT DATA BASE

HISTORY

May present a total healthy picture except for memory/behavioral changes.

Family members may report a gradual decrease in cognitive abilities, impaired judgment, impaired recent memory but good remote memory, behavioral changes.

Decreased interest in usual activities/hobbies and impaired motor skills may be noted.

History of recent viral illness or head trauma, drug toxicity, stress, nutritional deficits may be associated with confusion.

Seizure activity, secondary to the brain damage in Alzheimer's disease, may be reported/noted.

Patient may deny symptoms, especially cognitive changes, and/or describe vague, hypochondriacal complaints of fatigue, diarrhea, dizziness, or occasional headaches.

May be suspicious or fearful of imaginary people/situations, misperceive environment, misidentify objects and people, hoard objects, cling to significant other(s), claim misplaced objects are stolen.

May conceal inabilities, e.g., makes excuses not to perform task, may thumb through a book without reading it. May be content watching others; main activity may be hoarding inanimate objects, repetitive motions (fold-unfold-refold linen), hiding articles or wandering.

May forget mealtime; be dependent on others for meals; show changes in taste; lose ability to chew, feed self, use utensils; or may conceal lost skills by refusing to eat.

Elimination: urgency may indicate loss of muscle tone; may be incontinent of urine/feces as disease progresses, or may be prone to constipation; may forget to go to bathroom, forget steps involved in toileting self, or be unable fo find the bathroom.

May have been forced to retire. Prior psychosocial factors, individuality and personality influence present altered behavioral patterns.

Incidence of primary degenerative dementia is more common in women (who live longer) than in men; multi-infarct dementia occurs more often in men than in women.

PHYSICAL EXAMINATION

Neurological status:

May laugh at or feel threatened by these exams. Usually oriented to person until late in the disease.

Impaired recent memory, intact remote memory is characteristic of Alzheimer's. May change answers during the interview. Unable to do simple calculations or repeat the names of three objects.

Impaired motor skills with tremors, rigidity, unsteady gait.

Speech may be fragmented; aphasia and dysphasia may be present.

Primitive reflexes (e.g., positive snout, suck, palmar) may be present.

May have impaired communication: difficulty with finding correct words, especially nouns, conversation repetitive or scattered with substituted meaningless words, speech may become inaudible. Gradually loses ability to write or read (fine motor skills).

Emotional lability: cries easily, laughs inappropriately, variable mood changes (apathy, lethargy, restlessness, short attention span, irritability), sudden angry outbursts (catastrophic reactions), sleep disturbances.

Multiple losses, changes in body image, self-esteem, may show strong, depressive overlay.

DIAGNOSTIC STUDIES

Note: While no diagnostic studies are specific for Alzheimer's, they are used to rule out reversible problems which may be confused with these dementias.

CBC, RPR, electrolytes, thyroid studies: May determine and/or eliminate treatable/reversible dysfunctions, e.g., metabolic disease processes, fluid/electrolyte imbalance, neurosyphilis.

B_{12}: May disclose a nutritional deficit if low.

Dexamethasone suppression test (DST): To rule out treatable depression.

ECG: May be normal; to rule out cardiac insufficiency.

EEG: May be normal or show some slowing (aids in establishing treatable brain dysfunctions).

Skull X-rays: Usually normal.

Vision/hearing tests: To rule out deficits which may be the cause of or contribute to disorientation, mood swings, or altered sensory perceptions rather than cognitive impairment.

Positron-emission transaxialtomography (PET) scan, Brain electrical activity mapping (BEAM), Magnetic resonance imaging (MRI): May show areas of decreased brain metabolism characteristic of Alzheimers.

CT scan: May show widening of ventricles, cortical atrophy.

NURSING PRIORITIES

1. Provide safe environment, prevent injury.
2. Promote socially acceptable responses, limit inappropriate behavior.
3. Maintain reality orientation/prevent sensory deprivation/overload.
4. Encourage participation in self-care within individual limitations.
5. Facilitate communication with client/significant other(s).
6. Promote coping mechanisms of client/significant other(s).
7. Support client/family in grieving process.

DISCHARGE CRITERIA

1. Adequate supervision/support systems are available.
2. Achieves maximal level of independent functioning.
3. Family/S.O.(s) verbalize understanding of disease process/prognosis and client expectations/needs.
4. Family/S.O.(s) developing/strengthening coping skills and using available resources.

NURSING DIAGNOSIS:	**INJURY, POTENTIAL FOR, TRAUMA**
MAY BE RELATED TO:	**Inability to recognize/identify danger in environment**
	Disorientation, confusion
	Impaired judgment
	Weakness, muscular incoordination
POSSIBLY EVIDENCED BY:	**Wandering, forgetful**
	Misidentification of objects
	Perceptual difficulties (missing chairs, steps, etc.)
	Shuffling gait, stumbling, frequent falls
FAMILY OUTCOMES/EVALUATION CRITERIA:	**Caregiver(s) recognizes potential risks in the environment. Identifies/implements steps to correct them. Injury to client is prevented.**

INTERVENTIONS	RATIONALE
Independent	
Assess for degree of impairment in ability/competence. Assist family/significant other(s) to identify risks/	Enhances functions that are present. Identifies potential risks in the environment and heightens awareness

95

INTERVENTIONS	RATIONALE

Independent

potential hazards that may cause harm.	of risks so caregivers are more alert to dangers.
Eliminate/minimize identified hazards in the environment.	A person with cognitive impairment and perceptual disturbances is prone to accidental injury, because of the inability to take responsibility for basic safety needs or to evaluate the unforseen consequences, e.g., may light a stove/cigarette and forget it, mistake plastic fruit and eat it, misjudge chairs, stairs.
Provide with an identification bracelet showing name, phone number, and diagnosis.	Facilitates safe return if lost. Because of poor verbal ability and confusion, these persons may be unable to state address, phone number, etc. It is likely that they may be detained by police for confused, wandering, irritable/violent outbursts and poor judgment.
Dress according to physical environment/individual need.	The general slowing of metabolic processes results in lowered body heat. The hypothalamic gland is affected by the disease process, causing person to feel cold. Client may have seasonal disorientation and may wander out in the cold. Note: Leading causes of death are pneumonia/accidents.
Be attentive to nonverbal physiological symptoms.	Due to sensory loss and language dysfunction, may express needs in nonverbal manner, e.g., thirst by panting; pain by sweating, doubling over.
Be alert to underlying meaning of verbal statements.	May direct a question to another, such as, "Are you cold/tired?" meaning they are cold/tired.
Use "child-proof" locks; lock medications, poisonous substances, tools, sharp objects, etc. Remove stove knobs, burners.	As the disease worsens, the client may fidget with objects/locks (hypermetamorphosis) or put small items in mouth (hyperorality) which potentiates accidental injury/death.
Avoid continuous use of restraints.	Endangers the individual who succeeds in partial removal of restraints. May increase agitation and potentiate fractures in the elderly who have reduced calcium in the bones.

NURSING DIAGNOSIS:	**THOUGHT PROCESSES, ALTERED**
MAY BE RELATED TO:	**Neuronal degeneration**
	Loss of memory
	Sleep deprivation
	Psychologic conflicts
POSSIBLY EVIDENCED BY:	**Inability to interpret stimuli accurately and evaluate reality**

	Disorientation and difficulty in grasping ideas/commands
	Paranoia, delusions, confusion/frustration and changes in behavioral responses
CLIENT OUTCOMES/EVALUATION CRITERIA:	Recognizes changes in thinking/behavior and causative factors when able. Demonstrates a decrease in undesired behaviors, threats and confusion.

INTERVENTIONS	RATIONALE
Independent	
Assess degree of cognitive impairment.	Provides accurate information on which to base care.
Maintain a pleasant, quiet environment.	Reduces distorted input whereas crowds, clutter, noise generate sensory overload that stresses the impaired neurons.
Approach in a slow, calm manner.	This nonverbal gesture lessens the chance of misinterpretation and potential agitation. Hurried approaches can startle and threaten the confused client who misinterprets or feels threatened by imaginary people and/or situations.
Face the individual.	Maintains reality, expresses interest, and arouses attention, particularly in persons with perceptual disturbances, e.g., unable to focus or perceive by sound.
Call by name.	Names are the basis of self-identity, establish reality and individual recognition. Client may respond to own name long after failing to recognize significant other(s).
Decrease tone and rate when speaking.	Increases the chance for comprehension. High-pitched, loud tones convey stress and anger, which may trigger memory of previous confrontations and provoke an angry response.
Give simple directions, one at a time, or step-by-step instructions, using short words and simple sentences.	As the disease progresses, the communication centers in the brain become impaired, hindering the individual's ability to process and comprehend complex messages. Simplicity is the key to communicating (both verbal and nonverbal) with the cognitively impaired person.
Pause between phrases or questions, give hints, and use open-ended phrases when possible.	Invites a response and may increase comprehension. Hints stimulate communication and give the person a chance for a positive experience.
Listen with regard.	Conveys interest and worth to the individual who has difficulty processing and decoding messages.
Interpret statements, meanings, and words. If possible, supply the correct word.	Assisting the client with word processing aids in decreasing frustration.

INTERVENTIONS	RATIONALE
Independent	
Reduce provocative stimuli: negative criticism, arguments, confrontations.	Any provocation decreases esteem and may be interpreted as a threat that may trigger agitation or increase inappropriate behavior.
Use distraction. Talk about real people and real events when client begins ruminating about false ideas.	Rumination serves to promote disorientation. Reality orientation increases client's sense of reality, self-worth, and personal dignity.
Refrain from forcing activities and communications.	Force decreases cooperation and may increase suspiciousness, delusions.
Use humor with interactions.	Laughter can assist in communication and help reverse emotional lability.
Focus on appropriate behavior, give positive responses, a pat on the back, praise, applause. (Note: Use touch judiciously. Respect individual's personal space/response.)	Reinforces correctness, appropriate behavior. A focus on inappropriate behavior can stimulate that kind of behavior. While touch frequently transcends verbal interchange, conveying warmth, acceptance, and reality, the individual may misinterpret the meaning of touch. Intrusion into personal space may threaten the client's distorted world.
Respect individuality and evaluate individual needs.	Persons experiencing a cognitive decline deserve respect, dignity, and worth as an individual. Individual past and background is important in maintaining self-concept, planning activities, communicating, etc.
Allow personal belongings.	Familiarity enhances security, sense of self and avoids increased feelings of loss/deprivation.
Permit hoarding of safe objects.	An activity that preserves security and counterbalances irrevocable losses.
Assist with finding misplaced items or label drawers.	Decreases defensiveness when client believes s/he is being accused of stealing a misplaced, hoarded, or hidden item. To refute the accusation won't change the belief and may invite anger.
Monitor phone use closely.	Impaired judgment does not allow for distinguishing long distance numbers, makes client easy prey for phone sales pitches, may call dead relative, forget time of day when making calls, etc.
Monitor for medication side effects, signs of overmedication.	Drugs can easily build up to toxic levels in the elderly, and dosages/drug choice may need to be altered.
Collaborative	
Administer medications as individually indicated:	
Antipsychotic: e.g., haloperidol (Haldol); thioridazine (Mellaril);	Small dosages may be used to control agitation, delusions, hallucinations. Mellaril is being used widely because there are fewer extrapyramidal signs, visual problems, and especially gait disturbances. Client is at risk for side effects, e.g., extrapyramidal symptoms such as dystonia, akathisia, and increased confusion.
Vasodilators: e.g., cyclandelate (Cyclospasmol);	May improve mental function but requires further research.

INTERVENTIONS	RATIONALE
Collaborative	
Hydergine;	A metabolic enhancer (increases brain's ability to metabolize glucose and use oxygen). May make client more alert and less anxious, rather than increase cognition and memory, and has few side effects. Because of the small magnitude of the improvement, it is of little value in dementia therapy. This is an expensive drug and families need accurate information in order to make informed therapy decisions and avoid false hopes, disappointment, and lack of dramatic results.
Anxiolytic agents: diazepam (Valium), chlordiazepoxide (Librium).	More useful in early/mild stages for relief of anxiety. Can increase confusion in the elderly.

NURSING DIAGNOSIS:	**SENSORY-PERCEPTUAL ALTERATION (SPECIFY)**
MAY BE RELATED TO:	**Irreversible neuronal degeneration**
	Socially restricted environment (homebound/institutionalization)
	Sleep deprivation
POSSIBLY EVIDENCED BY:	**Memory loss**
	Changes in usual response to stimuli, e.g., spatial disorientation, confusion
	Exaggerated emotional responses, e.g., anxiety, paranoia, and hallucinations
	Inability to tell position of body parts
	Diminished/altered sense of taste
CLIENT OUTCOMES/EVALUATION CRITERIA:	**Demonstrates improved/appropriate response to stimuli. Caregivers identify/control external factors that contribute to alterations in sensory-perceptual abilities.**

INTERVENTIONS	RATIONALE
Independent	
Assess degree of impairment and how it affects the individual.	May affect how the client locates body within the environment. While brain involvement is usually global, a

INTERVENTIONS	RATIONALE
Independent	
	small percentage may exhibit asymmetric involvement, which may cause the client to neglect one side of the body (unilateral neglect). May not be able to locate internal cues, recognize hunger, thirst, or perceive external pain.
Maintain a reality-oriented relationship and environment.	Reduces confusion and promotes coping with the frustrating struggles of misperception, being disoriented/confused.
Provide clues for 24-hour reality orientation with calendars, clocks, notes, cards, signs, music, seasonal hues/color-code rooms, scenic pictures.	Clues are tangible reminders that aid recognition and may permeate memory gaps, increasing independence. Dysfunction in visual-spatial perception interferes with the ability to recognize directions and patterns, and the client may become lost, even in familiar surroundings.
Use sensory games to stimulate reality, e.g., smell Vick's and tell of the time mother used it on you; use of spring-fall nature boxes.	Communicates reality through every possible channel.
Indulge in periods of reminiscence (old music, historical events, photos, mementoes).	Stimulates recollections, awakens memories, aids in the preservation of self/individuality via past accomplishments, increases feelings of security, while easing adaptation to a changed environment.
Provide quiet, nondistracting environment when indicated, e.g., soft music, plain but colorful wallpaper/paint, etc.	Emphasizes qualities of calmness, consistency and helps to avoid situation in which capacity for dealing with visual/auditory information is overloaded. (Note: Patterned wallpaper may be disturbing to the client.)
(Refer to ND: Sleep Pattern, disturbance in)	
Collaborative	
Involve in activities with others as dictated by individual situation, e.g., one-to-one visitors, socialization groups at Alzheimer center, occupational therapy.	Provides opportunity for participation with others and may maintain some level of socialization.

NURSING DIAGNOSIS:	**FEAR**
MAY BE RELATED TO:	**Decreased ability in function**
	Public disclosure of disabilities
	Further mental/physical deterioration
POSSIBLY EVIDENCED BY:	**Social isolation**
	Aggressive behavior
	Apprehension

Irritability

Defensiveness

Suspiciousness

| CLIENT OUTCOMES/EVALUATION CRITERIA: | Demonstrates more appropriate range of feelings and lessened fear. |

INTERVENTIONS

Independent

INTERVENTIONS	RATIONALE
Note change of behavior, suspiciousness, irritability, defensiveness.	Change in moods may be one of the first signs of cognitive decline, and the client, fearing helplessness, tries to hide the increasing inability to remember and do normal activities.
Identify strengths the individual had previously.	Facilitates assistance with communication and management of current deficits.
Deal with aggressive behavior by imposing calm, firm limits.	Acceptance can reduce fear and aggressive behavior.
Provide clear, honest information about actions/events.	Assists in maintaining trust and orientation as long as possible. When the client knows the truth about what is happening, coping is often enhanced and guilt over what is imagined is decreased.

NURSING DIAGNOSIS:	DIVERSIONAL ACTIVITY, DEFICIT
MAY BE RELATED TO:	Physical limitations of degenerative process
	Premature retirement (sense of loss) which may not have been chosen
POSSIBLY EVIDENCED BY:	Decreased attention span
	Restlessness
	Statements of feeling confined
	Expressions of boredom
CLIENT OUTCOMES/EVALUATION CRITERIA:	Participates in activities with some satisfaction, compatible with ability.

INTERVENTIONS	RATIONALE
Independent	
Provide simple outings, short walks.	Motor functioning may be decreased as nerve degeneration results in weakness, decreasing stamina. Outings refresh reality, provide sensory stimuli which may reduce suspiciousness and hallucinations caused by feelings of imprisonment.
Promote balanced physiologic functions, using colorful nerf/beach balls, arm dancing with music.	Preserves mobility and reduces the potential for bone and muscle atrophy.
Create simple, noncompetitive activities paced to the individual's speed.	May be threatened by activities that could lead to failure. Motivates client in ways that will reinforce usefulness, stimulate reality, and enhance self-worth.
Make useful activities out of hoarding and repetitive motions, e.g., collect junk mail, scrapbook, folding/unfolding linen, bouncing balls, dusting, sweep floors.	May decrease restlessness.
(Refer to NDs: Thought Processes, altered, and Sensory-Perceptual alteration)	

NURSING DIAGNOSIS:	**SLEEP PATTERN, DISTURBANCE IN**
MAY BE RELATED TO:	**Disorientation (day/night reversal)**
	Irritability
	Poor judgment potentiated by neurological impairment
POSSIBLY EVIDENCED BY:	**Wakefulness and increased aimless wandering**
	Inability to identify need/time for sleeping
CLIENT OUTCOMES/EVALUATION CRITERIA:	**Establishes adequate sleep pattern, wandering is reduced. Reports/appears rested.**

INTERVENTIONS	RATIONALE
Independent	
Provide for rest/naps; reduce mental activity late in the day.	Physical and mental activity results in fatigue; confusion increases with fatigue.
Avoid use of continuous restraints (particularly when in room alone).	Potentiates sensory deprivation, increases agitation, and restricts rest.
Adhere to regular bedtime schedule and rituals.	Reinforces that it is bedtime and maintains stability of environment.
Reduce fluid intake in the evening.	Decreases need to get up to go to the bathroom during the night.

Collaborative

Administer medications as indicated for sleep;

Antidepressant: e.g., amitriptyline (Elavil);

Avoid use of diphenhydramine (Benadryl).

May be effective in treating pseudodementia, depression. However, the anticholinergic properties can induce confusion, worsen cognition. Orthostatic hypotension and other side effects limit their usefulness.

Once used for sleep, is now contraindicated because it interferes with the production of acetylcholine. The brains of Alzheimer victims have a deficit with acetylcholine production being inhibited.

NURSING DIAGNOSIS:	HOME MAINTENANCE MANAGEMENT, IMPAIRED
MAY BE RELATED TO:	Progressive impaired cognitive functioning
	Insufficient family organization or planning
	Unfamiliarity with resources
	Inadequate support systems
POSSIBLY EVIDENCED BY:	Household members express difficulty and request help in maintaining home in comfortable fashion.
	Disorderly surroundings
	Lack of necessary equipment or aids to care for client
	Overtaxed family members, e.g., exhausted, anxious
FAMILY OUTCOMES/EVALUATION CRITERIA:	Caregiver(s) identify and correct factors related to difficulty in maintaining a safe environment for the client. Demonstrate appropriate, effective use of resources, e.g., respite care, homemakers, Alzheimer groups.

INTERVENTIONS	RATIONALE

Independent

Assess level of cognitive/emotional/physical functioning.

Identifies strengths, areas of need. (Refer to ND: Self-Care Deficit.)

INTERVENTIONS

Independent

Assess environment, noting unsafe factors and ability for client to care for self.

Identify support systems available to client/significant other(s), e.g., other family members, friends.

Evaluate coping abilities, effectiveness, commitment of caregiver(s)/support persons.

Collaborative

Refer to alternate care sources, such as sitter/day care facility, senior care services, e.g., Meals on Wheels/respite care.

RATIONALE

To determine what changes need to be made to accommodate disabilities. (Refer to ND: Injury, potential for: Trauma.)

Assistance with planning and constant care is necessary to maintain this client at home. May help to have someone come in to provide relief from constant care.

Progressive debilitation taxes caregiver(s) and may alter ability to meet client/own needs. (Refer to ND: Coping, ineffective, Family: Compromised/Disabling.)

As condition worsens, may need additional help or may not be able to maintain client at home.

NURSING DIAGNOSIS:	HEALTH MAINTENANCE, ALTERED
MAY BE RELATED TO:	Deterioration can affect ability in all areas, e.g., significant alteration in communication skills, complete or partial lack of gross and/or fine motor skills.
	Cognitive impairment
	Ineffective individual/family coping
	Dysfunctional grieving
POSSIBLY EVIDENCED BY:	Reported or observed inability to take responsibility for meeting basic health practices
	Reported or observed lack of equipment, financial or other resources
	Reported or observed impairment of personal support system.
FAMILY OUTCOMES/EVALUATION CRITERIA:	Caregiver(s) assume responsibility for and adopt lifestyle changes supporting client health care goals. Caregivers verbalize ability to cope adequately with existing situation.

INTERVENTIONS	RATIONALE
Independent	
Assess level of dependence/independence. Reassess frequently.	Important to know how much responsibility to expect the individual to assume.
Identify support systems and level of functioning.	If family system is unavailable/unaware, such needs as nutrition, dental care, eye exams can be neglected.
Assist family/client to develop plan for keeping track of/dealing with health needs.	Helpful to maintain schedule for managing routine health care.
Collaborative	
Refer to supportive services as need indicates.	Consultant such as VNA may be helpful in developing ongoing plan/identifying resources as needed.

NURSING DIAGNOSIS:	**SELF-CARE DEFICIT (SPECIFY LEVEL)**
MAY BE RELATED TO:	**Physical limitations**
	Psychosocial problems
	Cognitive decline
	Frustration over loss of independence
	Depression
POSSIBLY EVIDENCED BY:	**Increasing inability to cope with simple daily activities**
	Frustration
	Misuse/misidentification of objects
	Forgetfulness
	Ability to manage tasks may fluctuate from time to time as deterioration occurs
CLIENT OUTCOMES/EVALUATION CRITERIA:	**Performs self-care activities within level of own ability. Identifies and uses personal/community resources that can provide assistance.**

INTERVENTIONS	RATIONALE
Independent	
Supervise but allow as much autonomy as possible.	Eases the frustration over lost independence.
Identify hygienic needs and provide assistance as needed. Need to include: care of hair/nails/skin, clean glasses, brushing teeth.	As the disease progresses, basic hygienic needs may be forgotten. Harm, infection, or exhaustion may occur when client/caregivers become frustrated, irritated, or intimidated by these problems.
Identify reason for difficulty in dressing/self-care, e.g., physical limitations in motion, apathy/depression, cognitive decline such as apraxia, or room temperature (too cold to get dressed).	Underlying cause affects choice of interventions/ strategies. Problem may be minimized by changes in environment or adaptation of clothing or may require consultation from other specialists.
Allot plenty of time to perform tasks.	Tasks once easy (e.g., dressing, bathing) are now complicated by decreased motor skills or cognitive and physical change. Time and patience reduce chaos.
Assist with neat dressing/provide colorful clothes.	Enhances esteem, may diminish sense of sensory loss and convey aliveness.
Offer one item of clothing at a time, in sequential order.	Simplicity reduces frustration and the potential for rage and despair.
Talk through each step one at a time.	Guidance reduces confusion and allows autonomy.
Allow to sleep in shoes/clothing or wear two sets of clothing if client demands.	Providing no harm is done, altering the ''normal'' lessens the rebellion and allows rest.
Wait and/or change the time to approach dressing/ hygiene if a problem arises.	Because anger is quickly forgotten, another time or approach may be successful.

NURSING DIAGNOSIS:	**NUTRITION, ALTERED: *LESS/MORE* THAN BODY REQUIREMENTS [POTENTIAL]**
MAY BE RELATED TO:	**Sensory changes**
	Impaired judgment and coordination
	Agitation
	Forgetfulness
	Regressed habits and concealment
CLIENT OUTCOMES/EVALUATION CRITERIA:	**Ingests nutritionally balanced diet. Maintains appropriate weight.**

INTERVENTIONS	RATIONALE
Independent	
Assess family/client's knowledge of nutrition.	Provides a base for teaching. A role-reversal situation

INTERVENTIONS

Independent

Determine amount of exercise/pacing client does.

Offer/provide assistance in menu selection.

Provide privacy, when eating habits become an insoluble problem. Accept eating with hands, tolerate spills without scolding, and expect whimsical mixtures, e.g., salad dressing in milk, salt and pepper on ice cream. (Note: Caution not to separate client from other people too soon or frequently.)

Offer small feedings and/or snacks.

Provide ample time for eating.

Simplify/break down steps of eating, serve food in courses, anticipate needs: cut foods, provide soft/finger foods. Offer a spoon. Allow time for chewing.

Avoid baby and hot foods.

Stimulate oral-suck reflex by gentle stroking of the cheeks or stimulating the mouth with a spoon.

Collaborative

Refer to dietician.

RATIONALE

can occur which increases the need for information.

Nutritional intake may need to be adjusted to meet needs related to individual amount of exercise.

Client may be indecisive/overwhelmed by choices or unaware of the need to maintain elemental nutrition. Metabolic rate decreases with age, requiring caloric adjustment. Poor judgment may lead to poor choices.

Aids esteem. Socially unacceptable and embarrassing eating habits develop as the disease progresses. May be unable to locate food on plate due to perceptual difficulties. Acceptance preserves esteem, decreases frustration or not wanting to eat as a result of anger, frustration. Early separation can result in client feeling upset and rejected.

Large feedings may overload the client, resulting either in complete abstinence or gorging.

A leisurely approach aids digestion, decreases the chance of anger precipitated by rushing, and allows time for chewing when motor functioning is impaired.

Promotes autonomy and independence. Decreases potential frustration/anger over lost abilities. Coordination decreases with the progression of the disease process. The ability to chew and handle utensils becomes impaired.

Baby foods lack fiber, taste and add to humiliation. Hot foods may burn or result in refusal to eat.

As the disease progresses, the client may clench teeth and refuse to eat. Stimulating the reflex may increase compliance. These methods usually work with regressed clients. Such primitive reflexes are more apparent in later stages of the disease.

May need assistance in developing nutritional balanced diet for individual client needs.

NURSING DIAGNOSIS:	BOWEL ELIMINATION, ALTERED, CONSTIPATION AND/OR URINARY, ELIMINATION, ALTERATION IN PATTERNS
MAY BE RELATED TO:	Urgency
	Disorientation

MAY BE RELATED TO— *continued*	Lost neurological functioning/muscle tone
	Inability to locate the bathroom/recognize need
POSSIBLY EVIDENCED BY:	Inappropriate toileting behaviors
	Incontinence/constipation
CLIENT OUTCOMES/EVALUATION CRITERIA:	Establishes adequate/appropriate pattern of elimination.

INTERVENTIONS

Independent

Assess prior pattern.

Locate near a bathroom; make signs for/color-code door.

Provide adequate lighting, particularly at night.

Take to the toilet at regular intervals. Dictate each step one at a time and use positive reinforcement.

Encourage adequate fluid intake during the day, diet high in fiber and fruit juices; limit intake during the late evening and at bedtime.

Avoid a sense of hurrying.

Be alert to nonverbal cues, e.g., restlessness, holding self, or picking at clothes.

Be discreet.

Convey acceptance when incontinence occurs. Do not delay changing.

Record frequency of voidings/bowel movements.

Collaborative

Administer stool softeners, Metamucil, glycerin suppository, as indicated.

RATIONALE

Information is useful for planning care.

Location, signs (pictures of toilet), and/or color-coding enhances orientation.

Promotes orientation. Incontinence may be attributed to inability to find a toilet.

Adherence to a daily and regular schedule may prevent accidents. Frequently the problem is forgetting how to do, e.g., pushing pants down, position, etc.

Essential for bodily functions and prevents potential dehydration/constipation. Restricting intake in evening may reduce frequency during the night.

Hurrying may be perceived as intrusion, which leads to anger and lack of cooperation.

May signal urgency/toileting need.

Although the client is confused, a sense of modesty is often retained.

Acceptance is important to esteem. May decrease the embarrassment and feelings of helplessness during the changing process.

Provides visual reminder of elimination and may indicate need for intervention.

May be necessary to facilitate/stimulate regular bowel movement.

| NURSING DIAGNOSIS: | SEXUAL DYSFUNCTION [POTENTIAL] |
| MAY BE RELATED TO: | Confusion |

Forgetfulness and disorientation to place or person

Altered body function

Decrease in habit/control of behavior

Lack of/sexual rejection by significant other

Lack of privacy

CLIENT OUTCOMES/EVALUATION CRITERIA:

Meeting sexuality needs in an acceptable manner.

INTERVENTIONS	RATIONALE
Independent	
Assess individual needs/desires/abilities.	Alternative methods need to be designed for the individual situation to fulfil the need for intimacy and closeness.
Show affection/acceptance.	The cognitively impaired person retains the basic needs for affection, love, acceptance, and sexual expression.
Assure privacy.	Sexual expression or behavior may differ. The individual may masturbate, expose self. Privacy allows sexual expression without embarrassment and the objections of others.
Use distraction, as indicated.	Distraction can be a useful tool when there is inappropriate/objectionable behavior.
Make time to listen/discuss concerns of significant other(s).	May need information and/or counseling about alternatives for sexual activity/aggression.

NURSING DIAGNOSIS:

COPING, INEFFECTIVE FAMILY: COMPROMISED OR DISABLING

MAY BE RELATED TO:

Client's disruptive behavior

Family grief about their helplessness watching their loved one deteriorate

POSSIBLY EVIDENCED BY:

Family becoming embarrassed and socially immobilized

Home maintenance becomes extremely difficult and leads to difficult decisions with legal/financial considerations.

FAMILY OUTCOMES/EVALUATION CRITERIA:	Identifies/verbalizes resources within themselves to deal with the situation. Acknowledges loved one's condition and demonstrates positive coping behaviors in dealing with situation. Uses outside support systems effectively.

INTERVENTIONS	RATIONALE

Independent

Include significant other(s) in teaching and planning for home care.	Can ease the burden of home management and increase adaptation. Comfortable and familiar lifestyle at home is helpful in preserving the need for belonging for the affected individual.
Encourage unlimited visitation.	Can provide a reassuring freedom from loneliness. Contact with familiarity forms a base of reality for the family/affected person.
Provide time to listen to concerns/anxieties of significant other(s).	The self-sacrificing, painful nature of the care in this disease requires support and comfort to let them know they are doing their best and to ease the process of adaptation and grievance.
Listen with regard to concerns/anxieties.	Significant others require constant support with the multifaceted problems that arise during the course of this illness.
Assist with problem-solving. Establish priorities.	Helps in facing the many uncertainties that lie ahead. Helpful to establish goals and plans when dealing with the many behavioral and cognitive changes.
Be realistic and honest in all matters.	Decreases stress that surrounds false hopes, e.g., may regain past level of functioning from advertised or unproven medication.
Focus on specific problems as they occur, the "here and now."	A premature focus on the possibility of long-term care or possible incontinence, for example, impairs the ability to cope with present issues. Disease progression follows no set pattern.
Continually reassess family's ability to care for client at home.	Behaviors like hoarding, clinging, unjust accusations, angry outbursts, etc., can precipitate family burnout and interfere with ability to provide effective care.
Help caregiver/family understand the importance of maintaining psychosocial functioning	Embarrassing behavior, the demands of care, etc., may cause psychosocial withdrawal.

Collaborative

Refer to local resources: adult day care, respite care, homemaker services, or a local chapter of ADRDA (Alzheimer's Disease and Related Disorders Association).	Coping with this individual is a full-time, frustrating task. Respite/day care may lighten the burden, reduce potential social isolation, and prevent family burnout. ADRDA is a national organization with many local chapters that provide group support and family teaching and promotes research. Local groups provide a social outlet for sharing grief and promotes problem-solving with such matters as financial/legal advice, home care, etc.

INTERVENTIONS

Collaborative

Support concerns generated by consideration/decision to place in Long Term Care facility.

RATIONALE

Constant care requirements may be more than can be managed. Support aids this difficult, guilt-producing decision that may become a financial burden as well.

NURSING DIAGNOSIS:	**GRIEVING, ANTICIPATORY**
MAY BE RELATED TO:	**Client awareness of something "being wrong" with changes in memory/family reaction, physiopsychosocial well-being**
	Family perception of potential loss of significant other
POSSIBLY EVIDENCED BY:	**Expressions of distress/anger at potential loss**
	Choked feelings, crying
	Alteration in activity level, communication patterns, eating habits, and sleep patterns
CLIENT OUTCOMES/EVALUATION CRITERIA:	**Expresses concerns openly. Discusses loss and participates in planning for the future.**

INTERVENTIONS

Independent

Assess degree of deterioration/level of coping.

Provide open environment for discussion. Use therapeutic communication skills of active listening, acknowledgment, etc.

Note statements of despair, hopelessness, "nothing to live for," expressions of anger.

Respect client's desire not to talk.

Be honest; do not give false reassurances or dire predictions about the future.

RATIONALE

Helpful to understand how much the client is capable of doing in order to maintain highest level of independence.

Encourages client to discuss feelings and concerns realistically.

May be indicative of suicidal ideation. Angry behavior may be client's way of dealing with feelings of despair.

May not be ready to deal with grief.

Honesty promotes a trusting relationship. Expressions of gloom, such as "You'll spend the rest of your life in a nursing home," are not helpful. (No one knows what the future holds.)

INTERVENTIONS	RATIONALE

Independent

Discuss with client/significant other(s) ways they can plan together for the future.

Having a part in problem-solving/planning can provide a sense of control over anticipated events.

Assist client/significant other(s) to identify positive aspects of the situation.

Ongoing research, possibility of slow progression may offer some hope for the future.

Collaborative

Refer to other resources, counseling, clergy, etc.

May need additional support/assistance to resolve feelings.

CHAPTER 5

PSYCHOACTIVE SUBSTANCE USE DISORDERS

Alcoholism (Acute)

DSM III-R: 303.00 Intoxication
291.40 Idiosyncratic intoxication
291.80 Uncomplicated alcohol withdrawal

ETIOLOGIC THEORIES

PSYCHODYNAMICS

The individual remains fixed in a lower level of development, with retarded ego and weak superego. The person retains a highly dependent nature, with characteristics of poor impulse control, low frustration tolerance, and low self-esteem.

BIOLOGIC THEORY

Enzymes, genes, brain chemistry, and hormones create and contribute to an individual's response to alcohol. There are two types: (1) familial, which is largely inherited, and (2) acquired. A childhood history of attention deficit disorder or conduct disorder also increases a child's risk of becoming alcoholic. There are physiologic changes that cause addiction to alcohol, or alcoholism.

FAMILY DYNAMICS

One in 12 to 15 persons has serious problems from drinking. In a dysfunctional family system, alcohol may be viewed as the primary method of relieving stress. Children of alcoholics are four times more likely to develop alcoholism than children of nonalcoholics. The child has negative role models and learns to respond to stressful situations in like manner. The use of alcohol is cultural, and many factors influence one's decision to drink, how much, and how often. Denial of the illness can be a major barrier to identification and treatment of alcoholism and alcohol abuse.

CLIENT ASSESSMENT DATA BASE

HISTORY

History of alcohol and/or drug use/abuse. Determine amount of alcohol consumed in last 24–48 hours, previous periods of abstinence/withdrawal.

Three times as many men as women become alcoholic, and men are more likely to develop the illness earlier in life. Average age is 25–35, though many children in grade school experiment with alcohol and alcohol is becoming a major problem among adolescents.

May report previous hospitalizations for alcoholism/alcohol-related diseases, e.g., cirrhosis, esophageal varices.

Presence of psychopathology, e.g., paranoid schizophrenia, major depression, may indicate combined substance abuse (dual diagnosis).

May report suicidal ideation/suicide attempts (alcoholic suicide attempts are 30% higher than national average, according to some research).

History of recurrent accidents, such as falls, fractures, lacerations, burns, blackouts, or automobile-related.

Mortality from alcohol intoxication is usually secondary to complicating illnesses; infections due to deteriorated defense mechanisms; injury due to falls, fires, motor vehicle accidents, fights; aspiration of vomitus; and respiratory depression.

May report frequent sick days off work/school, fighting with others, arrests (disorderly conduct, motor vehicle violations/DUIs), mood changes. (Client will likely deny that alcohol intake has any significant effect on the present condition.)

May report/exhibit visual, tactile, olfactory, and auditory hallucinations.

May complain of nausea/vomiting, diarrhea, vision problems, "internal shakes," headache, dizziness.

May report constant upper abdominal pain and tenderness radiating to the back (pancreatic inflammation).

May display an ignorance and/or denial of addiction to alcohol; reports inability to cut down or stop drinking despite repeated efforts.

May report difficulty sleeping and eating.

PHYSICAL EXAMINATION

May present with intoxication, overdose, or in various stages of withdrawal. Concurrent use of other drugs can compound symptoms/reactions.

Level of consciousness/orientation: Confusion, stupor, hyperactivity, distorted thought processes, slurred/incoherent speech may be noted. Memory loss/confabulation may occur.

Affect/mood/behavior: may be fearful, anxious, easily startled, inappropriate, silly, euphoric, irritable, physically/verbally abusive, depressed, and/or paranoid.

Hallucinations: May be picking items out of air or responding verbally to unseen person/voices.

Eye movements: Nystagmus may be present associated with cranial nerve palsy; blurred vision may be noted.

Pupil reaction: Constriction may indicate CNS depression.

Arcus senilis: Ring-like opacity of the cornea (normal in aging populations) may be seen.

Neuromuscular: Fine motor tremors of face, tongue, and hands are often present; seizures may occur (grand mal most common).

Gait: Unsteady walk (ataxia) may be due to thiamine deficiency or cerebellar degeneration (Wernicke's encephalopathy).

Skin: Flushed face/palms of hand, scars, ecchymotic areas, cigarette burns on fingers, spider nevi (impaired portal circulation); fissures at corners of mouth (vitamin deficiency) may be present.

Skeletal: Healed or new fractures (signs of recent/recurrent trauma).

Edema: Generalized tissue edema may be noted due to protein deficiencies.

Respirations: May be tachypneic in hyperactive state of alcohol withdrawal. Cheyne-Stokes respirations or respiratory depression may also occur.

Temperature: Elevation is common due to dehydration and sympathetic stimulation accompanied by flushing/diaphoresis, may indicate presence of infection.

Abdomen: Vomiting, gastric distention may be present; ascites, liver enlargement occasionally seen in clients with cirrhosis.

Nutritional state: Wasted muscles, dry/dull hair, swollen salivary glands, inflamed buccal cavity, capillary fragility may be noted if malnutrition is present.

Peripheral pulses: May be weak, irregular, rapid.

Blood pressure: Hypertension is common in early withdrawal stage but may become labile/progress to hypotension.

Breath sounds: Presence of diminished/adventitious sounds suggests pulmonary complications, e.g., respiratory depression, pneumonia.

Heart sounds: Tachycardia common during acute withdrawal; numerous dysrhythmias may be identified. (Other abnormalities depend on underlying heart disease.)

Bowel sounds: Alterations may occur related to gastric complications such as gastric hemorrhage or distention.

DIAGNOSTIC STUDIES

Blood alcohol/drug levels: Alcohol level may/may not be severely elevated depending on amount consumed and length of time between consumption and testing. In addition to alcohol, numerous controlled substances may be identified in a polydrug screen, e.g., morphine, Percodan, Quaalude.

CBC: May reflect such problems as iron-deficiency anemia or acute/chronic gastrointestinal (GI) bleeding. White blood cell count may be increased with infection or decreased, if immunosuppressed.

Glucose: Hyperglycemia/hypoglycemia may be present, related to pancreatitis, malnutrition, or depletion of liver glycogen stores.

Electrolytes: Hypokalemia and hypomagnesemia are common.

Liver function tests: SGOT, SGPT, and amylase may be elevated, reflecting liver or pancreatic damage.

Nutritional tests: Albumin may be low and total protein decreased. Vitamin deficiencies are usually present, reflecting malnutrition/malabsorption.

Urinalysis: Infection may be identified; ketones may be present related to breakdown of fatty acids in malnutrition (pseudodiabetic condition).

Chest x-ray: May reveal right lower lobe pneumonia (malnutrition, depressed immune system, aspiration) or chronic lung disorders associated with tobacco use.

ECG: Dysrhythmias, cardiomyopathies, and/or ischemia may be present owing to direct effect of alcohol on the cardiac muscle and/or conduction system, as well as effects of electrolyte imbalance.

Addiction Severity Index (ASI): An assessment tool that produces a "problem severity profile" of the client, including chemical, medical, psychologic, legal, family/social and employment/support aspects, indicating areas of treatment needs.

NURSING PRIORITIES

1. Maintain physiologic stability during acute withdrawal phase.
2. Promote patient safety.
3. Provide appropriate referral and follow-up.
4. Encourage/support family involvement in "Intervention" (confrontation) process.

DISCHARGE CRITERIA

1. Physiologic stability achieved.
2. Sobriety is being maintained on a day-to-day basis.
3. Transferred to rehabilitation program/attending group therapy, e.g., Alcoholics Anonymous.
4. Family/significant other(s) participate in Intervention process.

NURSING DIAGNOSIS:	BREATHING PATTERN, INEFFECTIVE [POTENTIAL]
MAY BE RELATED TO:	Direct effect of alcohol toxicity on respiratory center
	Sedative drugs given to decrease alcohol withdrawal symptoms
	Decreased energy/fatigue
	Tracheobronchial obstruction

115

INTERVENTIONS	RATIONALE

Independent

Monitor respiratory rate/depth and pattern as indicated. Note periods of apnea, Cheyne-Stokes respirations.	Frequent assessment is important as toxicity levels may change rapidly. Marked respiratory depression can occur due to CNS depressant effects from alcohol. This may be compounded by drugs used to control alcohol withdrawal symptoms. Hyperventilation is common during acute withdrawal phase. Kussmaul respirations are sometimes present due to acidotic state associated with vomiting and malnutrition.
Elevate head of bed.	Decreases possibility of aspiration; lowers diaphragm, enhancing lung inflation.
Encourage cough/deep breathing exercises and frequent position changes.	Facilitates lung expansion and mobilization of secretions to reduce risk of atelectasis/pneumonia.
Auscultate breath sounds. Note presence of adventitious sounds, e.g., rhonchi, wheezes.	Client is at risk for atelectasis related to hypoventilation and pneumonia. Right lower lobe pneumonia is common in alcohol-debilitated patients and is often due to aspiration. Chronic lung diseases are also common, e.g., emphysema, chronic bronchitis.
Have suction equipment, airway adjuncts available.	Sedative effects of alcohol/drugs potentiates risk of aspiration, relaxation of oropharyngeal muscles, and respiratory depression, requiring intervention to prevent respiratory arrest.

Collaborative

Administer supplemental oxygen if necessary.	Hypoxia may occur with CNS/respiratory depression.
Review/obtain chest x-rays, ABGs as indicated.	Monitors presence of secondary complications such as atelectasis/pneumonia; evaluates effectiveness of respiratory effort, identifies therapy needs.

NURSING DIAGNOSIS:	**CARDIAC OUTPUT, DECREASED [POTENTIAL]**
MAY BE RELATED TO:	**Direct effect of alcohol on the heart muscle**
	Altered systemic vascular resistance
	Electrical alterations in rate; rhythm; conduction

CLIENT OUTCOMES/EVALUATION CRITERIA:	Verbalizes understanding of the effect of alcohol on the heart. Displays vital signs within expected norms; absence of/reduced frequency of dysrhythmias. Demonstrates an increase in activity tolerance.

INTERVENTIONS	RATIONALE
Independent	
Monitor vital signs frequently during acute withdrawal.	Hypertension frequently occurs in acute withdrawal phase. Extreme excitability accompanied by catecholamine release and increased peripheral vascular resistance raises blood pressure (and heart rate), but may become labile/progress to hypotension. (Note: may have underlying cardiovascular disease that is compounded by alcohol withdrawal.)
Monitor cardiac rate/rhythm. Document dysrhythmias.	Long-term alcohol abuse may result in cardiomyopathy/congestive heart failure. Tachycardia is common due to sympathetic response to increased circulating catecholamines. Irregularities/dysrhythmias may develop with electrolyte shifts/imbalance. All of these may have an adverse effect on cardiac function/output.
Monitor body temperature.	Elevation may occur due to sympathetic stimulation, dehydration, and/or infections, increasing the vascular bed (vasodilation) and compromising venous return/cardiac output.
Monitor intake/output. Note 24-hour fluid balance.	Preexisting dehydration, vomiting, fever, and diaphoresis may result in decreased circulating volume, which can compromise cardiovascular function. (Note: Hydration is difficult to assess in the alcoholic because the usual indicators are not reliable and overhydration is a risk in presence of compromised cardiac function.)
Be prepared for/assist in cardiopulmonary resuscitation.	Causes of death during acute withdrawal stages include cardiac dysrhythmias, respiratory depression/arrest, oversedation, excessive psychomotor activity, severe dehydration (or overhydration), and massive infections. Mortality for unrecognized/untreated delirium tremens (DTs) may be as high as 15–25%.
Collaborative	
Note initial serum electrolyte levels.	Electrolyte imbalance, e.g., potassium/magnesium, potentiates risk of cardiac dysrhythmias and CNS excitability.
Administer medications as indicated, e.g., clonidine (Catapres);	Provides for greater mean reductions in heart rate and systolic blood pressure with less nausea and vomiting than chlordiazepoxide.
potassium.	Corrects deficits that can result in life-threatening dysrhythmias.

NURSING DIAGNOSIS:	INJURY, POTENTIAL FOR: (SPECIFY)
MAY BE RELATED TO:	Cessation of alcohol intake with varied autonomic nervous system responses to the system's suddenly altered state
	Involuntary clonic/tonic muscle activity (seizures)
	Equilibrium/balancing difficulties, reduced muscle and hand/eye coordination
CLIENT OUTCOMES/EVALUATION CRITERIA:	Demonstrates absence of untoward effects of withdrawal, and physical injury is prevented

INTERVENTIONS

Independent

Identify stage of alcohol withdrawal, i.e., Stage I is associated with signs/symptoms of hyperactivity (e.g., tremors, sleeplessness, nausea/vomiting, diaphoresis, tachycardia, hypertension). Stage II is manifested by increased hyperactivity plus hallucinations and/or seizure activity. Stage III symptoms include delirium tremens (DTs) and extreme autonomic hyperactivity with profound confusion, anxiety, insomnia, fever.

Monitor/document seizure activity. Maintain patent airway. Provide environmental safety, e.g., padded side rails, bed in low position.

Check deep tendon reflexes. Assess gait, if possible.

Provide for environmental safety when indicated. (Refer to ND: Sensory-Perceptual Alteration: specify.)

Collaborative

Administer IV/po fluids with caution, as indicated.

RATIONALE

Prompt recognition and intervention may halt progression of symptoms and enhance recovery/improve prognosis. In addition, reoccurrence/progression of symptoms indicates need for changes in drug therapy/more intense treatment.

Grand mal seizures are most common and may be related to decreased magnesium levels, hypoglycemia, elevated blood alcohol, or previous history of seizures. (Note: In absence of previous history of seizures, they usually stop spontaneously, requiring only symptomatic treatment.)

Reflexes may be depressed, absent, or hyperactive. Peripheral neuropathies are common, especially in malnourished patient. Ataxia (gait disturbance) is associated with Wernicke's syndrome (thiamine deficiency) and cerebellar degeneration.

May be required when equilibrium, hand/eye coordination problems exist.

Corrects dehydration and promotes renal clearance of toxins. Overhydration may occur.

INTERVENTIONS	RATIONALE

Collaborative

Administer medications as indicated:

Benzodiazepines, e.g.,
  chlordiazepoxide (Librium), diazepam (Valium);

Commonly used to control neuronal hyperactivity that occurs as alcohol is detoxified. I.V./oral administration is the route preferred, as intramuscular absorption is unpredictable. The muscle-relaxant qualities are particularly helpful to the client in controlling "the shakes," trembling, and ataxic quality of movements. Clients may initially require large doses to achieve desired effect, and then the drugs may be tapered and discontinued, usually within 96 hours. (Note: These agents must be used cautiously in client with hepatic disease, as they are metabolized by the liver.)

oxazepam (Serax);

Although less dramatic for control of withdrawal symptoms, may be drug of choice in client with liver disease because of its shorter half-life.

Phenobarbital;

Useful in suppressing withdrawal symptoms as well as an effective anticonvulsant. Use must be monitored to prevent exacerbation of respiratory depression.

Magnesium sulfate

Reduces tremors and seizure activity by decreasing neuromuscular excitability.

NURSING DIAGNOSIS:	SENSORY-PERCEPTUAL ALTERATION (SPECIFY)
MAY BE RELATED TO:	Chemical alteration: exogenous (e.g., alcohol consumption/sudden cessation) and endogenous (e.g., electrolyte imbalance, elevated ammonia, and BUN)
	Sleep deprivation
	Psychologic stress (anxiety/fear)
POSSIBLY EVIDENCED BY:	Disoriented in time/place or person
	Changes in usual response to stimuli
	Bizarre thinking
	Exaggerated emotional responses, change in behavior
	Altered sensory reception/integration
	Fear/anxiety

<table>
<tr><td>CLIENT OUTCOMES/EVALUATION
CRITERIA:</td><td>**Regains/maintains usual level of consciousness. Reports absence of auditory/visual hallucinations. Identifies external factors that affect sensory-perceptual abilities.**</td></tr>
</table>

INTERVENTIONS	RATIONALE
Independent	
Assess level of consciousness, ability to speak, response to stimuli/commands.	Speech may be garbled, confused, or slurred. Response to commands may reveal inability to concentrate, impaired judgment, or muscle coordination deficits.
Observe behavioral responses, e.g., hyperactivity, disorientation, confusion, sleeplessness, irritability.	Hyperactivity related to CNS disturbances may escalate rapidly. Sleeplessness is common due to loss of sedative effect gained from alcohol usually consumed prior to bedtime. Sleep deprivation may aggravate disorientation/confusion. Progression of symptoms may indicate impending hallucinations (Stage II) or DTs (Stage III).
Note onset of hallucinations. Document as auditory, visual, and/or tactile.	Auditory hallucinations are reported to be more frightening/threatening to client. Visual hallucinations occur more at night and often include insects, animals, or faces of friends/enemies. Clients are frequently observed "picking the air." Yelling may occur if client is calling for help from perceived threat (usually seen in Stage III).
Provide quiet environment. Speak in calm, quiet voice. Regulate lighting as indicated. Turn off radio/TV during sleep.	Reduces external stimuli during hyperactive stage. Client may become more delirious when surroundings cannot be seen, though some respond better to quiet, darkened room.
Provide care by same personnel whenever possible.	Promotes recognition of caregivers and a sense of consistency that may reduce fear.
Encourage family/S.O.(s) to stay with client whenever possible.	May have a calming effect and provide a reorienting influence.
Provide frequent reality orientation to person, place, time, and surrounding environment as indicated.	May reduce confusion/misinterpretation of external stimuli.
Minimize bedside discussion concerning client.	Client may hear and misinterpret conversation, which can aggravate hallucinations.
Provide environmental safety, e.g., place bed in low position, leave doors in full open or closed position, observe frequently, place call light/bell within reach, remove articles that can harm client.	Client may have distorted sense of reality, be fearful, or be suicidal, requiring protection from self-harm.
Collaborative	
Provide seclusion, restraints as necessary.	Clients with excessive psychomotor activity, severe hallucinations, violent behavior, and/or suicidal gestures may respond better to seclusion. Restraints are usually ineffective and add to client's agitation, but occasionally may be required to prevent self-harm.

INTERVENTIONS	RATIONALE

Collaborative

Monitor laboratory studies: e.g., electrolytes, liver function studies, BUN, ABGs, glucose, magnesium levels, ammonia.

Changes in organ function may precipitate or potentiate sensory-perceptual deficits. Electrolyte imbalance is common. Liver function is often impaired in the chronic alcoholic. Ammonia intoxication can occur if the liver is unable to convert ammonia to urea. Keto-acidosis is sometimes present without glycosuria; however, hyperglycemia or hypoglycemia may occur, suggesting pancreatitis or impaired gluconeogenesis in the liver. Hypoxemia and hypercarbia are common manifestations in chronic alcoholics who are also heavy smokers.

Administer minor tranquilizers as indicated. (Refer to ND: Anxiety (severe/panic)/Fear).

Reduces hyperactivity, promoting relaxation/sleep. This group of drugs has little effect on dreaming and allows dream recovery (REM rebound) to occur, which has been suppressed by alcohol use.

Administer medications as indicated: e.g.,

Thiamine; multivitamins high in C/B complex; Stresstabs.

Vitamins are depleted due to insufficient intake and malabsorption. Thiamine deficiency is associated with ataxia, loss of eye movement and pupillary response, palpitations, postural hypotension, and exertional dyspnea.

NURSING DIAGNOSIS:	**NUTRITION, ALTERED: LESS THAN BODY REQUIREMENTS**
MAY BE RELATED TO:	**Poor dietary intake (replaced by alcohol consumption)**
	Effects of alcohol on organs involved in digestion, e.g., pancreas/liver
	Alcohol interference with absorption and metabolism of nutrients and amino acids, while increasing the body's loss of vitamins in the urine
POSSIBLY EVIDENCED BY:	**Reports of inadequate food intake, altered taste sensation, abdominal pain, lack of interest in food**
	Body weight 20% or more under ideal
	Pale conjunctiva and mucous membranes
	Poor muscle tone, skin turgor

POSSIBLY EVIDENCED BY— *continued*	Sore inflamed buccal cavity/cheilosis
	Hyperactive bowel sounds, diarrhea
	Third spacing of circulating blood volume (e.g., edema of extremities, ascites)
	Presence of neuropathies
	Laboratory evidence of decreased red cell count (anemias), vitamin deficiencies, reduced serum albumin, and possible electrolyte imbalance
CLIENT OUTCOMES/EVALUATION CRITERIA:	Demonstrates progressive weight gain toward goal with normalization of laboratory values and absence of signs of malnutrition. Verbalizes understanding of effects of alcohol ingestion and reduced dietary intake on nutritional status. Demonstrates behaviors, lifestyle changes to regain/maintain appropriate weight.

INTERVENTIONS	RATIONALE
Independent	
Evaluate presence/quality of bowel sounds. Note abdominal distention, tenderness.	Irritation of gastric mucosa is common and may result in epigastric pain, nausea, and hyperactive bowel sounds. More serious effects of GI system may occur secondary to cirrhosis and hepatitis.
Note presence of nausea/vomiting, diarrhea.	Nausea and vomiting are often among the first signs of alcohol withdrawal and may interfere with achieving adequate nutritional intake.
Assess ability to feed self.	Tremors, altered mentation/hallucinations may interfere with ingestion of nutrients and indicate need for assistance.
Provide small, easily digested frequent feedings/snacks when oral feeding is begun. Advance as tolerated.	May limit gastric distress and enhance intake and toleration of nutrients. As appetite and ability to tolerate food increases, diet should be adjusted to provide the necessary calories and nutrition for cellular repair and restoration of energy.
Collaborative	
Review laboratory tests, e.g., SGOT, SGPT, LDH, serum albumin.	Assesses liver function, nutritional intake, and need for/effectiveness of supplemental therapy.
Refer to dietician/nutritional support team.	Useful in coordinating individual nutritional regimen.

INTERVENTIONS

Collaborative

Provide diet high in protein with at least half of calories obtained from carbohydrates.

Administer medications as indicated: e.g.,
    Antacids, antiemetics, antidiarrheals;

    Vitamins, thiamine.

Institute/maintain NPO status if GI bleeding or excessive vomiting is present.

RATIONALE

Stabilizes blood sugar, thereby reducing risk of hypoglycemia while providing for energy needs and cellular regeneration.

Reduces gastric irritation and effects of sympathetic stimulation.

Replace losses. (Note: All clients should receive thiamine and vitamins as deficiencies, clinical or subclinical, exist in most if not all chronic alcoholics.)

Provides gastrointestinal rest reducing potential harmful effects of gastric/pancreatic stimulation.

NURSING DIAGNOSIS:	ANXIETY (SEVERE/PANIC)/FEAR
MAY BE RELATED TO:	**Cessation of alcohol intake/physiologic withdrawal**
	Situational crisis (hospitalization)
	Threat to self-concept
	Perceived threat of death
POSSIBLY EVIDENCED BY:	**Feelings of inadequacy (shame, self-disgust, and remorse)**
	Increased helplessness/hopelessness with loss of control of own life
	Increased tension, apprehension
	Fear of unspecified consequences
CLIENT OUTCOMES/EVALUATION CRITERIA:	**Verbalizes reduction of fear and anxiety to an acceptable and manageable level. Expresses sense of regaining some control of situation/life. Demonstrates problem-solving skills and uses resources effectively.**

INTERVENTIONS

Independent

Indentify cause of anxiety, involving client in the pro-

RATIONALE

Person in acute phase of withdrawal may be unable to

INTERVENTIONS	RATIONALE

Independent

cess. Explain that alcohol withdrawal increases anxiety and uneasiness.

Develop a trusting relationship through frequent contact. Project an accepting attitude about alcoholism.

Inform client what you plan to do and why. Include client in planning process/provide choices when possible.

Reorient frequently. (Refer to ND: Sensory-Perceptual, alteration specify.)

Assess/reassess level of anxiety on an ongoing basis.

identify and/or accept what is happening. Anxiety may be physiologically/environmentally caused.

Provides client with a sense of humanness helping to decrease paranoia and distrust. Client will be able to detect biased or condescending attitude of caregivers.

Enhances sense of trust, and explanation increases cooperation/reduces anxiety. Feelings of self-worth are intensified when one is treated as a worthwhile person. Provides sense of control over self in circumstances where loss of control is a significant factor.

Client may experience periods of confusion (due to brain's response to decreased alcohol levels), resulting in increased anxiety.

Continued alcohol toxicity will be manifested by increased anxiety and agitation as effects of tranquilizers wear off.

Collaborative

Administer medications as indicated, e.g.,
    Benzodiazepines:
        chlordiazepoxide (Librium), diazepam (Valium);

    Barbiturates:
        phenobarbital, or possibly secobarbital, pentobarbital.

Arrange "Intervention" (confrontation) to assist client to accept that substance use is creating a problem.

Provide consultation for referral from detoxification/crisis center to ongoing treatment program as soon as medically stable, e.g., oriented to reality. (Refer to CP: Substance Dependence/Abuse Rehabilitation).

Minor tranquilizers given during acute withdrawal and then tapered off help client to relax, be less hyperactive, and feel more in control.

These drugs suppress alcohol withdrawal but need to be used with caution as they are respiratory depressants and REM sleep cycle inhibitors.

Process of Intervention, wherein family members, supported by staff, provide information about how the client's drinking and behavior has affected each one of them, helps the client to acknowledge that drinking is a problem and has resulted in current situational crisis.

Client is more likely to contract for treatment while still "hurting" and experiencing fear and anxiety from last drunk. Motivation decreases as well-being increases and person again feels able to control the problem. Direct contact with available treatment resources provides realistic picture of help. Decreases time for client to "think about it"/change mind or restructure and strengthen denial systems.

Depressants (Benzodiazepines, Barbiturates, Opioids)

DSM III-R 305.40 Sedative, hypnotic or anxiolytic intoxication
292.00 Uncomplicated sedative, hypnotic or anxiolytic withdrawal/delirium
305.50 Opioid intoxication
292.00 Opioid withdrawal

ETIOLOGIC THEORIES

PSYCHODYNAMICS

Individuals who abuse substances fail to complete tasks of separation-individuation, resulting in underdeveloped egos. The person has a highly dependent nature, with characteristics of poor impulse control, low frustration tolerance, and low self-esteem. The superego is weak, resulting in absence of guilt feelings. Underlying psychiatric status must be assessed, as these individuals may use stimulants for varying self-medication reasons.

BIOLOGIC THEORIES

A genetic link is thought to be involved in the development of substance use disorders. Although statistics are currently inconclusive, hereditary factors are generally accepted to be a factor in the abuse of substances.
Psychostructural factors (e.g., personality) are seen as significant. The defect is believed to precede the addiction, with the ego structure breaking down and the substance being used as a maladaptive coping mechanism.

FAMILY DYNAMICS

There is an apparent predisposition to substance abuse disorders in the dysfunctional family system. Factors such as the absence of a parent, one who is an overpowering tyrant, or one who is weak and ineffectual and the use of substances as the primary method of relieving stress appear to contribute to this dysfunction. These role models have a negative influence, and the child learns to handle stress in like manner. However, parents may be average, normal individuals with children who succumb to overwhelming peer pressure and become involved with drugs. Cultural factors such as acceptance of the use of alcohol and other drugs may also influence the individual's choice.

CLIENT ASSESSMENT DATA BASE

HISTORY

Temporary psychosis with acute onset of auditory hallucinations and paranoid delusions may occur.
Unexplained neuropsychiatric presentation may be indicative of drug use.
History from family member/significant other(s) may reveal dysfunctional patterns of interaction.
Preexisting physical/psychologic conditions may be noted.
May complain of nausea/vomiting, muscle aches, twitching, hot/cold flashes, continuous rhinorrhea, excessive lacrimation, sneezing, headache, or general malaise. (Note: Methadone abusers may complain of deep muscle/bone pain.)

PHYSICAL EXAMINATION

May present with intoxication, overdose, or in various stages of withdrawal. May be addicted to drug in question. Concurrent use of alcohol/other drugs can compound symptoms/reactions.
Mental status: impaired judgment with some affective change; alterations in consciousness may exist, from extreme agitation to coma. Speech may be slurred.
Behavior: Mood swings, aggression, combativeness may occur related to general "disinhibiting" effect of the drug (loss of impulse control).
Psychomotor activity: may be increased. Hypersensitivity, e.g., anxiety, tremors, hypotension, irritability, restlessness, and seizures may be noted.
Pupils: usually small; pinpoint constriction suggests heroin intoxication.
Pulse: Tachycardia suggests withdrawal syndrome; atrial fibrillation, ventricular dysrhythmias may be noted.

Respiratory: Depression may be noted in overdose, while increased rate is seen in withdrawal syndrome.
Thermoregulation: Instability with hyperpyrexia may occur.
Gait: may stagger, may exhibit loss of coordination, positive Romberg sign.
Skin: piloerection ("gooseflesh"); puncture wounds may be noted on arms, hands, legs, under tongue, indicating
    I.V. drug use.

DIAGNOSTIC STUDIES

Drug screen: Identifies drug(s) being used.
Addiction Severity Index (ASI): Produces a "problem severity profile" that indicates areas of treatment needs.

NURSING PRIORITIES

1. Achieve physiologic stability.
2. Protect client from injury.
3. Provide appropriate referral and follow-up.
4. Promote family involvement in the withdrawal/rehabilitation process.

DISCHARGE CRITERIA

1. Physiologic stability achieved.
2. Maintains abstinence from drug(s) on a day-to-day basis.
3. Transferred to rehabilitation program/attending group therapy, e.g., Narcotics Anonymous.
4. Family/S.O.(s) are participating in treatment program.

NURSING DIAGNOSIS:	**INJURY, POTENTIAL FOR (SPECIFY)**
MAY BE RELATED TO:	**CNS depression (effect of overdose)**
	CNS agitation (effect of abrupt withdrawal)
	Hypersensitivity to the drug(s)
	Psychologic stress (narrowed perceptual fields seen with anxiety)
	I.V. drug use techniques
CLIENT OUTCOMES/EVALUATION CRITERIA:	**Verbalizes understanding of risk factors of taking drugs. Refrains from acting upon hallucinations/impaired judgment. Completes withdrawal without injury to self development or complications.**

INTERVENTIONS	RATIONALE
Independent	
Identify drug(s) taken, when taken, and route used, if possible.	Helpful to identify interventions for specific drug. May be difficult to determine drug(s) taken as the client may not feel free to tell because of embarrassment or legal reasons or may not know what has been ingested.
Assess level of consciousness, e.g., agitated, stuporous, lethargic, confused, or unconscious. Note pinpoint pupils.	May be indicator of degree of intoxication and level of intervention required. Constricted pupils are a classic sign of opioid (heroin) ingestion.
Evaluate for evidence of head trauma.	Important to note for differential diagnosis to prevent permanent damage/death.
Determine when food was last eaten. Note complaints of nausea.	May slow absorption of drug(s) into the blood stream; however, may present risk of vomiting and aspiration if level of consciousness is depressed.
Monitor temperature as indicated. Observe for signs of dehydration.	Hypothermia may be seen in intoxication, and hyperpyrexia may occur with withdrawal or indicate infectious process. (Note: Dehydration often accompanies hyperpyrexia, requiring additional intervention/fluid replacement.)
Monitor vital signs (B/P, pulse, respirations).	Changes depend on drug taken, e.g., diazepam (Valium) may be evidenced by hypotension, tachycardia.
Provide quiet, lighted room. An isolation room with simple furniture may be needed.	Reduces stimuli, internal or external, which may lead to injury as the client responds.
Observe client at all times; use staff or family member as available.	Client with varying levels of consciousness should not be left alone because of the danger of accidental injury.
Provide orientation as needed.	Maintaining contact provides reassurance, reduces anxiety when consciousness returns.
Note presence of tremors.	Involuntary movements of one or more parts of the body may result from abrupt removal of drug.
Provide seizure precautions, e.g., padded side rails, bed in low position, airway adjunct/suction at bedside.	Precautions can prevent injury if seizures occur during withdrawal.
Note changes in behavior indicative of psychosis, e.g., distorted reality, altered mood, impaired language and memory.	Drug intoxication can precipitate an alteration in perceptions/psychotic behavior.
Assess emotional state, noting psychiatric history and suicide gestures/attempts. Note use/abuse of other substances.	Patterns of drug use will indicate likelihood of intentional or accidental overdose. Substance abuse/ suicidal attempts may be symptom or response to underlying psychiatric illness or to hallucinations caused by sensitivity to drug.
Determine history of hallucinations.	May be auditory, visual, tactile, and be very frightening. May also trigger suicidal/homicidal behavior.
Institute suicide precautions, as indicated.	May need environmental restraints to protect client until own coping abilities improve.
Collaborative	
Start/maintain IV line.	Provides an open line for emergency treatment.

Administer 50% glucose IV with thiamine added if client is comatose.	Acute thiamine deficiency and hypoglycemia may mimic drug intoxication.
Assist with gastric lavage, if indicated.	May be done when drug has been recently ingested, when consciousness is depressed, making vomiting hazardous, or when induced emesis has failed.
Administer medication per current treatment/protocol, e.g.,	
Emetics, e.g., apomorphine, syrup of ipecac;	Induced vomiting is an efficient and effective way to empty the stomach when the patient is fully conscious. It is of questionable value unless performed within a few hours of drug ingestion because of rapid gastrointestinal absorption.
Activated charcoal;	Binds with many substances in the GI tract, reducing absorption of ingested drug(s).
Phenobarbital;	Prolonged effect provides smoother sedation without "high" of more rapidly acting drugs and also has an anticonvulsant effect.
Methadone.	Replaces heroin or other narcotic analgesics in detoxification program, reducing/minimizing withdrawal symptoms.
Assist with barbiturate detoxification program.	Reintoxication should be done before drug withdrawal is attempted. This establishes an independent estimate of prior drug use and provides a base line to begin the detox schedule. The reintoxication should begin as soon as there are signs of intoxication, e.g., nystagmus, slurred speech, ataxia on backward and forward tandem gait.
Prepare for/assist with dialysis if indicated.	Occasionally effective for clearance of toxic/lethal levels of phenobarbital.

NURSING DIAGNOSIS:	**BREATHING PATTERN, INEFFECTIVE/ GAS EXCHANGE, IMPAIRED [POTENTIAL]**
MAY BE RELATED TO:	**Neuromuscular impairment**
	Decreased energy/fatigue
	Inflammatory process
	Decreased lung expansion
CLIENT OUTCOMES/EVALUATION CRITERIA:	**Establishes normal/effective breathing pattern with absence of cyanosis/ symptoms of respiratory distress.**

INTERVENTIONS	RATIONALE
Independent	
Monitor respiratory rate/depth/rhythm and breath sounds.	Sedative/depressant effects on CNS may result in loss of airway patency and/or respiratory depression. Prompt treatment is necessary to prevent respiratory arrest. Note: Acute pulmonary edema is a common complication in heroin overdose/intoxication.
Have suction equipment, airway adjuncts available.	Sedative effects of drugs, increased salivation, vomiting potentiates risk of aspiration, relaxation of oropharyngeal muscles, and respiratory depression, requiring prompt intervention to prevent respiratory arrest.
Collaborative	
Administer medications, as indicated, e.g., naloxone (Narcan).	Narcotic antagonist that may reverse effects of respiratory depression in opioid intoxication. Note: May trigger acute withdrawal syndrome.
Provide supplemental oxygen.	May be necessary to improve oxygen intake in presence of respiratory depression
Review chest x-ray.	Common complications of depressant (opiate) abuse include pneumonia, aspiration pneumonitis, lung abscess, atelectasis, which will require specific treatment.
Monitor ABGs, pulmonary function studies when indicated.	Chronic addiction may result in decreased vital capacity and pulmonary diffusion affecting gas exchange. Presence of septic pulmonary emboli or pulmonary fibrosis (from talc granulomatosis) may further compromise respiratory function.

NURSING DIAGNOSIS: **INFECTION, POTENTIAL FOR**

MAY BE RELATED TO: **I.V. drug use techniques**

Impurities in injected drugs

Localized trauma

Malnutrition

Altered immune state

CLIENT OUTCOMES/EVALUATION CRITERIA: **Verbalizes understanding of and demonstrates lifestyle changes to reduce risk factor(s). Achieves timely healing of infectious process if present or develops and is afebrile.**

INTERVENTIONS

Independent

Refer to CP: Stimulants, ND: Infection, potential for

NURSING DIAGNOSIS:	**COPING, INEFFECTIVE INDIVIDUAL**
MAY BE RELATED TO:	**Inadequate coping methods**
	Personal vulnerability
	Inadequate support systems
	Unmet expectations
POSSIBLY EVIDENCED BY:	**Impaired adaptive behavior and problem-solving skills**
	Addictive behaviors
	Poor self-esteem
	Chronic anxiety/worry/depression
	Emotional tension
CLIENT OUTCOMES/EVALUATION CRITERIA:	**Verbalizes individual reasons for abstinence. Demonstrates effective problem-solving skills as evidenced by not indulging in addictive substances.**

INTERVENTIONS

RATIONALE

Independent

Determine degree of impairment by talking to client/family and/or significant other(s), noting when person was last seen well, sleep patterns, and duration of problems.

CNS depressants are among the most widely used and abused drugs and have been prescribed for symptoms of anxiety, depression, and sleep disturbances. Therefore, these drugs are very likely to be abused when the underlying conditions remain untreated. Information provides an approximate time frame for impairment, with sleep disruption often the first observable sign of a problem. Prescription information provides clues to identity of drug(s) and amount taken.

Determine previous methods of dealing with life problems.

Identifies positive and/or negative coping skills client has used in the past and provides opportunity to discuss ways to use positive skills in current situation

INTERVENTIONS	RATIONALE

Independent

Active Listen client, noting verbal and nonverbal expressions of feelings.

Communicates message of confidence in client's ability to solve own problems and encourages expression of feelings.

Encourage client to look at own responsibility for what has happened. Confront difference between words and actions.

These clients often blame others and rationalize behavior to allow them to continue maladaptive behavior. Confrontation forces client to acknowledge reality of problem behavior.

Provide positive reinforcement when client acknowledges own responsibility for situation and displays new behavior.

Helps client to identify and accept new ways of coping with stressors as having value for developing a new lifestyle without the use of drugs.

Collaborative

Refer to rehabilitation program, involve in Intervention (confrontation) and/or therapy as indicated. (Refer to CP: Substance Dependence/Abuse Rehabilitation.)

Client will need ongoing assistance to acknowledge and maintain drug-free existence.

Stimulants (Amphetamines, Cocaine, Caffeine, Tobacco)

DSM III-R: Amphetamine or similarly acting sympathomimetic
      305.70 Amphetamine or similarly acting sympathomimetic abuse/intoxication
      305.60 Cocaine abuse/intoxication
      305.90 Caffeine intoxication

ETIOLOGIC THEORIES

PSYCHODYNAMICS

Individuals who abuse substances fail to complete tasks of separation-individuation, resulting in underdeveloped egos. The person retains a highly dependent nature, with characteristics of poor impulse control, low frustration tolerance, and low self-esteem. The superego is weak, resulting in absence of guilt feelings for behavior. Underlying psychiatric status must be assessed, as these individuals may use stimulants for varying self-medication reasons.

BIOLOGIC THEORIES

An apparent genetic link is involved in the development of substance use disorders. However, the statistics are currently inconclusive regarding abuse of stimulant drugs.

FAMILY DYNAMICS

Predisposition to substance use disorders occurs in a dysfunctional family system. There is often one parent who is absent or who is an overpowering tyrant, and/or one who is weak and ineffectual. Substance abuse may be evident as the primary method of relieving stress. The child has negative role models and learns to respond to stressful situations in like manner.

CLIENT ASSESSMENT DATA BASE

HISTORY

Note substance(s) used (aside from caffeine and nicotine, most commonly abused stimulants are amphetamine and cocaine).
Twice as many males appear to use stimulants as compared with females.
Primary use is in the age range of 21 to 44.
May be a dependent personality.
Pattern of habitual use of the particular drug/pathological abuse, with inability to reduce or to stop use, may be seen occurring for at least one month. Intoxication throughout the day, sometimes with daily involvement, may be noted.
Episodes of overdose wherein hallucinations and delusions occur may be repeated with cocaine.
Delirium with tactile and olfactory hallucinations, labile affect, violent or aggressive behavior, symptoms of a paranoid delusional disorder may be noted with amphetamine or similarly acting substances.
Amphetamine psychosis can occur with a one-time high dose, especially with intravenous administration, or with long-term use at moderate or high dose.
May have fixed delusional system of a persecutory nature, lasting weeks to a year or more.
Hallucinations of bugs or vermin crawling in/under the skin (formication) may be noted.
May express ideas of reference.
May exhibit aggressiveness, hostility, violence, quick response to anger; psychomotor agitation.
Stereotyped compulsive motor behavior, e.g., sorting, taking things apart and putting them back together, moving mouth from side to side in a stereotypic grimacing pattern may occur.
Anxiety may be present.
Impaired judgment and perception may be noted.
Impairment in social or occupational functioning may be observed/reported.

May be seen, or view self as, susceptible to influence by others, having an inability to say "no." May express need to feel elated, sociable, happy with self, a desire to prove self-worth, and a sense of low self-esteem. Inability to tolerate or to correct chronic fatigue, depression, and/or loneliness may be a factor.

May be compulsive regarding stimulant use or use the denial of powerlessness over the stimulant (use of drug for celebration or crisis, thinking can use in small quantities, often resulting in binge use). May think of recovery process as notion of will power, subject to impulse control.

While symptoms of intoxication may have passed, client may manifest denial, drug hunger, periods of "flare up" wherein there is a delayed reemergence of withdrawal symptoms, e.g., anxiety, depression, irritability, sleep disturbance, compulsiveness with food (especially sugars). (Reemergence may occur at three months, between nine and twelve months, and perhaps as late as 18 months after abstinence.)

May have been previously hosptialized or been in residential treatment program.

May report attendance at recovery groups, e.g., Narcotics/Alcoholics Anonymous or other drug-specific recovery groups.

PHYSICAL EXAMINATION

May present with intoxication/overdose or in various stages of withdrawal. May be addicted to drug in question. Concurrent use of alcohol/other drugs can compound symptoms/reactions. Acute allergic/anaphylactic reaction can occur in response to contaminants in drug "cut."

Physical symptoms of stimulant intoxication, e.g., tachycardia, pupillary dilation, elevated blood pressure, diaphoresis, chills, pyrexia, nausea/vomiting, anorexia, insomnia, may be present.

Emotional/psychological symptoms, e.g., elation, grandiosity, loquacity, hypervigilance, often occur.

DIAGNOSTIC STUDIES

Urine: Screen for presence of drug(s).
Addiction Severity Index (ASI): Produces a "problem severity profile," which indicates areas of treatment needs.

NURSING PRIORITIES

1. Maintain physiologic stability during acute withdrawal phase.
2. Promote safety and security of client's environment.
3. Provide support for learning of new coping skills through the withdrawal phase.
4. Provide appropriate referral and follow-up.
5. Support family involvement in "Intervention"/treatment process.

DISCHARGE CRITERIA

1. Physiologic stability is maintained.
2. Maintains abstinence from drug(s) on a day-to-day basis
3. Transferred to rehabilitation program/attending group
4. Family/significant other(s) are participating in treatment program.

NURSING DIAGNOSIS:	CARDIAC OUTPUT, DECREASED [POTENTIAL]
MAY BE RELATED TO:	Drug (cocaine) effect on myocardium (including purity/quantity used)
	Preexisting myocardiopathy (with or without previous prolonged drug abuse)

MAY BE RELATED TO—*continued*	Alterations in electrical rate/rhythm/conduction
CLIENT OUTCOMES/EVALUATION CRITERIA:	Reports decrease/absence of chest pain. Demonstrates adequate cardiac output free of signs of shock, dysrhythmias.

INTERVENTIONS	RATIONALE
Independent	
Monitor cardiac rate and rhythm. Document dysrhythmias.	Ventricular dysrhythmias/cardiac arrest may occur, especially in toxic levels of cocaine.
Investigate complaints of chest pain, indigestion/heartburn, etc.	Increased incidence of myocardial infarction in cocaine users.
Have emergency equipment/medications available.	Prompt treatment of dysrhythmias may prevent cardiac arrest.
Collaborative	
Administer medications as indicated, e.g., propranolol (Inderal);	Beta-adrenergic blocker that reduces cardiac oxygen demand by blocking catecholamine-induced increases in heart rate, blood pressure, and force of myocardial contraction.
lidocaine I.V.	Used in emergency situation to control/prevent ventricular dysrhythmias.

NURSING DIAGNOSIS:	VIOLENCE, POTENTIAL FOR: DIRECTED AT SELF OR OTHERS
MAY BE RELATED TO:	Aggressive behavior associated with amphetamine use
	Profound depression resulting from withdrawal from stimulants
	Paranoid ideation (may act provocatively and intrusively, rapidly and impulsively toward others)
	Perceptions of threats
	Altered perceptions/misidentifications
	Depressive behavior with expressions of suicidal ideas

POSSIBLE INDICATORS:	Overt and aggressive acts
	Increased motor activity
	Possession of destructive means
	Suspicious of others, paranoid ideation, delusions and hallucinations
	Expressed intent directly/indirectly
CLIENT OUTCOMES/EVALUATION CRITERIA:	Acknowledges fearfulness and realities of situation. Verbalizes understanding of behavior and precipitating factors. Demonstrates self-control.

INTERVENTIONS

Independent

Decrease stimuli; provide quiet in own room or place in stimulus-reduction room with supervision.

Remove potentially harmful objects from environment.

Explain consistent rules of unit, e.g., no violence, no threats.

Provide high staff profile in situations where potential violence can occur.

Allow chance for verbal expression of aggressive feelings.

Assist client in identifying what provokes anger.

Provide outlets for expression that involve physical activity, e.g., stationary bicycle, basketball/volleyball.

Discuss consequences of aggressive behavior.

Be alert to violence potential, increased pacing, verbalization of delusional persecutory content, hypervigilance regarding specific persons in the milieu, gesturing aggressively, threatening others verbally or physically.

Isolate immediately if client becomes violent, using adequate staff trained in assaultive management. An attitude of acceptance is important while refusing to tolerate the violent behavior.

RATIONALE

Reduces reactivity, enhances calm feelings. Observation allows for timely intervention.

Reduces opportunity for client to carry out suicidal ideas. Client may be suicidal when/if rebound CNS depression occurs secondary to stimulant withdrawal.

Secure environment enhances sense of safety, which can decrease perceived threat.

May prevent onset of violence. Enhances opportunity for client to learn ways to cope with aggressive feelings before reacting.

Encouragement of new avenue of expression helps client learn new coping skills.

Awareness of reaction is the first step in learning change.

Gross motor activity in protected environment can lessen aggressive drive.

Learning choices assists client to gain control of situation and self.

Recognizing potential and assisting client to gain control can be more effective prior to violent outbreak.

Client will feel safer if others take control until internal control can be regained by the client.

INTERVENTIONS	RATIONALE

Independent

Negotiate conditions for coming out of isolation when the client is calm, based on agreement of social appropriateness.

Clear expectations aid client in feeling secure about own control.

Build trust: follow through on commitments/agreements, maintain consistent staff and frequent brief contact with client.

Trust is essential to working with all clients. Brief contacts can prevent overstimulation.

Collaborative

Administer medications as indicated, e.g.,
    chlorpromazine (Thorazine), haloperidol (Haldol);

Short-term use of major tranquilizers during acute intoxication/psychosis assists client in gaining self-control; promotes sedation/rest when agitated, assaultive, over-stimulated. Note: Thorazine may cause postural hypotension; Haldol may provoke acute extrapyramidal reaction, requiring additional evaluation/medication.

    Diazepam (Valium), chlordiazepoxide (Librium);

Occasionally useful for treatment of acute cocaine intoxication. Either drug is useful for preventing delirium tremens when substance use is combined with alcohol.

    L-Tryptophan.

Useful in agitation and irritability; decreases anxiety.

Avoid the use of restraints/seclusion.

In stimulated state, may exacerbate hyperactivity.

NURSING DIAGNOSIS:	**SENSORY-PERCEPTUAL ALTERATION (SPECIFY)**
MAY BE RELATED TO:	**Altered sensory reception, transmission and/or integration: altered status of sense organs**
	Chemical alteration: exogenous (CNS stimulants or depressants, mind-altering drugs)
POSSIBLY EVIDENCED BY:	**Preoccupation with/appears to be responding to internal stimuli from hallucinatory experiences, e.g., "listening pose," laughing and talking to self, stops in mid-sentence and listens.**
	"Picks" at self and clothing

<table>
<tr><td>CLIENT OUTCOMES/EVALUATION CRITERIA:</td><td>Distinguishes reality from altered perceptions. States awareness that hallucinations may result from stimulant use.</td></tr>
</table>

INTERVENTIONS

Independent

Notice client's preoccupation, responses, gesturing, social skill.

Assist client in checking perceptions verbally, provide reality information.

Acknowledge client's emotional state, reassure regarding safety.

Explore ways of calming and relaxing client to enhance clarity of perception.

Be aware that altered sensation and perception may cause injury, e.g., be alert for client burning self with cigarette, excessive scratching at skin to rid self of bugs or drug (which may feel as though it is in the skin), accidentally harming self through poor judgment or misperceptions. (Refer to ND: Violence, potential for, directed at others.)

Inform client, if calm enough, of temporary nature of hallucinations that have resulted from stimulant use.

RATIONALE

Without overstimulating verbally, can assess whether or not client may be hallucinating.

Provides reassurance of safety, that formication (illusion of insects crawling on the body) or other misperceptions are not occurring. Can calm the client.

Empathetic response can diminish intensity of fear.

Relaxation can promote positive outlook, distracting from negativity of perceptions.

Amphetamine use causes impaired judgment, increasing risk of injury/self-harm.

Learning cause, effect, and possible temporary nature of misperceptions may reduce fear, anxiety, and negativity. May inject hope and positive attitude.

<table>
<tr><td>NURSING DIAGNOSIS:</td><td>NUTRITION, ALTERED: LESS THAN BODY REQUIREMENTS</td></tr>
<tr><td>MAY BE RELATED TO:</td><td>Anorexia secondary to stimulant use

Insufficient/inappropriate use of financial resources</td></tr>
<tr><td>POSSIBLY EVIDENCED BY:</td><td>Reported/observed inadequate intake

Lack of interest in food

Weight loss

Poor muscle tone

Signs/laboratory evidence of vitamin deficiencies</td></tr>
</table>

CLIENT OUTCOMES/EVALUATION CRITERIA:	Demonstrates progressive weight gain toward goal. Verbalizes understanding of causative factors and individual needs. Identifies appropriate dietary choices, lifestyle changes to regain/maintain desired weight.

INTERVENTIONS	RATIONALE
Independent	
Assess client's intake pattern over past several weeks.	Stimulants cause decreased appetite and impaired judgment regarding body needs.
Discuss needs/likes/dislikes about food choices.	Will be more likely to maintain desired intake if individual preferences are considered.
Anticipate hyperphagia and weigh every other day.	Often a consequence of stimulant withdrawal and may result in sudden/inappropriate weight gain.
Provide meals in a relaxed, nonstimulating environment.	Stimulus reduction aids relaxation and ability to focus on eating.
Encourage frequent nutritional snacks, small nutritious meals.	Small amounts of food frequently can prevent/reduce G.I. distress.
Collaborative	
Obtain/review routine lab work, e.g., CBC, UA.	Assessment of nutritional state is necessary to treat preexisting deficiencies and rule out anemia, dehydration, or ketosis.
Consult with dietitian.	Useful in establishing individual nutritional needs/dietary program.
Administer multivitamins as indicated.	Supplementation enhances correction of deficiencies.

NURSING DIAGNOSIS:	INFECTION, POTENTIAL FOR
MAY BE RELATED TO:	I.V. drug use techniques
	Impurities in drugs injected
	Localized trauma
	Nasal septum damage (from snorting cocaine)
	Malnutrition
	Altered immune state
CLIENT OUTCOMES/EVALUATION CRITERIA:	Verbalizes understanding of individual risk factors. Identifies interventions to prevent/reduce risk factors.

Demonstrates lifestyle changes to promote safe environment. Achieves timely healing of infectious process if present/develops and is afebrile.

INTERVENTIONS	RATIONALE
Independent	
Monitor vital signs. Assess level of consciousness.	Abnormal signs, including fever, can indicate presence of infection. Cerebral complications, e.g., meningitis, brain abscess, may occur.
Review physical assessment on a regular basis.	Can reveal daily changes and problematic areas. Provides recognition of pathology, identifies areas for providing information for health promotion and problem prevention.
Investigate complaints of acute/chronic bone pain, tenderness, guarding with movement, regional muscle spasm.	Occasionally, osteomyelitis may develop due to hematogenous spread of bacteria, most often affecting lumbar vertebrae.
Obtain information specific to pattern of drug use over past month, immunization history, allergies, medications used for other purposes.	Initial factual history can reveal information essential to physical treatment; where person obtained drug could assist in investigating possible "cut" with other drugs.
Assist as needed with body and oral hygiene; obtain clean clothes, properly fitting shoes.	Skin integrity requires cleanliness. Sores may need care to prevent infection.
Observe for nasal stuffiness, pain, bleeding, abnormal mucus production.	Cocaine snorting can cause erosion of the nasal septum requiring additional therapy/interventions.
Use blood/body fluid precautions per hospital policy, when appropriate.	Protects caregiver(s) from possible infection by infectious disease viruses, e.g., hepatitis/AIDS.
Ascertain health status of family members/S.O.(s) currently in contact with the client.	May expose client to diseases such as colds, hepatitis/AIDS, which could be problematic for the client.
Collaborative	
Review laboratory studies, e.g., UA, CBC, Bio-chem screen, VDRL (RPR), ESR.	May identify complications of IV cocaine and amphetamine use such as hepatitis, nephritis, tetanus, vasculitis, septicemia, subacute bacterial endocarditis, embolic phenomena, malaria, toxic allergic reactions resulting from other substances in the "cut." Immunologic abnormalities may occur due to repeated antigenic stimulation.
Review serum tests, if done, for infectious diseases, e.g., hepatitis, AIDS.	IV needle drug users are at high risk for contamination with AIDS and hepatitis viruses.

NURSING DIAGNOSIS:	SLEEP PATTERN DISTURBANCE
MAY BE RELATED TO:	CNS sensory alterations from stimulant use
POSSIBLY EVIDENCED BY:	Altered sleep cycle

POSSIBLY EVIDENCED BY— *continued*	Initial signs of insomnia and then hypersomnia
	Constant alertness
	Racing thoughts that prevent rest
	Denial of need to sleep or reports of inability to stay awake
CLIENT OUTCOMES/EVALUATION CRITERIA:	**Sleeping 6–8 hours at night. Resting minimally, appropriately, during the day. Verbalizes feeling rested when awakens.**

INTERVENTIONS	RATIONALE
Independent	
Establish sleep cycle in which client sleeps at night, awake during day with brief rest periods as needed.	Adequate rest and sleep can improve emotional state; restoration of regular pattern is a priority in a sleep-deprived stimulant user.
Decrease stimuli and enhance relaxation prior to bedtime; encourage use of presleep routines, e.g., hot bath, warm milk.	Client may need calming in order to attempt rest.
Provide opportunities for fresh air, mild exercise, non-caffeinated beverages, quiet environment as client can tolerate.	Promotes drowsiness/desire for sleep.
Collaborative	
Administer medications as indicated, e.g., L-Tryptophan at bedtime.	Client may initially require chemical assistance to attain proper sleep cycle.

NURSING DIAGNOSIS:	FEAR
MAY BE RELATED TO:	Paranoid delusions associated with stimulant use
POSSIBLY EVIDENCED BY:	Feelings/beliefs that others are conspiring against or are about to kill client
CLIENT OUTCOMES/EVALUATION CRITERIA:	Recognizes frightening feelings before preoccupying self or becoming violent. Discusses reality base of persecutory fears with staff. Demonstrates appropriate range of feelings and lessened fear.

INTERVENTIONS	RATIONALE
Independent	
Establish consistent staff. Build trust by being reliable, honest, genuine, prompt.	Trust and rapport are necessary for overcoming fear.
Be concrete, clear in communication. Assess client's readiness for humor and/or touch.	Fear negatively influences one's ability to laugh. Fear is serious to the perceiver and must be respected. Touch can be misinterpreted/increase anxiety.
Encourage verbalization of fears.	Ventilation and expression to trusted staff can lessen intensity of fearfulness.
Acknowledge awareness of client's feelings, e.g., fear, terror, overwhelmed, panic, anxiety, confusion.	Empathy can assist client to tolerate/deal with own feelings.
Assist client in reality-checking fears. Use gentle confrontation.	Client can reduce fear by understanding difference between reality and delusions. Should be used cautiously as reality-checking a delusional system puts trust at risk.

(Refer to CP: Substance Dependence/Abuse Rehabilitation.)

Hallucinogens (LSD, PCP, Cannabis)

Drugs that produce mood changes and perceptual changes varying from sensory illusion to hallucinations. The most popular and well-known are:

LSD and other LSD-like hallucinogenic drugs (e.g., MDA, MDMA (Ecstasy), mescaline, synthetic THC. DOM (STP), morning glory seeds, nutmeg), phencyclidine (PCP), cannabis (marijuana, hashish, THC).

DSM III-R: Hallucinogen (includes substances structurally related to 5-hydroxytryptamine, e.g., lysergic acid diethylamide (LSD) and dimethyltryptamine (DMT) and substances related to catecholamine, e.g., mescaline)

        305.30 Hallucinosis
        292.11 Delusional disorder
        292.84 Mood disorder

Phencyclidine (PCP) or similarly acting arylcyclohexylamine
        292.90 Organic mental disorder
        305.90 Intoxication
        292.81 Delirium
        292.11 Delusional disorder

Cannabis-induced organic mental disorders
        305.20 Cannabis intoxication
        292.11 Cannabis delusional disorder

ETIOLOGIC THEORIES

PSYCHODYNAMICS

Individuals who abuse substances fail to complete tasks of separation-individuation, resulting in underdeveloped egos. The person is thought to have a highly dependent nature, with characteristics of poor impulse control, low frustration tolerance, and low self-esteem. The superego is weak, and this results in absence of guilt feelings for their behavior.

BIOLOGIC THEORIES

A genetic link is thought to be involved in the development of substance use disorders. Although statistics are currently inconclusive, hereditary factors are generally accepted to be a factor in the abuse of substances.

FAMILY DYNAMICS

A predisposition to substance use disorders is found in the dysfunctional family system. There is often one parent who is absent or who is an overpowering tyrant, and/or one who is weak and ineffectual. Substance abuse may be evident as the primary method of relieving stress. The child has negative role models and learns to respond to stressful situations in like manner. However, parents may be average, normal individuals with children who succumb to overwhelming peer pressure and become involved with drugs.

CLIENT ASSESSMENT DATA BASE

HISTORY

Factors that can affect the kind of reaction (positive or negative) experienced by the hallucinogen user include individual circadian rhythms (fatigue), previous drug-taking experience, personality, mood, and expectations. Educational level can also cause different perceptions.

Social or occupational functioning impairment (fights, loss of friends, absence from work, loss of job, or legal difficulties) may be seen with drug use/tolerance.

Reports perceptions become increased (colors richer, music more profound, smells and tastes heightened), synesthesia (merging of senses, colors are "heard" or sounds are "seen"), changes in body image, alterations in time, hallucinations (usually visual), illusions and depersonalization. (Note: Hallucinations are rare with cannabis intoxication.)

Moods reflect depression or anxiety.

Feelings and thoughts that accompany the disturbance include self-reproach, excessive guilt, fearfulness, and preoccupation with the idea that their brains are destroyed and/or they will not return to a normal state.

Delusions may occur in a normal state of consciousness, due to a specific organic factor, and may persist beyond 24 hours after cessation of hallucinogen use. Persecutory delusions can follow cannabis use immediately or occur during the course of cannabis intoxication.

Delirium may occur within 24 hours after use or following recovery days after PCP has been taken.

A flashback is a spontaneous transitory recurrence of a drug-induced experience (LSD) in a drug-free state.

"Bad trips" are self-limiting and confined to period of intoxication and may occur with the use of hallucinogenic drugs:

LSD: 3 kinds: (a) bad body trip, e.g., "my body is purple"; (b) bad environment trip, visual distortions that are so real that person thinks s/he is going crazy; (c) bad mind trip, e.g., unexpected subconscious material bursts forth into consciousness, as in, "I'm responsible for my mother's death."

PCP: aggravates any underlying psychopathology.

Cannabis: rare; however, when they do occur, panic attacks are usually seen.

May complain of nausea/vomiting, increased salivation, dizziness, headache (LSD).

PHYSICAL EXAMINATION

May present with intoxication or overdose. Concurrent use of alcohol/other drugs can compound symptoms/reactions. Effects of PCP seem to be dose-related; high doses can lead to hypertensive crisis or coma/death from respiratory/cardiac failure.

Eyes: vertical and horizontal nystagmus (PCP), pupillary dilation, catatonic staring.

Vision: Blurring, altered depth perception may be reported.

Blood pressure: Hypertension may occur.

Pulse: tachycardia/palpitations.

Neuromuscular: muscle incoordination/tremors, seizures; increased muscle strength may be noted with PCP due to the anesthetic effect, which deadens pain perception.

Skin: diaphoretic.

Level of consciousness: usually responsive but coma may be noted (especially if intracranial hemorrhage occurs); slurred speech, mutism often present.

Mental status: sensation of slowed time, synesthesias, perceptual changes, including decreased response to pain, depersonalization.

Delirium: may also display clouded state of consciousness (sensory misperception, difficulty in sustaining attention, disordered stream of thought, disturbance of sleep-wakefulness and psychomotor activity), including misinterpretations, illusions, hallucinations, disorientation, and memory impairment.

Mood: euphoria/dysphoria, anxiety, emotional lability, apathy, grandiosity.

Behavioral findings: may include assaultiveness, bizarre behavior, impulsivity, unpredictability, belligerence, impaired judgment, paranoid ideation, panic attacks.

DIAGNOSTIC STUDIES

Drug screen/urinalysis: to identify drug(s) being used.

Addictive Severity Index (ASI): to assess substance abuse and determine treatment needs.

NURSING PRIORITIES

1. Promote physiologic/psychologic stability.
2. Protect client/others from injury.
3. Provide appropriate referral and follow-up.
4. Support client/family in "Intervention" (confrontation) process for decision to stop using drugs.

DISCHARGE CRITERIA

1. Achieves physiologic stability.
2. Maintains abstinence from drug(s) on a day-to-day basis.

3. Enrolled in/transferred to drug rehabilitation program.
4. Family/significant other(s) are participating in treatment programs.

NURSING DIAGNOSIS:	**VIOLENCE, POTENTIAL FOR: SELF-DIRECTED OR DIRECTED AT OTHERS**
MAY BE RELATED TO:	**Toxic reactions to drug(s)**
	Chemical alteration, exogenous (CNS stimulants/mind-altering drug)
	Organic brain syndrome (drug anesthetizes mind and body)
	Psychologic state (narrowed perceptual field)
POSSIBLE INDICATORS:	**Synesthesias, hallucinations, illusions, visual/auditory distortions**
	Panic state
	Decreased response to pain
	Increased motor activity, pacing, excitement, irritability, agitation
	Overt and aggressive acts
	Self-destructive behavior
	Hostile, threatening verbalizations
	Unpredictable behavior
	Suspiciousness of others, paranoid ideation, delusions, hallucinations
	Increasing anxiety, fear, and feelings of loss of control
	Change in behavior pattern
	Exaggerated emotional response
CLIENT OUTCOMES/EVALUATION CRITERIA:	**Acknowledges reality of situation and understanding of relationship of be-**

havior to drug use. Participates in program and demonstrates self-control as evidenced by relaxed posture, nonviolent behavior.

INTERVENTIONS	RATIONALE
Independent	
Place in darkened, quiet, nonthreatening environment with a nonintrusive observer.	Lowered stimulation decreases the likelihood of confusion and fear, thus there is less chance of violent behavior. Use of the observer promotes safety. Note: PCP users seek help only after the situation has gotten out of hand, and it is therefore important to take safe action immediately.
Speak in a soft, nonthreatening voice. Use "Talk-downs" when LSD has been taken. If technique is tried with other drugs (PCP) and agitation increases, stop immediately.	Nonthreatening communication may have a calming effect. However, "Talk-downs" (the use of orientation, support, and reassuring words/touch) may be deleterious, resulting in an increase in the user's agitation level in the presence of PCP intoxication.
Observe for increasing anxiety, fear, irritability, and agitation.	May indicate potential for change to violent behavior. Note: client has used a drug and therefore is not in complete control of self.
Accept client's anger without reacting on an emotional basis.	Responding emotionally on a personal level is not constructive and may be destructive.
Provide protection within the environment via constant observation and removal of objects that may be used to hurt self or others.	Reduces risk of injury to client and/or staff. Client may not feel pain and cannot follow directions.
Observe behavior without administering drugs.	A period of drug-free observation should precede any decision to administer medications, e.g., tranquilizers, so that a clear clinical picture can develop. In addition, because it is not known what other drugs may have been ingested, it is not advisable to add another drug, if avoidable.
Collaborative	
Administer medications as necessary, e.g., diazepam (Valium);	Used to reduce muscle spasms and/or restlessness in PCP user.
haloperidol (Haldol).	Preferred to control psychosis and assaultive behavior.
Avoid use of phenothiazine neuroleptics.	Drugs such as thorazine should probably be avoided because of the possibility of potentiating PCP anticholinergic effects.
Apply restraints, if needed and document reason(s) for use.	Restraints should be avoided in a frightened, hallucinating client but may be necessary because of potential injury to self or others, or where other dangerous drugs have been taken. PCP users are unpredictable, so it is best to err on the side of safety (using restraints with sufficient documentation) rather than risking injury.

NURSING DIAGNOSIS:	INJURY, POTENTIAL FOR: (SPECIFY)
MAY BE RELATED TO:	Muscle incoordination
	Reduced hand/eye coordination
	Decreased response to/perception of pain
	Reduced temperature/tactile sensation
	Clouded sensorium and impaired judgment
	Clonic movements, muscle rigidity, which may precede/occur with generalized seizure activity
	Unfamiliar environment
	Fear
	Internal factors, host: psychologic perception (hallucinations)
	Interactive conditions between individual and environment that impose a risk to the defensive and adaptive resources of the individual, e.g., placing hand in open flame, "flying" out of window.
CLIENT OUTCOMES/EVALUATION CRITERIA:	Verbalizes understanding of factors (e.g., drug use) that contribute to possibility of injury and takes steps to correct situation. Demonstrates behaviors and lifestyle changes necessary to minimize and/or prevent injury. Maintains/achieves physiologic stability evidenced by patent airway and adequate respiratory/cardiac function.

INTERVENTIONS

Independent

Ascertain drugs which have been taken when possible.

Anticipate some form of unpredictability and be prepared for the unexpected, including physiologic as well as psychologic emergencies.

Maintain client under close observation. Note precursors which might indicate increasing agitation, e.g., body tension, rising voice tone, quickening movements.

Provide a hockey/bicycle helmet as indicated.

Remove objects that may be used to hurt self or others and observe client constantly.

Monitor vital signs, respiratory rate/depth and rhythm.

Listen to character of respirations.

Encourage fluids frequently, if able to swallow safely.

Position client on side with head to the side as indicated.

Have emergency equipment (including airway adjunct/suction) and medications available.

Collaborative

Administer IV fluids and ammonium chloride or ascorbic acid, as indicated.

RATIONALE

Necessary for appropriate intervention/anticipation of needs. Lethal overdoses of hallucinogenic drugs (except for PCP) are rare; however, caution must be taken because adulterants such as sedative-hypnotics, anticholinergics, and PCP are often added. Note: The two biggest reasons for not finding out what drugs have been taken are: (1) the individual lies for legal reasons or may feel embarrassed and/or (2) the person who sold the drugs either did not know or lied about the drug. Either way, the client needs to be listened to, but know that the information may not be accurate.

These drugs can be dangerous as they can lead to bizarre thinking/harmful behavior. Also, because drugs are often mixed or "cut" with other drugs, it is difficult to know what drugs may actually be involved.

PCP alters thinking and is an anesthetic, and client may hurt self due to bizarre thinking, e.g., attempt to jump out window, or escape from restraints.

If client is banging head against hard objects, a helmet can decrease the potential for/severity of injury.

Provides protection within the environment.

Decreased diastolic blood pressure (cannabis) or hypertensive crisis (PCP) may develop. Bradypnea/respiratory arrest can occur, especially with PCP or heavy cannabis use.

Hypersalivation and vomiting, especially in the presence of ineffective cough and/or loss of muscle tone resulting in occlusion of airway, may cause crowing/gurgling/choked respirations, leading to respiratory arrest.

Adequate hydration keeps secretions loose and easier to expectorate and enhances renal clearance of drugs.

Facilitate drainage of vomitus and buildup of saliva and prevent choking in sedated/comatose client.

Toxic effects of PCP on the heart and respiratory system may result in cardiac/respiratory arrest requiring prompt intervention to prevent death.

Forced diuresis and acidifying urine enhances renal clearance of PCP. (Effects are dose related: >5 mg = low dose; >10 mg = high dose; >20 mg can lead to hypertensive crisis, coma/death due to respiratory/cardiac failure).

INTERVENTIONS	RATIONALE
Collaborative	
Apply restraints with caution when used.	May prevent injury to self or others. However, restraints should be avoided, if possible, in a frightened, hallucinating client.

NURSING DIAGNOSIS:	**TISSUE PERFUSION: ALTERED, CEREBRAL [POTENTIAL]**
MAY BE RELATED TO:	**Alterations in blood flow (hypertensive crisis)**
CLIENT OUTCOMES/EVALUATION CRITERIA:	**Regains/maintains usual level of consciousness free of adverse neurologic symptoms/complications.**

INTERVENTIONS	RATIONALE
Independent	
Elevate head of the bed; keep head in midline position.	Enhances venous drainage, thereby reducing risk of vascular congestion increasing intracranial pressure and possibility of hemorrhage in PCP intoxication.
Observe for pupillary or vital signs changes, decreased level of consciousness and/or motor function.	Provides for early detection and intervention to minimize intracranial pressure/injury.
Encourage rest and quiet. Reduce environmental stimuli.	Promotes relaxation and may assist with lowering of the blood pressure.
Collaborative	
Administer antihypertensive medications, e.g., diazoxide (Hyperstat) and hydralazine (Apresoline).	Effective in lowering blood pressure to prevent hypertensive crisis, which can be associated with PCP intoxication.

NURSING DIAGNOSIS:	**THOUGHT PROCESSES, ALTERED**
MAY BE RELATED TO:	**Physiologic changes (use of hallucinogenic substance)**
	Impaired judgment with loss of memory
POSSIBLY EVIDENCED BY:	**Inaccurate interpretation of environment, memory impairment, bizarre thinking, disorientation**
	Inability to make decisions

Unpredictable behavior

Cognitive dissonance

Distractibility

Inappropriate/non-reality-based thinking

Sleep deprivation

Inability to communicate needs/desires effectively (mutism or confusion)

CLIENT OUTCOMES/EVALUATION CRITERIA:

Observed return of memory and ability to function. Communicating effectively. Reports absence of visual/auditory distortions. Verbalizes understanding that the drug is the cause of/contributes to alteration in perception.

INTERVENTIONS

Independent

Observe closely, do not leave unattended, and make sure restraints are secure when used. Remove objects from the environment that could be used to harm self and others. (Refer to ND: Violence, potential for, self-directed or directed at others.)

Anticipate some form of unpredictable behavior and be prepared for the unexpected.

Tell client that current thoughts and feelings are a result of the PCP, if indicated.

Allow client to sleep whenever possible.

Observe for psychotic indicators of paranoia, delusions, hallucinations.

Note altered speech ability. Refer to loss of speech as temporary.

RATIONALE

PCP alters thinking and is an anesthetic, and client may hurt self via attempt to jump out window, jump in front of cars, escape from restraints, and so forth. Removal of potentially harmful objects provides for protection and safety.

Use of hallucinogens can lead to bizarre thinking/harmful responses.

This information may be helpful to the client who can accept it; however, it may cause agitation.

Sleep cycle is disturbed by PCP. Client will need sleep after being agitated and expending excessive amounts of energy; sleeping also provides time for drug(s) to clear system.

Overdose may precipitate a psychotic episode that will clear within hours to days. When psychosis remains, preexisting condition, e.g., schizophrenia, may have been precipitated.

Mutism and confusion may occur, and information may reassure client that problem is drug-induced and that it will improve with time. (Note: "Talk-down" approach may agitate the client and should be used with caution.)

Anticipate client's needs and allow more time for client to respond to any necessary questions and/or comments.

May reduce need to communicate in presence of confusion/interference with memory. Adequate time allows full expression. (Note: Be aware that touching and/or physical closeness may increase anxiety and agitation.)

Collaborative

Administer medications as indicated, e.g., diazepam (Valium or chlordiazepoxide (Librium).

Chronic PCP users who develop psychiatric complications may require further treatment for the thought disorder or depressive illness. The response may be very slow because of the persistence of PCP in the body tissues, sometimes for a period of several months.

NURSING DIAGNOSIS:	**ANXIETY (SPECIFY LEVEL)/FEAR**
MAY BE RELATED TO:	**Situational crisis**
	Threat to/change in health status
	Perceived threat of death
	Inexperience or unfamiliarity with the effect of drug(s) (e.g., PCP, LSD)
	Impaired thought processes
	Sensory impairment
POSSIBLY EVIDENCED BY:	**Assumptions of "losing my mind, losing control"**
	Verbalized concern of unknown consequences/outcomes
	Sympathetic stimulation, e.g., cardiovascular excitation, superficial vasoconstriction, pupil dilation, vomiting/diarrhea, restlessness, trembling
	Preoccupation with feelings of impending doom
	Apprehension
	Attack behavior

CLIENT OUTCOMES/EVALUATION CRITERIA:	Verbalizes/demonstrates lessened anxiety. Identifies the fear and verbalizes feelings of control of self and situation. Maintains anxiety at manageable level.

INTERVENTIONS

Independent

INTERVENTIONS	RATIONALE
Assess level of anxiety on an ongoing basis.	Increased anxiety may lead to agitation and violent behavior as client is not in complete control of actions/responses.
Place in darkened, quiet, nonthreatening environment with a nonintrusive observer.	Lowered stimulation decreases the likelihood of confusion and fear. Observer is used for safety (with other personnel available to help if needed).
Orient person to surroundings, time, and who is with the client. Speak in soft voice, with a nonthreatening manner.	Knowing where one is can increase the feeling of security when experiencing a "bad trip."
Use "Talk-down" with caution, telling the client that the ingested drug is the cause of feelings of anxiety, the effects are only temporary, and permanent damage should not occur.	Reassurance can be the single most important therapeutic intervention. "Talk-downs" are effective with persons who have taken LSD or similar substances. If the client can realize that the perceptions are drug-related, then an increase in control can take place. However, in some situations (e.g., PCP) "Talk-downs" can result in an increase in fear and agitation.
Encourage verbal expression of changes in perception that are occurring.	Can be used for assessment and provides guidance on direction for support.

Collaborative

INTERVENTIONS	RATIONALE
Administer sedatives if necessary, e.g., diazepam (Valium) or chlordiazepoxide (Librium).	Drugs of choice to be used in extreme cases in order to calm client. Note: Medications are often discouraged because "bad trips" are usually self-limiting, and time is the best remedy for treating the negative effects.

NURSING DIAGNOSIS:	SELF-CARE DEFICIT (SPECIFY)
MAY BE RELATED TO:	Perceptual/cognitive impairment
	Therapeutic management (restraints)
POSSIBLY EVIDENCED BY:	Inability to meet own physical needs
CLIENT OUTCOMES/EVALUATION CRITERIA:	Resumes/performs self-care activities within level of own ability. Verbalizes commitment to lifestyle changes to meet self-care needs.

INTERVENTIONS	RATIONALE
Independent	
Provide care as needed/permitted.	Client may be agitated, and care will need to be postponed until control is regained.
Involve client in formulation of care plan, as possible.	Enables client to participate at level of ability and enhances sense of control. (Note: PCP user is often unable to interact without getting agitated.)
Work with client's present abilities. Do not pressure to perform beyond capabilities.	Failure can produce discouragement, depression, and agitation.
Provide and promote privacy within limits of safety needs.	Important to enhance self-esteem.
Collaborative	
Problem-solve with client, using input from other team members as indicated.	Multidisciplinary approach with involvement of everyone who is caring for the client, along with the client, increases probability of plan being effective/successful.
Refer to CP: Substance Dependence/Abuse Rehabilitation	

Substance Dependence/Abuse Rehabilitation

DSM III R: Alcohol
     291.xx Alcohol-induced organic mental disorders
     303.90 Dependence; 305.00 Abuse
    Amphetamine or similarly acting sympathomimetic
     304.40 Dependence, 305.70 Abuse
     Cannabis: 304.30 Dependence; 305.20 Abuse
     Cocaine: 304.20 Dependence; 305.60 Abuse
    Hallucinogen
     304.50 Dependence; 305.30 Abuse
    Barbiturates
     Opioid: 304.00 Dependence; 305.50 Abuse
     Sedative/hypnotic/anxiolytic: 304.10 Dependence; 305.40 Abuse

CLIENT ASSESSMENT DATA BASE

Refer to appropriate acute care plan for alcohol, stimulants, hallucinogens, depressants.
Addiction Severity Index (ASI): an assessment tool that produces a "problem severity profile" of the client, including chemical, medical, psychologic, legal, family/social, and employment/support aspects, indicating areas of treatment needs.

NURSING PRIORITIES

1. Provide support for decision to stop substance abuse.
2. Strengthen individual coping skills and facilitate learning of new ways to reduce anxiety.
3. Provide information to meet physical/social needs.
4. Promote family involvement in rehabilitation program.
5. Facilitate family growth/development.

DISCHARGE CRITERIA

1. Assumes responsibility for own life and behavior.
2. Formulates plan to maintain substance-free life (e.g., identifies community resources/group support systems).
3. Resolves family relationships/co-dependency issues.
4. Completes treatment program successfully.

NURSING DIAGNOSIS:	**COPING, INEFFECTIVE INDIVIDUAL**
MAY BE RELATED TO:	**Personal vulnerability**
	Difficulty handling new situations
	Previous ineffective/inadequate coping skills with substitution of drug(s)
	Anxiety/Fear
POSSIBLY EVIDENCED BY:	**Denial (one of the strongest and most resistant symptoms of substance abuse)**

POSSIBLY EVIDENCED BY— *continued*	Lack of acceptance that drug use is causing the present situation
	Altered social patterns/participation
	Impaired adaptive behavior and problem-solving skills
	Decreased ability to handle stress of illness/hospitalization
	Financial affairs in disarray
	Employment difficulties (usually the last area to be affected), e.g., losing time on job/not maintaining steady employment
CLIENT OUTCOMES/EVALUATION CRITERIA:	Verbalizes awareness of relationship of substance abuse to current situation. Identifies ineffective coping behaviors/consequences. Uses effective coping skills/problem-solving and demonstrates necessary lifestyle changes. Attends support group (e.g., Cocaine/Narcotics/Alcoholics Anonymous) regularly.

INTERVENTIONS	RATIONALE
Independent	
Ascertain what name client would like to be addressed by.	Shows courtesy and respect. Gives sense of orientation and control.
Determine understanding of current situation and previous methods of coping with life's problems.	Provides information about degree of denial, identifies coping skills that can be used in present plan of care.
Confront and examine denial in peer group.	Since denial is the major defense mechanism in addictive disease, confrontation by peers can help the client accept the reality of what is happening and that drug use is a major problem.
Remain nonjudgmental. Be alert to changes in behavior, e.g., restlessness, increased tension.	Confrontation can lead to an increase in agitation that may compromise safety of client/staff.
Provide positive feedback for expressing awareness of denial in self and/or others.	Positive feedback is necessary to enhance self-esteem and to reinforce desired behavior.
Maintain firm expectation that client attend recovery support/therapy groups regularly.	Attendance is related to admitting need for help, working with denial, and for maintenance of a long-term drug-free existence.

INTERVENTIONS

Independent

Structure diversional activity that relates to recovery (e.g., social activity within support group) wherein issues of being chemical-free are examined.

Use peer support to examine ways of coping with drug hunger.

Provide information about addictive use versus experimental, occasional; biochemical/genetic disorder theory (genetic predisposition); use activated by environment; pharmacology of stimulant; compulsive desire as a life-long occurrence.

Encourage and support client's taking responsibility for own recovery (e.g., development of alternative behaviors to drug urge). Assist client to learn own responsibility for recovering.

Assist client to learn/encourage use of relaxation skills, imagery, visualizations.

Be aware of staff enabling behaviors and feelings.

Collaborative

Administer medications as indicated, e.g.,
    disulfiram (Antabuse);

    Methadone.

Encourage involvement with self-help associations, e.g., Alcoholics/Narcotics Anonymous.

RATIONALE

Discovery of alternative methods for coping with drug hunger can remind client that addiction is a life-long process and opportunity for changing patterns is available.

Addictive self-help groups are valuable for learning and promoting abstinence in each member, as well as in using peer pressure.

Progression of use in the addict is from recreational to addictive use. Comprehending this process is important in combating denial. Education may relieve client of blame, may help awareness of recurring addictive characteristics.

Denial can be replaced with responsible action when client accepts the reality of own responsibility.

Helps client to relax, develop new ways to deal with stress, problem-solve.

Lack of understanding of enabling and co-dependence can result in nontherapeutic approaches to addicts.

This drug can be helpful in maintaining abstinence from alcohol while other therapy is undertaken. By inhibiting alcohol oxidation (AldOH) the drug leads to an accumulation of acetaldehyde with a highly unpleasant reaction if alcohol is consumed.

This drug is thought to blunt the craving for/diminish the effects of heroin and is used to assist in withdrawal and long-term maintenance programs. It has fewer side effects and allows the individual to maintain daily activities and ultimately withdraw from drug use.

Puts client in direct contact with support systems necessary for continued sobriety/drug-free life.

NURSING DIAGNOSIS:	POWERLESSNESS
MAY BE RELATED TO:	Substance addiction with/without periods of abstinence
	Episodic compulsive indulgence
	Attempts at recovery
	Lifestyle of helplessness

POSSIBLY EVIDENCED BY:	Ineffective recovery attempts
	Continuous/constant thinking about drug and/or obtaining drug
	Alteration in personal, occupational, and social life
	Statements of inability to stop behavior/requests for help
CLIENT OUTCOMES/EVALUATION CRITERIA:	Admits inability to control drug habit, surrenders to powerlessness. Verbalizes awareness that will power alone cannot control abstinence and acceptance of need for treatment. Engages in peer support. Demonstrates active participation in program. Regains and maintains healthful status with a drug-free lifestyle.

INTERVENTIONS	RATIONALE
Independent	
Use crisis intervention techniques, e.g.:	Client is more amenable to acceptance of need for treatment at this time.
Assist client to recognize problem exists;	While client is hurting, it is easier to admit the drug(s) is a problem.
Identify goals for change;	Helpful in planning direction for care, promoting belief that change can occur.
Discuss alternative solutions;	Brainstorming helps to identify possibilities creatively and provides sense of control.
Assist in selecting most appropriate alternative;	As possibilities are discussed, the most useful solution becomes clear.
Support in decision and implementation of selected alternative(s).	Helps the client to persevere in process of change.
Discuss need for help in a caring nonjudgmental way.	A caring, confrontive manner is more therapeutic and client may respond defensively to a moralistic attitude, blocking recovery.
Discuss ways in which drug has interfered with life, occupation, personal/interpersonal relationships.	Important for client to identify how the drug has controlled life. Awareness can combat denial.
Explore support in peer group. Encourage sharing of drug hunger, situations that increase the desire to indulge, ways that substance has influenced life.	May need assistance in expressing self, speaking about powerlessness, and admitting need for help in order to face up to problem and begin resolution.
Assist client to learn ways to enhance health and structure healthy diversion from drug use, e.g., a balanced diet, adequate rest, acupuncture, biofeedback, deep	Learning to empower self in constructive areas can strengthen ability to continue recovery. These activities help restore natural biochemical balance; aid detoxifi-

156

INTERVENTIONS	RATIONALE

Independent

meditative techniques, exercise (walking, slow/long-distance running, etc.).

cation; manage stress, anxiety, use of free time. These diversions can increase self-confidence, thereby improving self-esteem. (Note: Release of endorphins from lengthy exercise can create a feeling of well-being.)

Assist client in self-examination of spirituality, faith.

Surrendering to and faith in a power greater than one-self has been found effective in substance recovery; may decrease sense of powerlessness.

Assist client to learn assertive communication.

Effective in assisting in ability to refuse use, to stop relationships with users and dealers, to build healthy relationships, regain control of own life.

Provide treatment information on an ongoing basis.

Helps client know what to expect. Creates opportunity for client to be a part of what is happening and make informed choices about participation/outcomes.

Collaborative

Refer to/assist with making appointment to treatment program for continuation after discharge, e.g., partial hospitalization drug treatment programs, Narcotics/Alcoholics Anonymous.

Follow-through on appointments may be easier than making the initial contact, and continuing treatment is essential to positive outcome.

NURSING DIAGNOSIS:	NUTRITION, ALTERED: LESS THAN BODY REQUIREMENTS
MAY BE RELATED TO:	Insufficient dietary intake to meet metabolic needs (psychologic, physiologic, or economic reasons)
POSSIBLY EVIDENCED BY:	Weight loss; weight below norm for height/body build
	Reported altered taste sensation
	Lack of interest in food
	Poor muscle tone
	Decreased subcutaneous fat/muscle mass
	Sore, inflamed buccal cavity
	Laboratory evidence of protein/vitamin deficiencies

| CLIENT OUTCOMES/EVALUATION CRITERIA: | Demonstrates progressive weight gain toward goal with normalization of laboratory values and absence of signs of malnutrition. Verbalizes understanding of effects of substance abuse and reduced dietary intake on nutritional status. Demonstrates behaviors and lifestyle changes to regain and maintain appropriate weight. |

INTERVENTIONS	RATIONALE
Independent	
Assess height/weight, age, body build, strength, activity/rest level. Note condition of oral cavity.	Provides information about individual on which to base dietary plan. Type of diet/foods may be affected by condition of mucous membranes and teeth.
Take triceps skinfold measurements.	Calculates subcutaneous fat and muscle mass to aid in determining dietary needs.
Note total daily calorie intake; maintain a diary of intake, times, and patterns of eating.	Information about client's dietary pattern will identify nutritional needs/deficiencies.
Evaluate energy expenditure (e.g., pacing or sedentary) and establish an individualized exercise program.	Activity level affects nutritional needs. Exercise enhances muscle tone, may stimulate appetite.
Provide opportunity to choose foods/snacks to meet dietary plan.	Enhances participation/sense of control and may promote resolution of nutritional deficiencies.
Weigh weekly and record.	Provides information regarding effectiveness of dietary plan.
Collaborative	
Review lab work as indicated, e.g., glucose, serum albumin, electrolytes, etc.	Identifies anemias, electrolyte imbalances, other abnormalities that may be present, requiring specific therapy.
Consult with dietician, as indicated.	Useful in establishing individual dietary needs. Provides additional source of learning.
Refer for dental consultation as necessary.	Teeth are essential to good nutritional intake and dental hygiene/care is often a neglected area in this population.

NURSING DIAGNOSIS:	**SELF-CONCEPT, DISTURBANCE IN: SELF-ESTEEM, PERSONAL IDENTITY, ROLE PERFORMANCE**
MAY BE RELATED TO:	**Social stigma attached to substance abuse**
	Social expectation that one control behavior

POSSIBLY EVIDENCED BY:	Biochemical body change (e.g., withdrawal from alcohol/drugs)

Situational crisis with loss of control over life events

Not taking responsibility for self/self-care

Lack of follow-through

Self-destructive behavior

Change in usual patterns or responsibility (family, job, legal)

Confusion about self, purpose, or direction in life

Denial that substance use is a problem |
| **CLIENT OUTCOMES/EVALUATION CRITERIA:** | Identifies feelings and methods for coping with negative perception of self. Verbalizes acceptance of self as is and an increased sense of self-esteem. Sets goals and participates in realistic planning for lifestyle changes necessary to live without drugs. |

INTERVENTIONS	RATIONALE
Independent	
Provide opportunity for and encourage verbalization/discussion of individual situation.	Client often has difficulty expressing self, even more difficulty accepting the degree of importance that substance has assumed in life and the relationship it has to the present situation.
Assess mental status. Note the presence of other psychiatric disorders (dual diagnosis).	Many clients use substances (alcohol and other drugs) to seek relief from depression or anxiety. Note: Approximately 60% of substance-dependent clients also have mental illness problems, and there is an increasing awareness that treatment for both is imperative.
Spend time with client. Discuss client's behavior/use of substance in a nonjudgmental way.	Presence of the nurse conveys acceptance of the individual as a worthwhile person. Discussion provides opportunity for insight into the problems abuse has created for the client.
Provide reinforcement for positive actions, and encourage the client to accept this input.	Failure and lack of self-esteem have been problems for this client, and the need to learn to accept self as an individual who has positive attributes is important.

INTERVENTIONS	RATIONALE
Independent	
Observe family/significant other(s) dynamics/support.	Substance abuse is a family disease, and how the members act and react to the client's behavior affects the course of the disease and how the client sees self. Many unconsciously become "enablers," helping the individual to cover up the consequences of the abuse.
Encourage expression of feelings of guilt, shame and anger.	The client often has lost respect for self and believes that the situation is hopeless. Expression of these feelings helps the client to begin to accept responsibility for own self and take steps to make changes.
Help the client to acknowledge that substance use is the problem and that problems can be dealt with without the use of drugs. Confront the use of defenses, e.g., denial, projection, rationalization.	When drugs can no longer be blamed for the problems that exist, the client can begin to plan a life without substance use. Confrontation helps the client accept the reality of the problems as they exist.
Ask the client to list past accomplishments and positive happenings.	There are things in everyone's life that have been successful. Often when self-esteem is low, it is difficult to remember these successes.
Use techniques of role rehearsal.	Assists client to practice the development of skills to cope with new role as a person who no longer needs drugs to deal with problems.
Collaborative	
Formulate plan to treat other mental illness problems. (Refer to appropriate CP as indicated.)	Clients who seek relief for other mental health problems through drugs will continue to do so once discharged. Both the substance use and the mental health problems need to be treated together to maximize abstinence potential.
Involve in group therapy.	Group sharing helps encourage verbalization as other members of group are in various stages of abstinence from drugs and can address the client's concerns/denial. The client can gain new skills, hope, and a sense of family/community from group participation.
Refer to other resources, such as Narcotics/Alcoholics Anonymous, which use a basic strategy known as the Twelve Steps.	One of the oldest and most popular forms of group treatment. The client admits powerlessness over drug and seeks help from a "higher power." Members help one another, and meetings are available at many different times and places in most communities. The philosophy of "one day at a time" helps attain the goal of abstinence.

NURSING DIAGNOSIS:	**COPING, INEFFECTIVE FAMILY, COMPROMISED/DYSFUNCTIONAL**
MAY BE RELATED TO:	**Personal vulnerability of individual family members**

Co-dependency issues

Situational crises

Compromised social systems

Family disorganization/role changes

Prolonged disease progression that exhausts supportive capability of family members

Significant person(s) with chronically unexpressed feelings of guilt, anger, hostility, despair

POSSIBLY EVIDENCED BY:

Denial (one of the strongest and most resistant symptoms)

Lack of acceptance that drinking/drug use is causing the present situation, or belief that **all** problems are due to substance use

Severely dysfunctional family, e.g., family violence, spouse/child abuse, separation/divorce, children displaying acting out behaviors

Financial affairs in disarray

Employment difficulties

Altered social patterns/participation

Significant other(s) demonstrating enabling or co-dependent behaviors, e.g., avoiding and shielding, attempting to control, taking over responsibilities, rationalizing and accepting, co-operating and collaborating, rescuing and subserving

FAMILY OUTCOMES/EVALUATION CRITERIA:

Verbalizes understanding of dynamics of co-dependence and participates in individual and family programs. Identifies ineffective coping behaviors/consequences. Demonstrates/plans for

FAMILY OUTCOMES/EVALUATION CRITERIA—*continued*

necessary lifestyle changes. Takes action to change self-destructive behaviors/alters behavior that contributes to partner's addiction.

INTERVENTIONS	RATIONALE
Independent	
Assess family history; explore roles of family members, circumstances involving drug use, strengths, areas for growth.	Determines areas for focus, potential for change.
Explore how the significant other has coped with the addict's habit, e.g., denial, repression, rationalization, projection.	Co-dependent also suffers from the same feelings as the client (e.g., anxiety, self-hatred, helplessness, hurt, loneliness, low self-worth, guilt) and needs help in learning new/effective coping skills.
Determine understanding of current situation and previous methods of coping with life's problems.	Provides information on which to base present plan of care.
Assess current level of functioning of family members.	Affects individual's ability to cope with situation.
Determine extent of "enabling" behaviors being evidenced by family members; explore with individual/client.	"Enabling" is doing for the client what s/he needs to do for own self. People want to be helpful and do not want to feel powerless to help their loved one to stop drinking and change the behavior which is so destructive. However, the substance abuser relies on others to cover up own inability to cope with daily responsibilities.
Provide information about enabling behavior, addictive disease characteristics for both user/nonuser co-dependent.	Awareness and knowledge provide opportunity for individuals to begin the process of change.
Provide factual information to client and family about the effects of addictive behaviors on the family and what to expect after discharge.	Many clients/families are not aware of the nature of addiction. If client is using legally obtained drugs, may believe this does not constitute abuse.
Encourage family members to be aware of their own feelings, look at the situation with perspective and objectivity. They can ask themselves: "Am I being conned? Am I acting out of fear, shame, guilt, or anger? Do I have a need to control?"	When the co-dependent family members become aware of their own actions that perpetuate the addict's problems, they need to decide to change themselves. If they change, the client can then face the consequences of the client's own actions and may choose to get well.
Provide support for co-dependent partner(s). Encourage group work.	Families/significant others need support as much as addicts in order to produce change.
Assist the co-dependent partner to become aware that client's abstinence and drug use is not the partner's responsibility.	Partners need to learn that user's habit may or may not change despite partner's involvement in treatment.
Help the recovering (former user) co-dependent to distinguish between destructive aspects of enabling behavior and genuine motivation to aid the user.	Enabling behavior can be partner's attempts at personal survival.
Note how the co-dependent partner relates to the treatment team/staff.	Determines enabling style. A parallel exists between how partner relates to user and to staff, based on partner's feelings about self and situation.

INTERVENTIONS

Independent

Assess co-dependent's conflicting feelings about treatment, e.g., may have similar feelings as abuser (blend of anger, guilt, fear, exhaustion, embarrassment, loneliness, distrust, grief, and possibly relief).

Involve family in discharge referral plans.

Be aware of staff enabling behaviors and feelings about particular clients and co-dependent partners.

Collaborative

Encourage involvement with self-help associations, Alcoholics/Narcotics Anonymous, Al-Anon, Alateen, etc.

RATIONALE

Useful in establishing co-dependent's need for therapy. Own identity may have been lost, may fear self-disclosure to staff, and may have difficulty giving up the dependent relationship.

Drug abuse is a family illness. Because the family has been so involved in dealing with the substance abuse behavior, they need help adjusting to the new behavior of sobriety/abstinence. Incidence of recovery is almost doubled when the family is treated along with the client.

Lack of understanding of enabling and co-dependence can create nontherapeutic approaches to addicts and their families.

Puts client/family in direct contact with support systems necessary for continued sobriety.

NURSING DIAGNOSIS:	SEXUAL DYSFUNCTION
MAY BE RELATED TO:	Altered body function: neurological damage and debilitating effects of drug use (particularly alcohol and opiates)
POSSIBLY EVIDENCED BY:	Progressive interference with sexual functioning
	In men, a significant degree of testicular atrophy is noted (testes are smaller and softer than normal); gynecomastia (breast enlargement); impotence/decreased sperm counts
	In women, loss of body hair, thin soft skin, and spider angioma (elevated estrogen); amenorrhea/increase in miscarriages
CLIENT OUTCOMES/EVALUATION CRITERIA:	Verbally acknowledges effects of drug use on sexual functioning/reproduction. Identifies interventions to correct/overcome individual situation.

INTERVENTIONS	RATIONALE
Independent	
Assess client's current information and have client describe problem in own words.	Determines level of knowledge, client needs.
Encourage and accept individual expressions of concern.	Most people find it difficult to talk about this sensitive subject and may not ask directly for information.
Provide education opportunity (e.g., pamphlets, consultation from appropriate persons) for patient to learn effects of drug on sexual functioning.	Much of denial and hesitancy to seek treatment may be decreased with sufficient and appropriate information.
Provide information about individual's condition.	Sexual functioning may have been affected by drug (alcohol) intake or physiologic and/or psychologic factors (such as stress). Information will assist client to understand own situation and identify actions to be taken.
Provide information about effects of drugs on the reproductive system/fetus (e.g., increased risk of premature birth, brain damage, and fetal malformation). Assess drinking/drug history of pregnant client.	Awareness of the negative effects of alcohol/other drugs on reproduction may motivate client to stop using drug(s). When client is pregnant, identification of potential problems aids in planning for future fetal needs/concerns.
Discuss prognosis for sexual dysfunction, e.g., impotence.	In about 50% of cases, impotence is reversed with abstinence from drug(s); 25% take a long time returning to normal functioning; approximately 25% remain impotent.
Collaborative	
Refer for sexual counseling, if indicated.	Client may need additional assistance to resolve more severe problems/situations. Client may have difficulty adjusting, if drug has improved sexual experience (heroin decreases dyspareunia in women/premature ejaculation in men). Further, the client may have engaged enjoyably in bizarre, erotic sexual behavior under influence of the stimulant; client may have found no substitute for the drug, may have driven a partner away, and may have no motivation to adjust to sexual experience without drugs.
Review results of sonogram, if pregnant.	Assesses fetal growth and development to identify possibility of fetal alcohol syndrome (FAS) and future needs.

NURSING DIAGNOSIS:	**KNOWLEDGE DEFICIT [LEARNING NEED], (SPECIFY)**
MAY BE RELATED TO:	**Lack of information regarding substance use, treatment and self-care needs, prognosis for individual situation**
	Misconception about use of drug(s)

	Interference with learning (other mental illness problems/organic brain syndrome)
POSSIBLY EVIDENCED BY:	Continued use in spite of complications/bad trips
	Statements of concern about disease, life style changes
	Questions/misconceptions about disease, treatment, and prognosis
CLIENT OUTCOMES/EVALUATION CRITERIA:	Verbalizes understanding of own disease process, treatment plan, and prognosis. Identifies/initiates necessary lifestyle changes to remain drug-free. Participates in treatment program.

INTERVENTIONS

Independent

INTERVENTIONS	RATIONALE
Assess client's knowledge of own situation, e.g., disease, complications, and needed changes in lifestyle.	Assists in planning for long-range changes necessary for maintaining sobriety/drug-free status. Client may have street knowledge of the drug but be ignorant of medical facts.
Time activities to individual needs.	Facilitates learning, as information is more rapidly assimilated when pacing is considered.
Discuss relationship of drug use to current situation.	Often client has misperception (denial) about real reason for admission to the psychiatric (medical) setting.
Discuss effects of drug(s) used, e.g., PCP is deposited in body fat and may reactivate (flashbacks) even after long interval of abstinence; alcohol use may result in mental deterioration/liver involvement/damage; cocaine can damage postcapillary vessels and increase platelet aggregation, promoting thromboses/and infarction of skin/internal organs, causing localized atrophie blanche or sclerodermatous lesions.	Information will help client understand possible long-term effects of drug use.
Inform client of effects of Antabuse with alcohol intake and importance of avoiding use of alcohol-containing products, e.g., cough syrups or foods/candy.	Interaction of alcohol and Antabuse results in nausea and hypotension, which may produce fatal shock. Individuals on Antabuse are sensitive to alcohol on a continuum, with some being able to drink on the drug while others can have a reaction with only slight exposure, e.g., alcohol-containing foods or products such as aftershave. Reactions appear to be dose-related as well.
Be aware of and deal with anxiety of client and family members.	Anxiety can interfere with ability to hear and assimilate information.

INTERVENTIONS	RATIONALE

Independent

Provide an active role for the client and family members in the learning process, e.g., discussions, group participation, role play.

Learning is enhanced when people are actively involved.

Provide written and verbal information as indicated. Include list of articles and books related to client/family needs and encourage reading and discussing what they learn.

Helps client and family to make informed choices about future. Bibliotherapy can be a useful addition to other therapy approaches.

Collaborative

Discuss variety of helpful organizations and programs that are available for assistance/referral.

Psychosocial needs may require addressing as well as other issues.

Review specific postcare needs, e.g., PCP user should drink cranberry juice and continue use of ascorbic acid; alcohol abuser with liver damage should refrain from drugs/anesthesias/household cleaning products detoxified in the liver.

Promotes individualized care related to specific situation. Cranberry juice and ascorbic acid enhance clearance of PCP from the system. Substances that have potential for liver damage are more dangerous in presence of already damaged liver.

CHAPTER **6**

SCHIZOPHRENIC DISORDERS

Schizophrenia

DSM III R: 295.1x Disorganized Type
295.2x Catatonic Type
295.3x Paranoid Type
295.9x Undifferentiated Type
295.6x Residual Type

ETIOLOGIC THEORIES

PSYCHODYNAMICS

Psychosis is the result of a weak ego. The development of the ego has been inhibited by a symbiotic parent/child relationship. Because the ego is weak, the use of ego defense mechanisms in times of extreme anxiety is maladaptive, and behaviors are often representations of the id segment of the personality.

BIOLOGIC THEORIES

Certain genetic factors may be involved in the development of this psychotic disorder. Individuals are at higher risk for the disorder if there is a familial pattern of involvement (parents, siblings, other relatives). Schizophrenia has been determined to be a "sporadic illness" (meaning you cannot currently follow genes from generation to generation). It is an autosomal dominant trait. However, most scientists agree that what is inherited is a vulnerability or predisposition, which may be due to an enzyme defect or some other biochemical abnormality, a subtle neurological deficit, or some other factor or combination of factors. This predisposition, in combination with environmental factors, results in development of the disease.

Some research exists that implies that these disorders may be a birth defect, occurring in the hippocampus region of the brain. The studies show a "disordering" of the pyramidal cells in the brains of schizophrenics, while the cells in the brains of nonschizophrenic individuals appear to be arranged in an orderly fashion. Ventricular brain ratio (VBR) or disproportionately small brain may be inherited and/or congenital. The cause can be a virus, lack of oxygen, or birth trauma.

A biochemical theory suggests the involvement of elevated levels of the neurotransmitter dopamine, which is thought to produce the symptoms of overactivity and fragmentation of associations that are commonly observed in psychoses.

FAMILY DYNAMICS

Family systems theory describes the development of schizophrenia as it evolves out of a dysfunctional family system. Conflict between spouses drives one parent to attach to the child. This overinvestment in the child

167

redirects the focus of anxiety in the family, and a more stable condition results. A symbiotic relationship develops between parent and child; the child remains totally dependent on the parent into adulthood and is unable to respond to the demands of adult functioning.

Interpersonal theory relates that the psychotic person is the product of a parent/child relationship fraught with intense anxiety. The child receives confusing and conflicting messages from the parent and is unable to establish trust. High levels of anxiety are maintained, and the child's concept of self is one of ambiguity. A retreat into psychosis offers relief from anxiety and security from intimate relatedness. Some research indicates that clients who live with families high in "expressed emotion" (e.g., hostility, criticism, disappointment, over-protectiveness, and overinvolvement) show more frequent relapses than clients who live with families who are low in expressed emotion.

CLIENT ASSESSMENT DATA BASE

HISTORY

General

Onset of symptoms usually occurs in adolescence or early adulthood (before 45 years of age).
Affects women and men equally.
Correlations with family history of psychiatric illness; lower socioeconomic groups, higher stressors, and premorbid personality described as "suspicious, introverted, withdrawn, or eccentric" have been noted.
History of alteration in functioning for at least six months, including an active phase of at least two weeks when psychotic symptoms were evident.
Family reports presence of psychologic symptoms (primarily in thought and perception) and deterioration from previous level of adaptive functioning. May report poor personal hygiene, interruption of sleep by hallucinations and delusional thoughts, early awakening, insomnia, and hyperactivity (e.g., pacing).
May have had previous acute episodes with impairment ranging from none to severe deterioration requiring institutionalization.

Disorganized

Incoherence; flat, incongruous, silly affect may be seen.
Usually correlated with extreme social impairment, poor premorbid personality; a chronic course with no significant remissions.

Catatonic

Reports of marked psychomotor disturbance, e.g., stupor, rigidity, mutism or excitement, negativism, and/or posturing.
The incidence of this type is rare in the western hemisphere although it was common several decades ago.
A potential for violence to self/others exists during catatonic stupor or excitement.
Malnutrition, exhaustion, hypochondriacal complaints, or oddities of behavior may be noted.

Paranaoid

Tends to occur in middle or late life.
Although the etiology is unclear, other family members may have had paranoid problems.
Systematized delusions and/or hallucinations of a persecutory or grandiose nature, usually related to a single theme, are common.
May become easily agitated, assaultive, and violent, if delusions are acted upon.
Impairment in functioning may be minimal, with gross disorganization of behavior relatively rare. Significant impairment may be noted in social/marital areas.
Affective responsiveness may be preserved but with a stilted, formal quality or extreme intensity in interpersonal interactions often observed. May express doubts about gender identity (e.g., fear of being thought of as, or approached by, a homosexual).
Symptoms characteristic of disorganized and catatonic types are absent.

Undifferentiated

Prominent delusions/hallucinations, incoherence, and grossly disorganized behaviors are seen.
This category is used when illness does not meet the criteria for any of the other schizophrenias or meets the criteria for more than one. It is also used when the course of the last episode is unknown.

Residual

Social withdrawal, eccentric behavior, and inappropriate affect are seen.
History of at least one episode of schizophrenia in which psychotic symptoms were evident, but the current clinical picture presents no psychotic symptoms.

PHYSICAL EXAMINATION

Mental status:
    Thought: delusions, loose association.
    Perception: hallucinations, illusions.
    Affect: blunted, flat, inappropriate, incongruous, or silly.
    Volition: cannot self-initiate or participate in goal-oriented activity.
    Capacity to relate to environment: mental/emotional withdrawal and isolation (''autism'') and/or psychomotor activity ranging from marked reduction to stereotypical, purposeless activity.
Speech: frequently incoherent.
Delusions:
    Disorganized type: Systematized delusions are absent; however, fragmentary delusions or hallucinations (disorganized, unthemitized [without theme] content) are common.
    Paranoid type: one or more systematized delusions with prominent persecutory or grandiose content; delusional jealousy may be observed.
    Undifferentiated type: Delusions are prominent.
Behaviors: grimaces, mannerisms, hypochondriacal complaints, extreme social withdrawal, as well as other odd behaviors. In disorganized type, behavior is incoherent and grossly disorganized.
Psychomotor: stupor, markedly decreased reactivity to milieu, and/or reduced spontaneity of movement/activity or mutism
    Negativism: resistance to all directions or attempts to move without apparent motive.
    Rigidity: rigid posture, maintained despite attempts to move client.
    Excitement: purposeless motor activity not caused by external stimuli.
    Posturing: voluntarily assuming inappropriate or bizarre posture.
Emotions: Unfocused anxiety, anger, argumentativeness, and violence may be observed.

DIAGNOSTIC STUDIES

(Usually done to rule out physical illness, which may be cause of reversible symptomatology.)
Computerized axial tomography (CT) scan: may show subtle abnormalities of brain structures in some schizophrenics.
Positron emission tomography (PET) scan: measures the metabolic activity of specific areas of the brain and holds some promise for future understanding of the structure and function of the brain in relation to these disorders.
Magnetic resonance imaging (MRI) and regional cerebral blood flow (rCBF): special imaging studies being used in research that may increase understanding of schizophrenia. There is a difference in the white and gray matter in the brains of schizophrenics and nonschizophrenics, when stimulated. The frontal lobe of the brain is less active and may be the source of negative symptoms.
Brain electrical mapping (BEAM): also being used in research.
Addiction Severity Index (ASI): determines problems of addiction, which may be associated with mental illness and indicates areas of treatment need.

NURSING PRIORITIES

1. Promote appropriate interaction between client and environment.
2. Enhance physiologic stability/health maintenance.

3. Provide protection, ensure safety needs.
4. Encourage family/significant other(s) to become involved in activities to promote independent, satisfying lives.

DISCHARGE CRITERIA

1. Physiologic well-being maintained with appropriate balance between rest and activity.
2. Demonstrates increasing/highest level of emotional responsiveness possible.
3. Copes effectively with social interactions.
4. Family displays effective coping skills and appropriate use of resources.

NURSING DIAGNOSIS:	THOUGHT PROCESSES, ALTERED
MAY BE RELATED TO:	Disintegration of thinking processes
	Psychologic conflicts
	Impaired judgment
	Sleep disturbance
	Disintegrated ego boundaries (confusion with environment)
	Ambivalence and concomitant dependence (part of need-fear dilemma interferes with ability to self-initiate fulfilling diversional activities)
POSSIBLY EVIDENCED BY:	Presence of delusional system (may be grandiose, persecutory, of reference, of control, somatic, accusatory)
	Symbolic and concrete associations
	Blocking
	Ideas of reference
	Inaccurate interpretation of environment
	Cognitive dissonance
	Commands, obsessions
	Impaired ability to make decisions

	Simple hyperactivity and constant motor activity (ritualistic acts, stereotyped behavior) to withdrawal and psychomotor retardation
	Interrupted sleep patterns
CLIENT OUTCOMES/EVALUATION CRITERIA:	Recognizes changes in thinking/behavior. Identifies delusions and increases capacity to cope effectively with them by elimination of pathological thinking. Maintains reality orientation. Establishes interpersonal relationships.

INTERVENTIONS

Independent

Assess the presence/severity of client's altered thought processes, noting form (dereistic, autistic, symbolic, loose, and/or concrete associations, blocking); content (somatic delusions, delusions of grandeur/persecution, ideas of reference); and flow (flight of ideas, retardation).

Establish a therapeutic nurse-client relationship.

Use therapeutic communications (e.g., reflection, paraphrasing) to effectively intervene.

Structure communications to reflect consideration of client's socioeconomic, educational, and cultural history/values.

Express desire to understand client's thinking by clarifying what is unclear, focusing on the feeling rather than the content, endeavoring to understand (in spite of the client's unclearness), listening carefully, and regulating the flow of the thinking as needed.

Reinforce congruent thinking. Refuse to argue/agree with disintegrated thoughts. Present reality and demonstrate motivation to understand client (model patience). Share appropriate thinking and set limits if client tries to respond impulsively to altered thinking.

Assess rest/sleep pattern by observing capacity to fall asleep, quality of sleep. Graph sleep chart as indicated until normal pattern returns.

RATIONALE

Identification of the symbolic/primitive nature of thinking/communications promotes understanding of the individual client's thought processes and enables planning of appropriate interventions.

Provides an emotionally safe milieu that enables interpersonal interaction and decreases autism.

Therapeutic communications are clear, concise, open, consistent and require use of self. This reduces autistic thinking.

Lack of consideration of these factors can cause misdiagnoses/inaccurate interpretation (otherwise normal thinking viewed as pathological).

Client is often unable to organize thoughts (easily distracted, can't grasp concepts or wholeness but focuses on minutiae). Flow of thoughts is often characterized as racing, wandering, or retarded. Active listening identifies patterns of client's thoughts and facilitates understanding. Expression of desire to understand conveys caring and increases client's feelings of self-worth.

Decreases altered (disintegrated, delusional) thinking as client's thoughts compensate in response to presentation of reality. Providing opportunity for the client to control aggressive behavior enhances self-esteem and promotes safety for the client and others.

Delusions, hallucinations, etc., may interfere with client's sleep pattern. Fears may alter ability to fall asleep. Sleep deprivation can produce behaviors such as withdrawal, confusion, disturbance of percep-

INTERVENTIONS

Independent

Structure appropriate times for rest and sleep; adjust patterns as needed.

Help client identify/learn techniques that promote rest/sleep, e.g., quiet activities, soothing music before bedtime, regular hour for going to bed, drinking warm milk.

Assess presence/degree of factors affecting client's capacity for diversional activities.

Monitor medication regimen, observing for therapeutic effect and side effects, e.g., anticholinergic (dry mouth, etc.), sedation, orthostatic hypotension, photosensitivity, hormonal effects, reduction of seizure threshold, agranulocytosis, and extrapyramidal symptoms. (Refer to ND: Knowledge Deficit [Learning Need], specify.)

Collaborative

Administer medications as indicated, e.g.,
    Neuroleptics (psychotropics, major tranquilizers):
        phenothiazines, such as
            chlorpromazine (Thorazine),
            thioridazine (Mellaril),
            trifluoperazine (Stelazine),
            perphenazine (Trilafon);
        thioxanthenes, such as
            chlorprothixene (Taractan),
            thiothixene (Navane);
        butyrophenones, such as
            haloperidol (Haldol);
        dibenzoxazepines, such as
            loxapine (Loxitane);

    Antiparkinsonism drugs, e.g.,

        Anticholinergics, such as
            trihexyphenidyl HCl (Artane),
            benztropine mesylate (Cogentin),
            procyclidine HCl (Kemadrin),
            biperiden HCl (Akineton);

        Antihistamines, such as
            diphenhydramine (Benadryl);

RATIONALE

tion. Sleep chart identifies abnormal patterns and is useful in evaluating effectiveness of interventions.

Consistency in scheduling reduces fears/insecurities, which may be interfering with sleep. Sleep is enhanced by balancing activity (physical, occupational) with rest/sleep.

Enhances client's ability to optimize rest/sleep, enhancing ability to think clearly.

Presence of hallucinations/delusions; situational factors such as long-term hospitalization (characterized by monotony, sensory deprivation); psychological factors such as decreased volition; physical factors such as immobility contribute to deficits in diversional activity.

Enables identification of the minimal effective dose to reduce psychotic symptoms with the least adverse effects. Identification of the onset of serious side effects, such as neuroleptic malignant syndrome, provides for appropriate interventions to avoid permanent damage.

Used for the reduction of psychotic symptoms. May be given orally or by injection. For long-term maintenance therapy, depot neuroleptics may be the drugs of choice, when available, to maintain medication adherence and prevent relapse. When given at bedtime, the sedative effects of psychotropic medication can enhance quality of sleep and reduce hypotensive side effects.

Used for relief of drug-induced extrapyramidal reactions and in treatment of all other forms of parkinsonism.

Block action of acetylcholine, thereby reducing excitation of the basal ganglia.

Suppresses cholinergic activity and prolongs action of dopamine by inhibiting its reuptake and storage.

INTERVENTIONS	RATIONALE
Collaborative	
Miscellaneous, such as amantadine (Symmetrel)	Releases dopamine from presynaptic nerve endings in basal ganglia.

NURSING DIAGNOSIS:	SENSORY-PERCEPTUAL, ALTERATION: (SPECIFY)
MAY BE RELATED TO:	Panic levels of anxiety
	Disturbance in thought, perception, affect, sense of self, volition, relationship to environment
	Psychomotor behavior
POSSIBLY EVIDENCED BY:	Illusions, delusions and hallucinations
	Disorientation
	Changes in usual response to stimuli
CLIENT OUTCOMES/EVALUATION CRITERIA:	Identifies self in relationship to environment. Recognizes reality and dismisses internal voices. Demonstrates improved cognitive, perceptual, affective, and psychomotor abilities.

INTERVENTIONS	RATIONALE
Independent	
Assess the presence/severity of alterations in client's perceptions. Note possible causative/contributing factors, e.g., anxiety, substance abuse, fever, trauma, or other organic illnesses/causes.	Provides information about client's behavior potentials regarding ADLs, sleep patterns, potential for violence (command hallucinations, homicide, suicide), nonverbal and verbal behaviors (content, form, style, flow).
Spend time with client, listening with regard and providing support for changes client is making.	Continued consistent support/acceptance will reduce anxiety and fears and enable client to decrease altered perceptions.
Provide a safe environment by not arguing with or ridiculing the client.	Altered perceptions are frightening to the client and indicate loss of control. Because of lack of insight, client views altered perceptions as reality. Arguing only leads to defensiveness and a regressive struggle with the client.
Orient to reality by communicating effectively (clear, concise); reinforcing reality (of client's altered perceptions); and clarifying time, place, and person.	Client's distortion of reality is a defense against actual reality, which is more frightening. Reality orientation assists client to correctly interpret stimuli within the milieu.

173

INTERVENTIONS	RATIONALE

Independent

Set limits on client's impulsive response to altered perceptions. Remain with the client and provide distraction when possible.

Client who is perceiving the environment incorrectly lacks internal controls to prevent impulsive response to misperceptions. Often client feels more in control if nurse remains in room. Distraction (music, TV, games) may also support client to regain capacity to control response to altered perceptions.

Be honest in expressing fears if potential for violence is perceived. (Refer to ND: Violence, potential for: self-directed or directed at others.)

Informing client when behaviors are frightening and providing anticipatory guidance (by verbalizing actions) focuses attention on reality and assists in reducing anxiety.

Collaborative

Provide external controls (quiet room, restraints; inform client of intent to use touch) as indicated.

External limits and controls must be provided to protect client and others until client regains control internally and is able to ignore altered perceptions.

NURSING DIAGNOSIS:	**COMMUNICATION, IMPAIRED: VERBAL**
MAY BE RELATED TO:	**Psychologic barriers, psychosis**
	Autistic and delusional thinking
	Alterations in perception
POSSIBLY EVIDENCED BY:	**Inability to verbalize rationally**
	Verbal expressions, such as neologisms, echolalia, associative/looseness, paralogical language
	Nonverbal expressions, such as echopraxia-stereotypical behaviors (bizarre gesturing, facial expressions, and posturing)
CLIENT OUTCOMES/EVALUATION CRITERIA:	**Verbalizes or indicates an understanding of communication problems. Employs strategies to communicate effectively both verbally and nonverbally. Establishes means of communication in which needs can be understood.**

INTERVENTIONS	RATIONALE
Independent	
Evaluate degree/type of communication impairment.	Degree of impairment of verbal/nonverbal communications (loose associations, neologisms, echolalia, and echopraxia) will affect client's ability to interact with staff and others and to participate in care.
Demonstrate a "listening attitude" within the nurse-client relationship.	A "listening attitude" enables the nurse to listen carefully, observe the client, and anticipate and watch certain patterns of client's communications that may emerge.
Acknowledge client's difficulty in communicating.	Recognition of client's difficulty expressing ideas and feelings demonstrates empathy, lessening anxiety and enabling client to concentrate on communicating.
Provide a nonthreatening environment/safe forum for client's communications.	Atmosphere in which a person feels free to express self without fear of criticism helps to meet safety needs, increasing trust and providing assurance for tolerance and validation of appropriate negative communications.
Accept use of alternative communications, such as drawing, singing, dancing, mime.	Increases client's feelings of security, provides avenues for expressing needs.
Avoid arguing or agreeing with inaccurate communications; simply offer reality view in nonjudgmental style (communiciate your lack of understanding to client).	Arguing is nontherapeutic and may cause the client to become defensive. Agreeing with the client's expression of inaccurate communication reinforces misinterpretation of reality.
Use therapeutic communications skills, such as paraphrasing, reflecting, clarification.	Client's flow of communications (too fast/too slow) may require regulation. These techniques assist with reality orientation, thereby minimizing misinterpretation and facilitating accurate communications.
Be open and honest in therapeutic use of verbal and nonverbal communications.	Client has increased sensitivity to nonverbal messages. Honesty increases sense of trust, a loss of which is at the base of client's problem. Openness and genuineness in expression of feelings provide a role model for client.
Use a supportive approach to client by communicating desire to understand (ask client to help you do so).	Recognizes that client's past experiences have created distrust, which produces attempt to maintain distance by being vague and unclear in sending messages.
Identify the symbolic, primitive nature of the client's speech/communications. Note: cultural beliefs (e.g., talking to dead relatives) may be accepted as normal within the client's culture.	Recognition of the symbolism of the client's primitive speech and thinking enables the nurse to better understand the client's feelings. Without this recognition, the actual communications may be vague and disorganized, indicating client's inability to focus and perceive clearly. Cultural attitudes need to be considered to avoid confusion with pathologic condition.

NURSING DIAGNOSIS:	COPING, INEFFECTIVE, INDIVIDUAL
MAY BE RELATED TO:	**Personal vulnerability**

175

MAY BE RELATED TO—*continued*	**Inadequate support system(s)**
	Unrealistic perceptions
	Inadequate coping methods
	Disintegration of thought processes
POSSIBLY EVIDENCED BY:	**Impaired judgment, cognition, and perception**
	Diminished problem-solving/decision-making capacities
	Poor self-esteem
	Chronic anxiety and depression
	Inability to perform role expectations
	Alteration in social participation
CLIENT OUTCOMES/EVALUATION CRITERIA:	**Identifies ineffective coping behaviors and consequences. Demonstrates understanding of and begins to use appropriate, constructive, effective methods for coping. Verbalizations of feelings are congruent with behavior.**

INTERVENTIONS	RATIONALE
Independent	
Assess the presence/degree of impairment of client's coping abilities.	Provides information about perceived and actual coping ability, life change units, anxiety level, stresses (internal, external), developmental level of functioning, use of defense mechanisms, and problem-solving ability.
Assist client to identify/discuss thoughts, perceptions, and feelings.	Client is able to view how perceptions/thinking/affect is processed and to strengthen reality orientation and coping skills.
Encourage client to express areas of concern. Support formulation of realistic goals and learning appropriate problem-solving techniques.	This disease first manifests itself at an early age, before the client has had an opportunity to learn effective coping skills. In a trusting relationship (a climate of acceptance), the client can begin to learn these skills, without fear of judgment.
Encourage client to identify precipitants that led to ineffective coping, when possible.	Knowledge of stressors that have precipitated deteriorated coping ability enables client to recognize and deal with these factors before problems occur.

INTERVENTIONS

Independent

Explore how client's perceptions are validated prior to drawing conclusions.

Assist client to recognize/develop appropriate/effective coping skills.

RATIONALE

With support, client has the opportunity to learn to validate perceptions before selecting ineffective/inappropriate coping methods (such as acting out behavior).

Increased/more flexible problem-solving/coping behaviors prevents decompensation (distorted reality, delusional system).

NURSING DIAGNOSIS:	SELF-CONCEPT, DISTURBANCE IN: SELF-ESTEEM; ROLE PERFORMANCE; PERSONAL IDENTITY
MAY BE RELATED TO:	Disintegrated thought processes (perception, cognition, affect)
	Loose/disintegration of ego boundaries
	Perceived threats to the self
	Disintegration of behavior, affect
POSSIBLY EVIDENCED BY:	Verbalized expressions of worthlessness, negative feelings about self
	Protective delusional systems
	Impaired judgment, cognition, and perception
	Role performance deterioration in family, social, and work areas
	Disturbed sense of self (depersonalization and delusions of control)
	Inadequate development of self-esteem and hopefulness
	Ambivalence and autism (interfering with acceptance of self and meaning of own existence)
CLIENT OUTCOMES/EVALUATION CRITERIA:	Demonstrates enhanced sense of self by decreasing depersonalization and

<table>
<tr><td>

CLIENT OUTCOMES/EVALUATION CRITERIA—*continued*

</td><td>

delusions. **Verbalizes feelings of value/ worthwhileness and views self as competent and socially acceptable (by self and others). Develops appropriate plans for improvement of role performance that promote highest possible level of adaptive functioning. Demonstrates self-directedness by expressing own needs and desires and making effective decisions. Participates in activities with others.**

</td></tr>
</table>

INTERVENTIONS	RATIONALE
Independent	
Assess the degree of disturbance in client's self-concept.	Documents own and others' perceptions, client's goals, significant losses/changes. Provides basis for evaluation of progress/therapy.
Spend time with client; listen with regard and acceptance.	Conveys empathy, acceptance, support, which enhances client's self-esteem. Personal identity is strengthened as client identifies with the nurse and experiences therapeutic caring within the relationship.
Encourage client to verbalize areas of concern/feelings.	Self-esteem is improved by increased insight into feelings. Insight is gained as client verbalizes/identifies feelings of inadequacy, worthlessness, rejection, loneliness.
Assist client to identify how negative feelings decrease self-esteem.	Negative feelings can lead to severe anxiety and/or suspiciousness. Increased awareness/perception of factors that cause negative feelings can assist client to recognize how negative feelings cause deterioration.
Encourage client to recognize positive characteristics related to self.	Discussion of positive aspects of the self-system, such as social skills, work abilities, education, talents, and appearance, can reinforce client's feelings of being a worthwhile/competent person.
Review personal appearance and things client can do to enhance hygiene/grooming. (Refer to ND: Self-Care, deficit, specify.)	Positive personal appearance enhances body image and respect for self.
Encourage client to participate in appropriate activities/exercise.	Enhances capacity for interpersonal relationships (in 1:1 and small groups). Activities that use the five senses increase the sense of self. Physical exercise promotes positive sense of well-being.
Assess client's capacity to tolerate use of touch carefully.	Use of touch can help client to reestablish body boundaries (if the experience can be tolerated).
Provide positive reinforcement for client's abilities/efforts.	Positive feedback increases self-esteem, provides encouragement, and promotes a sense of self-direction.
Determine current level of role performance and note causative/contributing factors that affect it.	Factors such as inadequate knowledge, role conflict, alteration of self/others' perceptions of role, and change in usual patterns of responsibility can affect

INTERVENTIONS

Independent

Assist the client to adapt to changing role performance by working with client/significant other(s) to develop strategies for dealing with disturbances in role and enhancing expectations of coping effectively.

Help client set realistic goals for managing life and performing own ADLs.

Assess the current sense of personal identity, considering if client acknowledges sense of self (observe how client addresses self, e.g., may refer to self in third person) or expresses feelings of unreadiness, merging with people/objects.

Analyze the presence/severity of factors that alter personal identity, e.g., paranoia, blunted affect.

Assess presence/severity of factors that affect client's religious/spiritual orientation. Note presence of religiosity.

Use therapeutic communication skills to support client's verbalization of sense of self and to discover its relationship to meaning of existence.

Facilitate early discharge for client when hospitalization has been required.

Collaborative

Administer appropriate tests, e.g., asking client to draw a stick figure of self, Body Image Aberration, Physical Anhedonia Scale.

Refer to resources such as occupational therapist/ movement therapy/Outdoor Education program; partial hospitalization program.

Initiate involvement in/refer to religious activities/ resources as desired/appropriate. Note overinvolvement in religious activity.

RATIONALE

the client's physical and psychologic capacity for effective role performance.

The client's eventual level of performance may be positively influenced by a support system that is responsive and caring.

Client needs to be productive and benefits from being given the responsibility for own life and direction within limits of ability.

Identifies individual needs, appropriate interventions. Inability to identify self poses a major problem that can interfere with person's interactions with others.

Disintegrated ego boundaries can cause a weakened sense of self. Clients often express fears of merging and losing personal identity.

Disintegrated behaviors create such factors as displaced anger toward God, expression of concern with meaning of life/death/values (may be expressed as delusions, hallucinations). These concerns may negatively affect the individual's sense of self-worth. Client may use religious beliefs as a defense against fears.

Therapeutic communications, such as active listening, summarizing, reflection, can support client to find own solutions.

Clients can increase their sense of self by early return to own milieu surrounded by personal possessions.

These tests demonstrate client's view, concept of self, and its correlation to many variables.

Provides activities that promote feelings of self-worth and accomplishment during involvement with others. Partial hospitalization may enhance return from hospital setting to community.

Spiritual resources such as a pattern of prayer, a sense of faith, or membership in an organized religious group may enhance the development of client's coping resources, sense of acceptance/self-worth. Strong attachment to an ideology (religiosity) may be used in an attempt to control feelings of anxiety.

NURSING DIAGNOSIS:	ANXIETY (SPECIFY LEVEL)/FEAR
MAY BE RELATED TO:	Disintegration of thought processes

SCHIZOPHRENIC DISORDERS: Schizophrenia

179

MAY BE RELATED TO—*continued*	Perception and affect occurring in response to overwhelming feelings of losing control
	Threat to self-concept
	Change in environment, role-functioning, interaction patterns
	Extremes in psychomotor activity (occurring with chronicity or severity)
POSSIBLY EVIDENCED BY:	Inappropriate response to such feelings (loss of control/approval)
	Inappropriate/regressed, or absent responses
	Poor eye contact
	Focus on self
	Increased perception of danger
	Decreased problem-solving ability
	Fear of perceived loss of control or approval from significant other(s); hurting self or others
	Psychomotor disturbances varying from excited motor behavior to immobility
CLIENT OUTCOMES/EVALUATION CRITERIA:	Responds appropriately to feelings of overwhelming anxiety (fears, loss of control, feelings of rejection) by decreasing regressive behaviors (disintegrated thinking/perception/affect). Communicates anxious feelings and problem-solves effectively. Orients to reality by interpreting milieu correctly. Perceives no danger in interactions with others.

INTERVENTIONS	RATIONALE

Independent

Note the level of the client's anxiety, considering severity, unfulfilled needs, misperceptions, present use of defense mechanisms, and coping skills.

The weakened ego of schizophrenia causes a decreased capacity to distinguish reality and a diminished capacity to problem-solve. This can result in a heightened sense of helplessness and anxiety.

Assess the degree and reality of the fears currently perceived by the client.

The client's experience of fear may contribute to decreased coping capacity and increased anxiety/fear.

Establish trust, through a patient, supportive, caring, and accepting relationship.

Trust, which is difficult for schizophrenic clients, is the basis of a therapeutic nurse-client relationship. The mutuality of the 1:1 experience enables clients to work through their fears and to identify appropriate methods for problem-solving by role-modeling within the 1:1.

Encourage the client to verbalize fears.

Verbalization of frightening perceptions (fears) reduces withdrawal and/or potential for violence (projection of aggressive impulses).

Assist client to identify/communicate sources of anxiety and areas of concern. Monitor for drug effectiveness/side effects.

Anxiety can arise from misperceived threats to self, unfulfilled needs, and perceived losses (of control/approval). Disintegration of thinking/perception/affect may be reduced as client verbalizes frightening feelings. Alertness for prevention of medication side effects can reduce frightening physiologic experiences that can escalate anxiety.

Demonstrate/encourage use of effective, constructive strategies for coping with anxiety, e.g., relaxation and thought-stopping techniques, meditation, and physical exercise. Use role modeling, positive reinforcement. (Refer to NDs: Communication, impaired: Verbal; Sensory-Perceptual alteration.)

Maladaptive coping needs to be examined with emphasis on ineffectiveness of outcomes. Reduces secondary gain and enables client to learn more adaptive, effective decision-making/problem-solving/coping skills.

Remain with the client and clarify reality.

Assists the client to achieve effective coping. The presence of a trusted individual can help client feel protected from external dangers and maintain contact with reality.

Involve client in planning treatment.

Participation in treatment increases client's sense of control and provides opportunity to practice problem-solving skills.

NURSING DIAGNOSIS:

MAY BE RELATED TO:

SOCIAL ISOLATION

Disturbed thought processes that result in mistrust of others/delusional thinking

Environmental deprivation, "institutionalization" (as a result of long-term hospitalization)

POSSIBLY EVIDENCED BY:	**Difficulty in establishing relationships with others**
	Expressions of feelings of rejection
	Dealing with problems by anger/ hostility and violence.
	Social withdrawal/isolation of self
CLIENT OUTCOMES/EVALUATION CRITERIA:	**Verbalizes willingness to be involved with others. Participates in activities/ programs with others. Develops 1:1 trust-based relationship.**

INTERVENTIONS	RATIONALE
Independent	
Assess presence/degree of isolation by listening to client's comments about loneliness.	Mistrust can lead to difficulty in establishing relationships and client may have withdrawn from close contacts with others.
Spend time with client. Make brief, short interactions that communicate interest, concern, and caring.	Establishes a trusting relationship. Consistent, brief, honest contact with the nurse can help the client begin to re-establish trusting interactions with others.
Plan appropriate times for activities (by limiting withdrawal, varying daily routine only as tolerated).	Consistency in 1:1 relationship and sameness of milieu is required initially to enable client to decrease withdrawn behavior. Motivation is stimulated by the humanistic sharing of a 1:1 experience.
Assist client to participate in diversional activities and limited/planned interaction situations with others in group meeting/unit party, etc.	With toleration of 1:1 relationship and strengthened ego boundaries, client will be able to increase socialization and enter small group situations. Brief encounters can help the client to become more comfortable in the company of others and provide an opportunity to try out new social skills.
Identify support systems available to the client, e.g., family, friends, co-workers, etc.	Support is an important part of the client's rehabilitation, providing a network to assist in social recovery.
Assess family relationships, communication patterns, knowledge of client condition.	Problems within family (poor social/relationship skills, high expressed emotion) may interfere with client's progress. Family therapy may be indicated.
Note client's sense of self-worth and belief about individual identity/role within family setting/milieu. (Refer to ND: Self-concept, disturbance in: Self-esteem; Role performance; Personal identity.)	When client feels good about self and own value, interactions with others are enhanced.

NURSING DIAGNOSIS:	**MOBILITY, IMPAIRED PHYSICAL [POTENTIAL]**
MAY BE RELATED TO:	**Disintegration of thought and behavior**

Psychomotor retardation

Sensory overload/deprivation

Perceptual impairment

Diminished muscle strength

Impaired coordination and limited range of motion/total immobility

Psychomotor activity (occurring with chronicity or severity) varying from excited motor behavior to immobility

CLIENT OUTCOMES/EVALUATION CRITERIA: Maintains optimal mobility and muscle strength. Demonstrates awareness of the environment (psychomotor behavior) and capacity to regulate psychomotor activity. Engages in physical activities.

INTERVENTIONS	RATIONALE
Independent	
Determine the level of impairment (rate from complete independence to dependence with social withdrawal) in relation to pre-illness capacity, considering age, meaning (motivation, desire, tolerance), onset, duration, coordination, range of motion, muscle strength, and control. Measure capacity for activity by observing endurance (attention span, psychomotor response, appropriateness of participation).	Provides information to determine the amount of nursing assistance required and client potentials.
Note the presence/severity of factors that affect the client's level of mobility, such as psychotic functioning, control needs, sensory overload/deprivation.	These factors need to be considered in planning nursing care, as they can affect client's ability to perform at appropriate activity level.
Encourage client to identify need for/plan resumption of activities/exercise.	As psychotic functioning decreases, the capacity to relate to milieu/others and to self-initiate increases. Involving client in scheduling activities provides client with sense of independence (control over environment).
Determine current activity level appropriate for client by assessing attention span, capacity to tolerate others in milieu.	Presence of psychotic features can cause mental/emotional withdrawal or agitation.
Structure appropriate times for exercise/activity (turning/moving unaffected body parts); monitor environmental stimulations such as radio, TV, visitors.	Movement reduces physiologic deterioration. Environmental stimulation can be used to maintain/promote sensory-perceptual capacity.

INTERVENTIONS	RATIONALE

Independent

Schedule adequate periods of rest/sleep. Monitor client's response and set limits as needed.

Establishing a regular sleep pattern helps client to become rested, reducing fatigue, and may improve ability to think. When client is able to think more clearly, participation in treatment program may be enhanced.

NURSING DIAGNOSIS:	VIOLENCE, POTENTIAL FOR: SELF-DIRECTED OR DIRECTED AT OTHERS
MAY BE RELATED TO:	Disintegrated thought processes stemming from ambivalence and autistic thinking
	Lack of development of trust and appropriate interpersonal relationships
POSSIBLE INDICATORS:	Disintegrated behaviors
	Perception of environmental and other stimuli/cues as threatening
	Irrational, threatening, or assaultive behavior
	Physical aggression to self
	Religiosity
CLIENT OUTCOMES/EVALUATION CRITERIA:	Resolves conflicts and/or copes with anxiety without the use of threats or assaultive behavior (to self or others). Participates in care and meets own needs in an assertive manner. Demonstrates self-control, as evidenced by relaxed posture, nonviolent behavior.

INTERVENTIONS	RATIONALE

Independent

Assess the presence/degree of client's potential for violence (at self or others) on a 1 to 10 scale. Determine suicidal/homicidal intent, indications of loss of control over behavior (actual or perceived), hostile verbal/nonverbal behaviors, risk factors, and prior/present coping skills.

Data base is essential for nursing care and documents degree of intent. (May be #1 nursing priority if score is high.) Prior history of violent behavior increases risk for violence as would factors such as command hallucinations.

INTERVENTIONS

Independent

Provide safe, quiet environment; tell client "you are safe."

Be careful in offering a pat on the shoulder/hug, etc.

Encourage verbalizations of feelings and promote acceptable verbal outlet(s) for expression, e.g., yelling in room.

Assist client to identify situations which trigger anxiety/aggressive behaviors.

Explore implications and consequences of handling these situations with aggression.

Assist client to define alternatives to aggressive behaviors. Initially engage in solitary physical activities, instead of group. Monitor competitive activities; use with caution.

Set limits, stating in a clear, specific, firm manner what is acceptable/unacceptable. Use demands only when situation requires.

Be alert to signs of impending violent behavior: increase in psychomotor activity; intensity of affect; verbalization of delusional thinking, especially threatening expressions; frightening hallucinations.

Accept verbal hostility without retaliation or defense. Nurse (caregiver) needs to be aware of own response to client behavior, e.g., anger/fear.

Isolate promptly in nonpunitive manner using adequate help if violent behavior occurs. Hold client if necessary. Tell client to "STOP" behavior.

Collaborative

Apply restraints or put in seclusion as indicated, documenting reasons for action.

Administer medications as indicated. (Refer to ND: Thought Processes, impaired.)

RATIONALE

Keeping environmental stimuli to a minimum and providing reassurance will help prevent agitation.

Touch may be misinterpreted as an aggressive gesture.

Ventilation of feelings may reduce need for physical action.

Promotes understanding of relationship between severe anxiety and situations that result in destructive feelings leading to aggressive actions.

Helps client to realize the possibility and importance of thinking through a situation before acting.

Enables client to learn to handle situations in a socially acceptable manner. Appropriate outlets will allow for release of hostility. Anxiety and fear may escalate during activities in which the client perceives self in competition with others and can trigger violent behavior.

Being clear and remaining calm increases chance that client will cooperate and potential for violence avoided. Having few but important limits enhances chances of having them observed.

Therapeutic interventions are more effective before behavior becomes violent.

Behavior is not usually directed at nurse personally and responding defensively will tend to exacerbate situations. Looking at meaning behind the words will be more productive. Awareness of own response allows nurse to express/deal with those feelings.

Removal to quiet environment can help calm client. Usually the individual is being self-critical and afraid of own hostility and does not need external criticism. Sufficient help will prevent injury to client/staff. Often holding client and/or saying "stop" is enough to help client regain control.

May be needed for short-term control until client regains control over self.

Used to reduce psychotic symptoms, decrease delusional thinking, and assist client to regain control of self.

NURSING DIAGNOSIS:	SELF-CARE DEFICIT: (SPECIFY)
MAY BE RELATED TO:	Perceptual and cognitive impairment
	Immobility resulting from social with-drawal, isolation, and decreased psychomotor activity
	Autonomic nervous sytem side effects of psychotropic medications
POSSIBLY EVIDENCED BY:	Inability to/or difficulty in areas of feeding self, keeping body clean, dressing appropriately and/or toileting self
	Urinary calculi formation
	Bladder stasis/paralysis
	Decreased bowel activity with constipation, fecal impaction, and/or paralytic ileus
CLIENT OUTCOMES/EVALUATION CRITERIA:	Performs self-care and ADL at highest level of adaptive functioning possible. Recognizes cues/maintains elimination patterns, preventing complications. Identifies/uses resources available for assistance.

INTERVENTIONS	RATIONALE
Independent	
Determine current versus pre-illness level of self-care (specify levels 0–4) re: feeding, bathing/hygiene, dressing/grooming, toileting.	Identifies potentials and determines degree of nursing care to be provided.
Assess presence/severity of factors which affect client's capacity for self-care, e.g., disintegrative perceptual/cognitive abilities, mobility status.	Impairment in these areas can alter client's ability/readiness for self-care.
Discuss personal appearance/grooming and encourage dressing in bright colors, attractive clothes. Give positive feedback for efforts.	Appearance affects how the client sees self. A run-down, disheveled appearance conveys a sense of low self-worth, while an attractive, well-put-together appearance conveys a positive sense of self to the client as well as to others.
Determine client's regular elimination patterns and compare with current pattern. Note contributing factors, e.g., anxiety, decreased attention span, disorien-	Identifies appropriate interventions as patterns of elimination are individually influenced by physiologic, cultural, and psychologic factors. These factors can affect

INTERVENTIONS

Independent

tation, reduced psychomotor activity, as well as use of psychotropic medications.

Encourage/provide diet high in fiber and at least 2 liters of fluid each day. (Refer to NDs: Fluid Volume deficit, potential; Nutrition, altered: Less/More than body requirements.)

Observe/record urinary output. Note changes in color, odor, clarity. Encourage client to observe/report changes.

Establish increasing daily activity level as client progresses. Include regular intervals for toileting.

Collaborative

Plan with client for effective use of community resources, such as nutritional programs, sheltered workshops, group/transitional/apartment homes, home health care.

Administer laxatives/stool softeners, as indicated.

RATIONALE

toileting, e.g., client does not pay attention to cues; dehydration from inadequate intake results in lessened urinary output and contributes to constipation; anticholinergic effect of medication may result in urinary retention.

A diet high in fiber and residue promotes bulk formation and at least 2 liters of fluid daily regulates stool consistency (facilitating bowel elimination) and renal function.

Bladder paralysis/retention can occur from psychotropic medications, increasing risk of infection.

Adequate exercise increases muscle tone; consistency in daily routine stimulates bowel elimination. A schedule prevents accidents that can occur due to polyuria from psychotropic medication or decreased attentiveness to cues and psychomotor activity.

Assists client to develop an effective plan for hygienic/self-care needs.

Used cautiously for brief period or as needed to enhance bowel function. Overuse promotes dependency.

NURSING DIAGNOSIS:	**FLUID VOLUME DEFICIT, POTENTIAL**
MAY BE RELATED TO:	**Disintegrated patterns of thinking and behavior**
	Altered eating/drinking patterns
	Excessive renal losses (side effects of some psychotropic medications)
CLIENT OUTCOMES/EVALUATION CRITERIA:	**Verbalizes understanding of need for fluid. Recognizes physical cues of thirst. Ingests individually appropriate amount of fluid. Demonstrates adequate fluid balance with appropriate urinary output, stable vital signs, moist mucous membranes, good skin turgor.**

INTERVENTIONS	RATIONALE
Independent	
Assess presence/severity of factors that affect client's fluid intake.	Factors such as physical immobility, psychotropic medications, mental status, can cause fluid volume imbalance.
Record intake/output; monitor mental status, vital signs, weight, skin turgor. Note medication interactions/side effects.	Careful monitoring and early recognition of symptoms can prevent complications. If oral intake is not adequate, orthostatic hypotension may develop. Dehydration/reduced circulating volume directly affects cerebral perfusion/mentation. Dry mucous membranes, decreased skin turgor can occur, increasing risk of tissue breakdown. Polyuria is a frequent side effect of psychotropics, further affecting fluid balance.
Structure/encourage appropriate times for fluid intake.	Scheduling of intake provides for an accurate record and helps to ensure adequate amounts are ingested.
Encourage measures such as frequent mouth care, chewing sugarless gum or sucking on hard (sugarless) candy, and drinking lemonade.	Reduces oral cavity discomfort associated with dehydration/effects of medication. Note: Omit sugarless gum for aged client because of danger of choking, as phenothiazines alter the swallowing reflex.

NURSING DIAGNOSIS:	**NUTRITION, ALTERATION IN: LESS/MORE THAN BODY REQUIREMENTS**
MAY BE RELATED TO:	**Imbalance between energy needs and intake**
	Disintegration of thought and perception
	Inability/refusal to eat
POSSIBLY EVIDENCED BY:	**Delusions or hallucinations related to food intake**
	Increased appetite (side effect of some psychotropic medications)
	Weight loss/gain
	Sore, inflamed buccal cavity
	Reported dysfunctional eating patterns e.g., eating in response to internal cues other than hunger
	Sedentary/excessive activity level

CLIENT OUTCOMES/EVALUATION CRITERIA:	Maintains adequate/appropriate nutritional intake. Demonstrates progressive weight gain/loss toward expected goal. Identifies behaviors/lifestyle changes to maintain appropriate weight.

INTERVENTIONS	RATIONALE

Independent

Assess presence/severity of factors that create altered nutritional intake.	Factors such as psychotic thinking or excessive activity to prevent frightening thoughts may cause inability/refusal to eat.
Review dietary intake via 24-hour recall/diary noting eating pattern and activity level.	Provides accurate information for assessment of client's nutritional status and needs. Alterations in dietary intake (decreased/increased calories, salt, fats, sugars) can aid in correcting faulty eating patterns. Lack of knowledge of appropriate dietary needs, perception of food and activity/exercise (immobility) can cause excessive caloric intake.
Encourage client to regulate caloric intake with activity/exercise program.	A balance of activity/exercise with appropriate caloric intake maintains weight loss/gain, improves nutritional status and can improve mental functioning.
Structure consistent times for eating and limit use of food for other than nutritional needs.	Positively reinforces client's appropriate eating behaviors. Limit behaviors (rituals, acting out) that allow client to withdraw/refuse meals or overeat. Secondary gains that may occur can be reduced by setting appropriate expectations.
Provide small, frequent feedings as indicated.	May enhance intake when psychotic thought/behavior interferes with eating.
Encourage client to choose own food, when possible.	Individual is more likely to eat chosen food than what has been arbitrarily given to client, especially when paranoid thoughts of poisoning are present.
Assess presence/severity of factors that affect client's oral mucous membranes. Identify strategies to relieve or minimize altered/irritated oral mucous membranes, such as: rinsing with water, chewing sugarless gum (unless aged), candy or glycerin-based cough drops, drinking lemonade, and mouth care before and after meals.	Altered nutrition can cause dehydration, edema, oral lesions, or altered salivation, which can adversely affect/restrict intake. With relief of "dry mouth," client's anxiety is reduced, medication compliance may be increased, and nutritional intake enhanced.

Collaborative

Arrange consultation with dietitian/nutritional team, as indicated.	May be necessary to establish/meet individual dietary needs.

NURSING DIAGNOSIS:	COPING, INEFFECTIVE FAMILY: DISABLING

MAY BE RELATED TO:	Ambivalent family system/relationships
	Difficulty family members have in coping effectively with client's maladaptive behaviors
POSSIBLY EVIDENCED BY:	Client's expressions of despair at family's lack of reaction/involvement
	Neglectful relationships with client
	Extreme distortion regarding client's health problem, including extreme denial about its existence/severity or prolonged overconcern
	Impaired restructuring of a meaningful life for individual family members
	Impaired individuation
FAMILY OUTCOMES/EVALUATION CRITERIA:	Verbalizes realistic perception of roles within limits of individual situation. Expresses feelings appropriately, honestly, and openly. Demonstrates improvement in communications (clear), problem-solving, behavior control, and affective spheres of family functioning.

INTERVENTIONS

Independent

Compare current and pre-illness level of family functioning.

Determine whether family is high in "expressed emotion," e.g., criticism, disappointment, hostility, solicitude, extreme worry, overprotectiveness, or emotional overinvolvement.

Assess readiness of family members/significant other(s) to participate in client's treatment.

RATIONALE

Provides information about client and family to assist in developing plan of care and choosing interventions. Note: Some family members may demonstrate psychopathologies that may make their influence detrimental to the client.

The emotional climate of the client's family has been shown to significantly affect the client's recovery. Relapse occurs significantly more often in families high in expressed emotion.

Family theorists believe that identified client also represents "disintegrated/enmeshed schizophrenogenic" family system. Aftercare of client must include family/significant others to raise level of interpersonal functioning.

INTERVENTIONS

Independent

Provide honest information about the nature and seriousness of the illness and enlist cooperation of family members to help client to remain in the community.

Promote family involvement with nurses/others to plan care and activities.

Encourage client/family/S.O.(s) to identify and change maladaptive behaviors.

Collaborative

Promote family involvement in behavioral management programs.

Promote involvement with mental health treatment team (e.g., mental health center, family physician/psychiatrist, psychiatric/public health nurse, social/vocational services, occupational/physical therapist), and respite care, when necessary.

Provide client/family/S.O.(s) with assistance to deal with current life situation, e.g., therapy (family/couples/1:1); aftercare services (day care centers, night hospitals, half-way houses, sheltered workshops, rehabilitation services).

RATIONALE

The family who already has maladaptive coping skills may have difficulty dealing with diagnosis and implications of a long-term illness. Client's behavior may be difficult and embarrassing for some families who have problematic coping skills themselves or who may have high profile in the community.

Involvement with others provides a role model for individuals to learn new behaviors/ways of handling stress.

Client's success in treatment is dependent on effective change of whole systems rather than treatment of client's behaviors as a separate entity.

Helps family members to realize that while they can have a positive or negative influence on the course of the illness, they are doing the best they can in a difficult situation, blame is to be avoided, and communication/problem-solving skills can be learned to reduce stress.

When bizarre behavior is difficult for family to manage, assistance may improve the situation and enable the client to remain in the community.

Aftercare may include efforts to enlarge social spheres and increase client's/family's level of functioning, enhancing ability to manage long-term illness.

NURSING DIAGNOSIS:	FAMILY PROCESS, ALTERED
MAY BE RELATED TO:	Situational crisis (schizophrenic disorder present in family which normally functions effectively)
	Change of roles
POSSIBLY EVIDENCED BY:	Deterioration in family functioning
	Failure to adapt to change/deal with crisis in a constructive manner and meet needs of its members
	Difficulty in relating to each other for mutual growth/development

191

POSSIBLY EVIDENCED BY— continued	Failure to send/receive clear messages
	Ineffective family decision-making process
	Family not meeting physical/emotional, security, spiritual needs of member(s)
FAMILY OUTCOMES/EVALUATION CRITERIA:	Expresses feelings regarding illness and altered coping openly and appropriately. Verbalizes understanding of illness, treatment regimen, and prognosis. Encourages and allows member who is ill to handle situation in own way. Engages in problem-solving for resumption of highest possible adaptive level of functioning.

INTERVENTIONS	RATIONALE
Independent	
Determine current and pre-illness level of family functioning. Note factors such as problem-solving skills, level of interpersonal relationships, outside support systems, roles, boundaries, rules, and communications.	These factors affect the family's capacity for returning to precrisis level of adaptive functioning as well as set the tone/expectations for a favorable prognosis.
Assess readiness of the family/S.O.(s) to reintegrate client into system, such as family's ability to use assistance or to cope with crisis appropriately by adaptation or change.	Ability to tolerate and assist with management of client behavior affects client's reentry into the family system.
Assist family to identify potential for growth of family system and individual members. Role model positive behaviors during this process.	Family who has previously functioned well has skills to build on and can learn new ways to deal with changed family structure and challenges of marginally functioning family member. The nurse can provide an example for learning new skills.
Collaborative	
Provide information about/referrals to therapy (family, couples, group) and supportive community resources (halfway houses, vocational counseling, day care centers, sheltered workshops, night hospitals).	Can provide assistance to help the family cope effectively with client's disintegrative behaviors. Having opportunity to take time away from situation enhances ability to manage long-term illness.

NURSING DIAGNOSIS:	HEALTH MAINTENANCE, ALTERED/ HOME MAINTENANCE MANAGEMENT, IMPAIRED
MAY BE RELATED TO:	Inadequate developmental task accomplishment

	Lower socioeconomic group with limited resources
	Lack of knowledge
	Inability or lack of cooperation
	Impaired or diminished family functioning
	Impaired perception, cognition, communication skills, and individual coping skills
POSSIBLY EVIDENCED BY:	Mistrust, lack of autonomy, and disturbed capacity for relationship formation
	Deteriorated family functioning
	Decreased capacity to identify and mobilize adequate support systems and maintain a safe, growth-promoting immediate environment
CLIENT OUTCOMES/EVALUATION CRITERIA:	**Maintains optimal health and family functioning through improved communications and coping skills. Returns home and maintains optimal wellness with minimal complications. Identifies and uses resources effectively.**

INTERVENTIONS	RATIONALE
Independent	
Assess present and pre-illness level of home/health maintenance. Consider deficits in communication, knowledge, decision-making, developmental tasks, support systems and their effect on client's basic health practices.	Dysfunction in family functioning (diminished problem-solving, financial, and support system; emotional impoverishment), lack of motivation to participate in treatment can impair home/health maintenance.
Identify readiness of client/S.O.(s) to maintain safe, growth-promoting environment that meets individual's needs.	Assisting client/significant others to develop a plan for a safe, well-ordered household can enable nurse to assess capacity for/compliance with home/health management needs.
Assist client/family to identify appropriate health care needs/practices, e.g., dental, physician/clinic, regular hygiene practices, as well as some social contacts.	Poor organizational capacity for ADLs and socialization as well as personal involvement can lead to neglect of these areas.

193

INTERVENTIONS

Independent

Involve client/S.O.(s) in the development of a long-term plan for optimal home health management, encouraging identification/use of resources.

Collaborative

Provide referrals to resources, e.g. appropriate support, health teams (mental health center group/day care, family, community, support systems).

RATIONALE

Involvement increases the potential for cooperation with the plan.

Ineffective coping requires support/teaching, which often necessitates referrals. Legal assistance may be required to provide conservatorships and client advocacy.

NURSING DIAGNOSIS:	**KNOWLEDGE DEFICIT, [LEARNING NEED], (SPECIFY)**
MAY BE RELATED TO:	**Chronic nature of the disorder**
	Cognitive limitation (altered thought process/psychosis)
	Misinterpretation/inaccurate information
	Unfamiliarity with information resources
	Suspiciousness and indecisiveness
POSSIBLY EVIDENCED BY:	**Ambivalence and dependency strivings**
	Need-fear dilemma and withdrawal (can lead to abrupt termination of treatment, therapy, medication)
	Inaccurate follow-through of instructions
	Inappropriate or exaggerated behaviors
	Recidivism
	Appearance of side effects of psychotropic medications

CLIENT OUTCOMES/EVALUATION CRITERIA:	Verbalizes understanding of disease and treatment. Participates in learning process/treatment regimen. Assumes responsibility for own learning within individual limits.

INTERVENTIONS

Independent

Determine the current level of knowledge about the disorder and its management.

Assess the presence/severity of factors that affect client's cognitive framework for decision-making about disorder and management, noting lack of recall, ignorance of resources and their use.

Instruct client/family about disorder, its signs and symptoms, management (medication, ADLs, vocational rehabilitation, socialization needs).

Identify/review risk factors of medications client is taking, e.g., sedation, postural hypotension, photosensitivity, hormonal effects, agranulocytosis, and extrapyramidal symtoms (tremors, akinesia/askathisia, dystonia, oculogyric crisis, and tardive dyskinesia).

Emphasize importance of immediate medical attention for onset of high fever and severe muscle stiffness and to discontinue the medication until seen by the doctor.

Have client verbalize/paraphrase knowledge gained.

Assist the client to develop strategies for continuing treatment. Make contract with client to provide for actions to take when problems arise.

Establish schedule for follow-up/postdischarge care. Assess client's verbalizations, refusal of medications, or other treatment strategies (socialization/vocation/exercise/diet).

Collaborative

Refer to group, family, and individual therapies and community support systems.

RATIONALE

Identifies areas of need and misperceptions. Communication skills such as validation of perceptions can assist in assessment of accuracy of client's knowledge base and readiness to learn.

Factors such as disintegrated thinking, cognitive deficits, ambivalence, denial, and dependency needs can limit learning/block utilization of knowledge base for management of disorder.

Provides information and can promote independent behaviors within client's ability.

The anticholinergic effects of psychotropics (and antiparkinsonian drugs that may be given concomitantly to decrease the incidence of extrapyramidal effects of neuroleptics) alter autonomic nervous system's functioning and may cause dry mouth (xerostomia), oral lesions, hemorrhagic gingivitis. Most side effects occur within the first few weeks of treatment and subside with time. However, signs indicative of agranulocytosis (sore throat, malaise), extrapyramidal symptoms, and tardive dyskinesia need immediate attention.

Severe muscle stiffness and high fever are the hallmarks of neuroleptic malignant syndrome, which can usually be effectively treated before it becomes life-threatening if it is detected early.

Evaluates comprehension of information regarding disorder's characteristics and management needs and may reduce recidivism.

Instructing the client/S.O.(s) that "feeling better" is no indication for discontinuing medication, that no addiction can develop with continued treatment, and providing for self-administration often enhances cooperation, reducing medication discontinuation.

Monitoring of client's behavior may reveal indications of willingness/ability to continue treatment.

Promotes trusting relationships and encourages further cooperation with treatment plan. Adequate man-

Collaborative

agement plans and organizing social supports for the family enable these clients to remain in the community.

NURSING DIAGNOSIS:	SEXUAL DYSFUNCTION
MAY BE RELATED TO:	Ego boundary disintegration
	Inability to distinguish between self and environment
	Weakened sexual identification
	Gender identity confusion, which interferes with normal sexual orientation formation
	Development of delusions around the primitive sexual orientation
	Lack of drive and energy, normal social inhibitions, and passivity
POSSIBLY EVIDENCED BY:	Uninhibited sexual behavior
	Preoccupation with sex or gender identity
	Inability to find sexual partner
	Involvement in multiple sexual liaisons
	Endocrine changes associated with antipsychotic drugs, e.g., ejaculatory inhibitions, impotence in men/amenorrhea in women
CLIENT OUTCOMES/EVALUATION CRITERIA:	Strengthens ego boundaries to enable identification and acceptance of sexual orientation. Verbalizes understanding of, identifies, and reports changes in body functions (if they occur) while taking antipsychotics. Demonstrates behavioral restraint in pub-

lic. Uses appropriate birth control device and does not contract STD.

INTERVENTIONS	RATIONALE
Independent	
Have client describe own perceptions of sexual/sexuality functioning.	When sexual/sexuality concerns/perceptions are shared, it provides an opportunity to understand the client's point of view and help the client to learn what is needed.
Assess presence/degree of factors that alter sexual/sexuality functioning.	Ego boundary disintegration can cause regressive behavior (withdrawal, preoccupation with self), which interferes with the formation of attachments and creates gender identity confusion. Antipsychotic medications can cause endocrine changes (amenorrhea, breast enlargement, lactation in women, and impotence, ejaculatory inhibition in men).
Provide information regarding medications, their effects and regulation, and counseling/teaching about problem-solving (expressing feelings of loss and seeking alternate solutions).	Lack of sufficient knowledge may be a contributing factor to the dysfunction. Information can provide assistance in the resolution of the problem(s).
Encourage client to identify/report any alterations in sexual/sexuality functioning.	Timely intervention may prevent future disintegration of ego boundaries and further side effects of medications.
Collaborative	
Counsel client about birth control, genetic implications of having children and the possibility of contracting sexually transmitted diseases (STD).	Severely ill clients have difficulty with relationships and do not make good partners or parents. Although higher functioning clients may find marriage supportive, they need to be aware that each child has a 12 to 15% chance of becoming schizophrenic. Premarital expert eugenic counseling is extremely important. The lack of social inhibitions places these clients at risk for the possibility of contracting a sexually transmitted disease, and a poor level of function may result in neglect of treatment.

Schizoaffective Disorder

DSM III-R: 295.70 Schizoaffective disorder (specify)
Term that emphasizes the temporal relationship of schizophrenic and mood symptoms and is used for conditions that do not meet the criteria for either schizophrenia or a mood disorder.

ETIOLOGIC FACTORS

PSYCHODYNAMICS

Refer to CP: Schizophrenia.

BIOLOGIC THEORIES

Refer to CP: Schizophrenia.

FAMILY DYNAMICS

Refer to CP: Schizophrenia.

CLIENT ASSESSMENT DATA BASE

HISTORY

Pronounced manic and depressive features are intermingled with schizophrenic features.
May report previous episode(s) and remission with no permanent defect.

PHYSICAL EXAMINATION/DIAGNOSTIC STUDIES

Refer to CP: Schizophrenia.

NURSING PRIORITIES

1. Provide protective environment; prevent injury.
2. Assist with self-care.
3. Promote interaction with others on a 1:1 basis and in group activities.
4. Identify resources available for assistance.
5. Support family involvement in therapy.

DISCHARGE CRITERIA

1. Improved sense of self-esteem, lessening depression, and elevated mood is noted.
2. Approaches and socializes appropriately with others, individually and in group activities
3. Signs of physical agitation are abating and no physical injury occurs.
4. Adequate nutritional intake is achieved/maintained.
5. Client/family displays effective coping skills and appropriate use of resources.

(Refer to CP: Schizophrenia for other NDs that apply, in addition to the following):

NURSING DIAGNOSIS:	VIOLENCE, POTENTIAL FOR: SELF-DIRECTED OR DIRECTED AT OTHERS
MAY BE RELATED TO:	Depressed mood

Feelings of worthlessness

Unsatisfactory parent/child relationship

Anger turned inward/directed at the environment

Punitive superego and irrational feelings of guilt

Numerous failures (learned helplessness)

Feelings of abandonment by significant other(s)

Hopelessness

Misinterpretation of reality

Extreme hyperactivity

POSSIBLE INDICATORS:

History of previous suicide attempts

Making direct/indirect statements indicating a desire to kill self/having a plan

Hallucinations

Delusional thinking

Self-destructive behavior (hitting body parts against wall/furniture)

Temper tantrums/aggressive behavior

Destruction of inanimate objects

Increased agitation and lack of control over purposeless movements

Vulnerable self-esteem

CLIENT OUTCOMES/EVALUATION CRITERIA:

Expresses improved sense of well-being/self-esteem. Manages behavior

CLIENT OUTCOMES/EVALUATION CRITERIA—continued

and deals with anger appropriately. Demonstrates self-control without harm to self or others.

INTERVENTIONS	RATIONALE
Independent	
Note direct statements of a desire to kill self; indirect actions, e.g., putting affairs in order, writing a will, giving away prized possessions; presence of hallucinations and delusional thinking; history of previous suicidal behavior/acts; statements of hopelessness regarding life situation.	Direct and indirect indicators of suicidal intent need to be attended to and addressed as being potentially acted on.
Ask client directly if suicide has been considered/planned and if the means are available to carry out the plan.	The risk of suicide is greatly increased if the client has developed a plan and particularly if means exist for the execution of the plan.
Provide a safe enviornment for the client by removing potentially harmful objects from access (e.g., sharp objects; straps, belts, ties; glass items; smoking materials).	Provides protection while treatment is being undertaken to deal with existing situation. Client's rationality is impaired and may harm self inadvertently.
Assign to quiet unit, if possible.	Milieu unit may be too distracting, increasing agitation and potential for loss of control.
Reduce environmental stimuli, e.g., private room, soft lighting, low noise level, and simple room decor.	In hyperactive state, client is extremely distractible, and responses to even the slightest stimuli are exaggerated.
Stay with the client. Provide supervision as necessary.	Provides support and feelings of security as agitation grows and hyperactivity increases.
Formulate a short-term verbal contract with the client that s/he will not harm self during specified period of time. Renegotiate the contract as necessary.	An attitude of acceptance of the client as a worthwhile individual is conveyed. Discussion of suicidal feelings with a trusted individual provides a degree of relief to the client. A contract gets the subject out in the open and places some of the responsibility for own safety with the client.
Ask client to agree to seek out staff member/friend if thoughts of suicide emerge.	The suicidal client is often very ambivalent about own feelings. Discussion of these feelings with a trusted individual may provide assistance before the client experiences a crisis situation.
Encourage verbalizations of honest feelings. Explore and discuss symbols of hope client can identify in own life.	Because of elevated anxiety, client may need assistance to recognize presence of hope in life situations.
Promote expression of angry feelings within appropriate limits. Provide safe method(s) of hostility release. Help client to identify true source of anger, and work on adaptive coping skills for continued use.	Depression and suicidal behaviors may be viewed as anger turned inward on the self, or anger may be expressed as hostile acting out toward others. If this anger can be verbalized and/or released in a nonthreatening environment, the client may be able to resolve these feelings, regardless of the discomfort involved.
Orient client to reality, as required. Point out sensory/environmental misperceptions, taking care not to belit-	Elevated level of anxiety may contribute to distortions in reality. Client may require assistance to distinguish

INTERVENTIONS

Independent

tle client's fears or indicate disapproval of verbal expressions.

Spend time with the client on a regular schedule and as indicated in response to client needs.

Provide structured schedule of activities that includes established rest periods throughout the day.

Provide physical activities as a substitute for purposeless hyperactivity, e.g., brisk walks, housekeeping chores, dance therapy, aerobics.

Observe for effectiveness and evidence of adverse side effects of drug therapy, e.g., anticholinergic (dry mouth, blurred vision), extrapyramidal (tremors, rigidity, restlessness, weakness, facial spasms).

Collaborative

Administer medication, as indicated, e.g.,
   Neuroleptics, e.g., chlorpromazine (Thorazine);

Antidepressants, e.g., imipramine (Tofranil);

Antimanics, e.g., lithium (Eskalith, Lithobid)

Assist with electroconvulsive therapy (ECT).

Identify community resources that client may use as support system and from whom help may be sought if suicidal thoughts/feelings occur.

RATIONALE

between reality and misperceptions of the environment.

Provides a feeling of safety and security, while also conveying the message, "I want to spend time with you because I think you are a worthwhile person."

Structured schedule provides feeling of security for the client. Additional rest promotes relaxation for the agitated client.

Physical exercise provides a safe and effective means of relieving pent-up tension.

Individual reactions to medications may vary, and early identification can assist with changes in dosage and/or drug choice, possibly preventing client from discontinuing drug therapy prematurely with potential loss of control.

Pharmacologic interventions need to be directed at the presenting symptoms and used on a short-term basis. Antipsychotics may be effective in reducing the hyperactivity associated with mania.

Allows the accumulation of neurotransmitters, norepinephrine and serotonin, potentiating their antidepressant effect.

The exact mechanism of action is not known; however, it is thought to alter chemical transmitters in the CNS, reducing manic behavior.

May be indicated to alter mood until neuroleptics or antidepressants become effective.

Having a concrete plan for seeking assistance during a crisis may discourage or prevent self-destructive behaviors.

NURSING DIAGNOSIS:	SOCIAL ISOLATION
MAY BE RELATED TO:	Developmental regression
	Depressed mood
	Feelings of worthlessness
	Egocentric behaviors (which offend others and discourage relationships)

MAY BE RELATED TO—*continued*	**Delusional thinking**
	Fear of failure
	Impaired cognition fostering negative view of self
	Unresolved grief
POSSIBLY EVIDENCED BY:	**Sad, dull affect**
	Absence of supportive significant other(s): family, friends, group
	Uncommunicative/withdrawn behavior; absence of eye contact
	Preoccupation with own thoughts; repetitive, meaningless actions
	Seeking to be alone
	Assuming fetal position
CLIENT OUTCOMES/EVALUATION CRITERIA:	**Verbalizes willingness to be with others. Spends time voluntarily with others, seeks out group activities. Develops 1:1 trust-based relationship.**

INTERVENTIONS	RATIONALE
Independent	
Spend time with client. (This may mean sitting in silence for a while.)	Nurse's presence helps improve client's perception of self as a worthwhile person.
Develop a therapeutic nurse/client relationship through frequent, brief contacts and an accepting attitude. Show unconditional positive regard.	The nurse's presence, acceptance, and conveyance of positive regard enhance the client's feeling of self-worth and facilitates trust and interaction with others.
Encourage attendance in group activities, after client feels comfortable in the 1:1 relationship. May need to attend with client the first few times to offer support. Accept client's decision to remove self from group situation if anxiety becomes too great.	The presence of a trusted individual provides emotional security for the client. Moving slowly into more threatening activity and accepting client's decision to leave promotes self-trust and sense of control.
Provide positive reinforcement for client's voluntary interactions with others.	Positive reinforcement enhances self-esteem and encourages repetition of desirable behaviors.
Verbally acknowledge client's absence from any group activities.	Knowledge that absence was noticed may reinforce the client's feelings of self-worth.
Assist client to learn assertiveness techniques.	Knowledge of the use of assertive techniques could improve client's relationships with others.

INTERVENTIONS

Independent

Devise a plan of therapeutic activities and provide client with a written time schedule.

Help client to learn skills that may be used to approach others in a socially acceptable manner. Practice these skills through role play.

Limit group activities, when agitated. Help client to establish one or two close relationships.

RATIONALE

The depressed client needs structure because of the impairment in decision-making/problem-solving ability. A structured schedule provides security until the client is able to do so independently.

With practice, these skills become easier in real-life situations, and client feels more comfortable performing them.

Client's ability to interact with others is impaired. More security is felt in a 1:1 relationship that is consistent over time.

NURSING DIAGNOSIS:	**NUTRITION, ALTERED: LESS THAN BODY REQUIREMENTS**
MAY BE RELATED TO:	**Energy expenditure in excess of calorie intake.**
	Refusal/inability to sit still long enough to eat meals
	Lack of attention to/recognition of hunger cues
POSSIBLY EVIDENCED BY:	**Lack of interest in food**
	Weight loss
	Pale conjunctiva and mucous membranes
	Poor muscle tone/skin turgor
	Amenorrhea
	Abnormal laboratory findings, e.g., anemias, electrolyte imbalances
CLIENT OUTCOMES/EVALUATION CRITERIA:	**Identifies and formulates plan to meet individual dietary needs. Demonstrates adequate intake to maintain individual nutritional balance/provide desired weight gain. Exhibits no signs of malnutrition.**

INTERVENTIONS	RATIONALE
Independent	
Determine individual daily caloric requirement, considering body structure, height, and activity level.	Important for the provision of adequate nutrition and realistic weight gain.
Have juice and snacks available at all times.	Nutritious intake is required on a regular basis to compensate for increased caloric requirements due to hyperactivity.
Maintain accurate record of intake, output, and calorie count.	Necessary to make an accurate nutritional assessment, identify individual needs, and maintain client safety.
Weigh daily.	Helpful in evaluating therapeutic needs and effectiveness of treatment plan.
Determine client's dietary likes and dislikes.	Client is more likely to eat foods that are particularly enjoyed.
Pace or walk with client as finger foods are taken. As agitation subsides, sit with client during meals. Offer support and encouragement.	Presence of a trusted individual may provide feeling of security and decrease agitation. Encouragement and positive reinforcement increase self-esteem and foster repetition of desired behaviors.
Assist client to learn the importance of adequate nutrition and fluid intake.	Client may have inadequate or inaccurate knowledge regarding the contribution of good nutrition to overall wellness.
Collaborative	
Consult with dietician as indicated.	Helpful in establishing individual needs/program and provides educational opportunity.
Provide high-protein, high-calorie, nutritious finger foods and drinks that can be consumed "on the run."	The client may have difficulty sitting still long enough to eat a meal because of hyperactive state. The likelihood is greater that food and drinks that can be carried around and eaten with little effort will be consumed.
Administer vitamin and mineral supplements, as indicated.	To improve and/or restore nutritional well-being.
Monitor laboratory values, and report significant changes.	Provides an objective assessment of nutritional status, therapeutic needs/effectiveness.

CHAPTER 7

DELUSIONAL (PARANOID) DISORDER

Delusional (Paranoid) Disorder

DSM III-R: 297.10 Specify type:
Erotomanic: Delusions that another person of higher status is in love with him or her
Grandiose: Delusions of inflated worth, power, knowledge, special identity, or special relationship to a deity or famous person
Jealous: Delusions that one's sexual partner is unfaithful
Persecutory: Delusions that one is being malevolently treated in some way
Somatic: Delusions that there is some physical disorder or abnormality of appearance

ETIOLOGIC THEORIES

PSYCHODYNAMICS

Emotional development is delayed due to a lack of maternal stimulation/attention. The infant is deprived of a sense of security and fails to establish basic trust. A fragile ego results in severely impaired self-esteem, a sense of "loss of control," fear, and severe anxiety. A suspicious attitude toward others is manifested and may continue throughout life. Projection is the most common mechanism used as a defense against feelings.

BIOLOGIC THEORIES

There appears to be a relatively strong familial pattern of involvement with these disorders. Individuals whose family members manifest symptoms of these disorders are at greater risk for development than the general population. Twin studies have also suggested genetic involvement.

FAMILY DYNAMICS

Some theorists believe that paranoid persons had parents who were distant, rigid, demanding, and perfectionistic, engendering rage, a sense of exaggerated self-importance, and mistrust in the individual. The clients become vulnerable as adults because of this early experience.

CLIENT ASSESSMENT DATA BASE

HISTORY

Onset most often occurs in middle or late adult life.

A nonbizarre delusional system of at least one month's duration is present.

Experiencing emotions and behavior appropriate to the content: fears that either client or significant others are in danger, are being followed, poisoned, infected; loved at a distance; having a disease; being deceived by one's spouse.

Exhibits controlled, cold, unemotional affect, guarded/evasive/distrustful behavior. Vigilant, looks for hidden motives, every person/event is under suspicion.

Significant impairment in social/marital functioning may be noted; usually behavior in all other areas of life appears normal.

May present with severe anxiety; inability to relax, exaggeration of difficulties, being easily agitated, and may display assaultive/violent behavior.

Expresses feelings of inadequacy, worthlessness, lack of acceptance and trust of others.

Demonstrates difficulty in coping with stress, uses maladjusted coping mechanisms, e.g., excessive use of projection and aggressive behavior, takes unnecessary precautions, and avoids accepting blame.

Perception is keen; will demonstrate impaired judgment about the perception.

Delusions of reference or control that may incorporate the "FBI, CIA," radio/TV.

Prominent auditory or visual hallucinations are not usually present.

May have history of substance abuse.

PHYSICAL EXAMINATION

Refer to CP: Schizophrenia.
Note: Paranoid symptoms can occur with physical illness and drug use.

DIAGNOSTIC STUDIES

Refer to CP: Schizophrenia.

NURSING PRIORITIES

1. Promote safe environment, safety of client/others.
2. Provide open, honest atmosphere in which client can begin to trust self and others.
3. Encourage client/family to focus on defining methods for coping with anxieties and life stressors and give up/live with delusional system.
4. Assist client to regain a sense of control.
5. Promote a sense of self-worth and increased self-esteem.

DISCHARGE CRITERIA

1. Coping with anxiety without the use of threats or assaultive behavior.
2. Reality is recognized and client agrees to give up or live with delusional system.
3. Client/family (S.O.s) are involved in therapy, e.g., behavioral, group.
4. Family/S.O.(s) are providing emotional support for the client.

NURSING DIAGNOSIS:	VIOLENCE, POTENTIAL FOR: DIRECTED AT SELF OR OTHERS
MAY BE RELATED TO:	Perceived threats of danger
	Increased feelings of anxiety
POSSIBLY EVIDENCED BY:	Acting out in an irrational manner
	Becoming threatening or assaultive in the face of perceived threat

CLIENT OUTCOMES/EVALUATION CRITERIA:	Verbalizes awareness of delusional system. Resolving conflicts, coping with anxiety without the use of threats or assaultive behavior.

INTERVENTIONS

Independent

Note prior history of violent behavior when under stress.

Assist client to identify situations that trigger anxiety and aggressive behaviors.

Explore implications and consequences of handling these situations with aggression.

Encourage to engage in solitary activity instead of group activities to begin with.

Be careful in offering a pat on the shoulder/hug, etc.

Assist client to define alternatives to aggressive behaviors. Engage in physical activities, such as ping pong, foosball. (Monitor competitive activities; use with caution.)

Encourage verbalizations of feelings and promote outlet for expression.

Be alert to signs of impending violent behavior, e.g., increase in psychomotor activity, intensity of affect, verbalization of delusional thinking, especially threatening expressions.

Accept verbal hostility without retaliation or defense. Nurse (caregiver) needs to be aware of own response to client behavior, e.g., anger/fear.

Provide safe, quiet environment; tell client s/he is "safe."

Isolate promptly in nonpunitive manner, using adequate help, if violent behavior occurs. Hold client if necessary. Tell to "STOP" behavior.

Collaborative

Administer medications, as indicated. (Refer to ND: Anxiety (severe).)

RATIONALE

Indicator of increased risk for recurrence of aggression/violent behavior.

Understanding relationship between severe anxiety and aggressive feelings can help client to identify options to avoid violent behavior.

Emphasizes importance of thinking through situations before acting.

Anxiety, fear, suspiciousness may escalate if involved in competitive/group activities.

Gestures involving touch may be misinterpreted as aggressive by the suspicious person.

Enables client to learn to handle situations in a socially acceptable manner. Appropriate outlets will allow for release of hostility. Competition can trigger violent behavior.

Ventilation of feelings reduces need for physical action.

Therapeutic interventions are more effective before behavior becomes violent.

Behavior is not usually directed at nurse personally and responding defensively will tend to exacerbate situation. Looking at meaning behind the words will be more productive. Awareness of own response allows nurse to confront/deal with those feelings.

Keeping environmental stimuli to a minimum will help reassure client and assist with prevention of agitation.

Removal to a quiet environment can help calm client. Sufficient help will prevent injury to client/staff. Usually the individual is being self-critical and afraid of hostility and does not need external criticism, and saying "stop" may be enough to allow client to regain control.

Antipsychotic/antianxiety drugs may decrease anxiety and delusional thinking, decreasing suspicious thoughts/aggressive behaviors and aiding client in maintaining control.

NURSING DIAGNOSIS:	ANXIETY (SEVERE)
MAY BE RELATED TO:	Inability to trust (has not mastered tasks of trust versus mistrust)
POSSIBLY EVIDENCED BY:	Rigid delusional system (serves to provide relief from stress that justifies the delusion) Frightened of other people and own hostility
CLIENT OUTCOMES/EVALUATION CRITERIA:	Acknowledges delusion and deals with it appropriately. Defines methods to decrease own anxiety level. Reports anxiety is reduced to a manageable level. Demonstrates a relaxed manner.

INTERVENTIONS	RATIONALE
Independent	
Develop primary nurse/client relationship.	The continuity of a primary care relationship can provide the time necessary to form an alliance with the suspicious person.
Assist client to identify sources of anxiety and concerns.	Increases awareness of problems/contributing factors. Client needs to become aware of how behavior affects others and take responsibility for it.
Explore present patterns of coping with anxiety and how effective they have been (e.g. threatening harm and/or shouting at others, believing they are "out to get me/my family").	Increases awareness that aggressive acts may have destructive outcome.
Provide education for learning effective, constructive strategies to handle fearful situations.	Client has been using maladjusted coping; needs to learn what is constructive.
Encourage implementation of new strategies, giving feedback on effectiveness.	Reinforces acceptable behaviors.
Avoid confrontation of delusion.	Logic does not work, and forcing the client to give up the delusion increases anxiety.
Observe for side effects of medications: note changes in behavior/response to environment; complaints of dry mouth, blurred vision; level of consciousness; intellectual responses/thought control. Monitor vital signs, intake/output/weight.	Adverse reactions such as extrapyramidal symptoms, tardive dyskinesia, orthostatic hypotension, decreased sensation of thirst, constipation, urinary retention, weight gain may occur; or paradoxical exacerbations of psychotic symptoms may develop and may actually heighten anxiety, suspiciousness.
Collaborative	
Institute behavioral therapy.	Hypersensitivity to the actions of others has been learned and can be unlearned. Breaking this cycle as-

INTERVENTIONS

Collaborative

Administer medications as indicated, e.g.,
    fluphenazine (Prolixin),
    haloperidol (Haldol).

RATIONALE

sists in reducing sensitivity to criticism and improving client's social skills.

Decreases anxiety and delusional thinking, which can increase ability to problem-solve. Note: decreased sensation of thirst, sensitivity to sun/photophobia are side effects of antipsychotic drugs requiring increased fluid intake and avoidance of prolonged exposure to sun.

NURSING DIAGNOSIS:	POWERLESSNESS
MAY BE RELATED TO:	**Feelings of inadequacies**
	Interpersonal interaction
	Sense of severely impaired self-esteem
	May believe has no control over situation(s)
POSSIBLY EVIDENCED BY:	**Use of paranoid delusions**
	Use of aggressive behavior to compensate
	Expressions of recognition of damage paranoia has caused self and others
CLIENT OUTCOMES/EVALUATION CRITERIA:	**States belief that outcome of situations causing concern can be significantly affected by own actions. Identifies individual actions to effect control. Demonstrates necessary behaviors/lifestyle changes to maintain control without use of aggression.**

INTERVENTIONS

Independent

Encourage client to do as much as possible for self, providing choices when possible.

Assist client to identify when feelings of "loss of control" began and events/situations that led to feeling "powerless" and aggressive acts.

RATIONALE

Permits/enables control of situation so suspicion can be reduced

Increases understanding of sources of stressful events and that aggression is an attempt to compensate for feeling powerless.

INTERVENTIONS

Independent

Review previous relationships/social contacts. If no longer involved in these relationships, have client describe what happened.

Discuss predelusional period and how events might precede panic state.

Explore alternate ways to regain control without resorting to aggression. (Refer to ND: Violence, potential for: Directed at self or others.)

Give positive feedback when client demonstrates use of constructive alternatives.

RATIONALE

Knowledge can be gained of how the client establishes relationships and why they deteriorated or remained intact, providing insight to change own behavior and enhancing future relationships.

Helps discern how much of delusion is real and how much relates to anxiety state.

Provides knowledge of constructive coping mechanisms.

Enhances self-esteem and reinforces acceptable behaviors.

NURSING DIAGNOSIS:	THOUGHT PROCESSES, ALTERATION IN
MAY BE RELATED TO:	**Psychologic conflicts**
	Increasing anxiety and fear (characteristic of the suspicious person)
POSSIBLY EVIDENCED BY:	**Difficulties in the process and character of thought**
	Interference with the ability to think clearly and logically
	Fragmentation and autistic thinking
	Delusions
CLIENT OUTCOMES/EVALUATION CRITERIA:	**Recognizes changes in thinking and behavior. Identifies the meaning of the delusion. Dealing with anxieties/ fears as evidenced by more logical/ reality-based thinking.**

INTERVENTIONS

Independent

Communicate in clear, concise terms with clearly stated rules about what client can/cannot do.

RATIONALE

The very suspicious/delusional client needs to have straight information that differentiates them from the seemingly dangerous surroundings. Knowledge of the "rules" can provide this person with a sense of control.

INTERVENTIONS

Independent

Note impulsive behaviors and request client to stop. If does not stop, evaluate basis of behavior and whether it is potentially harmful. (Refer to ND: Violence, potential for: Directed at self/others.)

Collaborative

Gradually involve in learning activities, occupational/recreational/activity therapies. (Refer to ND: Self-concept, disturbance in: Self-esteem.)

RATIONALE

These behaviors are often the result of psychotic thought/perceptual distortions and not willful actions.

As thought processes improve, task mastery opportunities can enhance self-esteem and enable the client to feel good about accomplishments.

NURSING DIAGNOSIS:	COPING, INEFFECTIVE INDIVIDUAL
MAY BE RELATED TO:	Maladjusted method of coping with stress
	Delusional system
POSSIBLY EVIDENCED BY:	Beliefs and behaviors of suspicion/violence
	Inappropriate ways of dealing with others
CLIENT OUTCOMES/EVALUATION CRITERIA:	Recognizes relationship of paranoid ideation to current situation. Verbalizes awareness of own coping abilities. Demonstrates appropriate, constructive, effective coping skills.

INTERVENTIONS

Independent

Provide outlet(s) for expression of fears/anxieties in 1:1 or group settings.

Assist in identifying/discussing thoughts, perceptions, and own conclusions of reality.

Encourage client to identify when fears/suspicions began and events that led to these feelings.

Explore how perceptions are validated prior to drawing conclusions. Discuss successes and failures of these attempts.

RATIONALE

In a trusting relationship, feelings can be freely expressed without fear of judgment.

Increases comprehension of what client sees as problems and gives insight into how information is being processed

Gaining knowledge of stressors that have precipitated deteriorations in coping ability may help prevent recurrence of these behaviors.

Validation of perceptions may prevent drawing the wrong conclusion and acting out behaviors.

INTERVENTIONS

Independent

Guide in defining methods to decrease anxiety, fears without distortion of reality or using delusional system. Encourage development of exercise programs/relaxation techniques.

RATIONALE

Increases repertoire of coping behaviors, preventing decompensation. Note: Use of guided imagery may exacerbate delusional thinking.

NURSING DIAGNOSIS:	**SELF-CONCEPT, DISTURBANCE IN: SELF-ESTEEM**
MAY BE RELATED TO:	**Underdeveloped ego**
	Lack of positive feedback
	Inability to trust
	Fixation in earlier level of development
POSSIBLY EVIDENCED BY:	**Delusional system (attempt to hurt or strike out at someone else in order to protect the self)**
	Self-destructive behavior
	Inability to accept positive reinforcement
	Not taking responsibility for self-care
	Nonparticipation in therapy
CLIENT OUTCOMES/EVALUATION CRITERIA:	**Verbalizes feelings of increased self-value/worth. Identifies self as a person capable of problem-solving and functioning in society in a manner acceptable to self and others. Demonstrates adaptation to changes by active participation in treatment program.**

INTERVENTIONS

Independent

Encourage to verbalize feelings of inadequacies, worthlessness, fear of rejection/need for acceptance by others.

RATIONALE

Must have insight into feelings in order to begin to improve self-esteem.

INTERVENTIONS

Independent

Explore how these negative feelings could lead to severe anxiety and suspiciousness.

Encourage to identify positive aspects about self related to social skills, work abilities, education, talents, and appearance.

Give positive feedback regarding abilities and how they can be used to increase self-esteem.

Engage in activities, increasing socialization and interaction with others as tolerated.

Provide clear, consistent verbal/nonverbal communication. Be truthful and honest; follow through on commitments.

RATIONALE

Increases awareness of internal factors that cause feelings of inadequacy and how these feelings lead to decompensation.

Reinforces own feelings of being a worthwhile person capable of adaptive functioning.

Provides encouragement and promotes a sense of self-direction.

Reduces social isolation, enhances feelings of self-worth and promotes social skills.

Helpful in establishing trust and reaffirming that the individual has value and worth.

NURSING DIAGNOSIS:	SOCIAL ISOLATION
MAY BE RELATED TO:	Disturbed thought processes
	Mistrust of others/delusional thinking
POSSIBLY EVIDENCED BY:	Difficulty in establishing relationships with others
	Expressions of feelings of rejection
	Isolation of self/withdrawal
	Dealing with problems with anger/hostility and violence
CLIENT OUTCOMES/EVALUATION CRITERIA:	Verbalizes willingness to be involved with others. Participates in activities/programs with others with lessened discomfort.

INTERVENTIONS

Independent

Assess degree of isolation, listening to client's comments about loneliness. Note sense of self-esteem. (Refer to ND, Self-concept, disturbance in: Self-esteem.)

Establish 1:1 relationship.

RATIONALE

Mistrust can lead to difficulty establishing relationships and client may have withdrawn from close contacts with others.

Consistent, brief, honest contact can help the client initiate and master tasks associated with learning to trust others.

213

INTERVENTIONS	RATIONALE
Independent	
Identify support systems available to the client: family, friends, co-workers, etc.	Can be an important part in the client's rehabilitation by improving socialization and diminishing sense of isolation.
Assess family relationships, communication patterns, knowledge of client condition.	Problems within the family may preclude their providing adequate support/continuing relationship and may interfere with client's progress. (Refer to ND: Coping, ineffective Family, Compromised/Family Process: altered.)
Collaborative	
Refer to family therapy as indicated.	Relationship with client and problems within the family may require professional assistance.

NURSING DIAGNOSIS:	**COPING, INEFFECTIVE, FAMILY: COMPROMISED/FAMILY PROCESS: ALTERED**
MAY BE RELATED TO:	**Temporary family disorganization/role changes**
	Inadequate or incorrect information or understanding by a primary person
	Prolonged progression of condition that exhausts the supportive capacity of significant other(s)
POSSIBLY EVIDENCED BY:	**Family system does not meet physical/emotional/spiritual needs of its members.**
	Inability to express or to accept wide range of feelings or feelings of members
	Inappropriate or poorly communicated family rules, rituals, symbols
	Inappropriate boundary maintenance
	Significant person describes preoccupation with personal reactions
	Significant person withdraws or enters into limited or temporary personal communication with client at time of need

FAMILY OUTCOMES/EVALUATION CRITERIA:	Expresses feelings freely and appropriately. Identifies/verbalizes resources within themselves to deal with the situation. Interacts appropriately with the client and provides opportunity for client to deal with situation in own way. Identifies need for outside support and uses appropriately.

INTERVENTIONS

Independent

Identify individual factors that may contribute to difficulty of family to provide needed assistance to the client.

Assess information available to and understood by family/significant other(s).

Discuss underlying reasons for client's behaviors, e.g., fear of loss of control, extreme sensitivity, use of projection and blame to avoid looking at own responsibility.

Encourage client/family to develop problem-solving skills.

Help individuals to look at own behavior in relation to the client's.

Collaborative

Refer to appropriate resources such as marital/family therapy, psychotherapy, support groups.

RATIONALE

Each member of a family system has an effect on other members, and this family may be in constant conflict with others.

Lack of understanding of illness can lead to anger responses in family members, resulting in continuing conflict.

Promotes understanding of client and provides opportunity for changing ineffective responses to positive, growth-promoting behaviors.

This client's behavior creates conflict among family members, and learning to resolve issues in an open, nonjudgmental manner lessens angry responses, allowing for resolution of the conflict.

Interaction among family members often enables the client to maintain suspicions and paranoid ideation, and when this behavior is acknowledged and dealt with, behavior can begin to change.

Since conflict is so prevalent in this family, and divorce is common, long-term assistance may be needed to maintain relationships or part amicably.

CHAPTER 8

MOOD (AFFECTIVE) DISORDERS

Bipolar Disorder

DSM III-R: 296.6x Bipolar disorder, mixed
 296.4x Bipolar disorder, manic
 296.5x Bipolar disorder, depressed (Refer to CP: Depressive Disorders)
 301.13 Cyclothymia

ETIOLOGIC THEORIES

PSYCHODYNAMICS

Psychoanalytic theory explains the cyclic behaviors of mania and depression as a response to conditional love from the primary caregiver. The child is maintained in a dependent position, and ego development is disrupted. This gives way to the development of a punitive superego (anger turned inward or depression) or a strong id (uncontrollable impulsive behavior or mania). In the psychoanalytic model, mania is viewed as the mirror image of depression—a "denial of depression."

BIOLOGIC FACTORS

There is increasing evidence to indicate that genetics plays a strong role in the predisposition to bipolar disorder. Incidence among relatives of affected individuals is higher than in the general population and highest among female relatives (occurs overall twice as frequently in women as in men). Biochemically there appear to be increased levels of the biogenic amine, norepinephrine, in the brain, which may account for the increased activity of the manic individual.

FAMILY DYNAMICS

Object loss theory suggests that depressive illness occurs if the person is separated from or abandoned by a significant other during the first six months of life. The bonding process is interrupted and the child withdraws from people and the environment. Rejection by parents in childhood or spending formative years with a family that sees life as hopeless and has a chronic expectation of failure make it difficult for the individual to be optimistic. The mother may be distant and unloving, the father a less powerful person, and the child expected to achieve high social and academic success.

CLIENT ASSESSMENT DATA BASE

HISTORY

Prevailing mood is remarkably expansive, "high," or irritable.

History of overinvolvement with other people and with activities; ambitious, unrealistic planning; acts of poor judgment regarding social consequences (uncontrolled spending, reckless driving, problematic or unusual sexual behavior)

Reports of activities that are disorganized and flamboyant or bizarre, with the individual denying their probable outcome and perceiving mood as desirable and potential as limitless

Mood is labile; irritability usually occurs when ideas are refuted or wishes denied.

Inflated self-esteem is typical, with unrealistic self-confidence.

Grandiosity may be expressed in a range from unrealistic planning and persistent offering of unsolicited advice (where no expertise exists) to grandiose delusions of a special relationship to important persons, including God, or persecution because of "specialness."

Reports disrupted sleep pattern or extended periods without sleep

May demonstrate a degree of dangerousness to self and others.

Grooming and clothing choices may be inappropriate, flamboyant, and bizarre.

PHYSICAL EXAMINATION

Mental Status: Concentration/attention are poor as client responds to multiple irrelevant stimuli in the environment, leading to rapid changes in topics (flight of ideas) in conversation and inability to complete activities. Delusions and psychotic phenomena may be noted. Poor judgment and irritability are usual.

Weight loss often occurs.

Physically hyperactive

Speech is rapid and pressured.

Inattention to ADLs is common.

DIAGNOSTIC STUDIES

Drug screen: to rule out possibility that symptoms are drug-induced

Electrolytes: Excess of sodium within the nerve cells may be noted.

Lithium level: done when client is receiving this medication to assure therapeutic range between 0.5 and 1.5 mEq/L.

NURSING PRIORITIES

1. Protect client/others from the consequences of hyperactive behavior.
2. Provide for client's basic needs.
3. Promote reality orientation and realistic problem-solving, and foster autonomy.
4. Support client/family participation in follow-up care/community treatment.

DISCHARGE CRITERIA

1. Oriented to reality with decreased occurrence of manic behavior(s)
2. Balance between activity and rest is restored.
3. Meeting basic self-care needs
4. Communicating logically and clearly
5. Client/family participating in ongoing treatment and understands importance of drug therapy/monitoring

NURSING DIAGNOSIS:	INJURY, POTENTIAL FOR, TRAUMA/ VIOLENCE, POTENTIAL FOR, DIRECTED AT OTHERS
MAY BE RELATED TO:	**Irritability and impulsive behavior**

POSSIBLE INDICATORS:	Delusional thinking Angry response when ideas are refuted or wishes denied Difficulty evaluating the consequences of own actions Overt and aggressive acts Hostile, threatening verbalizations History of assaultive behavior
CLIENT OUTCOMES/EVALUATION CRITERIA:	Demonstrates self-control with decreased hyperactivity. Verbalizes feelings (anger, etc.) in an appropriate manner. Uses problem-solving techniques instead of violent behavior/threats or intimidation. Expresses increased self-concept/esteem.

INTERVENTIONS	RATIONALE
Independent	
Decrease environmental stimuli, avoiding exposure to areas or situations of predictable high stimulation and removing stimulation from area if client becomes agitated.	Client may be unable to focus attention to only relevant stimuli and will be reacting/responding to *all* environmental stimuli.
Continually reevaluate the client's ability to tolerate frustration and/or individual situations.	Facilitates early intervention and assists client to manage situation independently, if possible.
Provide safe environment, removing objects and rearranging room to prevent accidental/purposeful injury to self or others.	Grandiose thinking, e.g., "I am superman," and hyperactive behavior can lead to destructive actions such as trying to run through the wall/into others.
Intervene when agitation *begins* to develop, with strategies such as verbally direct/prompt more effective behavior, redirect or remove from the provoking situation, voluntary "time out" in room or a quiet place, physical control, and/or use of seclusion and restraint (according to agency policy).	Intervention at earliest sign of agitation can assist client in regaining control, preventing escalation to violence and allowing treatment in least restrictive manner.
Defer problem-solving regarding prevention of violence and information collection about precipitating or provoking stimuli until agitation/irritability is diminished (e.g., no "why," analytical questions).	Questions regarding prevention increase frustration because agitation decreases ability to analyze situation.
Concretely communicate rationale for staff action.	Agitated persons are unable to process complicated communication.
Allow client to enter areas of increased stimuli gradually when client is ready to leave "time out" seclusion area.	Tolerance of environmental stimuli is reduced, and gradual reentry fosters coping ability.

INTERVENTIONS	RATIONALE

Independent

Avoid arguing when client verbalizes unrealistic or grandiose ideas or "put-downs."

Prevents triggering agitation in predictably touchy areas.

Ignore/minimize attention given to undesired behaviors, (e.g., bizarre dress, use of profanity), while setting limits on destructive actions.

Avoids giving reinforcement to these behaviors, while providing control for potentially dangerous activities.

Avoid unnecessary delay of gratification. Give concrete and nonjudgmental rationale if refusal is necessary.

In hyperactive state, client does not tolerate waiting or deal well with abstractions, and unnecessary delay can trigger aggressive behavior.

Offer alternatives when available ("I don't have any coffee; would you like a glass of juice?")

Uses client's distractibility to help decrease the frustration of being refused.

Provide information regarding more independent and alternative problem-solving strategies when client is not labile or irritable.

Improves retention, as agitated person will not be able to recall or use strategies discussed.

Encourage client, during calm moments, to recognize antecedents/precipitants to agitation.

Promotes early recognition of developing problem, allowing client to plan for alternative responses and intervene in a timely fashion.

Assist client in identifying alternative behaviors that are acceptable to both client and staff. Role play, if indicated. Intervene as necessary to protect client when behavior is provocative or offensive. (Refer to ND: Social Interactions, impaired.)

Client will be more apt to follow through on alternatives if they are mutually acceptable. Practice in a nonagitated time helps client learn new behavior. May become physically violent with others, when behavior is not socially acceptable.

Provide reinforcement/positive feedback when client attempts to handle frustrating incidents without violence.

Reinforcement/appreciation increases feeling of success and the likelihood of client trying that behavior again.

Collaborative

Analyze any violent incidents with involved staff/observers, identifying antecedents or provoking situations, client indicators of increasing agitation, client response(s) to interventions attempted, etc.

Information is used to develop individualized and proactive interventions based on experience.

Administer medications, as indicated
  Antimanic drugs, e.g., lithium carbonate (Eskalith);

Lithium is the drug of choice for mania. It is indicated for alleviation of hyperactive symptoms.

  Antipsychotic drugs, e.g., chlorpromazine (Thorazine), haloperidol (Haldol).

Useful in decreasing the level of hyperactivity and ameliorating accompanying thought disorder, if present.

NURSING DIAGNOSIS:	**NUTRITION, ALTERED: LESS THAN BODY REQUIREMENTS**
MAY BE RELATED TO:	**Inadequate intake in relation to metabolic expenditures**
POSSIBLY EVIDENCED BY:	**Body weight 20% or more below ideal weight**

	Observed inadequate intake
	Inattention to mealtimes
	Distraction from task of eating
CLIENT OUTCOMES/EVALUATION CRITERIA:	Verbalizes importance of adequate intake. Displays increased attention to eating behaviors. Demonstrates weight gain toward goal.

INTERVENTIONS	RATIONALE
Independent	
Assess nutritional and fluid intake on an ongoing basis, as indicated.	Establishes data base and monitors progress toward goal.
Weigh routinely.	Provides information about therapeutic needs/effectiveness.
Offer meals in area with minimal distracting stimuli.	Promotes focus on task of eating and prevents distractions from interfering with food intake.
Provide opportunity to select foods when client is ready to deal with choices.	If alternatives do not add confusion, can provide favored foods, sense of control.
Collaborative	
Offer high protein/carbohydrate diet. Provide interval feedings, using finger foods.	Maximizes nutritional intake and allows additional opportunity to "boost" dietary intake as client may eat foods that are easily picked up and/or carried around.

NURSING DIAGNOSIS:	**SLEEP PATTERN DISTURBANCE**
MAY BE RELATED TO:	Lack of recognition of fatigue/need to sleep
	Hyperactivity
POSSIBLY EVIDENCED BY:	Interrupted nighttime sleep
	One or more nights without sleep
	Changes in behavior and performance
	Increasing irritability/restlessness
	Dark circles under eyes

INTERVENTIONS	RATIONALE

Independent

Decrease environmental stimuli in room and from common areas; may need private room, seclusion.

Manic client is unable to relax and decrease attention to stimuli, affecting ability to fall asleep.

Restrict intake of caffeine, e.g., coffee, tea, cocoa, cola drinks.

May stimulate CNS, interferring with relaxation, ability to sleep.

Matter-of-factly reroute to bed without providing the distraction of other activities.

Avoids providing distracting stimuli or provoking irritability.

Offer small snack/warm milk at bedtime or when awake during the night.

Inattention to personal needs may have led to a less than adequate intake and hunger at night may distract from sleep.

Encourage engaging in physical activities/exercise during morning/afternoon. Restrict activity in the evening prior to bedtime.

Enhances sense of fatigue and promotes sleep/rest. Evening activity may actually stimulate client and interfere with/delay sleep.

Collaborative

Administer medications as indicated, e.g.,
    Sedatives;

Careful use may assist in reestablishing sleep pattern.

    Antipsychotics.

Produces a calming effect, reducing hyperactivity and promoting rest/sleep.

NURSING DIAGNOSIS:	SELF-CARE DEFICITS, GROOMING/ HYGIENE [MANAGEMENT OF PERSONAL BELONGINGS]
MAY BE RELATED TO:	Lack of concern
	Hyperactivity, impulsivity
	Poor judgment (including money and valuables)
POSSIBLY EVIDENCED BY:	Unkempt appearance, dirty, wearing inadequate and/or inappropriate clothing
	Giving away clothing, money, etc., spending or "charging" extravagantly
CLIENT OUTCOMES/EVALUATION CRITERIA:	Performs self-care activities within level of own ability. Uses resources/

assistance as needed. Takes responsibility for/manages personal belongings.

INTERVENTIONS	RATIONALE
Independent	
Assess current level of functioning; reevaluate daily.	Provides information about individual progress/deterioration necessary for planning/altering care.
Provide physical assistance, supervision and directions, reminders, encouragement, and support, as needed.	Providing only required assistance fosters autonomous functioning.
Acquire needed supplies, including clothing, if not immediately available. Obtain client's own toiletries/clothing as soon as possible.	May not have own, if disorganized prior to hospitalization or hospitalized as an emergency measure. Having own supplies/clothing supports autonomy, self-esteem.
Limit the selection of clothing available, as indicated.	May be necessary during time of extreme hyperactivity and distractibility until client is able to refrain from bizarre dress and/or care for personal belongings.
Monitor ability to manage money and valuables as well as other personal effects.	May give possessions away, spend money extravagantly, or become involved in grandiose plans, necessitating intervention.
Intervene to protect client from own impulsivity and from exploitation, if indicated, decreasing restrictions as soon as possible.	Provides protection from deleterious consequences of impulsivity without compromising or undue restriction of civil/personal liberties or autonomous functioning.
Set goals to establish minimum standards for self-care as condition improves, e.g., take a bath every other day, brush teeth twice a day.	Promotes idea that client can begin to assume responsibility for self, enhances sense of self-worth.

NURSING DIAGNOSIS:	**SENSORY-PERCEPTUAL ALTERATION: (SPECIFY)/[OVERLOAD]**
MAY BE RELATED TO:	**Decrease in sensory threshhold**
	Chemical alteration, endogenous
	Psychologic stress (narrowed perceptual fields caused by anxiety)
	Sleep deprivation
POSSIBLY EVIDENCED BY:	**Increased distractibility and agitation (in areas/times of increased environmental stimuli)**
	Anxiety

POSSIBLY EVIDENCED BY—*continued*	Disorientation; poor concentration
	Bizarre thinking
	Motor incoordination
CLIENT OUTCOMES/EVALUATION CRITERIA:	**Verbalizes awareness/causes of sensory overload. Demonstrates behaviors to reduce/manage sensory input, e.g., sits quietly, attends to simple tasks, and completes them. Initiates and/or takes "time out" in quieter area when prompted. Attends and is appropriately involved in activities (e.g., ward meeting, groups).**

INTERVENTIONS	RATIONALE

Independent

Orient to reality, e.g., identify primary caregiver, where room is. Keep communications simple.	May be disoriented/confused as a result of many distractions.
Assist client in focusing on input or task, e.g., address by name; use short, one-stage directions; provide a low-stimulus area for meals, tasks, interview.	Decreases distractions/choices that are available, helping to gain client's attention in presence of multiple distractions.
Avoid looking at watch, taking notes, talking to others when focusing on client.	Causes distracting stimuli, adding to stimulation, which can increase hyperactivity.
Remove to area of lower environmental stimulus level if client shows increasing agitation or distractibility.	Reduces distractions, thereby reducing stimulation and diminishing hyperactive behavior.
Explain upcoming events, necessary treatments in advance, giving reasons and using simple terms.	Stimuli may be less overwhelming when client is prepared.
Limit invasion of personal space, e.g., touching clothing, items in room. Use physical touch judiciously.	Reduces stimuli, shows respect for client, who may view touch as threatening.
Observe/monitor for indicators of improved tolerance for multiple sensory stimuli, and increase exposure to ward environment, people, activities accordingly.	Allows greatest possible participation in treatment milieu, personal freedom.

NURSING DIAGNOSIS:	**SOCIAL INTERACTIONS, IMPAIRED**
MAY BE RELATED TO:	**Poor judgment**
	Impulsivity
POSSIBLY EVIDENCED BY:	**Inappropriate behavior, e.g., interrupts, is intrusive, demanding, hypercritical and verbally caustic/hostile, provocative and/or teasing, does not respect others' personal space**

	Inappropriate and/or flamboyant social behavior with bizarre dress
	Problematic sexual behavior
CLIENT OUTCOMES/EVALUATION CRITERIA:	Listens/converses without consistent interruptions. Participates appropriately or constructively in 1:1, group, OT. Demonstrates social behavior and dress consistent with social norms of the client's peer group. Respects the privacy and personal property of others.

INTERVENTIONS	RATIONALE
Independent	
Redirect or suggest more appropriate behavior using low-key, matter-of-fact, nonjudgmental style.	Avoids triggering agitated/angry response.
Ask client to wait until a specified time and give rationale if gratification of a request is not possible.	When the client believes staff responses have reasons, refusals will provoke less agitation.
Maintain a nondefensive response to criticisms or suggestions regarding better ways to run things such as the ward. Use suggestions when appropriate.	A low-key response can reduce the volatility of the situation. (This may be frustrating when the client is either outrageous or partly correct.)
Act, as needed, to protect the client from harmful responses when behavior is provocative or offensive.	When the client is not taking this responsibility, the nurse needs to/is responsible to protect the client's safety.
Offer feedback (positive as well as negative) regarding the impact of social behavior, in 1:1, OT, group therapy.	The manic client is "outward oriented" and responsive to reinforcement.
Problem-solve with client (when able) regarding more effective ways to achieve goals.	When lability and poor concentration have improved, client will be able to focus and to control behavior enough to learn/"try out" new behaviors.

NURSING DIAGNOSIS:	SELF-CONCEPT, DISTURBANCE IN: SELF-ESTEEM
MAY BE RELATED TO:	Lack of positive feedback
	Unmet dependency needs
	Retarded ego development
POSSIBLY EVIDENCED BY:	Demonstration of exaggerated expectations or sense of own abilities

225

POSSIBLY EVIDENCED BY—*continued*	Unsatisfactory interpersonal relationships
	Imperious, demanding behavior
	Criticism of others
CLIENT OUTCOMES/EVALUATION CRITERIA:	Verbalizes appropriate/realistic evaluation of own abilities. Identifies feelings and methods for coping with negative perception of self. Formulates realistic plans for recovery.

INTERVENTIONS	RATIONALE

Independent

Avoid approaches that infer a different perception of the client's importance, use last name and appropriate title, ask how client would like to be addressed. Explain rationale for requests by staff, ward routine, etc. Maintain a nondefensive stance; strictly adhere to respectful/courteous approaches, matter-of-fact style, passive, friendly attitude.	Grandiosity is thought actually to reflect low self-esteem. Nursing approaches should reinforce patient dignity, worth.
Provide choices of activities, e.g., when to bathe, food desired, participation in social interactions, when possible.	This strategy reduces the client's sense of powerlessness.
Assist client, as reasonable, to maintain personal privacy.	Provides sense of appreciation for the client's dignity.
Offer matter-of-fact feedback regarding unrealistic plans, self-evaluation; utilize 1:1, group, OT, etc.	Provides an opportunity to cast doubt on unrealistic self-evaluation in the context of accepting relationships.
Identify and reinforce successes and gains made in 1:1, group, and OT settings.	Addressing issues of self-esteem allows the client to be positively reinforced for realistic successes.

NURSING DIAGNOSIS:	POWERLESSNESS
MAY BE RELATED TO:	Perceived lack of control in some aspect of life
	Experience of real or perceived failures
	Lifestyle of helplessness
	Feelings of hopelessness regarding chronicity of disease process
POSSIBLY EVIDENCED BY:	Verbalization of an inability to exert control over situation

	Denial of relationship between personal self-care behaviors and course of disease Nonparticipation in care
CLIENT OUTCOMES/EVALUATION CRITERIA:	Verbalizes sense of increased personal control. Describes strategies for minimizing future impact of and personal actions which can contribute to control of illness. Identifies symptoms of impending recurrence and plan of action.

INTERVENTIONS	RATIONALE
Independent	
Encourage verbalization and identification of feelings related to issues of chronicity, lack of control, etc.	Problem-solving begins with agreeing on "the problem."
Frame/reframe identified issues in terms of powerlessness and personal control, e.g., "You have control over what you do."	This framework allows the client the most personal power.
Frame adherence to medication and follow-up treatment, attention to lifestyle as ways of assuming personal control.	Linking follow-up treatment to the client's goals for self-control may enhance continued participation in care.
Draw parallel to other kinds of chronic illness, e.g., diabetes, epilepsy.	Supports the need for ongoing care and normalcy of lifelong medication.
Encourage client to identify aspects where control is possible in the hospital and encourage appropriate assertion of personal control/autonomy.	Allows client to "practice," provides experience of assuming control.
Encourage client to view life after discharge and identify aspects over which control is possible. Identify how the client will demonstrate that control.	Role rehearsal is helpful in returning client to level of independent functioning.
Frame relationship with health care provider after discharge as one of collaboration. Emphasize choices, decisions, personal control that will be possible.	Enhances the client's self-perception and sense of control in relation to "experts."
Assist client to identify a plan that will prevent/minimize severe recurrence of illness. Encourage identification of signs of recurrence and concrete response to symptoms, e.g., "If I go two nights without sleep, I will call my doctor."	Establishes some concrete guidelines and a plan that will allow community-based care providers to intervene, perhaps preventing an acute episode.

NURSING DIAGNOSIS:	INJURY, POTENTIAL FOR, POISONING [LITHIUM TOXICITY]
MAY BE RELATED TO:	Narrow therapeutic range of drug

227

MAY BE RELATED TO—*continued*	Client's ability (or lack of) to follow through with medication regimen
	Denial of need for information
CLIENT OUTCOMES/EVALUATION CRITERIA:	Recognizes the symptoms of lithium toxicity and appropriate actions to take. Identifies factors that can cause lithium level to change and ways of avoiding this.

INTERVENTIONS

RATIONALE

Independent

INTERVENTIONS	RATIONALE
Observe for/review signs of impending drug toxicity, e.g., blurred vision, ataxia, tinnitus, persistent nausea/vomiting, and severe diarrhea.	As there is a very narrow margin between therapeutic and toxic levels, toxicity can occur quickly and requires immediate intervention.
Assess current understanding, perceptions about medications. Evaluate ability to self-administer medication correctly.	Identifies misinformation/misconceptions about drug therapy and establishes learning needs.
Provide information regarding lithium with a structured format and informational handout.	Structured client education is more effective. Handout provides a memory prompt.
Stress importance of adequate sodium and fluid in diet.	Sodium and fluid are required for appropriate lithium metabolism and excretion, which is necessary to the prevention of toxicity.
Encourage involvement of family in regimen/monitoring.	Enhances understanding of reason for/importance of drug therapy.
Provide opportunity for client to demonstrate learning after initial class and at least once again before discharge. Clarify misconceptions, confusion about drug use/follow-up care.	Determines success of client education and helps to plan appropriate follow-up.
Document information that has been given and how client/family demonstrates learning.	Provides continuity, communicates to other providers the level of client's/family's knowledge.

Collaborative

Monitor serum lithium levels at least twice a week upon initiation of drug therapy until serum levels are stable, then weekly to bimonthly, as indicated.	Narrow therapeutic range increases risk of developing toxicity. Early detection and prompt intervention may prevent serious complications.
Provide a schedule for regular laboratory testing and follow-up appointments at discharge.	Assists client to stay on medication and maintain improved state.

NURSING DIAGNOSIS:	FAMILY PROCESSES, ALTERED
MAY BE RELATED TO:	Situational crises, illness, economic, change in roles
	Euphoric mood and grandiose ideas/actions

	Manipulative behavior and limit-testing
	Client's refusal to accept responsibility for own actions
POSSIBLY EVIDENCED BY:	Statements of difficulty coping with situation
	Lack of adaptation to change or not dealing constructively with illness
	Ineffective family decision-making process
	Failure to send and to receive clear messages
	Inappropriate boundary maintenance
FAMILY OUTCOMES/EVALUATION CRITERIA:	Expresses feelings freely and appropriately. Demonstrates individual involvement in problem-solving processes directed at appropriate solutions. Verbalizes understanding of illness, treatment regimen, and prognosis. Encourages and allows member who is ill to handle situation in own way, progressing toward independence.

INTERVENTIONS	RATIONALE
Independent	
Determine individual situation and feelings of individual family members, e.g., guilt, anger, powerlessness, despair, and alienation.	Living with a family member with bipolar illness engenders a multitude of feelings and problems that can affect interpersonal relationships/functioning and may result in dysfunctional responses/family disintegration.
Assess patterns of communication, e.g., are feelings expressed freely? Who makes decisions? What is the interaction between family members?	Provides clues to degree of problem being experienced by individual family members and coping skills being used to handle crisis of illness.
Assess boundaries of family members, e.g., Do members share family identity and have little sense of individuality or do they seem emotionally distant?	Degree of symbiotic involvement/distancing of family members affects ability to resolve problems related to behavior of identified patient.
Determine patterns of behavior displayed by client in relationships with others, e.g., manipulation of self-esteem of others, perceptiveness to vulnerability and conflict, projection of responsibility, progressive limit-testing, and alienation of family members.	These behaviors are typically used by the manic individual to manipulate others. These clients are sensitive to others' vulnerability and can intentionally escalate conflict, shifting responsibility from self to others and putting the other person on the defensive. Family

229

INTERVENTIONS	RATIONALE
Independent	
	members assume blame and continually try to keep peace at any cost. The client will test limits, constantly getting concessions from others and creating feelings of guilt and ambivalence. The result of these behaviors is alienation, and high rates of divorce occur.
Assess role of client in family, e.g., nurturer, provider, and how illness affects the roles of other members.	When the role of the ill person is not filled, dissonance and family disintegration can occur. The spouse and children of the manic individual may not understand what is happening and react in an adversarial manner, escalating the conflicts that exist.
Acknowledge difficulties observed while reinforcing that some degree of conflict is to be expected and can be used to promote growth.	Provides support for family members who may feel helpless to change the client and/or what is happening in their lives.
Provide information about behavior patterns and expected course of the illness. Encourage discussion of the acute episode with the client.	Assists families to understand normal aspects of bipolar illness. This knowledge may relieve guilt and promote family discussion of the problems and solutions. Family members tend to hide the illness of the client and excuse the manic's behavior with a variety of rationalizations.
Encourage the family members to confront the client's behavior.	May be afraid to discuss the behavior because of the client's volatile temper. Confrontation can promote insight into the dynamics of the illness and bring about a positive resolution of the family situation.
Encourage use of stress management techniques, e.g., appropriate expression of feelings, use of relaxation exercises, imagery.	Assists individuals to develop coping skills to deal with the client and difficult situation.
Collaborative	
Involve client and family members with support groups, clergy, psychologic counseling/family therapy.	Use of these support systems can assist individuals to cope with illness, which creates problems of relationships and daily living.

Depressive Disorders

DSM III-R: 293.2x Major depression, single episode
293.3x Major depression, recurrent
300.40 Dysthymia

These clients present with a disturbance of mood, characterized by a full or partial depressive syndrome. The focus is on issues of chronicity, preventive self-care, continuity of care, and symptoms of recurrence.

ETIOLOGIC THEORIES

PSYCHODYNAMICS

Psychoanalytic theory focuses on an early unsatisfactory parent/child relationship, with an unresolved grieving process. This results in the individual remaining fixed in the anger stage of the grieving process and turning it inward on the self. The ego remains weak, while the superego expands and becomes punitive.

Cognitive theory projects a belief that depression occurs as a result of impaired cognition, fostering a negative evaluation of self through disturbed thought processes. The individual views self as inadequate and worthless and life as pessimistic and hopeless.

Learning theorists propose that depressive illness arises out of the individual's having experienced numerous failures (either real or perceived). A feeling of inability to succeed at any endeavor ensues. This "learned helplessness" is viewed as a predisposition to depressive illness.

The behavioral model states that the cause of depression is believed to be in the person-behavior-environment interaction. Although people are seen as capable of exercising control over their behavior, they are not totally free of environmental influence.

BIOLOGIC THEORIES

There may be a family history of major affective disorders, and recently the disease has been found to have a genetic marker as shown by numerous studies that support the involvement of heredity in depressive illness.

Biochemical factors, e.g., electrolyte imbalances, appear to play a role in depressive illness. An error in metabolism results in the transposition of sodium and potassium within the neuron. Another theory implicates the biogenic amines norepinephrine, dopamine, and serotonin. The levels of these chemicals are deficient in individuals with this illness. Controversy remains as to whether these changes cause the illness or if the biochemical changes occur because of the depression.

FAMILY DYNAMICS

Object loss theory suggests that depressive illness occurs if the person is separated from or abandoned by a significant other during the first six months of life. The bonding process is interrupted, and the child withdraws from people and the environment.

CLIENT ASSESSMENT DATA BASE

HISTORY

Dejected or sad mood with loss of interest/enjoyment in usual activities

Expressed sadness, hopelessness, not caring about anything, not seeing any future for self. Sighing and tearfulness are common.

May experience irritability, fatigue, malaise, headache

Decreased appetite may be accompanied by weight loss, but occasionally the reverse may occur. Constipation may be present.

Sleep disturbances, e.g., insomnia, occurs in 90 percent of cases, either anxiety insomnia (when falling asleep is difficult) or depressive insomnia (where early morning awakening occurs, accompanied by painful ruminations). Some individuals may experience hypersomnia.

May report feeling best early in the morning, then continually feels worse as the day progresses in less severe levels of depression (dysthymia). In severe depression, the opposite may be true.

Disinterest in sexual activities and/or impotence may occur.

Feelings of worthlessness may be evidenced in self-derogatory statements, expressions of guilt, or exaggeration of minor inadequacies but may assume delusional proportions with presentations of unrealistic evidence of self-worth, e.g., feeling oneself responsible for major tragedies and catastrophes or persecuted for a failure.

May have difficulty starting activities, withdraw, be housebound, or remain in a single room or in bed

May have experienced an actual loss or life stressor perceived as a loss (e.g. retirement, job loss, divorce, illness, aging, etc.). May or may not see a connection between these occurrences and the onset of the depression.

Psychotic features with prominent delusions and/or hallucinations may be evident in major depression.

PHYSICAL EXAMINATION

Psychomotor retardation may be noted. May present a "slow motion" picture with slowed speech and latencies (long pauses before responding), decreased amount of speech, and slowed body movements, as if it were all just too much effort.

Thinking is characterized by poor concentration and decreased memory, indecision, pessimism, self-derogation, a sense of powerlessness, and, often, ideas of suicide. Thoughts of suicide or wanting to die may be frequent and occur at variable times in the course of the illness. May range in severity from indifference about the consequences of behavior, e.g., lack of cooperation with medical treatment or dangerous driving, to wishing it were "over" or for death, to specific suicide plans and attempts.

Posture may be bent/slouched (defeated-looking)

Weight may be less than desired for body size.

DIAGNOSTIC STUDIES

(The several biochemical alterations in depression are not, by themselves, indicative of depression but, combined with clinical observation, may indicate best pharmacologic response.)

Thyroid-stimulating hormone response to thyrotropin-releasing hormone: may reflect depression.

Dexamethasone-suppression test (DST) (an indirect marker of melancholia): If postdexamethasone cortisol levels exceed 5 μg/dl, the test is considered abnormal/positive.

EEG sleep profile: shows reduced latency of rapid eye movement sleep (REM).

Other tests that may be included:

Platelet monoamine oxidase activity (MAO): increased

Biogenic amines (especially norepinephrine and serotonin levels): decreased (Clients with low serotonin levels are 10 times more likely to commit suicide within a year)

Urinary 3-methoxy-4-hydroxyphenylglycol (MHPG): low levels indicate decreased norepinephrine output

Cerebrospinal fluid level of 5-hydroxytryptamine (5HIAA): reduced

NURSING PRIORITIES

1. Promote physical safety with special focus on suicide prevention.
2. Provide for client's basic needs, promoting highest possible level of independent functioning.
3. Provide experience/interactions that enhance self-esteem, sense of personal power.
4. Support client/family participation in follow-up care/community treatment.

DISCHARGE CRITERIA

1. Absence of suicidal ideation/risk
2. Physiologic stability with balance between rest and activity is maintained.
3. Expressing feelings appropriately with some optimism and hope for the future
4. Self-esteem/dignity is enhanced.
5. Resumes independent activity/responsibility for self
6. Client/family participating in follow-up care/community treatment

NURSING DIAGNOSIS:	VIOLENCE, POTENTIAL FOR: SELF-DIRECTED
MAY BE RELATED TO:	Depressed mood
POSSIBLE INDICATORS:	Feelings of worthlessness and hopelessness Verbalization of suicidal ideation/plan or futility of trying ("what's the use?") Giving possessions away/making a will Sudden mood elevation/appears more energized, or displays calmer, more peaceful manner Refusal/reluctance to sign a "no harm" contract
CLIENT OUTCOMES/EVALUATION CRITERIA:	Voluntarily complies with suicide precautions. Signs "no harm" contract. Verbalizes a decrease/absence of suicidal ideas. States two reasons for not harming self.

INTERVENTIONS	RATIONALE
Independent	
Identify degree of risk/potential for suicide. Assess seriousness of suicidal tendency, noting behaviors, e.g., gestures, threats, giving away possessions, previous attempts, presence of hallucinations or delusions. (Use scale of 1–10 and prioritize according to severity of threat, availability of means.)	The degree of hopelessness expressed by the client is an important indicator of the severity of the depression and suicide risk. Eight of 10 clients who state an intention to commit suicide, do. The more thought-out the plan, the higher the chances of completing it. The chances of suicide increase if there was a previous attempt or if a family history of suicide and depression is present. Impulsive clients are more likely to attempt suicide without giving clues, including those with psychotic thinking who are especially at risk when hallucinations or delusions encourage self-harm.
Reevaluate potential for suicide periodically at key times (e.g., mood changes, increasing withdrawal, as well as when discharge planning becomes active, before sending out on pass, before discharge).	Suicide risk is the greatest during the first month of admission. Over half of suicides by hospitalized patients occur out of the hospital, on leave or unauthorized absence. (The highest risk is when the client has both suicidal ideation and sufficient energy with which to act, e.g., at the point when the client begins to feel better.)

233

INTERVENTIONS	RATIONALE

Independent

Implement suicide precautions, such as:
Explain to client that you are concerned for client safety and that you will be helping client to stay "safe."

Communicates caring and provides sense of protection.

Provide close observation (1:1 or 15-minute checks for most acute risk). Place in room close to nurse's station; do not assign to a single room. Accompany to off-ward activities if attendance is indicated.

Being alert for suicidal and escape attempts facilitates being able to prevent or interrupt harmful behavior.

Be alert to use of hazardous equipment; remove hazardous personal items (e.g., scarves, belts, razor blades, scissors).

Provides environmental safety; removes objects that may prompt suicidal thoughts/attempts.

Check all items brought in to or by the client as indicated. Ask family, visitors to avoid bringing hazardous items.

Suicidal clients may bring harmful items back from pass or may ask family for items with a plan in mind.

Maintain special care in administration of medications.

Prevents saving up to overdose or discarding and not taking.

Be alert when client is using bathroom.

While decreasing the client's privacy may seem awkward, it is essential that the suicidal client be within easy reach at all times to prevent self-harm, e.g., hanging.

Make rounds at frequent, irregular intervals (especially at night, toward early morning, at change of shift or other predictably busy times for staff).

Prevents staff surveillance from becoming predictable. To be aware of client's location is important, especially when staff is busy and least available/observant.

Routinely check environment for hazards. Provide for environmental safety, e.g., relating to construction areas, lock doors/windows when not supervised, block access to stairways/roof, monitor cleaning chemicals/ repair supplies.

Minimizing opportunities for self-harm is an ongoing issue requiring constant attention and consideration of the unusual.

Create a contract with client on what client and nurse will do to provide for client's safety. Place a copy of the "contract," signed by client and staff, in the chart and give a copy to the client to keep.

Documents actions taken to prevent suicide and client response. Also promotes communication and can be helpful to the client to realize others care what happens.

Review medical regimen, including ECT, allowing client/family to ask questions and express feelings freely.

Antidepressant drugs may take three or more weeks to lift mood. In the meantime, other forms of therapy may be required to provide protection for suicidal client. ECT is generally a second line of treatment, used if depression has not responded to pharmacologic treatment and/or client continues to display suicidal ideation, sleeplessness, refusal to eat and drink. Client may fear ECT, and nurse needs to empathize with client's fears while being supportive of ECT as a positive treatment alternative.

Be aware of staff attitudes toward the use of electroconvulsive therapy and avoid influencing client negatively.

When nurses/others have negative/ambivalent feelings toward this treatment, these feelings can be communicated to the client, causing confusion/reluctance to accept appropriate therapy.

INTERVENTIONS

Collaborative

Administer drug trial of tricyclic antidepressants (TCA) or monoamine oxidase inhibitors (MAOI).

Assist with electroconvulsive therapy, as indicated.

RATIONALE

TCAs are generally considered safer and easier to manage and so are started first. If response is not noted in four to six weeks, an MAOI may be the drug of choice.

ECT becomes essential and in some cases life-saving when depression does not respond to other treatments and suicide is a major risk. (Eighty to 90 percent of clients with major depression show marked improvement after ECT.)

NURSING DIAGNOSIS:	INJURY, POTENTIAL FOR [EFFECTS OF THERAPY]
MAY BE RELATED TO:	Electroconvulsive effects on the cardiovascular, respiratory, musculoskeletal, and nervous systems
	Pharmacologic effects of anesthesia
CLIENT OUTCOMES/EVALUATION CRITERIA:	Maintains physiologic stability, free of injury/complications

INTERVENTIONS

Independent

Review medical testing, e.g., CBC, electrocardiograph, chest x-ray, urinalysis, and x-rays of lateral aspects of the spine.

Discuss what will be done, e.g., anesthesia, muscle relaxants, oxygenation, drugs used, who will be with the client, and how the client is likely to feel after ECT.

Have client empty bladder, remove jewelry and hair decorations before treatment.

Orient client upon awakening after the treatment, and support client until immediate confusion clears.

Monitor vital signs q 15 minutes until stable.

Have emergency equipment, suction, ambu bag, etc., available.

RATIONALE

A complete medical workup can identify preexisting problems and the potential for problems, which should be reported to personnel involved with procedure.

Knowledge can reduce anxiety and decrease fear response and is necessary for informed consent to procedure. Client will feel more secure knowing nurse will be there upon awakening.

Reduces risk of injury from external objects.

Short-term memory may be affected and client awakens confused. May be frightened by amnesia. Confusion increases with each treatment and knowledge that aftereffects disappear will be reassuring.

Premedication, muscle relaxants, and anesthesia may produce dysrhythmias and respiratory depression, which need immediate intervention.

Prompt treatment of respiratory depression/airway obstruction can prevent/correct life-threatening complications.

INTERVENTIONS	RATIONALE
Collaborative	
Administer supplemental oxygen as necessary.	Provides for optimum oxygenation during period of reduced ventilation.

NURSING DIAGNOSIS:	**COPING, INEFFECTIVE INDIVIDUAL**
MAY BE RELATED TO:	**Personal vulnerability**
	Inadequate support systems
	Unrealistic perceptions
	Multiple life changes
	Inadequate coping method
	Unmet expectations
	Actual/perceived loss
	Loss of physiopsychosocial well-being, e.g., poor nutrition, little or no exercise
POSSIBLY EVIDENCED BY:	**Perception of events and stressors in a manner that precipitates depressive episode**
	Perception of areas in life as unfulfilled or as losses
	Denial of loss
	Verbalization of inability to cope or ask for help
	Expression of guilt
	Crying/labile affect
	Chronic anxiety/depression
	Difficulty meeting basic needs/problem-solving

CLIENT OUTCOMES/EVALUATION CRITERIA:	Verbalizes understanding of relationship between feelings and antecedent events. Identifies coping patterns previously used and alternative strategies to cope with this/other situations.

INTERVENTIONS

Independent

Encourage verbalization of and assist in identification of feelings and relationship between feelings and event/stressor, when the event is known.

Assist client to identify need to address problem differently. Describe all aspects of the problem through the use of therapeutic communication skills.

Use crisis or social skills model to teach and appropriately reinforce more effective problem-solving/coping strategies.

Encourage anticipatory problem-solving, identifying potential future trouble areas, and coping strategies to implement. Have client write down coping strategies so they are available for immediate recall.

Assess losses that have occurred in the client's life. Discuss meaning these have had for the client.

Identify cultural factors and ways individual has dealt with previous loss(es).

Encourage to use appropriate expressions of anger and promote discussion of ways to identify and cope with underlying feelings, e.g., hurt, rejection.

Assist the client to recognize early symptoms of depression and plan ways to alleviate them. Help client to formulate steps to take for outside support if symptoms continue. Reinforce the positive aspects of being able to reach out for help.

Collaborative

Involve in activities, e.g., occupational/recreational therapy (including brisk walks, volleyball, punching bag), outdoor education program.

RATIONALE

Talking about and labeling the feelings helps client begin to deal with them more effectively. Assists client in realizing response (feeling) is connected to the stressor or precipitating event.

Contracting for change begins with agreeing on "the problem." Helps the client to consider all aspects of the problem in order to clearly define what the client is dealing with.

Begins to increase the client's repertoire of coping strategies. Learning that choices are available for behaving differently can often decrease the feeling of being stuck. "Storytelling" of how others have handled situations may be helpful, not only in providing potential solutions, but also in giving the idea that the problem is manageable.

Involves the client actively, and rehearsal promotes generalization of recently learned coping strategies to new situations. May help to minimize recurrence of depressive feelings.

Denial of the impact/importance of a loss may be contributing to severity of depression.

Cultural beliefs affect how people express and accept grieving processes.

Verbalization of feelings in a nonthreatening environment can help client begin to deal with unrecognized/unresolved issues that may be contributing to depression.

Helps the client to learn how to manage/take care of self. It is important that the client has support available, should help be needed, and experiences needing to reach out as positive, reflecting own self-worth.

Participation in individually prescribed activities and large motor exercises provide safe, effective methods for discharging pent-up tensions, learning to trust self, and enhancing self-esteem.

237

NURSING DIAGNOSIS:	ANXIETY, SPECIFY LEVEL/THOUGHT PROCESSES: ALTERED
MAY BE RELATED TO:	Negative perception of self
	Feelings of guilt
	Statements of self-deprecation
	Psychologic conflicts
	Impaired judgment
POSSIBLY EVIDENCED BY:	Complaints of nervousness or fearfulness
	Agitation
	Restlessness, hand-rubbing or wringing
	Tremulousness
	Angry or tearful outbursts
	Rambling and discoordinated speech
	Circumstantiality (unable to get to the point)
	Poor memory and concentration
	Numerous, repetitious physical complaints without organic cause
	Ideas of reference, hallucinations/delusions
	Decreased ability to grasp ideas
	Inability to follow
	Impaired ability to make decisions
CLIENT OUTCOMES/EVALUATION CRITERIA:	Verbalizes awareness of feelings of anxiety. Reports anxiety is reduced to manageable level. Attends to and

completes tasks (ADL, occupational therapy projects, etc.) of increasing length and difficulty. Converses appropriately with staff or in groups. Acknowledges changes in thinking/behavior. Identifies ways to deal effectively with decision-making.

INTERVENTIONS	RATIONALE
Independent	
Evaluate/reevaluate level of anxiety.	Approaches are different dependent upon level of anxiety. (Refer to CP: Generalized Anxiety Disorder.)
Moderate to Severe Anxiety	
Recognize and deal with own feelings in response to client's anxiety.	Anxiety is highly communicable. If the nurse becomes anxious (or impatient, irritable, etc.), this will be communicated and feed client's anxiety.
Listen nonjudgmentally to client's expressions; convey empathy; acknowledge or label feelings for client.	Helps client identify basis for anxious feelings, communicates acceptance, and assists in reducing current level of anxiety.
Use short, concrete communication. Assume calmed, "in-control-of-things" manner. Let client know about safety and supportive attentions of the staff/facility.	Attention, concentration, and problem-solving are compromised by anxiety. Benign attentions/monitoring by staff may be interpreted in a paranoid manner by the client.
Decrease environmental stimulation; remove to quiet area away from other clients. Suggest activity that may be relaxing, e.g., warm bath, back rub. Involve in a quiet activity when calmer.	Reduces anxiety-provoking stimuli and distractions. Helps client refocus away from anxiety.
Maintain a calm attitude and use physical touch, if acceptable to client.	May prove helpful if anxiety stems from delusions/hallucinations; touch can restore client to reality. Caution is required with suspicious clients who may interpret touch as aggression.
Defer problem-solving, assessment of precipitating factors until anxiety is reduced.	Ability to problem-solve is compromised, and such requests may increase anxiety.
Analyze incident with client and staff to identify precipitating factors, early signs of building anxiety, previously helpful interventions.	Develops an individualized plan that will help decrease anxiety, and establish/reestablish previous coping skill. Client needs to learn how to manage own anxiety by recognizing the signs and then acting to lower the anxiety.
Decrease decision-making for client by offering only a choice between two options, for example, whether to have cereal or eggs rather than a full menu.	Decreasing options to two lessens the amount of information to process and enhances decision-making. As ability to think through incoming information increases, more options can be added.
Choose for the client when necessary, based on knowledge of the client's interest and activity level, telling client how the choice was decided.	Choosing for the client may decrease sense of inadequacy and role-model decision-making process.
Discourage use of caffeine.	Can produce anxiety-like symptoms, compounding clinical picture and client's perception of situation

INTERVENTIONS	RATIONALE

Independent

Assist client to learn relaxation/imagery exercises. Use tapes of relaxation exercises and calm music. Reinforce practice of these, and prompt client to use them when becoming anxious. (Note: It may be necessary to stay with anxious client.)

> Develops skills for coping with anxiety responses. Staying with the client can keep client focused on the relaxation exercises and provide sense of worth and confidence.

Encourage practice sessions when not feeling anxious.

> Enables client to use skill more effectively (automatically) as needed.

Encourage creative activities and development of greater leisure skills.

> Helps expand positive energy and attention. Enhances self-esteem.

Involve in group settings, encouraging and reinforcing appropriate participation. Redirect into activities, e.g., interaction with others, as indicated.

> Increases opportunities for/reinforcement of desired, productive interaction style. Sharing with others decreases sense of being the only one. Client may learn new coping styles from stress of participation as well as from peers who have experienced similar stressors.

Deal with physical complaints in matter-of-fact style. Investigate appropriately if new; redirect if not new or validated. Do not ask how patient is or feels. Help client recognize physical symptoms as anxiety signals when appropriate. Note history of mitral valve prolapse.

> Detection of physical problems and prevention of discounting of client's discomfort are important. Reduces reinforcement for focusing on self and symptoms while providing opportunity and reinforcement for other-directed, more appropriate interaction style. (Note: Focus on physical complaints occurs in depressed persons in about 25 percent of cases.) Palpitations resulting from MVP may increase anxiety to panic state and require medical evaluation/treatment.

NURSING DIAGNOSIS:	MOBILITY IMPAIRED: PHYSICAL/SELF-CARE DEFICIT, SPECIFY
MAY BE RELATED TO:	Disinterest or unconcern
	Psychomotor retardation
	Lack of energy/inertia
	Impaired self-concept
POSSIBLY EVIDENCED BY:	Impaired ability to make decisions, such as whether to get out of bed, what to wear/eat
	Inactivity
	Altered sleep patterns
	Reports of "I can't/don't want to" or "Wait until later" to perform self-care activities

CLIENT OUTCOMES/EVALUATION CRITERIA:

Requests for help in the absence of physical incapacity

Disheveled appearance

Verbalizes understanding of own situation and individual treatment regimen. Demonstrates resumption of activities, increased concern/attention to grooming and hygiene, and behaviors to begin to direct own life. Initiates/performs self-care/other activities independently.

INTERVENTIONS	RATIONALE
Independent	
Speak directly to client; respect individuality and personal space as appropriate.	Promotes sense of worthwhileness of the person.
Provide structured opportunities for client to make choices of care, e.g., what to wear today, what activity to participate in.	Begins to establish own ability to make decisions and accept/deal with consequences.
Be aware of the amount of time client *actually* spends in bed/chair, especially those who appear in a poor nutritional state.	This immobility places client at risk for impaired skin integrity.
Examine skin over bony prominences for redness (include heels) after client has been in bed/chair awhile.	Identifies compromised tissues receiving decreased circulation (due to prolonged pressure) and requiring intervention.
Provide skin care with attention to cleanliness, massage, and lotion every two to three hours. Change position every two hours, including bed to chair or to stroll "once around the day room."	Until etiologic factors are remedied (immobility and nutritional status) these actions are helpful in preventing skin breakdown by alleviating pressure and promoting circulation.
Set progressive activity goals with client.	Reduces risks of complications related to sedentary lifestyle/immobility. Activity also releases natural endorphins, which aid in elevating mood.
Monitor intake and output. Note color/concentration of urine. Observe for complications of reduced fluid intake, e.g., dry mucous membranes and lips, poor skin turgor, constipation, and treat accordingly.	Direct indicators of individual needs/presence of problems. Poor hydration directly affects tissues, increasing risk of damage/breakdown in face of decreased mobility.
Offer fluids frequently/leave small amounts of fluid within easy reach.	Improves overall intake in depressed person to whom *everything* seems too difficult. Client may drink because it is available. Small amounts prevent guilt over things being "wasted" if not consumed. Prevents options for negative self-reinforcement, e.g., "nothing available," "can't drink that much."
Perform/assist with needed self-care activities for client, as necessary. Note frequency of elimination pattern. (Refer to ND: Bowel elimination, altered: Constipation)	Ensures that needed activities are accomplished if client is unable/unwilling to perform alone.

241

INTERVENTIONS

Independent

Provide/obtain needed equipment, client's own supplies, clothing.

Choose one self-care activity and plan with client how to implement in a simple, concrete fashion.

Provide low-key reinforcement for improved functioning in this area.

Give low-key reminder regarding need to perform a self-care activity.

Collaborative

Refer to occupational/recreational therapy involving motor activities, e.g., walking, working with clay, aerobic exercise, crafts, activities of daily living.

Encourage beautician/barber appointments, if available.

RATIONALE

Availability may prompt performance; having one's own things enhances self-esteem, autonomy.

Assisting client toward self-care in a slow and achievable manner is important. Depressed clients feel overwhelmed, and it is important that success is experienced one task at a time.

Enhances self-esteem; low-key style to avoid provoking discounting, self-derogation.

Gentle prodding can be helpful to the client; however, reminders may be perceived as criticism and can feed into self-derogatory thinking.

These activities help to discharge anger and aggression and relieve guilt, as well as build self-confidence and prepare client for return to previous occupation/leisuretime activities.

Can enhance self-image, stimulate participation in self-care activities.

NURSING DIAGNOSIS:	NUTRITION, ALTERED: LESS THAN BODY REQUIREMENT
MAY BE RELATED TO:	Inadequate nutritional intake to meet metabolic needs
	Lack of interest in eating or food
POSSIBLY EVIDENCED BY:	Refusal to eat
	Recent weight loss
	Poor muscle tone
	Decreased subcutaneous fat/muscle mass
	Pale conjunctiva and mucous membranes
CLIENT OUTCOMES/EVALUATION CRITERIA:	Demonstrates progressive weight gain toward goal with normalization of laboratory values and free of signs

of malnutrition. Identifies actions/ lifestyle changes to regain and/or to maintain appropriate weight.

INTERVENTIONS	RATIONALE
Independent	
Monitor/record amount and type of food intake.	Provides data base and documents change/progress toward goal.
Monitor body weight, depending on the seriousness of the problem and the client's response to being weighed.	Provides information about therapeutic needs/ effectiveness. Increased appetite is one of the earliest responses to antidepressants.
Avoid getting into a "power struggle" about these issues.	Focuses attention on food and weight, overemphasizing them (possibly providing secondary gain) rather than underlying dynamics.
Explain to client that malnutrition itself decreases energy levels and ability to think cohesively (e.g., decreased protein and vitamin B affect and may deepen depression).	May provide incentive to eat, increasing cooperation and intake.
Feed client if indicated by physical condition and refusal/inability to eat.	Assisting client to eat can help to meet nutritional needs.
Provide small meals and interval feedings, emphasizing high protein-carbohydrate choices.	A full meal may look like an insurmountable challenge, especially for client who is depressed.
Identify and obtain foods client thinks would be interesting/appealing. Use family/friends as resources as indicated.	May enhance desire to eat and promote increased intake. Family can provide information about client's likes and dislikes, other helpful ideas to increase food intake.
Increase calorie intake as activity level increases.	Caloric requirements need to be adapted to provide sufficient energy to meet expenditures/maintain weight.
Collaborative	
Consult with dietician as necessary.	Helpful in determining individual needs, alternate dietary therapy.
Provide tube feeding, as indicated.	May be necessary when client refuses or is unable to eat and client safety/condition requires.

NURSING DIAGNOSIS: **BOWEL ELIMINATION, ALTERED: CONSTIPATION**

MAY BE RELATED TO: **Decreased physical mobility**

Altered daily routine

Decreased intake of fluids/bulk

MAY BE RELATED TO—*continued*	Side effects of antidepressant medications
	Inattention to cues
POSSIBLY EVIDENCED BY:	Decreased frequency of bowel movement
	Passage of hard-formed stool
	Pain on defecation
CLIENT OUTCOMES/EVALUATION CRITERIA:	*Verbalizes understanding of causative factors. Identifies/practices appropriate interventions related to individual situation. Produces soft, formed stools that are passed without pain or undue straining.*

INTERVENTIONS

Independent

Ascertain usual pattern of bowel elimination and related routine. Compare with current situation.

Investigate possible causes, e.g., dietary inadequacies, reduced fluid intake, decreased activity.

Examine rectum for hard stool, impaction, as indicated. Note complaints of pain on defecation/inability to pass stool.

Implement individual dietary changes, e.g., increase roughage; provide fruit juices, stimulant beverages (hot or caffeine-containing, if tolerated).

Promote fluid intake of 1500–2000 cc/day.

Encourage regular exercise, increased activity.

Collaborative

Administer stool softener/bulk preparation.

Provide glycerine suppository or laxative product according to protocol if no bowel movement occurs.

RATIONALE

Useful in establishing goals, identifying appropriate interventions.

Identify problem areas where corrective actions can be taken.

Determines extent of problem and degree of intervention required.

Fiber stimulates peristalsis. Some juices, such as prune, have byproduct that stimulates intestinal mobility. Caffeine has a cholinergic effect, stimulating peristalsis.

Increases water available in the colon to keep stool soft and reduce effort required to defecate.

Stimulates peristalsis, enhancing elimination.

May be used to supplement dietary inadequacies/soften stool until normal stool is established.

Prevents impaction and helps to restore regular pattern.

| **NURSING DIAGNOSIS:** | **SLEEP PATTERN DISTURBANCE** |
| **MAY BE RELATED TO:** | **Biochemical alterations (decreased serotonin)** |

POSSIBLY EVIDENCED BY:	Unresolved fears and anxieties Inactivity Difficulty in falling/remaining asleep Early morning awakening Complaints of not feeling rested Dark circles under eyes
CLIENT OUTCOMES/EVALUATION CRITERIA:	Identifies interventions to promote/enhance sleep. Reports falling asleep within an hour of retiring and sleeping 4–6 hours before awakening. Verbalizes having had a satisfactory night's sleep/feeling well rested.

INTERVENTIONS	RATIONALE
Independent	
Identify nature of sleep disturbance and variation from usual pattern, e.g., may have difficulty falling asleep, may awaken early and be unable to fall asleep again, may have insomnia or hypersomnia.	Patterns provide clues to help client and nurse to work together to solve the problem.
Assess what client does when awake and plan with client to change pattern as indicated.	Clients often awaken and ruminate about themselves in a hopeless/helpless manner. Having client set aside a period during the day to ruminate may extinguish this behavior at night.
Establish with client a realistic goal.	Some individuals have unrealistic ideas of a "normal" night's sleep.
Identify previous bedtime rituals that may have been interrupted by illness or hospitalization and reestablish when possible.	Restoring familiar, successful rituals may allow the client to reestablish usual pattern.
Decrease afternoon and evening caffeine intake (coffee, tea, chocolate, colas).	Avoids stimulants, which may affect ability to fall/stay asleep.
Restrict evening fluids and have client void before retiring.	Reduces need to rise at night to void.
Provide *light* bedtime nourishment, such as milk if client likes it and it is not otherwise contraindicated.	Milk (with L-tryptophan) is thought to be helpful in promoting sleep. Snack prevents awakening during night due to hunger.
Reduce environmental stimuli, e.g., lights, noises, loudspeakers, etc.	Decreases distracting stimuli that may interfere with sleep.
Provide night lights, environmental control (room adequately warm or cool), appropriate nightwear/bedding, including special blanket/pillow, which can be brought from home.	May prevent confusion upon awakening. Insures personal comfort, promotes sleep, sense of security.

245

INTERVENTIONS	RATIONALE

Independent

Schedule treatments, procedures, assessments, medications during the daytime.

Prevents unnecessary interruption during sleep.

Increase daytime activity and discourage returning to bed during the day; nap before rather than after lunch, if needed.

Increased activity without overexertion promotes sleep. Morning napping disrupts sleep less than afternoon naps.

Collaborative

Give hypnotic or sedative only if other methods fail.

Products may suppress REM sleep, resulting in not feeling rested upon awakening.

Administer/recommend that antidepressants or other medication with sedative side effects be taken at HS when possible.

Decreases daytime drowsiness and aids sleeping at night.

NURSING DIAGNOSIS:	**COMMUNICATION, IMPAIRED VERBAL**
MAY BE RELATED TO:	**Psychologic barriers, indecision**
	Psychomotor retardation
	Anxiety
POSSIBLY EVIDENCED BY:	**Slowed speech, latencies, decreased amount of speech**
	Muteness
CLIENT OUTCOMES/EVALUATION CRITERIA:	**Responds to questions and makes needs known. Participates in 1:1 interaction for specified number of minutes. Demonstrates congruent communication with others in group interaction in OT, group therapy, ward meetings, and so forth.**

INTERVENTIONS	RATIONALE

Independent

Use client's name in beginning statement.

Reinforces individuality, gets attention.

Keep input fairly short and concrete.

Requires less effort for client to attend to and retain.

Ask only one question (about *one* thing) at a time. Avoid asking "yes-no" and "why" questions.

Promotes focus and requires that client put thinking into response. '"Why" questions are often perceived as threatening.

Take adequate time; wait patiently for responses.

Indicates interest, enhances self-esteem.

INTERVENTIONS	RATIONALE
Independent	
Observe and give feedback regarding the feeling tone conveyed.	Recognition of these feelings demonstrates empathy, sensitivity. Promotes understanding of how client is perceived by others, providing opportunity for insight/ change.
Start conversation and "give" client a topic, ward or world event, OT project, etc.	Initiating activity is often very difficult for client, and having an assignment helps get the activity started.
Determine what the client's interests/activities were and ask client to share those. Let client teach others about past skills by asking questions, indicating desire to learn about client's contributions to job and family.	Revitalizes memories from a time when client felt better. Indicates client's individuality and sense of offering self to others.
Reinforce attendance at activities (OT, group, ward events).	Attendance precedes participation.
Greet routinely with personal comment on clothing; share pertinent information from shift report, observations, etc., without concern for response by client.	Provides a "no-demand" acceptance, opportunity to interact if client chooses. Matter-of-fact manner prevents demand for client to provide a response when depressed feelings interfere.
Use touch, unless contraindicated.	Touch is a basic form of communication and can help client in interactions, demonstrates caring, and reinforces sense of self-worth.
Avoid taking client's difficulty in responding or negative/hostile responses personally.	Client will try to reinforce feeling of "worthlessness" by trying to create negative responses from others. Working with depressed client requires much patience and ability to recognize small goals as improvement.

NURSING DIAGNOSIS:	**SOCIAL ISOLATION/SOCIAL INTERACTION IMPAIRED**
MAY BE RELATED TO:	**Alterations in mental status/thought processes (depressed mood)**
	Inadequate personal resources; decreased energy/inertia
	Difficulty engaging in satisfying personal relationships
	Feelings of worthlessness/low self-concept
	Inadequacy in or absence of significant purpose in life
	Knowledge/skill deficit about social interactions

POSSIBLY EVIDENCED BY:	Decreased involvement with others
	Expressed feelings of difference from others
	Remaining in home/room/bed
	Refusing invitations/suggestions of social involvement
	Verbalization/demonstration of awareness that interpersonal or social interactions do not have desired, satisfactory, or reinforcing outcomes
	Dysfunctional interaction with peers, family, and/or others
CLIENT OUTCOMES/EVALUATION CRITERIA:	Remains out of bed except for one rest period daily. Attends/then participates in specific number of activities per day/week. Completes errands, initiates socialization activities a specific number of times per week. Reinstates two previously enjoyed activities involving others, or develops new ones. Verbalizes increased satisfaction with outcomes of social interactions.

INTERVENTIONS	RATIONALE
Independent	
Involve in interpersonal situations where interaction style can be observed.	Provides information about interaction style/skills and helps client recognize where discomfort and feelings of inadequacy have been experienced.
Assist individual to assess own satisfaction with outcome(s) of interpersonal interactions	Helps client plan what is to be expected from interacting and how client can behave to realize those expectations. Involves the client in problem identification and helps to evaluate whether goals are realistic.
Provide feedback regarding observations of verbal/nonverbal interactions.	Develops client's awareness of positive actions that are already being used and identifies problem areas.
Emphasize attendance at routine ward activities as well as nondemanding activities (e.g., movies).	Starting with achievable goals gives client the ability to succeed and enhance self-esteem.
Gradually increase activity schedule, still initially emphasizing attendance rather than participation or enjoyment to be gained.	Enhances chances of cooperation, diminishes threat, promotes progression of interaction.
Contract with client (e.g., one hour of attendance at an activity is rewarded by an hour in room without being "pestered" for nonsuicidal client).	Involving client in decision-making increases sense of control over situation and may promote cooperation.

INTERVENTIONS	RATIONALE
Independent	
Encourage visits by friends, relatives, other social contacts identified/located by family member.	Helps reestablish neglected, previously rewarding relationships.
Obtain hobby equipment from home, if indicated. Have client teach nurse or others this hobby.	Encourages resumption of previously enjoyed activities and reduces sense of isolation. Increases sense of purpose while providing 1:1 interaction.
Contact frequently. Greet consistently. Involve with one other person or in quiet activity in day area.	Acknowledges sense of self-worth.
Involve family, friends to escort, transport on outings, functional (shopping, business, obtaining belongings at home) or social activities (a brief meal, church or temple service, etc.).	Events such as these require little of client but increase social involvement and yield social reinforcement. Decreases sense of isolation from outside world.
Request feedback on outings and activities from *both* client and others involved (therapists, companions).	The goal is to increase involvement, and because client will likely report a less successful event than a more objective observer, input is important from both. The client can also hear other's perception of an event, which can serve to validate/add to the client's perception.
Avoid asking client if activities are "enjoyable" or "fun."	Keep staff and client expectations realistic. Avoid cheerfulness, as it may be interpreted as false.
Keep feedback regarding performance (e.g., increased involvement in groups, etc.) matter-of-fact and low key, but *always* acknowledge and reinforce attendance, performance.	Client is unable to discount reinforcement and is thus reinforced for participation. Positive reinforcement encourages repetition of desired behaviors.
Be consistent and on time in planned meetings with client.	Client will experience lateness as further evidence of decreased self-worth. In building trust, client needs to know that the nurse will follow through on previously agreed meetings/commitments.
Use social skills training model to assist client to identify alternative strategies; role-play/rehearse new (more effective) behavior; obtain feedback and reinforcement; try new behavior in a "real situation."	Client may need to learn social skills and practice new behaviors. Improved social skills are more likely to have results that satisfy/reinforce interactions.
Provide positive reinforcement for demonstration of more effective social skills.	Increases the reward for trying the new tactics.
Assist in identifying the natural reinforcers that occur with more effective interactions.	These reinforcers will increase the client's confidence and strengthen the behavior.
Use group situations for maximum impact/reinforcement, e.g., group therapy, OT, RT, etc.	The group provides more opportunity for interaction, feedback, reinforcement.
Have client anticipate "post-hospital" situations and plan/rehearse ways to use new behavior. Accompany client on a field trip as indicated.	Provides opportunity for support and feedback. Helps generalize the newly learned behavior to future situations.
Provide "as needed" or ongoing updates to social skills enhancement, adding information and/or reinforcing what has been learned.	Provides for continuing growth/therapy.

249

NURSING DIAGNOSIS:	SEXUAL DYSFUNCTION/SEXUALITY PATTERNS, ALTERED
MAY BE RELATED TO:	Biopsychosocial alteration of sexuality
	Decreased energy and concern, apathy
	Loss of sexual desire
	Decreased self-esteem
	Psychosocial abuse, e.g., harmful relationships
POSSIBLY EVIDENCED BY:	Reported difficulties, limitations, or changes in sexual behaviors/activities
	Verbalization of problem (e.g., women may express a loss of interest; men may experience impotence and loss of libido)
	Actual or perceived limitation imposed by depression
	Alteration in relationship with partner
	Misinformation/misconceptions about sexual functioning/behavior
CLIENT OUTCOMES/EVALUATION CRITERIA:	Verbalizes understanding of effect of depression on sexual functioning. Identifies stresses that contribute to dysfunction. Resumes sexual functioning at level desired/as agreed upon by client and partner.

INTERVENTIONS	RATIONALE
Independent	
Assess client's sexual history and degree of satisfaction prior to depression.	Establishes a baseline and elicits client's feelings about previous sexual satisfaction. (Note: may need to discuss this when client is well into recovery, as feelings of self-worth are intertwined with feelings about sexual satisfaction.)

INTERVENTIONS	RATIONALE

Independent

Assist client to define expectations for sexual satisfaction and decide what can be done to attain these.

Planning can help the client identify more clearly what own desires are and whether they are reasonable/attainable.

Provide sex education as necessary. Include significant other/partner as indicated.

Often sexual problems are partly ignorance and misconceptions about sexual facts, and knowledge can assist with problem resolution.

Review medication regimen; observe for side effects of drugs prescribed.

Many medications can affect libido and/or cause impotence. Evaluation of drug and individual response is important to ascertain whether drug is responsible for the problem.

Collaborative

Refer for further counseling/sex therapy as indicated.

May need additional/in-depth assistance if problems are severe/unresolved as depression lifts.

NURSING DIAGNOSIS:	**FAMILY PROCESSES, ALTERED**
MAY BE RELATED TO:	**Situational crises of illness of family member**
POSSIBLY EVIDENCED BY:	**Expressions of confusion**
	Statements of difficulty coping with situation
	Family system not meeting needs of its members
	Difficulty accepting or receiving help appropriately
	Ineffective family decision-making process
	Failure to send and to receive clear messages
FAMILY OUTCOMES/EVALUATION CRITERIA:	**Expresses feelings freely and appropriately. Demonstrates individual involvement in problem-solving processes directed at appropriate solutions for the situation/crisis. Encourages and allows member who is ill to handle situation in own way,**

```
┌─────────────────────────────────────────────────────────────────┐
│ FAMILY OUTCOMES/EVALUATION        progressing toward independence. │
│         CRITERIA—continued        Identifies/uses community resources │
│                                   appropriately.                   │
└─────────────────────────────────────────────────────────────────┘
```

INTERVENTIONS

RATIONALE

Independent

Assess degree of family dysfunction and current coping methods of individual members.

Identifies problems of individual family members, provides direction for intervention.

Identify family developmental stage (e.g., newly married couple/divorced, children leaving home); components of family and client's role in the family constellation.

Developmental stage may be a factor in current situation and client's depression. Disruption of client's role may contribute to family disorganization/strain on other family members who have to step in and assume duties client usually takes care of.

Identify patterns of communication within the family. Are feelings freely expressed? Is blame or fault assigned? What is the process of decision-making in the family and who makes the decisions? What is the interaction between family members?

Dysfunctional communication contributes to feelings of inadequacy, rejection, and inability to cope on the part of the members of the family.

Acknowledge difficulties observed while giving permission to express feelings and discussing more effective methods of communication.

Reassures family that feelings are acceptable and can be dealt with appropriately.

Provide information as necessary in verbal, written and/or tape format as appropriate.

Provides opportunity for family members to review and incorporate new knowledge to assist in resolution of current situation.

Establish/discuss goals/expectations of family members/client after discharge. Let individuals know the importance of taking it slow and not pressuring each other to change.

Realistic expectations of abilities of client to assume place in the family are crucial to continued recuperation. Family needs to understand that members need to continue to work on new style of communication and changing ways of dealing with conflict issues.

Collaborative

Involve in group/family therapy, as indicated.

Opportunity to hear others discuss shared problems and ways of handling can encourage family members to look at new ways of interacting.

Provide information about resources available as needed, e.g., social services, homemaker assistance, counseling, visiting nurse association.

Assistance may be needed for family members to assimilate new skills and begin to make necessary lifestyle changes to promote wellness.

NURSING DIAGNOSIS:	KNOWLEDGE DEFICIT [LEARNING NEED] (SPECIFY)
MAY BE RELATED TO:	Lack of information about pathophysiology and treatment of depression
	Misconceptions about mental illness
POSSIBLY EVIDENCED BY:	Inaccurate statements about own situation and potential for recovery

	Lack of follow-through with treatment regimen
	Inappropriate behavior, apathy
CLIENT OUTCOMES/EVALUATION CRITERIA:	**Requests information. Verbalizes understandings of illness, prognosis, and therapeutic regimen. Participates in treatment program. Identifies/uses resources appropriately.**

INTERVENTIONS

Independent

Determine level of knowledge, mental/emotional readiness for learning.

Provide information about depression/treatment as indicated. Give written information as well as verbal.

Provide information about drug therapy and potential side effects, e.g., anticholinergic effects of antidepressants; possibility of hypertensive crisis if individual consumes foods containing tyramine while taking MAOI drugs.

Encourage frequent fluids, lip salve, ice chips, as indicated.

Suggest medication dosage be taken at bedtime, when appropriate.

Discuss importance of monitoring blood pressure as indicated. Suggest client rise slowly from sitting/lying position.

Review diet restrictions, e.g., tyramine-free diet, limitation of caffeine.

Discuss use of identification bracelet/card, notification of other health caregivers.

Reinforce importance of not stopping drugs abruptly.

Collaborative

Refer to resources/agencies, e.g., social services, homemaker/baby-sitting, support groups.

RATIONALE

May be first experience with illness/mental health system. Previous experience may or may not have provided accurate information. May be too depressed to access information accurately.

Provides opportunity for client to learn about own situation and enhances recall.

Client needs to know what to expect from drug trial. Knowledge can increase cooperation with drug regimen. Particularly, clients need to be aware that improvement may not occur until 4–6 weeks and that side effects will generally improve/disappear within two weeks.

Provides relief of dry mouth caused by anticholinergic effect of drug therapy.

Sedative effect may be helpful in promoting and maintaining sleep.

Most common side effect of antidepressants is orthostatic hypotension, which can result in dizziness, injury following sudden position change.

Necessary to avoid interaction (hypertensive crisis) when MAOI medications are used and for two weeks following discontinuation.

Provides information if needed in emergency situation to prevent sudden termination of medication, which could be detrimental.

Sudden cessation of drugs can result in untoward effects, e.g., may aggravate condition, deepening depression, and cause withdrawal with nausea/vomiting and diarrhea.

May be helpful to client for long-range planning for regaining/maintaining wellness.

253

CHAPTER **9**
Anxiety Disorders

Generalized Anxiety Disorder

DSM III-R: 300.02 Generalized anxiety disorder
Although some degree of anxiety is normal in life's stresses, it can be adaptive or maladaptive. Problems arise when coping mechanisms are inadequate to deal with the danger, which may be recognized or unrecognized. The essential feature is unrealistic or excessive anxiety and worry about life circumstances.

ETIOLOGIC THEORIES

PSYCHODYNAMICS

Freudian view is that of conflict between demands of the id and superego, with the ego serving as mediator. Anxiety occurs when the ego is not strong enough to resolve the conflict.
Sullivanian theory states that fear of disapproval from the mothering figure is the basis for anxiety. Conditional love results in fragile ego and lack of self-confidence. Individual has low self-esteem, fears failure, and is easily threatened.
Dollar and Miller believe anxiety is a learned response based on an innate drive to avoid pain. Anxiety results from being faced with two competing drives or goals.

BIOLOGIC THEORIES

Although biologic and neurophysiologic influences in the etiology of anxiety disorders have been investigated, no relationship has yet been established. However, there does seem to be a genetic influence with a high family incidence.
The autonomic nervous system discharge that occurs in response to a frightening impulse and/or emotion is mediated by the limbic system, resulting in the peripheral effects of the autonomic nervous system seen in the presence of anxiety.

FAMILY DYNAMICS

The individual exhibiting dysfunctional behavior is seen as the representation of family system problems. The "identified patient" is carrying the problems of the other members of the family, which are seen as the result of the interrelationships (disequilibrium) between family members rather than as isolated individual problems.

CLIENT ASSESSMENT DATA BASE

HISTORY

Chronic anxiety symptoms that are not punctuated by intermittent panic attacks
Client at least 18 years of age
Women twice as likely to be affected as men
May be pacing anxiously or, if seated, will restlessly move arms and legs about
Complains vociferously about inner turmoil and may demand help
Facial expression is in keeping with terror felt
May report history of threat to either physical integrity (illness, inadequate food and housing, etc.) or self-concept
    (loss of self esteem; loss of significant other; assumption of new role)
Absence of other mental disorder, such as depressive disorder or schizophrenia

PHYSICAL EXAMINATION

Manifests at least six of the following symptoms during anxious periods, which have been evident more often than
    not during the last six months:
    Motor tension: shakiness, jitteriness, jumpiness, trembling, tension, muscle aches, fatigability, inability to relax,
        eyelid twitch, furrowed brow, strained face, fidgeting, restlessness, easily startled, headaches
    Autonomic hyperactivity: sweating, heart pounding or racing, cold and clammy hands, dry mouth, dizziness,
        lightheadedness, tingling hands or feet, upset stomach, hot or cold spells, frequent urination, diarrhea,
        discomfort in the pit of the stomach, lump in the throat, flushing, pallor, high resting pulse and respiratory
        rate, increased blood pressure
    Apprehensive expectation: anxiety, worry, fear, rumination, anticipation of misfortune to self or others, inability
        to act differently (feeling stuck)
    Vigilance and scanning: hyperattentiveness resulting in distractibility, difficulty in concentrating, insomnia, feel-
        ing "on edge," irritability, impatience

DIAGNOSTIC STUDIES

Drug screen: to rule out drugs as contribution to cause of symptoms
Other diagnostic studies may be conducted to rule out physical disease as basis for individual symptoms, e.g.,
    ECG for severe chest pain.

NURSING PRIORITIES

1. Assist client to recognize own anxiety.
2. Promote insight into anxiety and related factors.
3. Provide opportunity for learning new, adaptive coping responses.
4. Involve client/family in educational/support activities.

DISCHARGE CRITERIA

1. Feelings of anxiety are recognized and handled appropriately.
2. Coping skills are developed to manage anxiety-provoking situations.
3. Identifies and uses resources effectively
4. Client/family participating in ongoing therapy program

NURSING DIAGNOSIS:	ANXIETY (SEVERE)/POWERLESSNESS
MAY BE RELATED TO:	Real or perceived threat to physical integrity or self-concept (may or may not be able to identify the threat)

Unconscious conflict about essential values (beliefs) and goals of life

Unmet needs

Positive or negative self-talk

POSSIBLY EVIDENCED BY:

Persistent feelings of apprehension and uneasiness (related to unidentified stressor or stimulus)

A general anxious feeling that client has difficulty alleviating

Sympathetic stimulation

Extraneous movements: foot shuffling; hand, arm fidgeting; rocking movements

Restlessness, poor eye contact

Focus on self

Impaired functioning

Verbal expressions of having no control or influence over situation, outcome, or self-care

Free-floating anxiety

Nonparticipation in care or decision-making when opportunities are provided

**CLIENT OUTCOMES/EVALUATION
CRITERIA:**

Verbalizes awareness of feelings of anxiety. Identifies effective coping mechanisms to successfully deal with stress. Reports anxiety is reduced to a manageable level. Demonstrates problem-solving skills/lifestyle changes as indicated for individual situation.

INTERVENTIONS	RATIONALE
Independent	
Establish and maintain a trusting relationship through the use of warmth, empathy, and respect. Provide adequate time for response. Communicate support of the client's self-expression.	The client may perceive the nurse as a threat, increasing the client's anxiety. Attending behaviors can increase the degree of comfort the client experiences with the nurse.
Be aware of any negative or anxious feelings nurse may have because of the client's conscious or unconscious resistance of nurse's helpful efforts.	Negative reactions to the client will block future progress. Anxiety is "contagious" and nurse needs to recognize and control own anxiety in order to help client.
Identify behaviors of the client that produce anxiety in the nurse. Explore these behaviors with the client when relationship is established.	Promotes growth and change and helps client realize how own behavior affects others.
Have client identify and describe the sensations of emotional and physical feelings. Assist the client to link behavior and feelings. Validate all inferences and assumptions with the client.	In order to adopt new coping responses, the client first needs to recognize anxiety and be aware of feelings, how they link to certain maladaptive coping responses, and own responsibility in learning to control behavior.
Help to explore conflictual issues by beginning with nonthreatening topics and progressing to more conflict-laden ones.	Anxious client does not think clearly, and beginning with simple topics promotes comfort level, increasing sense of success and progress.
Monitor the anxiety level of the nurse/client interaction on an ongoing basis.	Moderate anxiety may be productive/motivate client, but too high a level can interfere with the interaction and ability to attend to information.
Use supportive confrontation as indicated.	Confrontation can be useful when client progress is blocked but may heighten anxiety to a level that is detrimental to the therapy process; therefore, it should be used with caution.
Assist the client to identify the situations and interactions that immediately precede the anxiety. Suggest the client keep an anxiety notebook that focuses on feelings and what is going on in the environment when anxious feelings begin.	After the client recognizes feelings of anxiety, examination of the development of the anxiety (e.g., what precipitates it, the strength of the stressor(s), and what resources are available) can help the client develop new coping skills. Writing serves to decrease the anxiety while the client is learning about it, making it more tangible/controllable.
Help client to correlate cause and effect relationships between stressor and anxiety.	Gives more control over situation. Increases sense of power if client can identify cause of anxiety.
Note when complaints of anxiety move from one area to another (e.g., money, health, relationship), and help client recognize what is happening.	Feelings of anxiety can become "free-floating," becoming attached to one concern after another, and the client needs to recognize this so it can be dealt with.
Link the present experience with relevant ones from the past. Ask questions like "Does that seem familiar to you? What does it remind you of from the past?"	Provides opportunity for client to make connections between these events and development of current anxiety, promoting insight and learning experience.
Assist the client to learn new, adaptive coping mechanisms by exploring how the client dealt with anxiety in the past and what methods produced relief. Help to identify the maladaptive effects of present coping responses.	The client is capable of learning new, adaptive coping responses by analyzing coping mechanisms used previously, identifying available resources, and accepting personal responsibility for change.

INTERVENTIONS	RATIONALE
Independent	
Encourage use of adaptive coping responses that have worked in the past.	Increases confidence in own ability to deal with stress.
Keep the focus of responsibility for change on the client.	Increases feelings of self-control and self-esteem.
Use role-playing if appropriate.	Allows client to "practice" new coping responses in a safe setting.
Include significant others as resources and social supports in helping client learn new coping responses.	Enhances ability to cope when one does not feel alone. In addition, since anxiety may have an interpersonal basis, involvement of S.O.(s) can enhance the client's relationship skills, enabling the use of others as resources rather than withdrawal.
Expose client slowly to anxiety-provoking situations.	Allows the client time to identify/implement new, adaptive coping responses and to become comfortable in using them.
Assist to reevaluate goals, modify behavior, use resources, and test out new coping responses.	Goals may have been too rigid and may have set up client for anxiety that could be avoided by change in behavior/responses.
Develop regular physical activity program.	Excess energy is discharged in a healthful manner through physical exercise. Biochemical effects of exercise decrease feelings of anxiety.
Encourage client to use relaxation techniques, meditation, and biofeedback.	Relaxation is the ultimate stress management technique because it brings about a decreased heart rate, lowers metabolism, and decreases respiration. The relaxation response is the physiological opposite of the anxiety response.
Collaborative	
Administer tranquilizing medication as indicated, e.g., meprobamate (Equanil, Miltown), clorazepate (Tranxene), chlordiazepoxide (Librium), diazepam (Valium), oxazepam (Serax).	Anti-anxiety medication provides relief from the immobilizing effects of anxiety.

NURSING DIAGNOSIS:	**COPING, INEFFECTIVE INDIVIDUAL**
MAY BE RELATED TO:	**Level of anxiety being experienced by the client**
	Inadequate coping methods
	Personal vulnerability
	Inadequate support systems
	Little or no exercise
	Unmet expectations

259

MAY BE RELATED TO—*continued*	Multiple stressors, repeated over period of time
POSSIBLY EVIDENCED BY:	Maladaptive coping skills
	Verbalization of inability to cope
	Muscular tension/headaches
	Chronic worry, emotional tension
	Chronic fatigue, insomnia
	Inability to problem-solve
	Alteration in societal participation
	High rate of accidents
	Overeating/excessive smoking and/or drinking/drug use
CLIENT OUTCOMES/EVALUATION CRITERIA:	Identifies ineffective coping behaviors and consequences. Expresses feelings appropriately. Identifies options and uses resources effectively. Uses effective problem-solving techniques.

INTERVENTIONS	RATIONALE
Independent	
Assess current functional capacity, developmental level of functioning, and level of coping. Assess defense mechanisms used, e.g., denial, repression, conversion, dissociation, reaction formation, undoing, displacement, or projection.	Knowing how the individual's coping ability is being affected by current events determines need for/kind of intervention. People tend to regress during illness/crisis and need acceptance/support to regain/improve coping ability.
Identify previous methods of coping with life problems.	How client has handled previous life problems is a reliable predictor of how current problems will be handled.
Determine use of substances (e.g., alcohol, other drugs; smoking habits; eating patterns).	Substances are often used as coping mechanism to control anxiety and can interfere with client's ability to deal with current situation.
Observe and describe behavior in objective terms. Validate observations with client as possible. Note physical complaints.	Provides accurate picture of client situation and avoids judgmental evaluations. Anxious people may have increased somatic concerns. (Refer to CP: Somatoform Disorders.)
Assess for premenstrual tension syndrome when appropriate.	Increased progesterone may cause increased anxiety for women during the luteal phase of the menstrual cycle.

INTERVENTIONS	RATIONALE

Independent

Active-Listen client concerns and identify perceptions of what is happening.

Promotes sense of self-worth and value for beliefs and clarifies client view of situation.

Confront client behaviors in context of trusting relationship, pointing out differences between words and actions, when appropriate.

Helps client to become aware of distortions of reality resulting from anxiety state.

Provide information about different ways to deal with situations that promote anxious feelings, e.g., identification and appropriate expression of feelings and problem-solving skills.

Provides opportunity for client to learn new coping skills and incorporate these into own lifestyle.

Use role-play and rehearsal techniques as indicated.

Promotes practice of new skills in a nonthreatening environment.

Encourage and support client in evaluating lifestyle, noting activities, stresses of family, work, and social situations.

Helps client to look at difficult areas which may contribute to anxiety and to make changes gradually without undue/debilitating anxiety.

Collaborative

Refer to outside resources, e.g., groups, psychotherapy, counselor, religious resources, sexual counseling, as indicated.

May need additional assistance/support to maintain improvement/control.

NURSING DIAGNOSIS:	**SOCIAL INTERACTION, IMPAIRED/ SOCIAL ISOLATION**
MAY BE RELATED TO:	**Use of unsuccessful social interaction behaviors**
	Inadequate personal resources
	Self-concept disturbance
	Absence of available significant others or peers
	Altered mental status
POSSIBLY EVIDENCED BY:	**Verbalized/observed discomfort in social situations**
	Dysfunctional interactions with peers, family, staff, others
	Expression of feelings of difference from others
	Sad, dull affect

POSSIBLY EVIDENCED BY—*continued*	Uncommunicative, withdrawn behavior; absence of eye contact
	Preoccupation with own thoughts
CLIENT OUTCOMES/EVALUATION CRITERIA:	Recognizes anxiety and identifies factors involved with feelings of isolation/impaired social interactions. Participates in activities to enhance interactions with others. Gives self positive reinforcement for changes that are achieved.

INTERVENTIONS	RATIONALE
Independent	
Listen to client comments regarding sense of isolation. Differentiate isolation from solitude and loneliness.	Provides information about individual concerns/problems of feelings of aloneness. Client may not be aware of difference between being alone by choice and feeling of being alone even when others are around.
Spend time with client, discussing areas of concern, e.g., reasons anxious feelings interfere with ability to be involved with others. Express positive regard for the client; Active-Listen concerns.	Provides opportunity for learning ways to deal with feelings of anxiety in social situations. Communicates belief in client's self-worth and provides safe environment for self-disclosure.
Develop plan of action with client; look at available resources, risk-taking behaviors, appropriate self-care.	Involvement of client communicates sense of competence and ability to change behavior, even in presence of anxious feelings.
Assess client's use of coping skills and defense mechanisms.	Awareness of defenses individual is using provides for choice of changing behavior. Helps to develop skills that can be used to manage anxiety and promote social interaction.
Assist client to learn social skills and use role-playing for practice.	Provides for new ways to handle anxiety in interaction with others.
Encourage journal-keeping and recording social interactions of each day for review.	Noting the comfort/discomfort that is experienced and possible causes can provide insight, may reduce anxiety, and is useful in evaluating individual responses/coping behaviors. (Refer to ND: Coping, ineffective, individual.)
Collaborative	
Involve in classes/programs directed at resolution of problems, e.g., assertiveness training, group therapy, outdoor education program.	Developing positive social skills/behaviors provides opportunity for diminishing anxiety and promoting involvement with others.

NURSING DIAGNOSIS:	SLEEP PATTERN DISTURBANCE
MAY BE RELATED TO:	Psychologic stress

POSSIBLY EVIDENCED BY:	**Repetitive thoughts**
	Reports of difficulty in falling asleep/ awakening earlier or later than desired
	Complaints of not feeling rested
	Dark circles under eyes
	Frequent yawning
CLIENT OUTCOMES/EVALUATION CRITERIA:	**Verbalizes understanding of relationship of anxiety and sleep disturbance. Identifies appropriate interventions to promote sleep. Reports improvement in sleep pattern, increased sense of well-being, and feeling well-rested.**

INTERVENTIONS	RATIONALE
Independent	
Determine type of sleep pattern disturbance present, including usual bedtime, rituals/routines, number of hours of sleep, time of arising, environmental needs, and how much of a problem it is to client.	Identification of individual situation/degree of interference with functioning determines need for/appropriate interventions.
Provide quiet environment, comfort measures (e.g., back rub, wash hands/face/bath), and sleep aids, such as warm milk. Restrict use of caffeine and alcohol before bedtime.	Promotes relaxation and cues for falling asleep. Stimulating effects of caffeine/alcohol interfere with ability to fall asleep.
Discuss use of relaxation techniques/thoughts, visualization.	Promotes reduction of anxious feelings, resulting in improved sleep/rest.
Suggest ways to handle waking/not sleeping, e.g., don't lie in bed and think, get up and remain inactive, or do something boring.	Having a plan can reduce anxiety about not sleeping.
Involve in exercise program, but do not exercise within two hours of going to sleep.	Increases fatigue, promotes sleep but avoids excess stimulation from activity before bedtime.
Avoid use of sedatives, when possible.	Sedative drugs interfere with REM sleep and affect quality of rest. A rebound effect may lead to intense dreaming, nightmares, and more disturbed sleep.

NURSING DIAGNOSIS:	**COPING, INEFFECTIVE, FAMILY: COMPROMISED [POTENTIAL]**
MAY BE RELATED TO:	**Inadequate or incorrect information or understanding by a primary person**

263

MAY BE RELATED TO—*continued*	Temporary family disorganization and role changes
	Prolonged disability that exhausts the supportive capacity of significant other(s)
FAMILY OUTCOMES/EVALUATION CRITERIA:	**Identifies resources within themselves to deal with situation. Interacts appropriately with the client, providing support and assistance as needed. Recognizes own needs for support, seeks assistance, and uses resources effectively.**

INTERVENTIONS	RATIONALE
Independent	
Assess information available to and understood by family/significant others.	Lack of information/understanding of client's behavior can lead to dysfunctional interactional patterns, which contribute to anxiety in family members.
Identify role of the client in family and how the illness has changed the family organization, e.g., mother who does not maintain household, father who does not go to work.	Degree of disability suffered by the client that interferes with performance of usual family role can contribute to family stress/disorganization.
Note other factors besides illness that affect the abilities of family members to provide needed support, e.g., anxiety, personality disorders.	Systems theory maintains that other members of the family also exhibit dysfunctional behavior, but the client is the "identified patient."
Discuss underlying reasons for client's behaviors.	Helps family understand and accept behaviors that may be difficult to handle.
Assist family and client to understand "who owns the problem" and who is responsible for resolution.	Promotes responsibility of knowing that whoever has the problem has to solve it. The individual can ask for help, but others do not "rescue" or try to solve it for the person.
Encourage development of problem-solving skills.	Assists family in learning new ways to deal with conflicts and reduce anxiety-provoking situations.
Collaborative	
Refer to appropriate resources as indicated, e.g., counseling, psychotherapy, financial, spiritual.	May need additional assistance to maintain family integrity.

Panic Disorders (/Phobias)

DSM III-R: 300.21 Panic disorder with agoraphobia
300.01 Panic disorder without agoraphobia
300.22 Agoraphobia without history of panic disorder
300.23 Social phobia, specify
300.29 Simple phobia

ETIOLOGIC THEORIES

PSYCHODYNAMICS

Phobic object may symbolize the underlying conflict, although there is not always a clear connection. Personal perceptions, life experiences, cultural values color the meaning of the symbol for the client.
Freudian view is that anxiety feelings stem from loss of love and support from mothering figure, which increases the client's dependency needs. The client combats the diffuse intolerable anxiety by an exaggerated use of *displacement* on a particular object or situation, which makes the anxiety more manageable.
Phobic partners may develop in the family; these are "helpers" who stand by and participate in maintaining phobic behavior, protecting phobic client from acute panic and anxiety. Participation of partner furthers the unconscious wish of phobic client to be taken care of and to be in control.

BIOLOGIC THEORIES

Refer to CP: Generalized Anxiety Disorder.

FAMILY DYNAMICS

Refer to CP: Generalized Anxiety Disorder.

CLIENT ASSESSMENT DATA BASE

HISTORY

At least three panic attacks occur within a three-week period in circumstances other than during marked physical exertion or in a life-threatening situation and are not precipitated only by exposure to a circumscribed phobic stimulus.
Occurs more frequently in women than in men
Usually begins in late teens or early adulthood
More common among people who have experienced an early traumatic loss, such as the death of a parent
Onset is usually sudden, heralded by an attack of anxiety in the face of what is destined to be the phobic object or situation.
Reports a persistent fear of some object/situation that poses no actual danger or in which the danger is magnified out of proportion to its seriousness; tries to avoid or escape contact with the feared object or situation
May be unable to move, speak, or identify ways of decreasing anxiety or may begin running about aimlessly and shouting
Degree of discomfort may vary from mild anxiety to incapacitation.
May express a sensation of dread and a certain knowledge that death is at hand or may fear dying, going crazy, or doing something uncontrolled
May be preoccupied with bodily symptoms and feelings of terror
May experience brief periods of delusional thinking, hallucinations, inability to test reality.
May exhibit one of three types of phobias:
Agoraphobia: fears *any* situation where client may feel helpless or humiliated by frequent panic attacks, not only open places but any place where client can not readily escape from public view
Simple phobia: involves a specific object such as spiders or snakes or situations such as heights, darkness, or closed spaces

Social phobia: fears talking or writing in public and/or eating, blushing, or urinating; fears that these behaviors will result in public scorn. May avoid sexual involvement due to fear of arousal, particular sexual acts, and/or relationships.

Manipulates environment and depends on others to avoid confrontation with the object or situation

Some constriction of life activities is present.

No history of a physical disorder (e.g., hyperthyroidism, hypoglycemia). However, mitral valve prolapse may be present. May occur in conjunction with other disorders such as major depression, somatization disorder, or schizophrenia.

PHYSICAL EXAMINATION

Panic attacks are manifested by discrete periods of apprehension or fear. At least four of the following symptoms appear during each attack:

Shortness of breath (dyspnea), smothering sensations, choking, hyperventilation
Palpitations or tachycardia
Chest pain or discomfort
Sweating, hot flashes, or chills
Feelings of faintness, dizziness, or lightheadedness; trembling/shaking
Nausea/abdominal distress
Depersonalization or derealization
Paresthesias (numbness or tingling sensations)

DIAGNOSTIC STUDIES

Drug screen: Identify drugs that may be used by client to reduce anxiety or drugs that may produce symptoms.

Other diagnostic studies may be conducted to rule out physical disease as basis for individual symptoms, e.g., EKG for severe chest pain.

NURSING PRIORITIES

1. Provide for physical safety.
2. Assist client to recognize onset of anxiety.
3. Help client learn alternative responses.
4. Assist with desensitization to phobic object/situation.
5. Promote involvement of client/family in group/community support activities.

DISCHARGE CRITERIA

1. Stays in feared situation even when discomfort is experienced
2. Identifies techniques to lower/keep fear at manageable level
3. Confronts the phobia and is desensitized to the stimulus
4. Demonstrates greater independence and an increasingly freer lifestyle.

(Refer to CP: Generalized Anxiety Disorder for needs/concerns in addition to the following NDs.)

NURSING DIAGNOSIS:	**FEAR**
MAY BE RELATED TO:	**Unfounded morbid dread of a seemingly harmless object/situation, e.g., fear of being alone in public places, snakes, spiders, dark, heights (virtually any object/situation)**
POSSIBLY EVIDENCED BY:	**Physiologic symptoms, mental/cognitive behaviors indicative of panic**

	Withdrawal from or total avoidance of situations that place client in contact with feared object
CLIENT OUTCOMES/EVALUATION CRITERIA:	Acknowledges and discusses fears. Demonstrates understanding through use of effective coping behaviors and active participation in treatment regimen. Resumes normal life activities.

INTERVENTIONS	RATIONALE
Independent	
Encourage discussion of the phobia. Investigate sexual concerns, noting problems expressed, e.g., sex is a duty/obligation, which is not enjoyed by the client.	Only when a difficulty is acknowledged can it be dealt with. (Note: Phobic reaction to sex may indicate a problem of incest.)
Provide for client's safety, e.g., a secure environment, staying with the client, and letting the client know the nurse will provide for safety.	In severe anxiety, client fears total disintegration and loss of control.
Suggest that the client substitute positive thoughts for negative ones.	Emotion is hooked to thought and changing to a more positive one can decrease the level of anxiety experienced. This also gives the client an alternative way of looking at the problem.
Discuss the process of thinking about the feared object/situation before it occurs.	Anticipation of a future phobic reaction accelerates the physical manifestations of fear.
Encourage client to share the seemingly unnatural fears and feelings with others, especially nurse therapist.	Clients are often reluctant to share feelings for fear of ridicule and may have repeatedly been told to ignore feelings. Once the client begins to acknowledge and talk about these fears, it becomes apparent that the feelings are manageable.
Share own experience with client as indicated when relationship has been established.	If nurse therapist has successfully dealt with a phobia in own life, the client may be encouraged by the fact that someone has overcome a similar problem. Use judiciously to avoid meeting own needs rather than focusing on the client's needs.
Encourage to stop, wait, and not rush out of feared situation as soon as experienced. Support use of relaxation exercises.	Phobics fear "fear" itself. If client waits out the beginnings of anxiety and decreases it with relaxation exercises, then client may be ready to continue confronting the fear.
Explore things that may lower fear level and keep it manageable, e.g., use of singing while dressing, practicing positive self-talk while in a fearful situation.	Provides the client with a sense of control over the fear. Distracts the client so that fear is not totally focused on and allowed to escalate.
Use desensitization approach, e.g.:	Client fears disorganization and loss of control of body and mind when exposed to the fear-producing stimulus. This fear leads to an avoidance response, and reality is never tested. Gradual systematic exposure of the client to the feared situation under controlled conditions allows the client to begin to overcome the fear.

267

INTERVENTIONS	RATIONALE

Independent

Expose client to a predetermined list of anxiety-provoking stimuli graded in hierarchy from the least frightening to the most frightening;

Experiencing fear in progressively more challenging but attainable steps allows client to realize that dangerous consequences will not occur.

Pair each anxiety-producing stimulus with arousal of another affect of an opposite quality, strong enough to suppress anxiety, e.g., relaxation, exercise, biofeedback;

Helps client to achieve physical and mental relaxation as the anxiety becomes less uncomfortable.

Help client to learn how to use these techniques when confronting an actual anxiety-provoking situation. Provide for practice sessions (e.g., role play), deal with phobic reactions in real-life situations.

Phobic client needs continued confrontation to gain control over fear. Practice helps the body become accustomed to the feeling of relaxation, enabling the individual to handle feared object/situation.

Encourage client to set increasingly more difficult goals.

Develops confidence and movement toward improved functioning and independence.

Collaborative

Administer anti-anxiety medications as indicated, e.g., diazepam (Valium), chlordiazepoxide (Librium), alprazolam (Xanax), oxazepam (Serax), lorazepam (Ativan).

Biologic factors are thought to be involved in phobic/panic reactions, and these medications produce a rapid calming effect and may assist client to change behavior (particularly alprazolam) by keeping anxiety low during learning and desensitization sessions. Addictive tendencies of CNS depressants need to be weighed against benefit from the medication.

NURSING DIAGNOSIS:	**ANXIETY (SEVERE TO PANIC)**
MAY BE RELATED TO:	**Unidentified stressor(s)**
	Contact with feared object/situation
	Limitations placed on ritualistic behavior
POSSIBLY EVIDENCED BY:	**Attacks of immobilizing apprehension**
	Physical, mental, and cognitive behaviors indicative of panic
	Expressed feelings of terror and inability to cope
CLIENT OUTCOMES/EVALUATION CRITERIA:	**Verbalizes a reduction in anxiety to a manageable level. Demonstrates increasing tolerance to phobic object/situation without experiencing immobilizing attacks. Identifies and uses resources effectively.**

INTERVENTIONS	RATIONALE
Independent	
Establish and maintain a trusting relationship by listening to the client; displaying warmth, answering questions directly, offering unconditional acceptance; and being available and respecting the client's use of personal space.	Therapeutic skills need to be directed toward putting the client at ease because the nurse who is a stranger may pose a threat to the highly anxious client.
Be aware and in control of own feelings; explore the cause and use this understanding therapeutically.	The nurse's anxiety can be communicated to the client, which only adds to the client's sense of terror. Discussion of these feelings can provide a role model for the client and show a different way of dealing with them.
Support the client's defenses initially.	The client is using the defense in an attempt to deal with an unconscious conflict, and giving up the defense prematurely results in increased anxiety.
Verbally acknowledge the reality of the pain of the client's present coping mechanisms (panic) without focusing on the symptoms that are being expressed.	The symptoms that the client is using relieve some of the intolerable anxiety felt by the client. If client is unable to release this tension, the anxiety will only increase and client may lose control.
Provide feedback about behavior, stressors, and coping responses. Validate what you observe with the client.	Sets groundwork for dealing with anxiety when client is calmer. Includes client in plan of care, providing sense of control/self-worth.
Stress the relationship between physical and emotional health and reinforce that this is an area to be explored when client feels better.	Client needs to be aware of mind-body relationship and the physiologic changes that cause discomfort.
Observe for increasing anxiety. Assume a calm manner, decrease environmental stimulation, and provide temporary isolation, as indicated.	Early detection and intervention facilitates modifying client's behavior by changing the environment and the client's interaction with it to minimize the spread of anxiety.
Assist client/family to recognize and modify situations that cause anxiety when precipitating factor can be identified. (Note: Simple phobias are usually specific and object centered, not so with all phobic disorders.)	Recognition of causes/relationships provides opportunity to intervene before anxiety escalates/loss of control occurs.
Determine/discuss use of alcohol/other drugs.	May be used to reduce anxiety/avoid panic attacks and can lead to abuse. (Refer to Chap. 5, Psychoactive Substance Use Disorders.)
Be aware of diagnosis of mitral valve prolapse.	This cardiac abnormality affects between one-fourth and one-half of panic disorder clients. Heart palpitations resulting from the failure of the valves to close properly can increase anxiety and trigger panic attacks.
Note use of caffeine-containing beverages.	These clients may be more sensitive to the anxiety-producing effects of caffeine, which may precipitate panic/anxiety attacks.
Administer supportive physical measures, such as warm baths/whirlpool, massage.	Provides physical relaxation and helps client manage anxiety/maintain control.
Encourage interest in outside activity through the following actions:	Increases participation in life while decreasing the amount of time and energy available for maladaptive coping mechanisms.

269

INTERVENTIONS	RATIONALE

Independent

Share an activity with the client;	This is emotionally supportive and reinforces socially acceptable behavior.
Provide for physical exercise/activity of some type within client toleration;	Uses energy in constructive ways. Endorphins (the body's naturally produced "narcotics") induce feelings of wellness/euphoria and are thought to be released during exercise. (Note: One-half of clients have increased anxiety with exercise.)
Structure the client's day with a list of planned activities realistic to client's capabilities. Include others in client's care to provide support.	Provides opportunity to experience success, which enhances self-esteem and increases self-confidence.
Discuss side effects of medications, noting reactions that may occur, e.g., drowsiness, ataxia, confusion, headache, slurred speech, lethargy, giddiness, dizziness, vertigo, and impaired visual accommodation.	Side effects of anti-anxiety medications may cause concern/heighten anxiety and may require evaluation/treatment.

Collaborative

Administer medication as indicated (refer to ND: Fear):	Anti-anxiety drugs (especially alprazolam) provide relief from the immobilizing effects of anxiety and promote participation in ADLs and therapy program.
Monoamine-oxidase inhibitors (MAOIs), e.g., phenelzine sulfate (Nardil).	These drugs have been found to be effective in treating panic attacks. Side effects may be temporary, and caution needs to be exercised about food that should not be consumed while on these drugs.
Refer client/family to counseling, psychotherapy, or groups, as indicated.	May need additional assistance/long-term support to make lifestyle changes necessary to achieve maximum recovery.

Obsessive Compulsive Disorder

DSM III-R: 300.30 Obsessive compulsive disorder

An obsession is a repetitive thought that the individual is unable to control. A compulsion is an urge to perform an act that cannot be resisted without great difficulty.

ETIOLOGIC THEORIES

PSYCHODYNAMICS

Freud placed origin for obsessive-compulsive characteristics in the anal stage of development. The child is mastering bowel and bladder control at this developmental stage and derives pleasure from controlling own body and indirectly the actions of others.

Erikson's comparable stage is autonomy versus shame and doubt. The child learns that to be neat and tidy and to handle bodily wastes properly gains parental approval and to be messy brings criticism and rejection.

The obsessional character develops the art of the need to obtain approval by being excessively tidy and controlled. Frequently the parents' standards are too high for the child to meet, and the child continually is frustrated in attempts to please parents.

The defensive mechanisms used in obsessive-compulsive behaviors are unconscious attempts by the client to protect the self from internal anxiety. The greater the anxiety, the more time and energy will be tied up in the completion of the client's rituals. First, the client uses *regression*, a return to earlier methods of handling anxiety. Second, the obsessive thoughts are either devoid of feeling or are attached to anxiety. Thus *isolation* is utilized. Third, the client's overt attitude toward others is usually the opposite of the unconscious feelings. Thus *reaction formation* is being used. Last, compulsive rituals are a symbolic way of *undoing* or resolving the underlying conflict.

BIOLOGIC THEORIES

Although biologic and neurophysiologic influences in the etiology of anxiety disorders have been investigated, no relationship has yet been established. The mind-body connection is well accepted; however, it is difficult to establish whether the biologic changes cause anxiety or whether the emotional state causes physiologic manifestations.

FAMILY DYNAMICS

Refer to CP: Generalized Anxiety Disorder.

CLIENT ASSESSMENT DATA BASE

HISTORY

Most often seen in adolescence and early adulthood

Affects men as well as women equally

May be seen more frequently in upper-middle class and in individuals with higher levels of intellectual functioning

May be very controlled from within; have difficulty relaxing

Obsessive thoughts may be destructive or delusional.

May express belief that nonpurposeful and nondirected activity is unsafe and bad

Pleasurable activities cause anxiety.

Thinking processes are rigid, intellectual, and sharply focused toward tasks.

May focus on details but be unproductive in work situations because of narrow scope and rigidity of ideas

Often are poor problem-solvers

May exhibit difficulty in interpersonal relationships

Characteristic rituals that may be indulged in include dressing and undressing a number of times, placing articles in a specific order, repetitive hand-washing, and intensive cleanliness.

Ritualistic speech is often noted.

PHYSICAL EXAMINATION

Refer to CPs: Generalized Anxiety Disorder; Panic Disorder.

DIAGNOSTIC STUDIES

Refer to CPs: Generalized Anxiety Disorder; Panic Disorder.

NURSING PRIORITIES

1. Assist client to recognize onset of anxiety.
2. Explore the meaning and purpose of the behavior with the client.
3. Assist client to limit ritualistic behaviors.
4. Help client learn alternative responses to stress.
5. Encourage family participation in therapy program.

DISCHARGE CRITERIA

1. Anxiety is decreased to a manageable level.
2. Ritualistic behaviors are managed/minimized.
3. Environmental and interpersonal stress is decreased.
4. Client/family are involved in support group/community programs.
(Refer to CP: Generalized Anxiety Disorder for needs/concerns in addition to the following NDs.)

NURSING DIAGNOSIS:	**ANXIETY (SEVERE)**
MAY BE RELATED TO:	**Earlier life conflicts (may be reflected in the nature of the repetitive actions and recurring thoughts)**
POSSIBLY EVIDENCED BY:	**Repetitive action (e.g., hand-washing)**
	Recurring thoughts (e.g., dirt and germs)
	Decreased social and role functioning
CLIENT OUTCOMES/EVALUATION CRITERIA:	**Verbalizes understanding of significance of ritualistic behaviors and relationship to anxiety. Demonstrates ability to cope effectively with stressful situations without resorting to obsessive thoughts or compulsive behaviors.**

INTERVENTIONS	RATIONALE
Independent	
Establish relationship through use of empathy, warmth, and respect. Demonstrate interest in client as a person through use of attending behaviors.	Anything about which the client feels anxious will serve to increase the ritualistic behaviors. Establishing trust provides support and communicates that the

272

INTERVENTIONS

Independent

RATIONALE

nurse accepts the client as a person with the right to self-determination.

Acknowledge behavior without focusing attention on it. Verbalize empathy toward client's experience rather than disapproval or criticism. Better to say "I see you undress three times every morning. That must be tiring for you" rather than "Try to dress only one time today."

Ignoring ritualistic behaviors can result in diminishing them. As anxiety is reduced, the need for the behaviors is reduced. Reflecting the client's feelings may reduce the intensity of the ritualistic behavior.

Use a relaxed manner with the client; keep the environment calm.

Any attempts to decrease stress will help the client to feel less anxious, thus reducing the intensity of the ritualistic behaviors.

Assist client to learn stress management, e.g., relaxation exercises, imagery. Identify what the client perceives as relaxing, e.g., warm bath, music.

Stress management techniques can be used instead of ritualistic behaviors to break habitual pattern.

Engage in constructive activities such as quiet games that require concentration, as well as arts and crafts such as needlework, woodwork, ceramics, and painting.

Planned activities allow the client less time for compulsive behavior and serve to distract the client in a manner that allows creativity and positive feedback.

Give positive reinforcement for noncompulsive behavior. Avoid reinforcing compulsive behavior. Help significant other(s) learn the value of not focusing on the ritualistic behaviors.

This approach will prevent the client from obtaining secondary gains from the maladaptive behaviors.

Assist the client to find ways to set limits on own behaviors. At the same time allow adequate time during the daily routine for the ritual(s).

Encourages the client to problem-solve how to limit own behaviors while also recognizing that behaviors cannot be stopped by others or anxiety will be increased. If the time required for performing the rituals is not considered in planning care, then the client feels rushed and anxious in performing behaviors. A mistake is more likely to be made and the whole ritual will have to be started again, resulting in increased anxiety possibly to an unmanageable level.

Limit the amount of time allotted for the performance of rituals. Encourage client to gradually decrease this time.

Provides initial control of maladaptive behaviors until client is able to enforce own limits and substitute more adaptive response(s) to stress.

Encourage client to explore the meaning and purpose of behaviors; to describe the feelings when the behaviors occur, intensify, or are interrelated; and to examine the precipitating factors to the performance of the rituals.

This exploration provides an opportunity to begin to understand the process and gain control over the obsessive-compulsive sequence. Note: When opportunity for ritualistic behavior does not occur, the client fears that something bad will happen.

NURSING DIAGNOSIS:

SKIN/TISSUE INTEGRITY, IMPAIRMENT OF: POTENTIAL

MAY BE RELATED TO:

Repetitive behaviors related to cleansing, such as hand-washing, brushing teeth, showering

CLIENT OUTCOMES/EVALUATION CRITERIA:	Identifies risk factors. Verbalizes understanding of treatment/therapy regimen. Demonstrates behaviors/techniques to prevent skin/tissue breakdown.

INTERVENTIONS	RATIONALE

Independent

INTERVENTIONS	RATIONALE
Assess changes in skin/tissue, e.g., alterations in skin turgor, edema, dryness, altered circulation, and presence of infections.	Repetitive behaviors, such as hand-washing with detergents or cleaning with caustic substances, can damage the skin and underlying tissues.
Encourage use of mild soap and hand creams while using methods previously described in ND: Anxiety (severe) to decrease repetitive behaviors.	Helps to minimize tissue trauma until other forms of therapy reduce damaging behaviors.
Discuss measures client can take during/after cleaning behaviors, e.g., use of rubber gloves and application of antiseptic cream.	Protects skin and tissues in the presence of constant hand-washing, use of caustic substances.

Collaborative

INTERVENTIONS	RATIONALE
Administer anti-anxiety medications as indicated, e.g., clomiprimine (Anafranil).	Being used experimentally to decrease feelings of anxiety, reduce need for ritualistic behavior(s), and allow for learning of other methods of stress reduction.

Post-Traumatic Stress Disorder

DSM III-R: 309.89 Post-traumatic stress disorder, specify if delayed onset (onset of symptoms at least six months after the trauma)

ETIOLOGIC THEORIES

PSYCHODYNAMICS

The client's ego has experienced a severe trauma often perceived as a threat to physical integrity or self-concept. This results in severe anxiety, which is not controlled adequately by the ego and manifests in symptomatic behavior. Because the ego is vulnerable, the superego may become punitive and cause individual to assume guilt for traumatic occurrence; the id may assume dominance, resulting in impulsive, uncontrollable behavior.

BIOLOGIC THEORIES

Refer to CP: Generalized Anxiety Disorder.

FAMILY DYNAMICS

Refer to CP: Generalized Anxiety Disorder.

CLIENT ASSESSMENT DATA BASE

HISTORY

May present with various degrees of anxiety with symptoms lasting days, weeks, or months

May display cognitive disruptions and show difficulty concentrating and/or completing usual life tasks

May show excessive fearfulness of objects and/or situations in the environment that reminds the person of the trauma (e.g.: startle response to loud noises that sound like combat zone for someone who experienced combat trauma)

Persistent recollection/talk of the event, despite attempts to forget

Pain/physical discomfort of the injury may be exaggerated beyond expectation in relation to injury.

May show poor impulse control with unpredictable explosions of aggressive behavior or acting out of feelings (dudgeon).

May report sleep disturbances with recurrent intrusive dreams of the event, nightmares, and/or difficulty in falling asleep. (Note: Intrusive thoughts, flashbacks, and/or nightmares are the triad symptomatic of PTSD.)

May show social isolation or phobia with decreased responsiveness, psychic numbing, emotional detachment, and estrangement.

PHYSICAL EXAMINATION

Mental status examination: may reveal change in usual behavior, moody, pessimistic, brooding, irritable, a loss of self-confidence, depressed

Excessive autonomic arousal of the cardiovascular and/or respiratory system, e.g., excessive perspiration, hyperalertness, muscular tension, tremulousness, in addition to physical complaints noted in history.

(Note: a thorough physical examination should be done to rule out neurologic/organic problems. Occurrence of PTSD is often preceded or accompanied by physical illness/harm.)

DIAGNOSTIC STUDIES

Refer to CPs: Generalized Anxiety Disorder; Panic Disorders/(Phobias).

NURSING PRIORITIES

1. Provide safety for client/others.
2. Assist client to enhance self-esteem and regain sense of control over feelings/actions.

3. Encourage development of assertive, not aggressive behaviors.
4. Promote understanding that the outcome of the present situation can be significantly affected by own actions.
5. Assist client/family to learn healthy ways to deal with/realistically adapt to changes and events that have occurred.

DISCHARGE CRITERIA

1. Self-image is improved/enhanced.
2. Individual's feelings/reactions are acknowledged, expressed, and dealt with appropriately.
3. Physical complications are treated/minimized.
4. Appropriate changes in lifestyle are planned/made.

NURSING DIAGNOSIS:	**ANXIETY (SEVERE TO PANIC)/FEAR**
MAY BE RELATED TO:	**Current memory of past traumatic life event, such as natural disasters, accidental/deliberate man-made disasters and events such as rape, assault, or combat**
	Threat to self-concept/death, change in environment
	Negative self-talk (preoccupation with trauma)
POSSIBLY EVIDENCED BY:	**Increased tension/wariness**
	Sense of helplessness
	Apprehension, fearfulness, uncertainty/confusion, restlessness, increased tension
	Somatic complaints
	Sense of impending doom
	Fright, terror, panic, and/or withdrawal
	Sympathetic stimulation with cardiovascular excitement/palpitations, shortness of breath, diaphoresis, pupil dilation, nausea, diarrhea, etc.
CLIENT OUTCOMES/EVALUATION CRITERIA:	**Verbalizes awareness of feelings of anxiety/sense of control over fearful**

stimuli. **Identifies healthy ways to manage them. Demonstrates ability to confront situation using problem-solving skills. Reports/displays reduction of physiologic symptoms.**

INTERVENTIONS	RATIONALE
Independent	
Assess degree of anxiety/fear present, associated behaviors, and reality of threat perceived by client.	Identifies needs for developing plan of care/interventions. Need to clearly understand client's perception in order to provide appropriate assistance in overcoming the fear.
Develop trusting relationship with the client.	Trust is the basis of a therapeutic nurse/client relationship and enables them to work effectively together.
Identify whether incident has reactivated preexisting or coexisting situations (physical/psychologic).	Concerns/psychologic issues will be recycled every time trauma is reexperienced and affect how the patient views current situation.
Observe for and elicit information about physical injury and assess symptoms such as numbness, headache, tightness in chest, nausea, and pounding heart.	Physical injuries may have occurred during incident/panic of recurrence, which may be masked by anxiety of current situation. These need to be identified and differentiated from anxiety symptoms so appropriate treatment can be given.
Note presence of chronic pain or pain symptoms in excess of degree of physical injury.	Psychologic responses may enhance/exacerbate physical symptoms.
Evaluate social aspects of trauma/incident, e.g., disfigurement, chronic conditions, permanent disabilities.	Problems that occurred in the original trauma may have left visible reminders that have to be dealt with on a daily basis.
Identify psychologic responses, e.g., anger, shock, acute anxiety (panic), confusion, denial. Note laughter, crying, calm or agitation, excited (hysterical) behavior, expressions of disbelief and/or self-blame. Record emotional changes.	Although these are normal responses at the time of the trauma, they will recycle again and again until they are adequately dealt with.
Determine degree of disorganization.	Indicator of level of intervention that is required, e.g., may need to be hospitalized when disorganization is severe.
Note signs of increasing anxiety, e.g., silence, stuttering, inability to sit still/pacing.	May be indicative of inability to handle current happenings, e.g., feelings or therapy, suggesting need of more intensive evaluation/intervention.
Identify development of phobic reactions to ordinary articles, e.g., knives; situations, e.g., strangers ringing doorbell, walking in crowds of people; occurrences, e.g., car backfires.	These may trigger feelings from original trauma and need to be dealt with sensitively, accepting reality of feelings and stressing ability of client to handle them. (Refer to CP: Panic Disorder/(Phobias.)
Stay with client, maintaining a calm, confident manner. Speak in brief statements, using simple words.	Can help client to maintain control when anxiety is at a panic level.
Provide for nonthreatening, consistent environment/atmosphere.	Minimizes stimuli, reducing anxiety and calming the individual, and is helpful in breaking the cycle of anxiety/fear.

277

INTERVENTIONS	RATIONALE
Independent	
Gradually increase activities/involvement with others.	As anxiety (panic) level is decreased, client can begin to tolerate interaction with others. Activity further releases tension in an acceptable manner. (Refer to ND: Violence, potential: directed at self/others.)
Explore with client perception of what is causing anxiety.	Increases ability to connect symptoms to subjective feeling of anxiety, providing opportunity for client to gain insight/control and make desired changes.
Assist client to correct any distortions being experienced. Share perceptions with client.	Perceptions based on reality will assist to decrease fearfulness. How the nurse views the situation may help client to see it differently.
Assist client to identify feelings being experienced and focus on ways to cope with them.	Increases awareness of affective component of anxiety and ways to control and manage it.
Explore with client the manner in which the client has coped with anxious events before the trauma.	Helps client regain sense of control and recognize significance of trauma.
Engage client in learning new coping behaviors, e.g., progressive muscle relaxation, thought-stopping.	Replacing maladaptive behaviors can enhance ability to manage anxiety and deal with stress. Continuing to ruminate about the incident can retard recovery, while beginning to stop the obsessive thinking will help.
Give positive feedback when client demonstrates better ways to manage anxiety and is able to calmly and/or realistically appraise own situation.	Provides acknowledgment and reinforcement, encouraging use of new coping strategies. Enhances ability to deal with fearful feelings and gain control over situation, promoting future successes.
Collaborative	
Administer antianxiety/psychotropic medications as indicated: e.g.,	

benzodiazepines: diazepam (Valium), alprazolam (Xanax);
    propanediols: meprobamate (Equanil);
    antihistamines: hydroxyzine (Vistaril);
    barbiturates: phenobarbital (Luminal);
	Used to decrease anxiety, lift mood, aid in management of behavior, and ensure rest until client regains control of own self.

lithium carbonate (Eskalith);	Low-dose therapy may be used to reduce explosive behavior.
phenothiazines, chlorpromazine (Thorazine).	May be used for the reduction of psychotic symptoms when loss of contact with reality occurs.

NURSING DIAGNOSIS:	**POWERLESSNESS**
MAY BE RELATED TO:	**Being overwhelmed by symptoms of anxiety** **Lifestyle of helplessness/poor coping skills**

POSSIBLY EVIDENCED BY:	**Verbal expression of lack of control over present situation/future outcome**
	Reluctance to express true feelings
	Dependence on others
	Passivity and/or anger
	Nonparticipation in care or decision-making when opportunities are provided
CLIENT OUTCOMES/EVALUATION CRITERIA:	**Identifies areas over which individual has control. Expresses sense of control over present situation/future outcome. Demonstrates involvement in care and planning for the future.**

INTERVENTIONS	RATIONALE
Independent	
Identify present/past coping behaviors that are positive and reinforce use.	Awareness of past successes enhances self-confidence and increases options for current use, promoting a sense of control.
Note ethnic background, cultural/religious perceptions, and beliefs about the occurrence, e.g., retribution from God.	Sense of own responsibility (blame) and guilt about not having done something to prevent incident or not having been good enough to deserve surviving are strong beliefs in individuals, which are influenced by background and cultural factors.
Formulate plan of care with client, setting realistic goals for achievement.	Actively involves client, providing a measure of control over life situation.
Encourage client to identify factors under own control as well as those not within own ability to control.	Recognition of areas of control serves to decrease sense of helplessness. Confronting issues outside of client's control may encourage acceptance of that which cannot be changed.
Assist to identify when feelings of powerlessness and loss of control began.	Increases understanding of sources of stressful events that trigger these feelings.
Explore actions client can use during periods of stress, e.g., deep breathing, counting to ten, reviewing the situation.	Provides information to assist client with learning constructive ways to cope with feeling of powerlessness and to regain control.
Give positive feedback when client uses constructive methods to regain control.	Acknowledgment and reinforcement encourages repetition of desirable behaviors.
Promote involvement in group therapy.	Provides an opportunity for client to learn new coping behaviors from peers who have experienced similar traumatic events/reactions in the past.

279

NURSING DIAGNOSIS:	**VIOLENCE, POTENTIAL FOR: DIRECTED AT SELF/OTHERS**
MAY BE RELATED TO:	A startle reaction
	An intrusive memory of an event causing a sudden acting out of a feeling as if the event were occurring
	Use of alcohol/other drugs to ward off painful effects and produce psychic numbing
	Breaking through of rage that has been walled off
	Rage at the sense of helplessness/dependency or at those who were exempted from the trauma
	Response to intense anxiety or panic state and loss of control
POSSIBLE INDICATORS:	Vulnerable self-esteem
	Increased motor activity, pacing, excitement, irritability, agitation
	Increasing anxiety level
	Argumentative, dissatisfied, overreactive, hypersensitive, provocative behaviors
	Hostile, threatening verbalizations
	Overt and aggressive acts
	Goal-directed destruction of objects in environment
	Self-destructive behavior (including substance abuse) and/or active, aggressive suicidal/homicidal acts
CLIENT OUTCOMES/EVALUATION CRITERIA:	Verbalizes awareness of positive ways to cope with feelings. Demonstrates

self-control as evidenced by relaxed posture/manner, use of problem-solving rather than threats or assault-ive behavior to resolve conflicts and/or cope with anxiety.

INTERVENTIONS	RATIONALE
Independent	
Evaluate for presence of self-destructive and/or suicidal/homicidal behaviors, e.g., mood/behavior changes, increasing withdrawal. Assess seriousness of threat, e.g., gestures, previous attempts. (Use scale of 1–10 and prioritize according to severity of threat, availability of means.)	Client may be in such despair or esteem may be so low that behaviors may be engaged in that are violent towards self/others with conscious or unconscious wish for suicide. (Note: If scale is high, this may be #1 nursing priority.)
Encourage client to identify and verbalize triggering stimuli, causative/contributing factors that lead to po-tential or actual violence by client. Negotiate contract with client regarding actions to be taken when feeling out of control.	Client needs to learn to recognize what precipitates anger and tension. Early recognition and prompt inter-vention may prevent occurrence of violence. Contract-ing to let nurse/significant person know when feeling overwhelmed helps the client obtain assistance as needed and maintain a sense of control.
Assist client to understand that feelings of anger may be appropriate in the situation but need to be ex-pressed verbally or in an acceptable manner rather than acted upon in a destructive way.	Needs to learn to discharge anxiety and affect in a socially acceptable manner.
Tell the client to stop with any violent behaviors. Use environmental controls (such as providing a quiet place for client to go, holding the client) if behavior continues to escalate.	Saying "Stop" may be sufficient to assist client to re-gain control but external controls may be required if client is unable to call up internal controls. (Note: Phys-ical holding can provide a sense of contact and caring to help the client to regain control.)
Give client as much control as possible in other areas of life, helping to identify more appropriate solutions and responses to tension and anxiety.	Learning new ways of responding to impulsive ten-dencies increases capacity for controlling impulses.
Encourage exercise program; involve in outdoor edu-cation program.	Relieves tension and increases sense of well-being.
Collaborative	
Use seclusion or restraints until control is regained, as indicated.	Provides external control to prevent injury to client/staff/others.
Administer medications, as indicated. Refer to ND: Anxiety (severe to panic)/Fear.	Used to decrease anxiety, lift mood, and aid in man-agement of behavior/assist in regaining control of im-pulses.

NURSING DIAGNOSIS:	**COPING, INEFFECTIVE, INDIVIDUAL**
MAY BE RELATED TO:	**Personal vulnerability**
	Inadequate support systems

281

MAY BE RELATED TO—*continued*	Unrealistic perceptions
	Unmet expectations
	Inadequate coping method(s)
	Overwhelming threat to self
	Multiple stressors, repeated over period of time
POSSIBLY EVIDENCED BY:	Verbalization of inability to cope or difficulty asking for help
	Muscular tension/headaches
	Chronic worry
	Emotional tension
CLIENT OUTCOMES/EVALUATION CRITERIA:	Identifies ineffective coping behaviors and consequences. Verbalizes awareness of own coping abilities. Expresses feelings appropriately. Identifies options and uses resources effectively.

INTERVENTIONS	RATIONALE
Independent	
Assess degree of dysfunctional coping, including use/abuse of chemical substances.	Identifies needs/depth of interventions required. Individuals display different levels of dysfunctional behavior in response to stress, and often the choice of alcohol and/or other drugs is a way of deadening the psychic pain.
Be aware of and assist client to use ego strengths in a positive way and acknowledge ability to handle what is happening.	Often the firm statement of the nurse's conviction that the client can handle what is happening connects with the inner belief in self that is inherent in people.
Permit free expression of feelings at client's own pace. Do not rush client through expressions of feelings too quickly; avoid reassuring inappropriately.	Nonjudgmental listening to all feelings conveys acceptance of the worth of the client. Taking own time to talk about what has happened and allowing feelings to be fully expressed aids in the healing process. Client may believe pain and/or anguish is misunderstood if rushed. Statements such as "You don't understand, you weren't there" are a defense, a way of pushing others away.
Encourage client to become aware and accepting of own feelings and reactions when identified.	There are no bad feelings, and accepting them as signals that need to be attended to and dealt with can help the client move toward resolution.

INTERVENTIONS	RATIONALE

Independent

Give "permission" to express/deal with anger at the assailant/situation in acceptable ways.

Being free to express anger appropriately allows it to be dissipated so underlying feelings can be identified and dealt with, strengthening coping skills.

Keep discussion on practical and emotional level, rather than intellectualizing the experience.

When feelings (the experience) are intellectualized, uncomfortable insights and/or awareness are avoided by the use of rationalization, blocking resolution of feelings impairing coping abilities.

Identify supportive persons available for the client.

Having unconditional support from loving/caring others can assist the client to confront situation, cope with it, and move on to live more fully.

Collaborative

Provide for sensitive, trained counselors/therapists, and use therapies such as psychotherapy (in conjunction with medications), implosive therapy, flooding, hypnosis, relaxation, Rolfing, memory work, or cognitive restructuring.

While it is not necessary for the helping person to have experienced the same kind of trauma, sensitivity and listening skills are important to helping the client confront fears and learn new ways to cope with what has happened. Therapeutic use of desensitization techniques (flooding, implosive therapy) provides for extinction through exposure to the fear. Body work can alleviate muscle tension. Some techniques (Rolfing) help to bring blocked emotions to awareness as sensations of the traumatic event are reexperienced.

Refer to occupational therapy, vocational rehabilitation.

Assistance with new activities and learning new skills may be needed to help the client develop coping skills to reintegrate into the work setting. New activities/work skills, while generating some anxiety, will help with the process of desensitization and reduction/elimination of anxiety.

NURSING DIAGNOSIS: GRIEVING, DYSFUNCTIONAL

MAY BE RELATED TO: Actual/perceived object loss (loss of self as seen before the traumatic incident occurred, as well as other losses incurred in/after the incident)

Loss of physiopsychosocial well-being

Thwarted grieving response to a loss

Lack of resolution of previous grieving response

Absence of anticipatory grieving

POSSIBLY EVIDENCED BY: Verbal expression of distress at loss

POSSIBLY EVIDENCED BY—*continued*	Expression of unresolved issues
	Denial of loss; anger, sadness, crying; labile affect
	Alterations in eating habits, sleep and dream patterns, activity level, libido
	Reliving of past experiences
	Expression of guilt
	Difficulty in expressing loss
	Alterations in concentration and/or pursuit of tasks
CLIENT OUTCOMES/EVALUATION CRITERIA:	Demonstrates progress in dealing with stages of grief. Participates in work and self-care/activities of daily living as able. Verbalizes a sense of progress toward resolution of the grief and hope for the future.

INTERVENTIONS

Independent

Note verbal/nonverbal expressions of guilt or self-blame.

Acknowledge reality of feelings of guilt, and assist client to take steps toward resolution.

Assess signs/stage of grieving for self and/or others, e.g., denial, anger, bargaining, depression, acceptance.

Be aware of avoidance behaviors, e.g., anger, withdrawal.

Provide information about normalcy of feelings/actions in relation to stages of grief.

Give "permission" to be at this point, when the client is depressed.

Encourage verbalization without confrontation about realities.

RATIONALE

"Survivor's guilt" affects most people who have survived trauma in which others have died, and client questions, "Why was I spared?" or perhaps believes, "I am not worthy, and others may have been."

Acceptance of feelings and support of new coping skills allows for taking risk of new behaviors.

Identification and understanding of stages of grief assist with choice of interventions, plan of care, and movement toward resolution.

Client has avoided dealing with the feelings, leading to current situation. Recognition at this time can help with beginning new approach to solving the problem(s).

Individual may believe it is unacceptable to have these feelings, and knowing they are normal can provide sense of relief.

Provides opportunity for the client to accept self and feel satisfied with current progress.

Helps client to begin resolution and acceptance. Confrontation may convey lack of acceptance and impede progress.

INTERVENTIONS	RATIONALE

Independent

Identify cultural factors and ways individual has dealt with previous loss(es). Point out individual strengths/ positive coping skills.

Different cultures deal with loss in different ways, and it is important to allow client to deal with situation in own way. How the client has dealt with losses in the past can be a reliable predictor of how these losses are currently being dealt with and how they may be dealt with in the future, effectively or ineffectively. Client may discount own capabilities.

Reinforce use of previously effective coping skills.

Identification of helpful ways client is already dealing with problems allows client to feel positive about self.

Assist significant other(s) to cope with client response.

Support and understanding of reasons for client's behavior provides opportunity for family to work with client in development of new coping skills to resolve grief.

Collaborative

Refer to other resources, e.g., peer/support group, counseling, psychotherapy, spiritual.

May need additional help in order to resolve situation/ concomitant problems.

NURSING DIAGNOSIS:	**SLEEP PATTERN DISTURBANCE**
MAY BE RELATED TO:	**Psychologic stress (anxiety, depression with recurring disruptive dreams)**
POSSIBLY EVIDENCED BY:	**Verbal complaints of difficulty in falling asleep/not feeling well rested**
	Insomnia that causes awakening
	Reports of sleep disturbances, e.g., nightmares, dreams of personal death, disaster-related dreams, flashbacks, intrusive/trauma images, fear of reexperiencing the event
	Hypersomnia (as a way of avoiding behaviors, events, or situations that arouse recollections)
CLIENT OUTCOMES/EVALUATION CRITERIA:	**Verbalizes understanding of sleep disorder/problem. Identifies behaviors to promote sleep. Sleeping adequate/ appropriate number of hours for individual needs. Reports increased sense of well-being and feeling rested.**

INTERVENTIONS

Independent

Assess sleep pattern disturbance by observation and reports from client and/or significant others.

Identify causative and contributing factors, e.g., intrusive/repetitive thoughts, nightmares, severe anxiety level. Note use of caffeine and/or alcohol.

Provide a quiet environment; arrange to have uninterrupted sleep as much as possible.

Encourage client to develop behavior routine when insomnia is present, e.g., no napping after noon, having warm bath/milk before bed, relaxing thoughts, getting out of bed 10 minutes after awakening if unable to fall asleep again, limiting sleep to 7 hours each night.

Collaborative

Administer sedative, hypnotic, or anti-anxiety drugs as indicated. (Refer to ND: Anxiety (severe to panic)/Fear.)

RATIONALE

Subjective and objective information provides assessment of individual problems and direction for interventions.

These factors interfere with ability to fall asleep and with the REM cycle of sleep, affecting quality of rest.

Assists in establishing optimal sleep/rest routine.

Rituals assist in decreasing anxiety and fear of facing a sleepless night. (Note: Tryptophan in milk is believed to induce sleep.)

May require short-term drug therapy to decrease sense of exhaustion/fear and promote relaxation to enhance sleep. (These drugs should be used sparingly to avoid dependence and addiction.)

NURSING DIAGNOSIS:	SOCIAL ISOLATION/SOCIAL INTERACTION, IMPAIRED
MAY BE RELATED TO:	Difficulty in establishing and/or maintaining relationships with others
	Reduced involvement with the external world
	Numbing of responsiveness to the environment/affective numbing (which blocks relating to others)
	Feelings of guilt and shame/survivor's guilt
	Unacceptable social behaviors/values
POSSIBLY EVIDENCED BY:	Conflicts with family, significant others
	Withdrawal and avoidance of others/absence of supportive others
	Alcohol/drug abuse

Expressed feelings of rejection/alienation

Chronic loss of interest and energy for work and relationships

Sense of vulnerability over fear of loss of control of aggressive impulses

Sense of responsibility (guilt) for inciting event or failing to control it; rage at those exempted from loss or injury

Observed discomfort in social situations/use of unsuccessful social interaction behaviors

CLIENT OUTCOMES/EVALUATION CRITERIA:

Verbalizes recognition of causes of isolation. Acknowledges willingness to be more involved with others. Demonstrates involvement/participation in appropriate activities and programs.

INTERVENTIONS	RATIONALE
Independent	
Assess degree of isolation. Note withdrawn behavior and use of denial.	Indicates need for/choice of interventions. Withdrawing and denial can inhibit/sabotage participation in therapy.
Assess support systems available to client (e.g., family, friends, co-workers).	Involvement of significant others can help to build and/or reestablish support system and reintegrate client into a social network.
Acknowledge any positive efforts client makes in establishing contact with others.	Positive reinforcement of movement toward others can decrease sense of isolation and encourage repetition of behaviors enhancing socialization.
Collaborative	
Encourage client to continue and/or seek outside or outpatient therapy/peer group activities.	May need ongoing support, encouragement to reestablish social connections and develop/strengthen relationships.
Refer for employment counseling, if indicated. (Refer to ND: Coping, ineffective, individual.)	Interpersonal difficulties may have affected work relationships and performance, and client may need help to reintegrate into current job or relocate.

NURSING DIAGNOSIS: **FAMILY PROCESS: ALTERED**

MAY BE RELATED TO: **Situational crises**

POSSIBLY EVIDENCED BY:	Expressions of confusion about what to do and that they are having difficulty coping
	Family system does not meet physical/emotional/spiritual needs of its members
	Difficulty accepting/receiving help appropriately
	Not adapting to change or dealing with traumatic experience constructively
	Difficulty expressing individual and/or wide range of feelings
	Ineffective family decision-making process
FAMILY OUTCOMES/EVALUATION CRITERIA:	Expresses feelings freely and appropriately. Verbalizes understanding of trauma, treatment regimen, and prognosis. Demonstrates individual involvement in problem-solving processes directed at appropriate solutions for the situation.

INTERVENTIONS

Independent

Determine family members' understanding of client's illness/PSTD.

Identify patterns of communications in the family, e.g., Are feelings expressed clearly and freely? Do they talk to one another? Are problems resolved equitably? What are interactions among/between members?

Encourage family members to verbalize feelings (including anger) about client's behavior.

Acknowledge difficulties each member is experiencing while reinforcing that conflict is to be expected and can be used to promote growth.

RATIONALE

Family members/spouse often do not recognize that client's present behavior is the result of trauma that has occurred.

How family members communicate provides information about their ability to problem-solve, understand one another, cooperate in making decisions, and resolve problems resulting from trauma.

Spouse may feel angry/unloved and believe client is rejecting, rather than recognizing behaviors as a sign of client's pain.

Recognition of what the person is feeling/going through provides a sense of acceptance. Most people have the fantasy that once the conflict has been resolved, everything will be fine. Discussing conflict as an ongoing problem that can be resolved so all parties win can help family members begin to believe a new method of handling it can be learned.

INTERVENTIONS	RATIONALE

Independent

Identify and encourage use of previous successful coping behaviors.

In the stress of current situation, family members tend to focus on negative behaviors, feel hopeless, and neglect looking at positive behaviors used in the past.

Encourage use of stress management techniques, e.g., appropriate expression of feelings, relaxation exercises, guided imagery.

Reduction of stress enables individuals to begin to think more clearly/develop new behaviors to cope with client.

Provide educational information about PSTD and opportunity to ask questions/discuss concerns.

These materials can help family members learn more about client's condition and assist in resolution of current crisis.

Collaborative

Refer to other resources as indicated, e.g., support groups, clergy, psychologic counseling/family therapy.

Additional/ongoing support and/or therapy may be needed to help family resolve family crisis and look at potential for growth.

NURSING DIAGNOSIS:	SEXUAL DYSFUNCTION/SEXUALITY PATTERNS: ALTERED
MAY BE RELATED TO:	Biopsychosocial alteration of sexuality (stress of post-trauma response)
	Loss of sexual desire
	Impaired relationship with a significant other
POSSIBLY EVIDENCED BY:	Alterations in achieving sexual satisfaction/relationship with significant other
	Change of interest in self and others
	Irritation, lack of affection
	Preoccupation with self
CLIENT OUTCOMES/EVALUATION CRITERIA:	Verbalizes understanding of reasons for sexual problems/changes that have occurred. Identifies stresses involved in lifestyle that contribute to the dysfunction. Demonstrates improved communication and relationship skills. Participating in program designed to resume desired sexual activity.

INTERVENTIONS	RATIONALE

Independent

Inquire in a direct manner if there has been a change in sexual functioning/if problems exist, preferably in a conjoint session.

Client may prefer to dwell on reliving details of trauma and may not complain about this area of life. Spouse may not recognize relation of trauma to marital discord/sexual problems, and being with the client provides an opportunity for them to begin to talk realistically about what is happening. (Note: Men typically have loss of sexual desire and occasional impotence; women experience lack of sexual pleasure and anorgasmia.)

Determine intimate behavior/closeness between couple recently and in comparison to quality of sexual relationship before the trauma when appropriate.

May reveal problems that have not been acknowledged previously by the couple. Client may deny existence of difficulties, excusing self as being "sick," "needing time to recover from trauma."

Provide information about the effect anxiety and anger have on sexual desire/ability to perform.

When spouse/significant other does not know this, it is easy to feel unloved and not cared about or believe mate is having an affair. With understanding/insight into cause(s), spouse's anxiety may be relieved, and support and affection can be extended to the client.

Encourage expression of feelings openly and appropriately, as well as appropriate expression of emotions, e.g., crying.

Client/spouse may believe they are helping by being stoic and not expressing feelings of powerlessness, helplessness, fear, etc., to each other.

Help client who has been the victim of sexual assault to understand relationship of reluctance to have mate touch/make sexual advances to the event that occurred.

Client may have difficulty recognizing and feel embarrassed by the fact that mate's advances serve as reminder(s) of the trauma.

Discuss substance use and relationship to sexual difficulties.

Some clients use alcohol and other drugs to dull the pain of PSTD, and these substances interfere with sexual functioning, causing diminished desire, inability to achieve and maintain an erection. (Note: It is not known what effect chronic use of alcohol has on female sexual functioning.)

Review relaxation skills. (Refer to ND: Coping, ineffective Individual.)

Learning to relax assists with reduction of anxiety and allows client/spouse to focus on learning skills to regain sexual functioning.

Collaborative

Refer to other resources as indicated, e.g., sex therapist.

Specific techniques may be used to assist the couple in regaining comfort level/ability to engage in nongenital/genital activity and intimacy.

NURSING DIAGNOSIS:	**KNOWLEDGE DEFICIT [LEARNING NEED], (SPECIFY)**
MAY BE RELATED TO:	**Lack of exposure to/misinterpretation of information**
	Unfamiliarity with information resources

POSSIBLY EVIDENCED BY:	Lack of recall
	Statement of misconception
	Verbalization of the problem
	Inaccurate follow-through of instruction
	Inappropriate or exaggerated behaviors, e.g., hysterical, hostile, agitated, apathetic
CLIENT OUTCOMES/EVALUATION CRITERIA:	Participates in learning process. Assumes responsibility for own learning and begins to look for information/ask questions. Identifies stress situations and specific action(s) to deal with them. Initiates necessary lifestyle changes and participates in treatment regimen.

INTERVENTIONS	RATIONALE
Independent	
Provide information about what reactions client may expect and let client know these are common reactions. Phrase in neutral terms, e.g., ". . . may or may not happen."	Knowing what to expect can reduce anxiety and help the client in learning new behaviors to handle stressful feelings/situations. Having information about the commonality of experiences helps the individual feel less alone/strange, aiding in acceptance of these feelings.
Assist client to identify factors that may have created a vulnerable situation and that s/he may have power to change to protect self in the future. Avoid making value judgments.	Factors such as body stance, carelessness, and not paying attention to negative cues may provide opportunity for tragic consequences that could possibly have been avoided/minimized. However, any inference that client is responsible for the incident is not therapeutic.
Discuss contemplated changes in lifestyle and how they will contribute to recovery.	Client needs to be able to look at these changes, what will be accomplished and whether they are realistic.
Assist with learning stress management techniques.	Relaxation is a useful coping skill for dealing with stress of recurrent fears/stress response.
Discuss recognition of and ways to manage "anniversary reactions," letting client know normalcy of recurrence of thoughts and feelings at this time.	Planning ahead and knowing some skills to handle this time can help to avoid severe regression.
Collaborative	
Suggest support group for significant other(s).	Assists with understanding of and ways to deal with/help client.

INTERVENTIONS	RATIONALE
Collaborative	
Encourage psychiatric consultation/group participation.	Additional assistance may be required if client is overly violent or inconsolable or does not seem to be making an adjustment.
Refer to family/marital counseling if indicated.	Client problems affect others in family/relationships, and further counseling may help resolve issues of enabling behavior/communication problems.

CHAPTER 10
SOMATOFORM DISORDERS

Somatoform Disorders

DSM III-R: 300.81 Somatization disorder
300.11 Conversion disorder
307.80 Somatoform pain disorder
300.70 Hypochondriasis

This group of disorders is characterized by the expression of physical symptoms suggesting the presence of physiologic disorder, but for which there are no demonstrable organic findings or known pathologic mechanisms. There does exist, however, positive evidence, or a strong presumption, that the symptoms are linked to psychologic factors or conflicts.

ETIOLOGIC THEORIES

PSYCHODYNAMICS

It is thought that this disorder represents an unconscious transformation of internal conflicts into physical symptoms that can be explained in terms of the ego's ability to control the sensory and motor apparatus, which may have specific meaning for the client.

Dependency is common in individuals with somatoform disorders, and fixation in an earlier level of development may be evident.

Repression is the primary defense mechanism, as severe anxiety is repressed and manifested by the presence of physical symptoms.

BIOLOGIC FACTORS

Although biologic and neurophysiologic influences in the etiology of anxiety have been investigated, no relationship has yet been established. However, there does seem to be a genetic influence with a high family incidence.

The autonomic nervous system discharge that occurs in response to a frightening impulse and/or emotion is mediated by the limbic system, resulting in the peripheral effects of the autonomic nervous system seen in the presence of anxiety. These manifestations of anxiety may be related to physiologic abnormalities.

FAMILY DYNAMICS

The family contributes to these conditions by initiating, reinforcing, and perpetuating the behavior patterns. The children learn (overtly or covertly) that physical complaints are acceptable ways of coping with stress and obtaining attention, care, and gratification of dependency needs. The client may gain attention and meet these needs by overdramatization of the symptoms, with resultant overinvolvement of other family members in enmeshed patterns of behavior.

CLIENT ASSESSMENT DATA BASE

HISTORY

Somatization Disorder

Recurrent and multiple somatic complaints of several years' duration for which medical attention has been sought but that are apparently not caused by any physical disorder.
The disorder begins before age 30 and runs a chronic course.

Conversion Disorder

A loss of, or alteration in, physical functioning that suggests physical disorder, but for which no organic pathology can be determined. The most common conversion symptoms are those that suggest neurologic disease.

Somatoform Pain Disorder

The preoccupation with pain for a duration of at least six months. There is either an absence of organic pathology, or if present, the pain is grossly in excess of what would be expected from the physical findings.

Hypochondriasis

Unrealistic misinterpretation of physical signs or sensations as abnormal, leading to preoccupation with the fear or belief of having a serious disease.
Predisposing factors are largely unknown, although various particular past experiences may be linked to the specific disorders.
May be preceded by a physical disorder that provides a prototype for the symptoms (e.g., pseudoseizures in an individual with epilepsy)
History of a past experience with true organic disease, either personally or with a close family member, may predispose an individual to hypochondriasis.

General

These disorders are more common in women than in men.
Severe psychologic stress often precedes and exacerbates appearance of the physical symptoms.
Complaints of physical symptoms of several years' duration beginning before the age of 30
Misinterpretation of physical sensations/signs, leading to preoccupation with fear of having a serious disease
History of frequent visits to physicians (doctor-shopping) to obtain relief despite medical reassurance of absence of organic pathology
Evidence of anger and frustration toward physicians for "inability to determine cause of physical symptoms"
Report of behaviors associated with lower level of development (e.g., obvious secondary gain, such as unfulfilled dependency need, derived from sick role)
Evidence of a psychologic stressor in the individual's environment that preceded the onset or exacerbation of the physical symptom
Evidence that presence of the symptom alleviates or promotes avoidance of the psychologic conflict
Absence of emotional concern regarding the physical impairment or dysfunction ("la belle indifference")
History of severe organic disease in self or close family member
Excessive use of analgesics without relief from pain
Observed/reported impairment in social or occupational functioning as a result of preoccupation with physical complaints
May report psychosexual dysfunction (impotence; dyspareunia; sexual indifference); excessive dysmenorrhea

PHYSICAL EXAMINATION

Apparent loss or alteration in physical functioning that suggests neurologic disease. Examples include blindness, deafness, paralysis, anosmia, aphonia, seizures, and coordination disturbances.
Conversion symptoms: may represent endocrine malfunction, with symptoms such as vomiting and pseudocyesis (false pregnancy).

Vital signs: Heart and respiratory rates may be elevated if symptoms mimic those of cardiopulmonary disease (similar to those experienced during panic attack).

Mental Status Exam:

    Fearful; preoccupation with belief of having serious disease

    Depressed (may include suicidal ideations)

    Anxious (symptoms associated with moderate to severe level) or "la belle indifference" (lack of concern over loss of physical functioning)

    Communication patterns: ruminating about physical symptoms

Patterns of elimination: may be evidence of constipation or diarrhea

Eating/drinking patterns: may be manifested by anorexia/weight loss/dehydration or behaviors associated with excessive intake

DIAGNOSTIC STUDIES

Virtually any diagnostic procedure (including exploratory surgery) may be performed as deemed appropriate to rule out organic pathology in light of the physical symptom(s) presented by the client.

Urine and/or serum toxicology screen: to determine evidence of substance use/abuse

NURSING PRIORITIES

1. Control/minimize chronic pain.
2. Promote client safety.
3. Resolve potentially dysfunctional areas of client/family dynamics.
4. Promote independence in self-care activities.
5. Provide information and support for lifestyle changes necessary to prevent recurrence of physical symptom(s).

DISCHARGE CRITERIA

1. Relief from admitting physical symptom(s) is obtained.
2. Client/family recognizes relationship between psychologic stressors and onset/exacerbation of physical symptom(s).
3. Demonstrates stress management techniques that may be used in order to prevent the occurrence/exacerbation of the physical symptom(s).

NURSING DIAGNOSIS:	VIOLENCE, POTENTIAL FOR SELF-DIRECTED
MAY BE RELATED TO:	Depressed mood
	Feelings of powerlessness over physical condition
	Belief that s/he has a serious illness
	Hysterical response to chronic pain
POSSIBLE INDICATORS:	Statements regarding hopelessness for improvement of life situation
	Making direct or indirect statements indicating a desire to kill self

POSSIBLE INDICATORS—continued	Has suicide plan and the means to carry it out
	Putting business affairs in order; writing a will; giving away prized possessions
	Self-destructive behavior and/or active, aggressive suicidal acts
	History of previous suicide attempts
CLIENT OUTCOMES/EVALUATION CRITERIA:	Refrains from self-harm. Verbalizes need for change within dysfunctional system. Expresses feeling of hope for the future. Demonstrates control over life situation by meeting needs in an assertive manner.

INTERVENTIONS

Independent

Ask client direct questions regarding intent, plan, and availability of means for self-harm. Evaluate risk on a scale of 1–10.

Provide a safe environment and place potentially harmful objects, such as straps, belts, ties, sharp objects, glass items, and drugs, in a secured area.

Secure a verbal or written contract from client not to harm self and to seek help if suicidal ideations emerge.

Encourage verbalizations of honest feelings. Help client identify symbols of hope in own life through exploration and discussion.

Encourage client to express angry feelings within appropriate limits. Provide safe method of hostility release, e.g., pounding pillows. Help client to identify true source of anger and work on adaptive coping skills for use outside the hospital setting.

Collaborative

Administer anti-anxiety and/or antidepressant medication as indicated. (Refer to ND: Coping, ineffective individual.)

RATIONALE

Direct questions, if presented in a caring, concerned manner, provide the necessary information to assist the nurse in formulating an appropriate plan of care for the suicidal client. Determination of risk establishes level of concern/nursing priority.

Harmful objects should be removed to provide a safe environment and allow time for the client to develop internal controls to prevent impulsive gestures.

A contract allows the client to share in the responsibility for own safety. A degree of control is experienced, and the attitude of acceptance of the client as a worthwhile individual is conveyed.

Verbalization of feelings in a nonthreatening environment may help the client come to terms with unresolved issues and find reasons for wanting to continue living.

Depression and suicidal behaviors may be viewed as anger turned inward on the self. When this anger is verbalized in a nonthreatening environment, the client may resolve these feelings, regardless of the discomfort involved.

Anti-anxiety medications may provide needed relief from anxious feelings. Antidepressant medication may elevate the mood as it increases level of energy and decreases feelings of fatigue. Note: Potential for suicide increases as energy level improves.

NURSING DIAGNOSIS:	COMFORT, ALTERED: PAIN, CHRONIC
MAY BE RELATED TO:	Severe level of anxiety, repressed
	Low self-esteem
	Unmet dependency needs
	History of self or loved one having experienced a serious illness
	Fixation in earlier level of development
	Retarded ego development
	Inadequate coping skills
POSSIBLY EVIDENCED BY:	Multiple somatic complaints of several years duration
	Absence of physiologic evidence for physical symptoms
	Narcissistic tendencies, with total focus on self and physical symptoms
	History of seeking assistance from numerous health-care professionals
	Demanding behaviors
	Refusal to attend therapeutic activities
	Denial of correlation between physical symptoms and psychologic problems
CLIENT OUTCOMES/EVALUATION CRITERIA:	Verbalizes relief from physical complaints. Recognizes correlation between physical symptoms and psychologic problems. Demonstrates adaptive coping strategies in the face of stressful situations, discontinuing use of physical symptoms as a response.

CLIENT OUTCOMES/EVALUATION CRITERIA:	Verbalizes relief from pain. Acknowledges relationship between emotional problems and onset/exacerbation of pain. Demonstrates techniques to interrupt escalating anxiety/pain. Client/family cooperate in pain management program.

INTERVENTIONS	RATIONALE

Independent

Note and record the duration and intensity of the pain. Assess factors that precipitate the onset of pain.	The correlation of these factors provides client with information to become aware of cause/effect relationship and to gain control of outcome.
Convey to client your belief that the pain is indeed real, even though no organic pathology can be found.	Denying or belittling the client's feelings is nontherapeutic and interferes in the development of a trusting relationship.
Provide nursing comfort measures with a matter-of-fact approach that does not provide added attention to the pain behavior (e.g. backrub, warm bath, heating pad).	May serve to provide some temporary relief of pain for the client. Secondary gains from solicitious behavior may provide positive reinforcement and can actually prolong use of maladaptive behaviors.
Assist client with activities that distract from focus on self and pain. Use these distractors to facilitate initiation of discussion of unresolved psychological issues, e.g., open expression of feelings such as guilt, fear about life events.	Helps the client to focus on adaptive behavior patterns and serves as a transition to higher levels of therapy. Unresolved psychologic issues must be dealt with before maladaptive patterns can be eliminated.
Help client connect times of onset/exacerbation of pain to times of increased anxiety. Identify specific situations that cause anxiety to rise, and demonstrate techniques to interrupt the pain response, e.g., visual or auditory distractions, guided imagery, breathing exercises, massage, application of heat or cold, relaxation techniques.	Client ability to connect pain to times of increased anxiety helps to decrease denial and is the first step in resolution of the problem. Use of techniques described may help to maintain anxiety at manageable level and prevent the pain from becoming disabling.
Provide positive reinforcement for times when client is not focusing on pain.	Positive reinforcement, in the form of the nurse's presence and attention, may encourage a continuation of these more adaptive behaviors by the client.

Collaborative

Review ongoing assessments by physician and laboratory and other diagnostic results. Observe and report any new or different pattern of pain behavior to physician.	The possibility of organic pathology needs to be continually ruled out.
Administer pain medication as indicated.	Short-term use may be necessary when pain is severe and other measures do not provide adequate relief.
Refer to chronic pain clinic.	May be helpful to learn ways to manage pain on a long-term basis.

NURSING DIAGNOSIS:	COPING, INEFFECTIVE INDIVIDUAL
MAY BE RELATED TO:	Severe level of anxiety, repressed
	Low self-esteem
	Unmet dependency needs
	History of self or loved one having experienced a serious illness
	Fixation in earlier level of development
	Retarded ego development
	Inadequate coping skills
POSSIBLY EVIDENCED BY:	Multiple somatic complaints of several years duration
	Absence of physiologic evidence for physical symptoms
	Narcissistic tendencies, with total focus on self and physical symptoms
	History of "doctor-shopping"
	Demanding behaviors
	Refusal to attend therapeutic activities
	Denial of correlation between physical symptoms and psychologic problems
CLIENT OUTCOMES/EVALUATION CRITERIA:	Verbalizes relief from physical complaints. Recognizes correlation between physical symptoms and psychologic problems. Demonstrates adaptive coping strategies in the face of stressful situations, discontinuing use of physical symptoms as a response.

INTERVENTIONS

Independent

Review laboratory and diagnostic results with the client in simple, easy-to-understand terminology. Answer any questions that may have arisen from discussions with the physician.

Show unconditional positive regard. Convey that you understand the symptom is real to the client, even though no organic pathology can be found.

Be available to assist the client with basic dependency needs in the initial stages of the relationship. Recognize, however, that the client may be using the physical condition to preserve the dependency role.

Gradually decrease response to time and assistance requested by the client as the trusting relationship is established. Encourage independent behaviors and respond with positive reinforcement.

Encourage client to verbalize fears and anxieties. Withdraw attention if rumination about physical symptoms begins.

Help client correlate appearance of physical symptoms with times of stress through exploration of past experiences.

Discuss possible alternative coping behaviors client may use in response to stress (e.g., relaxation techniques, deep breathing, physical activities, such as jogging, aerobics, brisk walks, housekeeping chores, sex). Offer positive reinforcement for use of these alternatives.

Report/investigate any new physical complaint.

Collaborative

Administer anti-anxiety medication, e.g., diazepam (Valium), chlordiazepoxide (Librium), alprazolam (Xanax), as indicated.

RATIONALE

Client has the right to knowledge about own care. Honest explanation may help client to understand psychologic implications. Anxiety is high, so learning is difficult, thus explanations need to be kept simple and concrete.

Denial of the client's feelings is nontherapeutic and interferes with establishment of a trusting nurse/client relationship.

To deny client this need at this time would result in an increased anxiety level and intensification of maladaptive behaviors.

Positive reinforcement enhances self-esteem and encourages repetition of desirable behaviors. Doing things for oneself helps to develop independence and improves coping ability.

Verbalization of feelings with a trusted individual may help client come to terms with unresolved issues. Lack of response to maladaptive behaviors may discourage their repetition.

Until denial defense is eliminated, change required for improvement will not occur.

Because of high level of anxiety, client may require assistance in problem-solving and the ability to recognize available alternatives. Positive reinforcement enhances self-esteem and encourages repetition of desirable coping behaviors.

Although physical symptoms have been used as a way of coping by the client, the possibility of organic pathology must always be considered to prevent jeopardizing client safety.

Anti-anxiety medications have a calming effect on the patient, masking the feelings of anxiety, which may minimize physical response.

NURSING DIAGNOSIS:	**SELF-CONCEPT, DISTURBANCE IN: BODY IMAGE**
MAY BE RELATED TO:	**Severe level of anxiety, repressed**
	Low self-esteem
	Unmet dependency needs

POSSIBLY EVIDENCED BY:	Negative feelings about body
	Preoccupation with real or imagined change in bodily structure and/or function
	Verbalizations about physical appearance that are out of proportion to any actual physical abnormality that may exist
	Fear of negative reaction or rejection by others
	Change in social involvement
CLIENT OUTCOMES/EVALUATION CRITERIA:	Verbalizes realistic perception of bodily structure and/or function. Expresses positive feelings about body. Functions independently and interacts socially without experiencing discomfort.

INTERVENTIONS

Independent

Obtain accurate assessment of client's perception of own body image. Recognize that disability is real to the client, even in the absence of evidence of organic pathology.

Encourage and give positive feedback for independent self-care behaviors, while gradually withdrawing attention from dependent behaviors.

Help client to see that image is distorted and out-of-proportion to reality of actual change in structure and/or function.

Assist client to recognize normal feelings associated with the grieving process and offer support as the client progresses toward acceptance of change in self.

Explore with client stressful life situations that may have symbolic correlation to the loss when the loss of function has no organic etiology, e.g., blindness in response to witnessing a traumatic event; aphonia in response to inner conflict associated with verbal expression of rage.

Encourage verbalization of fears and anxieties associated with identified stressful life situations. Discuss

RATIONALE

Information about the way in which the individual views self aids in developing accurate plan of care. Denial of client's feelings is nontherapeutic and impedes the development of trust.

Lack of attention to maladaptive behaviors discourages their repetition. Positive reinforcement enhances self-esteem and promotes repetition of desirable behaviors.

Recognition that a misperception exists is necessary before client can accept reality and reduce significance of impairment.

May need to deal with actual loss/impairment as well as problematic behavior. Progress through the grieving process is facilitated by client's recognition of feelings as acceptable and own ability to acknowledge ownership of those feelings.

If improvement is to occur, client needs to recognize and accept that there is a relationship between the loss of function and anxiety associated with stressful life situations. Denial of psychologic implications impedes positive change.

Verbalization of feelings with a trusted individual may help the client come to terms with unresolved issues.

301

INTERVENTIONS

Independent

ways in which client may respond more adaptively in the future.

Involve family/S.O. (s) in treatment plan, assisting them to understand underlying reasons for client's behavior.

RATIONALE

A plan of action formulated with assistance and at a time when anxiety is low may prevent later dysfunctional response by client.

Having understanding support from significant other(s) can help client to accept reality of situation and make required changes.

NURSING DIAGNOSIS:	SELF-CARE DEFICIT: (SPECIFY)
MAY BE RELATED TO:	Paralysis of body part
	Inability to see, hear, speak
	Pain, discomfort
POSSIBLY EVIDENCED BY:	Inability to bring food from a receptacle to the mouth; obtain or get to water sources; wash body or body parts; regulate temperature or flow of water
	Impaired ability to put on or take off necessary items of clothing, obtain or replace articles of clothing, fasten clothing, maintain appearance at a satisfactory level
	Unable to get to toilet or commode (impaired mobility); manipulate clothing for toileting; flush toilet or empty commode; sit on or rise from toilet or commode; carry out proper toilet hygiene
CLIENT OUTCOMES/EVALUATION CRITERIA:	Feeds, dresses, and grooms self without assistance. Maintains optimal level of personal hygiene by bathing as indicated and carrying out essential toileting procedures without assistance.

INTERVENTIONS

Independent

Assess degree of impairment; note level of disability as well as areas of strength.

RATIONALE

Establishes client needs as well as identifying individual potentials.

INTERVENTIONS	RATIONALE

Independent

Encourage client to perform ADL to own level of ability. Intervene only when client is unable to perform.

Loss of function may be related to unfulfilled dependency needs. Intervening when client is capable of performing independently serves to foster dependency in the client.

Convey a nonjudgmental attitude as nursing assistance with self-care activities is provided. Remember that the physical symptom is real to the client and is not within the client's conscious control.

A judgmental attitude interferes with the nurse's ability to provide therapeutic care for the client, provoking defensiveness that blocks client's willingness to look at own behavior/dynamics.

Provide positive reinforcement for ADL performed independently.

Positive reinforcement enhances self-esteem and encourages repetition of desirable behaviors.

Encourage client to discuss feelings regarding the disability and the need for dependency it creates. Help the client to see the purpose this disability is serving.

Self-disclosure and exploration of feelings with a trusted individual may help client fulfill unmet needs and come to terms with unresolved issues, thus eliminating the need for maladaptive physical responses.

Involve family in care at level of their ability/willingness.

Feelings of anger toward the client may interfere with ability to provide care in a therapeutic/nonjudgmental manner.

Collaborative

Refer to occupational/physical therapy, community resources/supports.

Involvement with these programs enhances client's self-esteem, promoting ability to care for self.

NURSING DIAGNOSIS:	SLEEP PATTERN DISTURBANCE
MAY BE RELATED TO:	**Severe level of anxiety, repressed**
	Fears associated with malfunction of body systems
	Preoccupation with physical symptoms
	Chronic pain
POSSIBLY EVIDENCED BY:	**Verbalizations of difficulty falling asleep**
	Verbal complaints of not feeling well rested
	Observed/reported wakefulness during the night
	Verbalizations of inability to sleep
	Dark circles under eyes

POSSIBLY EVIDENCED BY—*continued*	Lethargy
CLIENT OUTCOMES/EVALUATION CRITERIA:	**Reports 6–8 hours of uninterrupted sleep each night. Falls asleep within 30 minutes of retiring without the use of medication. Verbalizes feeling of being rested.**

INTERVENTIONS	RATIONALE

Independent

Observe sleep patterns closely and keep accurate records. Compare observations with client's perceptions of how sleep has been.	Even though client appears to be sleeping, if REM sleep is not achieved, client will not feel rested. Identifies need for intervention and helps in formulation of an appropriate plan of care.
Discourage excessive sleep during the day, and encourage establishment of a routine pattern of sleep and activity.	Ritualistic patterns and a realistic balance of activity and rest promote achievement of adequate sleep.
Identify individual activities to use prior to retiring, e.g., warm baths, massage, warm/nonstimulating drinks or reduction of fluid intake, light snacks.	These measures induce relaxation, promote inducement of sleep, and decrease interruptions of sleep.
Limit client's intake of caffeinated drinks, such as tea, coffee, and colas.	Caffeine is a CNS stimulant and may interfere with the client's achievement of rest and sleep.
Discourage client's participation in stimulating activities and discussion of fears and anxieties associated with physical symptoms just prior to hour of sleep.	These activities may agitate the client and increase anxiety to a level that interferes with achievement of sleep and rest.

Collaborative

Administer sedative medications at bedtime, as indicated, e.g., triazolam (Halcion).	These medications assist client to achieve sleep until normal sleep pattern is restored. Sedatives should not be used for longer than a 3-week period, as they eventually interfere with/rather than promote sleep.
Administer anti-anxiety and narcotic analgesic medications judiciously, and as deemed necessary, during the daytime hours. May give dose at hs.	These medications have sedative side effects that may induce sleep during the day and interfere with client's sleep at night. Pain transmission centers in the brain are close to the sleep center and may interfere with attainment of sleep.

NURSING DIAGNOSIS:	SOCIAL ISOLATION
MAY BE RELATED TO:	**Severe level of anxiety**
	Low self-esteem
	Fixation in lower level of development
	Preoccupation with self and physical symptoms

POSSIBLY EVIDENCED BY:	Chronic pain
	Fear of having a serious illness
	Rejection by others due to focus on self/physical symptoms
	Sad, dull affect
	Absence of supportive significant other(s)—family, friends, social contacts
	Uncommunicative, withdrawn; no eye contact
	Preoccupation with own thoughts; repetitive verbalization about self/physical symptoms
	Seeking to be alone
CLIENT OUTCOMES/EVALUATION CRITERIA:	Voluntarily spends time with others in group activities. Interacts with others without apparent discomfort. Demonstrates interest in others, while discontinuing use of statements that focus on self/physical symptoms.

INTERVENTIONS	RATIONALE
Independent	
Spend time with client after setting limits on attention-seeking behaviors. Withdraw presence if ruminations about physical symptoms begin.	The nurse's presence conveys a sense of worthwhileness to the client. Lack of reinforcement of maladaptive behaviors may help to decrease their repetition.
Increase amount of time/attention given during times when client is not focusing on physical symptoms.	This separates the person from the behavior and increases feelings of self-worth as unconditional acceptance is experienced by the client without need for the physical symptoms.
Objectively describe client's interpersonal behaviors and how the focus on self/physical symptoms discourages relationships with others.	Client may not realize how own behavior is perceived by others/results in alienation.
Assist client in learning assertiveness techniques, especially the ability to recognize the difference between passive, assertive, and aggressive behaviors and the importance of respecting the human rights of others while protecting one's own basic human rights.	Use of these techniques enhances self-esteem and facilitates communication and mutual acceptance in interpersonal relationships.

305

INTERVENTIONS

Independent

Encourage attendance in group activities after client is interacting appropriately in the 1:1 relationship. Accompany the client the first few times.

Provide positive feedback for any attempts at social interaction in which the client's focus is on others rather than self/physical symptoms.

RATIONALE

As a trusted individual, the nurse provides objective feedback about client's behavior in the group. Subsequent discussion and role play on a 1:1 basis may help prepare client for future group encounters and may promote success with this endeavor.

Positive feedback enhances self-esteem and encourages repetition of desirable behaviors.

NURSING DIAGNOSIS:	**KNOWLEDGE DEFICIT [LEARNING NEED] (SPECIFY)**
MAY BE RELATED TO:	**Strong denial defense system**
	Severe level of anxiety, repressed
	Preoccupation with self and pain
	Lack of interest in learning
POSSIBLY EVIDENCED BY:	**Verbalization of denial statements, such as, "I don't know why the doctor put me on the psychiatric unit. I have a physical problem."**
	History of "doctor-shopping" for evidence of organic pathology to substantiate physical symptoms
	Lack of follow-through with psychiatric treatment plan
CLIENT OUTCOMES/EVALUATION CRITERIA:	**Verbalizes understanding of psychologic implications of physical symptoms. Reports relief from physical symptoms. Demonstrates more appropriate coping mechanisms to employ in response to stress.**

INTERVENTIONS

Independent

Assess client's level of knowledge regarding effects of psychologic problems on the body. Be aware of degree to which denial defense controls client's behavior.

RATIONALE

Knowing what information the individual already has provides a base that is necessary to develop an effective plan of care for the client. Strong denial system needs to be penetrated before learning can begin.

INTERVENTIONS

Independent

Assess client's level of anxiety and readiness to learn.

Explain purpose and review results of laboratory and diagnostic testing, as well as aspects of the physical examination.

Have client keep two separate records: (1) a diary of the appearance, duration, and intensity of physical symptoms, and (2) documentation of situations that the client finds especially stressful.

Help client identify needs that are being met through the sick role (e.g., dependency needs, attention-seeking, and cover-up for painful conflicts in life situation). Help client recognize and accept more adaptive means for fulfilling these needs. Practice through role-playing.

Demonstrate/encourage use of adaptive methods of stress management, e.g., relaxation techniques, physical exercises, meditation, breathing exercises, autogenics.

Collaborative

Consult with occupational/recreational therapists to establish a treatment plan for the client to learn adaptive coping mechanisms.

Encourage participation in outdoor education program.

RATIONALE

Learning does not take place when level of anxiety is moderate to severe.

Client has basic right to knowledge about care. Objective knowledge about physical condition may help to break through the strong denial defense.

Comparison of these records may provide objective data from which to observe the relationship between physical symptoms and stress.

Client usually does not realize that the physical symptoms are fulfilling unmet needs. Recognition needs to be achieved before change can occur. Role-playing can relieve anxiety by helping client anticipate responses to stressful situations.

These techniques may be employed in an attempt to relieve anxiety and discourage the use of physical symptoms as a maladaptive response.

Can provide specialized techniques for coping with stress (e.g., decision-making, problem-solving, housekeeping, art therapy, plant therapy, bowling, volleyball, weight-lifting).

Involvement in activities that challenge physical and psychologic abilities can help the client learn to become more self-aware and confident and increase self-esteem.

NURSING DIAGNOSIS:	SEXUAL DYSFUNCTION [ACTUAL/POTENTIAL]
MAY BE RELATED TO:	Severe level of anxiety, repressed
	Low self-esteem
	Perceived or actual loss of bodily structure or function
	Preoccupation with physical symptoms
	Total focus on self/chronic pain response
	Fear of contracting a serious disease

POSSIBLY EVIDENCED BY:	Complaints of alterations in achieving perceived sex role
	Sexual indifference
	Lack of pleasure during intercourse
	Pain during intercourse (dyspareunia)
	Inability to achieve or maintain erection
	Desire to achieve greater satisfaction in sexual role
CLIENT OUTCOMES/EVALUATION CRITERIA:	Verbalizes achievement of sexual functioning at a desired level. Demonstrates techniques to control stresses in current lifestyle that may contribute to dysfunction.

INTERVENTIONS	RATIONALE
Independent	
Obtain sexual history, including previous pattern of functioning and client's perception of current problem.	Identifies individual problem(s) in order to develop an appropriate plan of care for the client.
Determine pattern of drug use, including type, amount, and frequency of use.	Certain types of drugs can interfere with sexual functioning, e.g., alcohol, tranquilizers, narcotics, antihypertensives, antidepressants.
Identify stressors in client's life. Explore correlation of stressful situations to onset of sexual dysfunction.	Recognition and acceptance of psychologic implications (progression beyond the denial defense) need to occur before positive change can be effected.
Be aware of pathophysiology that could negatively affect sexual functioning, e.g., hypertension, diabetes.	Organic pathology as an etiologic factor needs to be considered in the problem-solving when setting goals and identifying appropriate interventions.
Provide education regarding sexual functioning and alternative methods of fulfillment, as client indicates need and desire for this type of information.	Client may have misinformation about normal bodily functioning that may interfere with sexual fulfillment. Alternative methods may help to meet a need until desired level of functioning is attained.
Include significant other in as many sessions as seems appropriate and is possible.	Input from client's sexual partner will have a significant influence on client's progress. The couple should be treated as a unit. An absence of mutual trust and unwillingness to discuss each other's needs interferes with the goals of remediation.
Collaborative	
Refer to appropriate resources, such as clinical specialist, professional sex therapist, or family counselor.	May require individuals with a greater degree of knowledge and expertise in this specialty area to achieve resolution of persistent problem(s).

CHAPTER 11
DISSOCIATIVE DISORDERS

Multiple Personality; Dissociative Disorders

DSM III-R: 300.14 Multiple personality disorder
300.13 Psychogenic fugue
300.12 Psychogenic amnesia
300.60 Depersonalization disorder
300.15 Dissociative disorder NOS

ETIOLOGIC THEORIES

PSYCHODYNAMICS

The essential feature of dissociative disorders is an alteration in the normally integrative functions of consciousness, identity, or memory, which may be sudden or gradual and transient or chronic. Part of the individual's life is blocked off from consciousness during periods of intolerable stress. The stressful emotion becomes a separate entity, as the individual "splits" from it and mentally drifts into a fantasy state. Intrapsychic conflict thus uses denial and "ego-splitting" to decrease anxiety.

BIOLOGIC THEORIES

Research on the bases of these disorders is increasing as more recognition of the mind-body connection is accepted. It is difficult to determine whether the biologic changes that accompany severe anxiety precede or precipitate the emotional state. Biochemical, physiologic, and endocrine systems have an intimate connection with actual physical changes occurring in all body systems via the autonomic nervous system. Some studies have shown EEG abnormalities that have been associated with cerebral mechanisms in the temporal and limbic regions of the brain, which mediate identity formation and a sense of personal boundaries and may affect development of gender and generation boundaries.

FAMILY DYNAMICS

Systems theory sees the family as a system in which the process (interaction between members of the family) is the prime determinant. Level of differentiation and level of anxiety determine the degree of pathology.

Psychosocial theory states that individuals who develop dissociative disorders have often experienced severe physical, sexual, and/or emotional abuse early in life, stress so severe that the only way to cope with the painful emotions is to detach from them. The child learns to respond to stressful situations in this manner. One parent may be abusive, with the other being a passive participant, not taking care of the child. Psychiatric diagnoses (especially alcoholism) in close relatives is common, although multiple personality diagnosis is not. Certain

309

behaviors observed in childhood, while considered normal, may be identified as dissociative, including construction of imaginary playmates, use of different names or ages for themselves, taking on the role of an animal, imagining themselves as having been adopted or coming from another family, separation from the past, gender confusion, and regressive behavior. Responding to stressful situations with dissociative behaviors then becomes a method of coping for some individuals into adulthood, when there is less control over the dissociative states. The response becomes maladaptive in that the individual escapes from the stressful situation rather than facing it.

CLIENT ASSESSMENT DATA BASE

HISTORY

Age of onset is early childhood, although the disorder is most often not diagnosed until the third decade. Seldom diagnosed upon initial clinical contact (accurate diagnosis may be delayed by a period of months to years).

Multiple Personality

More common in women than in men, in persons with some higher education, and in white-collar workers. Presence of two or more distinct personalities within the individual. Each personality may be a fully integrated, complex unit with unique memories, behaviors, and relationships or may be a personality state that does not have as wide a range of patterns. Transition from one personality to another is sudden, often associated with psychosocial stress.

Alternate personalities within one individual may range in number from 1 to 60, with a mean of approximately 13. Most commonly, alternate personalities are children, although personalities stated to be older than the individual are not uncommon. Opposite gender personalities are also common. Alternate personalities vary in their awareness of others. Fugue states or memory lapses represent a lack of awareness in the presenting personality.

May exhibit symptoms more frequently seen in psychosis.

Other Dissociative Disorders, Such as Psychogenic Fugue/Amnesia and Depersonalization

Typically brief episodes, with recovery occurring quickly and recurrence uncommon.

PHYSICAL EXAMINATION

Meticulous initial physical assessment necessary to rule out organic causes of the dissociative symptoms.

Usually present with symptoms related to depression (> 90 percent), in order of occurrence, followed by mood swings, suicidal feelings/behaviors, insomnia, amnesia, sexual dysfunction, conversion symptoms, fugue states, panic, depersonalization, and substance abuse (50 percent). If questioned, the client will likely admit to memory lapses.

DIAGNOSTIC STUDIES

Evaluations to rule out an underlying or concurrent disease process are based on individual symptoms.

Neurologic testing, for example, EEG, CT scan, and MRI, to rule out organic brain conditions related to trauma, tumor, congenital defects, and temporal lobe epilepsy, symptoms of which often parallel manifestations of multiple personality disorder.

Psychosocial assessment, such as Rorschach, Thematic Apperception Test (TAT), Minnesota Multiphasic Personality Inventory (MMPI), WAIS, and hypnosis or pentothal interviews as indicated, as these clients are frequently misdiagnosed initially because of blurring of symptoms that parallel other psychiatric problems, commonly, depression, neuroses, personality disorders, and schizophrenia. Behavioral observation and documentation describing the character, duration, frequencing, and precipitation of behavioral changes and client comments or complaints are essential to the diagnostic process.

Drug screen: Assess for concomitant substance use.

NURSING PRIORITIES

1. Assist client to recognize anxiety.
2. Provide safe environment; protect client/others from injury.
3. Promote insight into relationship between anxiety and development of other personalities.
4. Support client/family in developing effective coping skills and participating in therapeutic activities.

DISCHARGE CRITERIA

1. Recognizes potentially violent personality and controls behavior.
2. Client/family are participating in therapeutic regimen.
3. Effective coping skills/understanding of underlying dynamics of condition are demonstrated.
4. Major/emerging personality has been chosen and accepted.

NURSING DIAGNOSIS:	**ANXIETY (SEVERE/PANIC)/FEAR**
MAY BE RELATED TO:	**Maladaptation of ineffective coping continuing from early life**
	Unconscious conflict(s), threat to self-concept
	Unmet needs
	Phobic stimulus
	Threat of death, perceived or actual
POSSIBLY EVIDENCED BY:	**Fragmentation of the personality**
	Maladaptive response to stress
	Increased tension
	Apprehension, fright
	Feelings of inadequacy; focus on self/ "it, out there" (projection)
	Sympathetic stimulation: cardiovascular excitation, superficial vasoconstriction, pupil dilation
CLIENT OUTCOMES/EVALUATION CRITERIA:	**Verbalizes awareness of feelings of anxiety. Acknowledges and discusses fear. Identifies ways to manage anxiety/fear effectively. Demonstrates problem-solving skills. Uses resources effectively.**

INTERVENTIONS	RATIONALE

Independent

Develop rapport and trust; accept verbal expression of feelings/anxieties.

A trusting alliance with the nurse/caregiver facilitates early identification of the underlying sources of anxiety and development of an appropriate treatment approach. Learning to turn to trusted others for support assists the client to develop healthy methods of dealing with anxiety.

Discuss with the client the availability of assistance in maintaining safety.

Avoids a false assurance of safety, which can increase the feeling of isolation and the likelihood of destructive behaviors. The nurse needs to recognize that internal threats to safety may not be readily apparent. Expressions of anxiety may represent a very real threat to or from alternate personalities and/or others.

Maintain a neutral approach when confronted by an alternate personality.

A neutral response allows essential observation and documentation and promotes a trusting relationship. It also avoids the caregiver consciously or unconsciously promoting fragmentation of the personality. Because this disorder remains rare and has been sensationalized, personnel may be intrigued by manifestations and respond to the client in ways that reinforce the behaviors manifesting the disorder.

Reduce alterable sources of stress. Provide calm environment; minimize external stimuli. Identify causes/precipitators of anxiety/stress.

Manipulation of the environment to reduce extraneous sources of stress allows the client to recognize and develop skills in managing internal sources of conflict.

Provide positive reinforcement and expectations, and role-model desired behaviors.

This client is commonly very suggestible and responsive to the positive expectations and attention of trusted others. Development of healthy coping mechanisms helps in reducing anxiety.

Prepare client for the testing procedures; provide information about the reason for the test and what is to be expected from the results. Review test results as indicated.

An explanation of the processes of each test can allay anxiety. Care needs to be taken that the physical assessment is presented as routine because the client may misperceive the test as indicative of the presence of a physical disorder and may be prone to a psychosomatic or conversion disorder. Receiving the results in a timely manner relieves anxiety. Once organic causes have been ruled out, it is unlikely that extensive examinations and/or testing will have to be repeated, reducing the likelihood that the client might adopt physical symptoms providing secondary gain.

Observe for/review with client untoward effects/adverse reaction to medication regimen. Monitor level of alertness, vital signs; note urinary retention, dry mouth, blurred vision, Parkinson's-like symptoms, rigidity, or atypical response (excitability, restlessness, agitation).

Psychoactive medications (sedatives, minor tranquilizers, antipsychotic agents, and antidepressants) frequently produce hypotension and anticholinergic and extrapyramidal symptoms, in addition to the desired effect. Early intervention will alleviate prolonged difficulties and/or serious physical complications and may prevent/lessen anxiety about their presence.

Collaborative

Coordinate and develop a combined treatment plan. Facilitate communication among team members.

It is essential that all members of the treatment team work together in the plan of care to ensure that goals and objectives are in agreement and continuity of care

INTERVENTIONS

Collaborative

RATIONALE

exists. A cohesive treatment plan prevents dissension between disciplines. These clients are prone to manipulative behaviors and may be resistant to therapy; they do better when dealing with one primary provider supported by a cohesive treatment team.

Administer anti-anxiety medications as indicated, e.g., alprazolam (Xanax), diazepam (Valium).

Anti-anxiety medications are given with caution for brief periods to allay panic states or disabling anxiety. Caution is essential as substance abuse is a common complication and also because of the potential for self-destruction.

NURSING DIAGNOSIS:	**VIOLENCE, POTENTIAL FOR: DIRECTED AT SELF/OTHERS**
MAY BE RELATED TO:	**Depressed mood**
	Conflicting personalities
	Panic states
	Suicidal behaviors
POSSIBLE INDICATORS:	**Serious suicide threats**
	"Internal homicide" (in which one personality attempts to kill another personality)
	Increased motor activity, pacing, excitement, irritability, agitation
	Self-destructive behaviors/active aggressive suicidal acts
CLIENT OUTCOMES/EVALUATION CRITERIA:	**Verbalizes understanding of why behavior occurs. Demonstrates self-control as evidenced by relaxed posture, nonviolent behavior. Expresses increased self-esteem and meets needs in an assertive manner. Uses resources and support systems effectively.**

INTERVENTIONS

Independent

Remain vigilant to behavioral changes that may signal

RATIONALE

Client behavior may change abruptly and dramati-

INTERVENTIONS	RATIONALE

INTERVENTIONS

Independent

destructive actions. Assess seriousness of suicidal tendency, gestures, threats, or previous attempts. (Use scale of 1–10 and prioritize according to severity of threat, availability of means.)

Help client identify/recognize precipitants to destructive behaviors.

Structure the environment to reduce stressors that precipitate destructive behavior. Assist the client to reduce exposure to external stressors by avoidance when practical.

Active-Listen and encourage the client to seek restraint and/or support when self-destructive or violent impulses are present.

Arrange protection for personality that is prone to violent behavior(s). Another personality, usually the primary one, can be appointed to monitor/control the behavior(s) of the suspect personality.

Assist the client to identify alternatives to aggression or self-destructive behaviors, e.g., verbal expression, physical activity, written expression.

Take immediate and decisive action when danger is imminent. Tell client to "stop" and/or hold as necessary, until client calms down.

Note presence/degree of depression and reassess periodically, noting suicidal ideation.

Collaborative

Hospitalize as necessary.

Place in isolation and provide physical restraint in a nonpunitive manner. Observe closely/stay with client.

Administer anti-anxiety medication, as indicated.

RATIONALE

cally. Impulse control may be impaired. May be #1 nursing priority if score is high on the scale.

Early detection permits timely intervention, allowing environmental manipulation to reduce the occurrence of injurious behaviors.

Calm surroundings permit the client to recognize personally distressing factors, thereby reducing externally disruptive behaviors.

A therapeutic alliance promotes client responsibility for behavioral restraint while supplementing internal controls. Ventilation will reduce the need for action.

Usually one personality can be identified as having these behaviors, and use of another personality may keep the violence from occurring.

Provides a substitute activity in response to overwhelming impulse to enable client to respond to impulses in a nondestructive manner.

The organized approach of a concerned response by caregivers allows for rapid resolution and minimizes potential for injury to the client/staff/others.

Client may become discouraged and depressed, as treatment is a long-term process, possibly in excess of 10 years.

Usually instituted for differential diagnosis, in response to self-destructive thoughts/behavior, violence or potential violence, and/or psychosomatic complaints or conversion reaction.

Punishment has no therapeutic value, but external controls are necessary to ensure safety/provide reassurance to client when internal controls fail. Close observation following initial restraint will be necessary to assure the effectiveness of the restraints and that the client is not injured by the restraint, e.g., strangulation, impaired circulation, suffocation, aspiration.

May be required to reduce anxiety until internal controls are achieved.

NURSING DIAGNOSIS:	COPING, INEFFECTIVE, INDIVIDUAL
MAY BE RELATED TO:	Overwhelming trauma to the client as a small child, occurring in the family of origin
	Personal vulnerability
	Unmet expectations
	Inadequate support systems
	Inadequate coping methods
	Memory loss
POSSIBLY EVIDENCED BY:	Fragmentation of the personality
	Small child's inability to cope effectively (the disorder is a maladaptive mechanism that persists into adulthood)
	Fear, confusion, anger, frustration, guilt, and embarrassment
	Divorce and alienation
	Inability to meet role expectations
	Inappropriate use of defense mechanisms (fugue, amnesia, dissociative states)
CLIENT OUTCOMES/EVALUATION CRITERIA:	Identifies ineffective coping behaviors and consequences that are creating problems for the client. Meets psychologic needs as evidenced by appropriate expression of feelings, identification of options, and use of resources. Demonstrates positive coping mechanisms.

INTERVENTIONS	RATIONALE
Independent	
Identify stressor(s) that precipitate severe anxiety. (Re-	Helps in recognition of individual factors precipitating

INTERVENTIONS	RATIONALE
Independent	

fer to ND: Self-concept, disturbance in: Personal identity.)	dissociative symptoms (e.g., splitting, fugue, amnesia, which interfere with development of adequate coping skills).
Provide support and encouragement during times of depersonalization.	Client experiences fear and anxiety at these times and may fear "going crazy." Acknowledging these feelings will help client deal appropriately with them.
Discuss measures being taken to protect client. Stay with client as needed.	Reassures client of psychologic safety/security when dissociative behaviors/therapy are frightening to the client. Presence of a trusted person can provide sense of security.
Encourage discussion and verbalization of stressful situation and exploration of feelings associated with those times. Help client to understand that disequilibrium is to be expected, is understandable, and will resolve as integration occurs.	Ventilation in a nonthreatening environment may help the client to come to terms with issues that may be contributing to the dissociative process.
Demonstrate acceptance during disclosure of painful experiences.	Fear of condemnation and criticism makes such disclosure difficult, even in a trusting relationship, and support provides reassurance that information will be treated tactfully.
Have client identify methods of coping with stress in the past, the purpose served, and consequences, and determine whether the response was adaptive or maladaptive.	As anxiety decreases, client can begin to develop insight into the appropriateness of the response and develop a plan of action for the future.
Remain alert to possibility of substance use.	A significant percentage of these clients use substances, such as alcohol, as a means of coping, clouding symptomatology, and interfering with progress.
Assist the client to explore alternative coping strategies, evaluating benefits and consequences of each.	Helps the client to learn new ways to problem-solve and make decisions, which will promote development of independence and use of adaptive coping skills.
Reinforce positive coping mechanisms.	Promotes repetition of adaptive behaviors. These clients are very responsive to positive attention.
Provide supportive, insight-oriented therapy: encourage expression of anxieties, fear, guilt, anger, frustration, and disappointment; accept verbal expressions without judgment; encourage recognition of strengths, positive attributes, and progress toward wellness.	Dissociative symptoms arise from internal conflict. The behaviors protect the client from psychic pain. Subsequently, any stressor can precipitate a like reaction. Insight-oriented therapy in a supportive setting allows the client to confront and resolve past and present painful or fear-inducing events.
Discuss problems of discouragement with lengthy treatment.	Discouraged feelings are inevitable in face of treatment that may last for years, and client may resort to old, maladaptive coping mechanisms and feel like giving up. (Refer to ND: Violence, potential for: directed at self/others.)
Identify specific conflicts that remain unresolved and problem-solve possible solutions.	When these underlying conflicts are not resolved, any improvement in coping behaviors may be regarded as temporary.

316

INTERVENTIONS	RATIONALE
Collaborative	
Encourage client to develop a network of support systems through family, friends, community resources, and school and church affiliations, as well as health and mental health care providers and internal resources.	The tendency to overdependency present in these individuals is antitherapeutic and draining to family, friends, and therapy providers. Development of a support network and internal resources promotes autonomy.

NURSING DIAGNOSIS:	**SELF-CONCEPT, DISTURBANCE IN: PERSONAL IDENTITY**
MAY BE RELATED TO:	**Psychologic conflicts (dissociative state(s))**
	Childhood trauma/abuse
	Threat to physical integrity/self-concept
	Underdeveloped ego
POSSIBLY EVIDENCED BY:	**Confusion about sense of self, purpose or direction in life**
	Memory loss (unable to recall selected events/own identity)
	Alteration in perception or experience of the self
	Loss of one's own sense of reality/the external world
	Poorly differentiated ego boundaries
	Presence of more than one personality within the individual
CLIENT OUTCOMES/EVALUATION CRITERIA:	**Verbalizes acceptance of the disorder. Engages in a therapeutic alliance. Verbalizes awareness of all personalities, their thoughts and behaviors (development of co-consciousness). Displays cooperation among the personalities. Demonstrates more stable personalities with resolution of traumatic events, moving toward partial to full**

integration into one personality. Verbalizes acceptance of positive feelings toward emerging personality.

INTERVENTIONS	RATIONALE
Independent	
Determine client's perception of the extent of the threat to self-integrity and current response.	Degree of distress perceived by the client will assist in determining actions necessary for intervention.
Help client understand/accept reality of the other personality(ies) and meaning of lapses in memory.	May be unaware/lack understanding of condition, resulting in increased anxiety and confusion about self.
Obtain information about client from family members as well as from other personalities and what client does recall.	Helps in orienting to realities of past events and assists client toward memory integration.
Share information in small amounts over a period of time, avoiding giving too much (flooding) at any one time.	Enables client to begin to deal with painful information for which the amnesia has provided protection in the past. Too much material at any one time can be difficult for client to handle, and decompensation could occur.
Encourage client to identify the need each subpersonality serves in the overall identity of the individual.	In multiple personality disorder, knowledge of these unfulfilled needs is the first step toward integration of the personalities and the client's ability to face unresolved issues without dissociation.
Facilitate identification of stressful situations that precipitate transition from one personality to another. (Refer to ND: Coping, ineffective, Individual.)	Assists client to respond more adaptively and to eliminate the need for transition to another personality.
Discuss integration of subpersonalities into a unified identity within the individual, and help client understand that all personalities will contribute to the whole.	The idea of total elimination generates fear and defensiveness within subpersonalities who function as separate entities.
Provide psychotherapy with feedback relative to behavioral observations. Encourage journal-keeping and other methods designed to allow gradual insight.	Decreases denial and amnesia, providing an opportunity for the client to accept the presence of the disorder and begin to own behaviors and personality components. Acceptance and ownership assist the client toward cooperation within the individual, and subsequent integration can take place.
Collaborative	
Plan use of confrontive methods with all team members. Use cautiously.	These methods need to be paced with the individual's ability to benefit therapeutically and planned within the team conference to avoid overstressing the individual and precipitating exacerbation or decompensation.
Use/assist with hypnosis as indicated.	May help client work through and accept realities of positive aspects of each personality.
Engage in activities that reflect life experiences, using occupational/vocational/recreational/physical therapy. Begin with pleasurable stimuli (as identified by the client), e.g., events, smells, pets, or music, associated with pleasurable activities.	Presents additional stimulation, which may encourage recall of repressed material. Provides opportunity to experience positive feelings that have also been repressed and work toward beginning to deal with negative feelings/occurrences.

NURSING DIAGNOSIS:	**COPING, INEFFECTIVE, FAMILY: COMPROMISED**
MAY BE RELATED TO:	**Multiple stressors, repeated over period of time**
	Prolonged progression of disorder that exhausts the supportive capacity of significant people
	Temporary family disorganization and role changes
POSSIBLY EVIDENCED BY:	**Significant person describes inadequate understanding or knowledge base that interferes with effective assistive or supportive behaviors**
	Marital conflict (separation/divorce)
FAMILY OUTCOMES/EVALUATION CRITERIA:	**Identifies/verbalizes resources within themselves to deal with the situation. Provides opportunity for client to deal with situation in own way. Remains intact, or separates in healthy way, is supportive of the client, and one another.**

INTERVENTIONS	RATIONALE
Independent	
Identify contributing factors within the family or environment.	Family and marital dysfunction are extremely likely to occur. These factors contribute to ongoing emotional stress.
Provide client/family education relative to the disorder and treatment plan.	An understanding of the problem and the fact that the disorder can be treated reduces anxiety, frustration, and guilt and allows the client to progress within a supportive environment.
Explore family dynamics. Note enabling/sabotage behaviors, e.g., failure to attend therapy/keeping client from attending.	Other family members may be invested in keeping the "sick" member symptomatic in order to camouflage their own problems.
Provide for client safety within the family setting or arrange for alternative living arrangements if abuse (or neglect in children's cases) are at issue.	If the client remains in the family of origin, a diagnosis of multiple personality disorder should alert personnel to the possibility of abuse/neglect. As the "responsible adult," client may be unable to consistently meet needs of child(ren).
Assist the family to respond to the client in a manner that reinforces positive behaviors.	Without assistance, the family may provide secondary gain for continued illness versus wellness.

319

INTERVENTIONS	RATIONALE

Independent

Encourage the family to ventilate negative feelings and continue as much as possible with usual daily activities. Discourage family from allowing client to escape responsibilities due to the illness.

Family members are less likely to abandon the affected member if they have an outlet for anger/frustration and are not overburdened in caretaking. Positive expectations from family members promote hope for recovery and self-esteem and decreases the likelihood of secondary gain.

Collaborative

Refer for additional individual, family, or marriage counseling.

Concurrent psychiatric problems in other family members are common. If the client's symptoms are the most florid, that individual has likely been identified as the "sick" family member and others have not sought/received help.

CHAPTER **12**
GENDER AND SEXUAL DISORDERS

Gender Identity Disorders

DSM III-R: 302.60 Gender identity disorder of childhood
302.50 Transsexualism (specify: asexual, homosexual, heterosexual, unspecified)
302.85 Gender identity disorder of adolescence or adulthood, nontranssexual type (specify asexual, homosexual, heterosexual, unspecified)
302.85 Gender identity disorder NOS

ETIOLOGIC THEORIES

PSYCHODYNAMICS

The libido is seen as the force that expresses sexual instinct and develops gradually during the oral stage, focusing on the mouth and lips. The central concern of the anal stage is the anus and the elimination/retention of feces. During the phallic stage, the male is concerned with love of mother, is jealous of father, and has castration anxiety (Oedipus complex). The female has penis envy, loves her father, and rejects her mother. This theory focuses on the biologic inferiority of women because they do not have penises, with subsequent envy of the male.

Developmental theories suggest that sexuality develops throughout life and especially during the formative years. Confusion in relation to one's individual personality and sexual identity affects the ability to be intimate, interfering with sexual development.

BIOLOGIC THEORIES

Some research sources report that there is a neuroendocrine factor, for example, that the fetus was exposed to large amounts of androgenic hormones or that the mother may have received synthetic hormones at a crucial developmental period, preventing adequate stimulation for neural differentiation.

Androgen is necessary for masculinization in the fetal male, with the fetus developing as female without the addition of this hormone. If androgenic influences in the fetal hypothalamus are decreased in the male or increased in the female, transsexualism may occur.

FAMILY DYNAMICS

Role-modeling is believed to play a part in the development of these disorders as well as in the context of a disturbed relationship with one or both parents. Imprinting and classic conditioning are thought by some to affect the development of gender identity.

321

In males, a symbiotic relationship appears to exist between mother and child. The father is usually absent, ineffectual, or hostile and is perceived as weak and distant, with the mother seen as strong and protective.

In females, the child may not be valued as a girl, or the mother may be absent, depressed, or suffer from other illness, resulting in inadequate mothering. The father may treat the daughter as his little boy, expecting "masculine" behavior.

CLIENT ASSESSMENT DATA BASE

HISTORY

May present at any age, but most often in late adolescence or early adulthood, although may have a later onset. The onset of the problem usually can be identified in childhood.

Higher occurrence in males than females (may be due to narrow study base)

Essential feature is an incongruence between assigned sex and the sense of knowing to which sex one belongs.

May report a persistent and intense distress about his/her assigned sex and the desire to be/insistence that s/he is of the other sex.

Exhibits a persistent marked aversion to wearing sex-appropriate clothing.

A preoccupation with stereotypical activities/toys of the opposite sex and/or repudiation of anatomical structures may be noted/reported in childhood.

Moderate to severe coexisting personality disturbance may be noted.

May complain of considerable anxiety and depression, attributable to difficulty of living in role of assigned sex.

May report impairment in social/occupational functioning and may have history of suicidal attempts.

PHYSICAL EXAMINATION

Mental Status:
>Abnormal findings may be indicative of intense distress (e.g., ego-dystonic homosexuality) about gender identity or coexisting psychiatric disorders.
>Mood and affect may reveal evidence of increased anxiety and depression.

No other significant findings.

DIAGNOSTIC STUDIES

Psychologic testing to rule out concomitant psychiatric conditions
Screen for sexually transmitted diseases (STD) including AIDS

NURSING PRIORITIES

1. Assist client to learn stress management techniques to reduce anxiety.
2. Promote sense of self-esteem.
3. Encourage development of social skills/comfort level with own sexual identity/preference.
4. Provide opportunities for client/family to participate in group therapy/other support systems.

DISCHARGE CRITERIA

1. Anxiety is reduced/managed effectively.
2. Self-esteem/image is enhanced.
3. Client accepts and is comfortable with identity as established.
4. Client/family are participating in ongoing treatment/support programs.

NURSING DIAGNOSIS:	ANXIETY (SEVERE)
MAY BE RELATED TO:	Ego-dystonic gender identification
	Unconscious conflicts about essential values/beliefs

POSSIBLY EVIDENCED BY:	**Threat to self-concept** **Unmet needs** **Increased tension/helplessness (hopelessness)** **Feelings of inadequacy, apprehension, uncertainty** **Increased wariness** **Insomnia** **Focus on self** **Impaired daily functioning**
CLIENT OUTCOMES/EVALUATION CRITERIA:	**Appears relaxed and reports anxiety is reduced to a manageable level. Verbalizes awareness of feelings of anxiety and healthy ways to deal with them. Demonstrates problem-solving skills and uses resources effectively.**

INTERVENTIONS	RATIONALE
Independent	
Assess level of anxiety and degree of interference with daily activities/life.	Necessary information to identify the extent of problem for the individual and plan appropriate interventions.
Review drug history (prescription/illicit), familial/physiologic factors, e.g., mental/physical illness, family disorganization.	Drugs may have been used to handle anxious feelings in the past. Other factors contribute to anxiety and may affect individual's ability to handle stress of dealing with own identity problems.
Assist client to identify feelings, conveying empathy and unconditional positive regard. Encourage free expression of feelings in appropriate ways.	Identification of feelings within a safe, therapeutic environment can help the client begin to explore causes of anxiety and begin to move toward acceptance of self as a worthwhile person.
Acknowledge reality of anxiety/fear. (Do not deny or reassure client that everything will be all right.)	Helps client accept own feeling(s) and learn trust in self. Denial of these feelings contributes to increased anxiety.
Provide accurate information to assist client to clarify reality base, reframe sexuality, and delineate boundaries.	Anxiety may be the result of misinterpretation or lack of knowledge about sexuality/gender identity and client may fantasize unrealistic ideation.
Accept the client as s/he is.	Lack of acceptance of own self is the basis of much anxiety, and when others project an atmosphere of unacceptance also, anxiety is increased.

INTERVENTIONS	RATIONALE

Independent

Identify things client has done previously when feeling nervous/anxious.	Assists the client to see which previous actions have been helpful and can be used in this situation, increasing sense of control/capability and allaying anxiety.
Assist with developing program of exercise, e.g., brisk walking, aerobic class.	Strenuous activity releases opiatelike endorphins, which create sense of well-being and decrease anxiety.

NURSING DIAGNOSIS:	**SELF-CONCEPT, DISTURBANCE IN: ROLE PERFORMANCE AND PERSONAL IDENTITY**
MAY BE RELATED TO:	**Crisis in development in which person has difficulty knowing to which sex s/he belongs**
	Sense of discomfort and inappropriateness about anatomical sex
POSSIBLY EVIDENCED BY:	**Confusion about sense of self, purpose or direction in life, sexual identification/preference**
	Verbalization of desire to be/insistence that person is the opposite sex
	Change in self-perception of role
	Conflict in roles
CLIENT OUTCOMES/EVALUATION CRITERIA:	**Verbalizes realistic perception and acceptance of self in role. Talking with family/significant other(s) about situation and changes that are occurring/have occurred. Developing realistic plans for adapting to new role/role changes.**

INTERVENTIONS	RATIONALE

Independent

Identify type of role dysfunction/distress client is expressing, e.g., ego-dystonic heterosexual/homosexual feelings, gender dysphoria.	Lack of self-acceptance and conflicting feelings regarding sexual expression may require therapeutic intervention. (When the individual views sexual expression/feelings/behavior as adaptive, a healthy attitude exists and intervention is unnecessary.)

INTERVENTIONS	RATIONALE
Independent	
Provide acceptance of the client as presented.	These clients are sensitive to others' beliefs and will pick up on prejudicial feelings. The client needs to be free to express any views/feelings in order to begin to solve the problems being faced.
Determine presence of support systems, e.g., family, social/work.	May feel "different" and isolate self from usual support systems. May be pressured by family/friends to be heterosexual, creating conflict within self.
Evaluate beliefs and values of the individual about hetero/homo/transsexuality. Discuss client's beliefs in detail, providing information as appropriate.	Client may be ignorant of the facts and base fears and ideas on hearsay, prejudice, and religious beliefs. Learning the facts and discussing them with an unbiased person provides an opportunity to make informed decisions.
Explore client's feelings about gender identity (transsexuality) and review options for change, e.g., hormonal therapy, psychotherapy, surgical reassignment.	The client who feels strongly that s/he is in the wrong body needs to have complete information about available choices to help them begin to accept self and feel comfortable with the decision. (Note: Not all transsexuals decide to have surgery.)
Assist client to develop strategies to cope with threat to identity.	Provides protection and gives client a sense of control to have thought about/decided on actions that can be taken when feeling threatened.
Assess response of family/significant others. (Refer to NDs: Coping, ineffective Family: Compromised and/or Coping, ineffective Family: Potential for Growth.)	May be in shock when first learning of client's concerns and then may either reject or rally to support client.
Encourage client to deal with situation in small steps.	Helps client cope with the larger picture when in stress overload.
Provide accurate information about threat to and potential consequences for the individual.	Knowledge about gender identity issues helps client assess own situation and make decisions based on fact.
Collaborative	
Refer to trained professionals who are expert in the field of human sexuality.	Client needs to be known to the therapist for a period of three to six months, demonstrate a sense of discomfort with self, and a desire to live in the opposite sex role before a major life-changing decision is finalized.
Refer to a therapist trained in the field of sexual reassignment for a second opinion when surgery is contemplated.	Because these procedures are not reversible, the client needs to be sure the correct decision has been made and demonstrate success in living in the opposite role for a period of one to two years.

NURSING DIAGNOSIS:	SEXUALITY PATTERNS, ALTERED
MAY BE RELATED TO:	**Ineffective or absent role models**
	Conflicts with sexual orientation and/ or preferences

MAY BE RELATED TO—*continued*	Impaired relationship with a significant other
POSSIBLY EVIDENCED BY:	Verbalizations of discomfort with sexual orientation and/or role
	Lack of information about human sexuality
CLIENT OUTCOMES/EVALUATION CRITERIA:	Verbalizes understanding of sexuality and acceptance of self. Demonstrates behaviors directed at lifestyle changes necessary to achieve desired effects.

INTERVENTIONS

Independent

Have client describe problem in own terms, noting comments of client/significant other that may reveal discounting by overt/covert sexual expressions.

Take sexual history, including perception of normal function, use of vocabulary, and concerns about sexual identity.

Note cultural and religious/value factors and conflicts that may exist.

Explore knowledge of alternative sexual responses and expressions.

Inquire about drug use, including OTC/prescription, illicit, and alcohol.

Provide atmosphere in which discussion of sexual problems is encouraged, promoting free expression of feelings.

Encourage discussion of possibilities and alternatives for client situation. (Refer to ND: Self-concept, disturbance in: Role performance/Personal identity.)

Review hormonal therapy as indicated.

Collaborative

Refer to resources as indicated, e.g., gender identity clinic; homosexual/lesbian support group; Homosexuals Anonymous Fellowship; LAMBDA, AA, Gay and Lesbian; Common Bond.

RATIONALE

It may be difficult for client to talk about situation/express feelings, and client may joke, make oblique remarks, or use sarcasm to convey/cover concerns.

Provides information about level of knowledge about anatomy/physiology of human sexuality and identifies/clarifies concerns to be dealt with by the client/nurse.

Provides opportunity to give information/discuss resources available to client who may believe thoughts and feelings are sinful and feel guilty.

May only have knowledge gained in discussions with friends, from myths, and misconceptions.

Drug use can affect sexual functioning. May use substances to dull pain of indecision/anxiety of identity.

Essential to identification and resolution of problems. Client may have concerns about sexual behavior and diseases, such as AIDS.

Full range of discussion can assist the client in reaching a decision about the identity that is comfortable and the course to pursue.

Transsexuals who elect to undergo surgical reassignment, as well as others who for economic or other reasons choose to live in the transsexual role, usually receive long-term, high-dose estrogen or testosterone therapy. The client needs to understand the implications before making the decision to pursue this course of therapy because it is irreversible.

Information from these groups can help client reach a decision about sexual preference and/or provide support once decision has been made. HAF is a Christian-based group that directs efforts to assisting the client

INTERVENTIONS	RATIONALE
Collaborative	toward a decision to become heterosexual. Other organizations are reference groups that provide information/support.

NURSING DIAGNOSIS:	**COPING, INEFFECTIVE FAMILY: COMPROMISED**
MAY BE RELATED TO:	**Inadequate/incorrect information or understanding**
	Temporary preoccupation by a significant person who is trying to manage emotional conflicts and personal suffering and is unable to perceive or to act effectively in regard to client's needs
	Temporary family disorganization and role changes
	Client providing little support in turn for the primary person
POSSIBLY EVIDENCED BY:	**Client expresses/confirms a concern or complaint about S.O.(s) response to client's gender-identity problem**
	S.O. describes preoccupation with own personal reactions to client's problem/confusion
	S.O.(s) attempt supportive behaviors with less than satisfactory results/ withdraw support when needed
FAMILY OUTCOMES/EVALUATION CRITERIA:	**Identifies resources within itself to deal with situation. Interacting appropriately with client and staff, providing support and assistance as indicated.**

INTERVENTIONS	RATIONALE

Independent

Determine individual situation and identify factors that may contribute to difficulty family is having in providing needed assistance/support for the client.

Individuals may have problems of their own that interfere with ability to extend themselves to the client. Problems of prejudice, myth/misinformation, values may also cause separation between family members.

Note behaviors of family members, e.g., withdrawn, supportive, rejecting, or willing to learn. (Refer to ND: Coping, Family: Potential for Growth.)

Identifies individual needs and steps to be taken to resolve family disorganization/assist the family in moving toward growth.

Discuss underlying reasons/behaviors client is expressing/exhibiting.

Helps family understand and accept the person as having different values.

Encourage each individual to be responsible for own self, not taking on the problem(s) of others.

The concept of "who owns the problem" can help clarify issues of who has responsibility for solution of specific problems.

Provide information about gender identity issues.

Because much of the problem may center around lack of knowledge, information can help individuals make informed decisions/choices about what is happening.

Encourage free expression of feelings and ideas about gender identity issues.

Promotes an atmosphere in which individual can reveal feelings of self-blame, revulsion, confusion, and anger, or blaming of other(s). Once these have been expressed, members can move on to resolution.

Discuss options for individuals in regard to client's decision about gender identity/surgical reassignment, e.g., separation/divorce for spouses, resolution of parent/child issues.

Family members may have difficulty accepting client's alternate sexual expression/sexual reassignment. Individual needs to make decision about willingness to accept other person in altered role. Children of transsexuals have questions such as "Who am I, as the daughter of a father who is now a woman?"

Provide time to talk with family to discuss views/concerns about situation.

Opportunity to ventilate feelings, ask questions, and express ideas helps resolve problems.

Assist members to develop effective communication skills, e.g., active-listening, "I-messages," problem-solving process. Provide role model with which the family may identify.

Helpful in dealing with current situation as well as providing skills that will assist with resolution of future problems. Role-modeling shows individuals that the skills can be helpful to them.

Collaborative

Identify/refer to support groups/classes that deal with similar problems, e.g., Gender Identity Clinic.

Talking with others who have been through similar experiences can provide opportunity for members to learn/accept client.

Refer for marriage counseling as appropriate.

May be needed to help couple decide whether separation or divorce is in the best interests of each person, or whether they want to work out the problems and stay together.

NURSING DIAGNOSIS:	COPING, FAMILY: POTENTIAL FOR GROWTH
MAY BE RELATED TO:	**Individual's basic needs are suffi-**

	ciently gratified and adaptive tasks effectively addressed to enable goals of self-actualization to surface
POSSIBLY EVIDENCED BY:	**Family members attempt to describe growth impact of crisis on their own values, priorities, goals, or relationships**
	Family member(s) are moving in direction of health-promoting and enriching lifestyle that supports client's search for self
	Choosing experiences that optimize wellness
FAMILY OUTCOMES/EVALUATION CRITERIA:	**Expresses willingness to look at their own role in family's growth. Verbalizes knowledge and understanding of client's gender choice. Expresses desire to undertake tasks leading to change.**

INTERVENTIONS	RATIONALE
Independent	
Listen to family's expressions of hope, planning, and effect on relationships/life.	Provides clues to opportunities that exist to help family move toward growth and positive relationships. When family members are doing this, client is free to move toward a positive resolution of own life.
Help the family in supporting the client in meeting own needs/making own decision.	Significant other(s) may not have skills/know how to give support even when desired, and giving information and providing support enables them to learn.
Note expressions of change of values, e.g., "He/she is still my son/daughter even though homosexual/ lesbian or contemplating sex-change surgery."	Indicators of beginning of acceptance of the situation as it is and willingness to learn and support child.
Provide a role model with which the family may identify.	Modeling of accepting behaviors/communication skills enables family members to learn new ways of interacting with the client.
Discuss importance of open communication and the harm secretive behavior produces.	Open communication allows all participants to have access to all information, enhancing resolution of problems/understanding of what is happening.
Encourage open discussions of concerns about lifestyle changes, fear of AIDS, and other sexually transmitted diseases.	Individuals may have unexpressed fears, and this provides the opportunity to ask questions and get accurate answers.
Provide experiences for the family, e.g., involvement with other families facing similar decisions.	Helps them learn ways of assisting/supporting client.

329

INTERVENTIONS	RATIONALE
Collaborative	
Refer to community resources, e.g., same gender, transsexual groups.	Provides ongoing support as client/family makes necessary lifestyle changes, go on with their lives.

Sexual Disorders

PARAPHILIAS

DSM III-R: 302.40 Exhibitionism
302.81 Fetishism
302.89 Frotteurism
302.20 Pedophilia
302.83 Sexual masochism
302.84 Sexual sadism
302.30 Transvestic fetishism

SEXUAL DYSFUNCTIONS (DESIRE DISORDERS)

302.71 Hypoactive sexual desire disorder
302.79 Sexual aversion disorder
302.72 Female sexual arousal disorder
302.72 Male erectile disorder
302.73 Inhibited female orgasm
302.74 Inhibited male orgasm
302.75 Premature ejaculation
302.76 Dyspareunia
302.51 Vaginismus
302.90 Sexual disorder NOS

ETIOLOGIC FACTORS

PSYCHODYNAMICS

Psychoanalytic theories state that paraphilias are the product of childhood desires that survive into adulthood in their immature forms because emotional development has been inhibited, distorted, and diverted. These wishes are believed to be universal and are used to achieve arousal and release when ordinary forms of sexual activity are not available. Deviations arise when these immature forms of libido dominate adult sexual life. Fixation is thought to occur in Freud's oral, anal, and phallic phases when corresponding body parts provide sources of instinctual gratification. Conflict arises when an imperfect compromise occurs between these impulses and reality, resulting in fear, which the unconscious perceives as castration.

Behavioral theorists believe any paraphilia/sexual dysfunction can be acquired through conditioning, in which an initial pairing of an object is accidentally associated with/then becomes necessary for sexual release. This need may become generalized to other situations of tension/anxiety.

BIOLOGIC THEORIES

Sometimes the cause is clearly biologic, e.g., temporal lobe epilepsy that may cause changes in sexual behavior between seizures. It has also been suggested that the problem arises out of interference with brain pathways governing rage and sexual arousal. Sex hormones have been studied. Rat studies have demonstrated that small, properly timed doses of androgens (male hormones) or estrogens (female hormones) in the fetus or newborn can influence sexual behavior.

It is generally accepted that abnormal hormonal activity and biologic (genetic) predisposition interacting with social and family factors influence the development of these fantasies/sexual acts, which may occur within normal sexual activity but that when they become the primary source of sexual satisfaction result in problems for the individual/others.

FAMILY DYNAMICS

There appears to be some evidence that paraphilias run in families and may be the result of dysfunctional family interactions and social learning.

Sexual dysfunctions are believed to be influenced by what the individual has learned/not learned as a child within the family system and by values and beliefs that may be based on myths and misconceptions.

CLIENT ASSESSMENT DATA BASE

HISTORY

Paraphilias

Occur mostly in males.

Some evidence of occurrence in families of paraphiliacs and of depressed patients. Pedophilia occurs at a high rate in the families of pedophiles.

May relate need for unusual or bizarre imagery or acts to achieve sexual arousal, often with unwilling partners.

Because some of these behaviors may be variants of normal sex, the unusual object/situation must be exclusive or at least the preferred source of sexual excitement.

May not view self as ill; however, behavior may cause distress for the individual or may bring suffering to others.

May be in conflict with partner or society due to behavior.

Interference with interpersonal/occupational functioning may be noted.

May express shame or guilt about behavior.

May or may not act on fantasies.

Personality disturbances frequently accompany sexual disorder(s).

Exhibitionism: The presence of recurrent, intense sexual urges and fantasies involving the exposure of one's genitals to a stranger. These have been acted on, cause severe distress, and may be accompanied by masturbation.

Fetishism: The use of nonliving object(s) to stimulate recurrent intense sexual urges and sexually arousing fantasies, e.g., female undergarments.

Frotteurism: Rubbing and touching against a nonconsenting person to invoke recurrent, intense sexual urges and fantasies. It is the touching, not the coercive nature of the act, that is sexually exciting.

Pedophilia: Sexual activity with a prepubescent child or children.

Sexual Masochism: Involves the act (real, not simulated) of being humiliated, beaten, bound, or otherwise made to suffer.

Sexual Sadism: Involves acts (real, not simulated) in which the psychological or physical suffering (including humiliation) of the victim is sexually exciting to the person.

Transvestic Fetishism: Cross-dressing.

Voyeurism: Observing unsuspecting person(s), usually a stranger, who is naked, in the process of disrobing, or engaging in sexual activity.

Sexual Desire Disorders

Most commonly occur in early adulthood, although male erectile disorder may surface later in life.

May be lifelong or acquired after a period of normal sexual functioning.

May complain of inhibition or interference with some part of the human response cycle, e.g., low sexual desire, aversion to genital sexual contact, arousal/erectile/orgastic disturbances, premature ejaculation; genital pain during or after sexual intercourse, and involuntary spasm of the outer third of the vagina interfering with coitus.

Impairment may be noted in marital relationships but rarely affect job performance.

May display negative attitude(s) toward sexuality.

Believed to be common, especially in milder forms.

PHYSICAL EXAMINATION

Mental Status:
    Findings may be indicative of intense distress about situation/condition or coexisting psychiatric disorders. Mood and affect may reveal evidence of increased anxiety and depression.

Serious physical damage may be seen when sadomasochism is present.

DIAGNOSTIC STUDIES

As indicated to rule out physical causes of sexual dysfunction.

Screen for sexually transmitted diseases (STD) including AIDS

332

NURSING PRIORITIES

1. Assist client to understand the nature of the behavior (disorder/dysfunction).
2. Encourage use of acceptable methods for reduction of anxiety.
3. Help to recognize the legal/interpersonal consequences of paraphilic behaviors.
4. Explore options for change.
5. Encourage involvement of client/family (significant other) in treatment regimen.

DISCHARGE CRITERIA

1. Client is aware of the nature of the problem and consequences for the individual/family.
2. Options have been explored and appropriate one(s) chosen.
3. Anxiety is reduced/managed in acceptable ways.
4. Client expresses confidence in own capabilities/sense of self-worth.
5. Participating in treatment program and using community/treatment resources effectively.

NURSING DIAGNOSIS:	**ANXIETY (MODERATE TO SEVERE)**
MAY BE RELATED TO:	**Unconscious conflict about sexual feelings**
	Threat to self-concept
	Threat to role-functioning
	Unmet needs
POSSIBLY EVIDENCED BY:	**Increased tension (sexual)**
	Feelings of inadequacy
	Fear of unspecified consequences
	Extraneous movements (foot-shuffling, hand/arm movements)
	Glancing about; poor eye contact
	Focus on self
	Impaired functioning; immobility
CLIENT OUTCOMES/EVALUATION CRITERIA:	**Verbalizes awareness of feelings of anxiety and reports reduction to a manageable level. Demonstrates problem-solving skills and uses resources effectively.**

INTERVENTIONS	RATIONALE

Independent

Determine degree and precipitants of anxiety.	Sexual activity is usually undertaken to reduce a state of inner tension and pressure. Fear of being found out and/or disapproved of also creates anxiety for these individuals. May have sought help because of these fears/coming to the attention of the legal system.
Note prodromal symptoms of irritability, restlessness, tension, and headache.	In the exhibitionist, these may be the response to abnormal discharges in the temporal lobes.
Identify client's perception of the threat represented by the situation.	The client may not perceive the behavior as a problem; however, it is the reaction of others and consequences that create anxiety. Circumstances that prevent the client from indulging in the behavior can lead to intense anxiety.
Assess withdrawn behavior and evaluate for substance use (alcohol, other drugs), sleep disturbances, limited/avoidance of interactions with others.	These behaviors may be used by the client to deal with anxiety/other feelings (e.g., guilt) instead of other, positive coping mechanisms. Substance use may be a factor in the occurrence of the dysfunction(s).
Encourage appropriate expression of feelings, e.g., crying (sadness), laughing (fear, denial), swearing (fear, anger).	Suppression of feelings has contributed to difficulties client has in dealing with anxiety and coping appropriately with sexual desires.
Confront the client's behavior without judgment.	Client needs to hear that behavior is not acceptable but that the individual is all right.
Assist the client to recognize a helpful degree of anxiety and ways to begin to use it.	Moderate degree of anxiety heightens awareness and permits the client to focus on dealing with the problems.

Collaborative

Administer medication as indicated, e.g., anti-androgen drugs: Depo-Provera.	These drugs have been useful for altering sexual behavior, but their use is limited because they suppress desired as well as unwanted sexual responses.
Refer to behavioral therapy/psychotherapy, marital/family therapy as indicated.	Aversion therapy, in which the unwanted sexual act/thought is linked to an unpleasant sensation such as an electric shock or nausea and/or imagining a frightening or disgusting event, is used as negative reinforcement and is designed to extinguish the desire. Desensitization to heterosexual coitus is used with limited long-lasting success. Psychotherapy may be used to help the client recognize the problems of sadness and isolation caused by the dysfunction/deal with emotional issues involved. May also be used to help client accept sexual nature when behavior is not damaging/dangerous, e.g., transvestism. Marital/family therapy may resolve problems of communication, which may be major factor in many sexual dysfunction problems.

NURSING DIAGNOSIS:	SELF-CONCEPT, DISTURBANCE IN: SELF-ESTEEM
MAY BE RELATED TO:	Emotional insecurity
	Lack of self-confidence
	Substance use
	Biophysical/psychosocial factors, e.g., achievement of sexual satisfaction in deviant ways
POSSIBLY EVIDENCED BY:	Verbalization of fear of rejection/reaction by others; negative feelings about body; feelings of helplessness, hopelessness, or powerlessness
	Change in social involvement
	Difficulty accepting positive reinforcement
	Lack of follow-through
	Self-destructive behavior
CLIENT OUTCOMES/EVALUATION CRITERIA:	Identifies feelings and methods for coping with negative perception of self. Verbalizes increased sense of self-esteem in relation to current situation, e.g., sees self as a worthwhile person. Demonstrates adaptation to events that have occurred by setting realistic goals and active participation in treatment program.

INTERVENTIONS	RATIONALE
Independent	
Determine individual situation that contributes to client's self-esteem, as well as client's perception of the threat to self and awareness of own responsibility for dealing with situation.	Even though client may not recognize sexual behavior as related to current problem(s), identification of individual circumstances helps in choosing appropriate interventions.
Assess type of sexual problem by asking direct questions, e.g., preference for nonliving objects, dressing in clothes of the opposite sex, use of physical/mental pain as a source of sexual arousal.	Client may not see sexual deviance as a problem but may seek help for feelings of guilt and sadness. Asking directly can promote client recognition of these factors.

INTERVENTIONS	RATIONALE

Independent

Ascertain if client has ever been arrested.	Pattern of involvement with the law can provide information about extent of the problem.
Provide information about sexual anatomy/physiology as needed.	Lack of information and myths/misconceptions are the basis of sexual functioning problems, and accurate knowledge may be crucial to resolution of the problems.
Determine client motivation for change.	When client accepts the fact that the sexual behavior is responsible for the problems that exist and makes the decision to change, therapy has more chance of being successful. If therapy is court-ordered, possibility for change is less likely.
Discuss what purpose (positive intention) the behavior serves for the client (e.g., sense of inadequacy as a male may be met by exhibitionistic behaviors), and what other options might be available to meet needs in more satisfying and socially acceptable ways.	Identification of the purpose allows opportunity for the client to examine whether the behavior meets the purpose in an adaptive or maladaptive manner.
Give positive reinforcement for progress noted.	Encouragement can support development of mature coping behaviors.
Permit client to progress at own rate.	Immaturity is believed to be involved in the development of paraphilias, and adaptation to a change in self-concept depends on the significance the individual attaches to the change, how long this behavior has been used, and necessary changes in lifestyle. Learning to see oneself as a capable, competent adult who interacts in an adult sexual manner takes a long time.
Assist client to incorporate changes accurately into self-concept.	Helps client recognize and cope with events/alterations and sense of loss of control.

Collaborative

Refer to classes, e.g., assertiveness training, positive self-image, communication.	Assists with learning skills to promote self-esteem.

NURSING DIAGNOSIS:	SEXUAL DYSFUNCTION/SEXUAL PATTERNS, ALTERED
MAY BE RELATED TO:	Biophysical alteration of sexuality: ineffectual or absent role models; vulnerability; misinformation; physical/sexual abuse
	Lack of significant other
	Loss of sexual desire
	Disruption of sexual response pattern, e.g., premature ejaculation, dyspareunia

POSSIBLY EVIDENCED BY:	Conflicts involving values Knowledge/skill deficit about alternative responses Conflicts with variant preferences Reported difficulties, limitations/changes in sexual behaviors or activities Difficulty achieving desired satisfaction in socially acceptable ways Alterations in achieving sexual satisfaction
CLIENT OUTCOMES/EVALUATION CRITERIA:	Verbalizes understanding of sexual anatomy/function and individual reasons for sexual problems. Identifies stressors involved in lifestyle that contribute to dysfunction; satisfying/acceptable sexual practices and some alternative ways of dealing with sexual expression. Demonstrates improved communication/relationship skills.

INTERVENTIONS	RATIONALE
Independent	
Take sexual history, noting when problem(s) began, degree of anxiety, displacement of pattern of arousal to other than the opposite sex, and client desire of/need for change.	Identification of individual situation promotes appropriate goal-setting and interventions.
Determine cultural/value conflicts, preexisting problems affecting current situation.	Stress in other areas of life will affect sexual functioning. Client may feel guilt and shame or feel depressed because of deviant behavior.
Explore possible drug use.	Substance/prescription use may affect sexual functioning/be used to relieve anxiety of sexual deviant behavior.
Avoid making value judgments.	Does not help client to deal with the situation or feel better about self.
Determine what client needs/wants to know and provide information accordingly. Review information regarding safety and/or consequences of actions.	Prevents unnecessary repetition of information/presenting information client is not willing to hear. Reviewing necessary information gives client message that it is important and serves as a reminder of own responsibility.

337

INTERVENTIONS	RATIONALE

Independent

Encourage open discussion of concerns and expression of feelings and assist with problem-solving.

Provide sex information/education, as necessary.

Collaborative

Refer for assessment of physical conditions, e.g., presence of diabetes, vascular problems.

Monitor penile tumescence during REM sleep, as indicated.

Refer to appropriate resources as necessary, e.g., clinical specialist psychiatric nurse, professional sex therapists/family counseling.

Promotes thinking about causes/results of behavior(s) and resolution of problem.

Lack of knowledge may be significant to underlying problem(s).

One-third to one-half of clients with sexual dysfunction have a physical cause.

Impotence can be assessed by noting erectile ability occurring during sleep. Physical conditions are ruled out when erection occurs.

Additional/in-depth counseling, sex therapy may help client come to terms with underlying problems that interfere with recovery.

NURSING DIAGNOSIS:	**FAMILY PROCESS, ALTERED**
MAY BE RELATED TO:	**Situational crisis (e.g., change in roles/revelation of sexual deviance/dysfunction)**
POSSIBLY EVIDENCED BY:	**Expressions of confusion about what to do/difficulty coping with situation**
	Inappropriate boundary maintenance
	Family system does not meet emotional/security needs of its members
	Difficulty accepting/receiving help appropriately
	Family does not adapt to change or deal with traumatic experience constructively
	Family does not demonstrate respect for individuality and autonomy of its members
FAMILY OUTCOMES/EVALUATION CRITERIA:	**Expressing feelings freely and appropriately. Demonstrates individual involvement in problem-solving processes directed at appropriate solutions for the situation. Encourages**

> and allows member who is involved to handle situation in own way, progressing toward independence.

INTERVENTIONS	RATIONALE
Independent	
Also refer to CP: Gender Identity, NDs: Coping, ineffective, Family: Compromised and Coping, Family: Potential for Growth	
Determine crisis that has occurred and individual members' perceptions of the situation.	Sexual behavior may have resulted in arrest and be new knowledge to family members. Dysfunction may be perceived as signaling the end of individual's sexual activity.
Identify patterns of communication in the family.	Interaction among family members provides information about family dynamics, boundaries and role expectations and may be indicative of support client may receive.
Assess energy direction: whether efforts at resolution/problem-solving are purposeful or scattered.	Indicative of degree of disorganization family is experiencing.
Note cultural and/or religious factors.	Strong beliefs about sexual expression and deviance/dysfunction influence acceptance or rejection by individuals involved.
Assess support systems available outside the family.	May be needed to help client as well as family members if disorganization is severe.
Acknowledge difficulties observed while reinforcing that some degree of conflict is to be expected and can be used to promote growth.	Acceptance of the reality of what is going on helps client and family to feel comfortable/begin to deal with situation.
Stress importance of continuous open dialogue between family members.	Promotes understanding of each other's point of view and allows for resolution of misunderstandings/misconceptions.
Identify and encourage use of previous successful coping behaviors.	Family has used these in the past and may have neglected them during the stress of current situation.
Encourage use of stress management techniques, e.g., appropriate expression of feelings, relaxation exercises/imagery.	Decreases anxiety and promotes opportunity to problem-solve in calm manner.
Collaborative	
Refer to additional resources as indicated, e.g., classes, psychologic counseling, family/multifamily group therapy.	Providing information, opportunity to share feelings/concerns with others can be helpful to positive resolution of problems.

CHAPTER 13

ADJUSTMENT DISORDER

Adjustment Disorder (Specify)

DSM III-R: Adjustment disorder *with*
> 309.24 Anxious mood
> 309.00 Depressed mood
> 309.30 Disturbance of conduct
> 309.40 Mixed disturbance of emotions and conduct
> 309.28 Mixed emotional features
> 309.82 Physical complaints
> 309.83 Withdrawal
> 309.23 Work (or academic) inhibition
> 309.90 Adjustment disorder NOS

The essential feature of adjustment disorder is a maladaptive reaction to an identifiable psychosocial stressor that occurs within three months after the onset of the stressor. The response is considered maladaptive because there is impairment in social or occupational functioning or because the behaviors are exaggerated beyond the usual, expected response to such a stressor. Duration of the symptoms is less than six months.

ETIOLOGIC THEORIES

PSYCHODYNAMICS

Factors implicated in the predisposition to this disorder include unmet dependency needs, fixation in an earlier level of development, and underdeveloped ego.

BIOLOGIC THEORIES

Refer to CP: Generalized Anxiety Disorder

FAMILY DYNAMICS

The individual's ability to respond to stress is influenced by the role of the mother (her ability to adapt to the infant's needs) and the child-rearing environment (allowing the child gradually to gain independence and control over own life). The mother's difficulty allowing the child to become independent leads to problems with adjustment in later life.

Individuals with adjustment difficulties have experienced negative learning through inadequate role-modeling in dysfunctional family systems. These dysfunctional patterns impede the development of self-esteem and adequate coping skills, which also contribute to maladaptive adjustment responses.

CLIENT ASSESSMENT DATA BASE

The following categories are identified by the predominant symptoms:

Depressed Mood: The major symptoms include depressed mood, tearfulness, and hopelessness. A differential diagnosis with the affective disorders must be considered.

Anxious Mood: The major symptoms include nervousness, worry, and jitteriness. A differential diagnosis with anxiety disorders must be considered.

Mixed Emotional Features: Symptoms of affective and anxiety disorders are manifested as the individual attempts to adjust to a stressful situation.

Disturbance of Conduct: The major response involves conduct in which there is a violation of the rights of others or of major age-appropriate societal norms and rules. A differential diagnosis with conduct disorder or antisocial personality disorder must be considered.

Mixed Disturbance of Emotions and Conduct: The predominant manifestations are both emotional (depression, anxiety) and disturbances in conduct.

Withdrawal: The predominant manifestation is social withdrawal without depressed or anxious mood.

Physical Complaints: Involves physical symptoms such as headache, backache, other aches and pains, and fatigue as the individual's maladaptive response to a stressful situation.

HISTORY

The disorder is apparently quite common; however, there is no information regarding distribution between the sexes.

Reports occurrence of personal stressor within past three months, resulting in impairment in social or occupational functioning that is in excess of a normal and expectable reaction.

May appear depressed and tearful, or nervous and jittery, or both

Anger may be expressed inappropriately, and there may be evidence that client has violated the rights of others or age-appropriate norms. (Client or family may report truancy, vandalism, reckless driving, fighting, defaulting on legal responsibilities.)

May report difficulties with performance at work/school setting, when no difficulties had been experienced prior to the occurrence of the stressor.

May be manipulative, testing limits and playing individuals/family members against each other in order to fulfill own desires.

May refuse to interact with others, preferring to isolate self in own room.

May report/observe substance use/abuse.

May complain of headache, backache, other aches and pains, fatigue.

PHYSICAL EXAMINATION

Vital signs: normal unless underlying physical disorder exists.

Mental Status Exam:

  Depressed (may include suicidal ideations), tearful, anxious, nervous, jittery.

  Attention and memory span may be impaired, depending on level of anxiety and/or evidence of substance use.

  Communication and thought patterns should reflect level of development. Impairment may be evidenced by negative ruminations of depressed mood or flight of ideas/loose associations of severely anxious condition.

DIAGNOSTIC STUDIES

As indicated to rule out underlying pathophysiologic condition.

Drug screen: to determine substance use.

NURSING PRIORITIES

1. Provide safe environment/protect client from self-harm.
2. Assist client to identify precipitating stressor and learn problem-solving techniques.
3. Provide information and support for necessary lifestyle changes.
4. Promote involvement of client/family in therapy process/planning for the future.

DISCHARGE CRITERIA

1. Relief from feelings of anxiety and/or depression is noted, with suicidal ideation reduced.
2. Anger is expressed in an appropriate manner.
3. Maladaptive behaviors are recognized and rechanneled into socially accepted actions.
4. Involved in social situations/interacting with others.
5. Displays ability and willingness to manage life situations.

NURSING DIAGNOSIS:	**VIOLENCE, POTENTIAL FOR: DIRECTED AT SELF**
MAY BE RELATED TO:	**Depressed mood, hopelessness, powerlessness**
	Low self-esteem
	Unresolved grief
	Lack of support systems
	Substance use/abuse
POSSIBLE INDICATORS:	**History of previous suicide attempts**
	Making direct or indirect statements indicating a desire to kill self
	Suicide plan with means to carry it out
	Self-destructive behavior and/or active, aggressive suicidal acts
	Putting business affairs in order; writing a will; giving away prized possessions
	Statements regarding hopelessness for improvement of life situation
	Unstable behavior and/or smell of alcohol on breath/other indicators of substance use
CLIENT OUTCOMES/EVALUATION CRITERIA:	**Verbalizes understanding of behavior and factors that precipitate violent behavior. Expresses increased self-concept/esteem. Participates in care and meets own needs in an assertive**

INTERVENTIONS	RATIONALE

Independent

Ask client direct questions regarding intent, plan, and availability of the means for self-harm. Evaluate and prioritize on a scale of 1 to 10 according to severity of threat, availability of means.

Direct questions, if presented in a caring, concerned manner, provide the necessary information to assist the nurse in formulating an appropriate plan of care for the suicidal client.

Provide a safe environment, making sure potentially harmful objects, such as straps, belts, ties, sharp objects, glass items, and drugs, are placed in a secured area.

Aids in preventing impulsive gestures at a time when client lacks own internal controls.

Secure a verbal or written contract from client that s/he will not harm self and will seek out staff member if suicidal ideations emerge.

A contract encourages the client to share in the responsibility of own safety. A degree of control is experienced, and the attitude of acceptance of the client as a worthwhile individual is conveyed.

Promote verbalizations of honest feelings. Through exploration and discussion, help client identify symbols of hope in own life.

Verbalization of feelings in a nonthreatening environment may help the client come to terms with unresolved issues and identify reasons for wanting to continue living.

Encourage client to express angry feelings within appropriate limits. Provide safe method of hostility release, e.g., pounding pillows, yelling.

Depression and suicidal behaviors may be viewed as anger turned inward on the self.

Help client identify true source of anger and feelings beneath anger, and work on adaptive coping skills for future use.

When anger is verbalized in a nonthreatening environment, the client may be able to resolve these feelings, regardless of the discomfort involved.

Be alert to increased potential for suicidal action as mood elevates.

Client may mobilize self for suicidal attempt as less depression is experienced.

Collaborative

Administer anti-anxiety or antidepressant medication as indicated, e.g.,
    Benzodiazepines: diazepam (Valium), chlordiazepoxide (Librium), alprazolam (Xanax);
    Tricyclic drugs: amitriptyline (Elavil), desipramine (Norpramin), doxepin (Sinequan), imipramine (Tofranil);
    Monoamine-oxidase inhibitors: isocarboxazid (Marplan), phenelzine (Nardil).

Anti-anxiety medication may provide needed relief from anxious feelings. Antidepressant medication may elevate the mood, as it increases level of energy and decreases feelings of fatigue.

NURSING DIAGNOSIS:	**VIOLENCE, POTENTIAL FOR: DIRECTED AT OTHERS**
MAY BE RELATED TO:	**Rage reactions**

POSSIBLE INDICATORS:

Negative role modeling

Interruption of client's attempt to fulfill own desires

Inability to tolerate frustration

Failure of/unresolved grieving (anger directed at the environment)

Vulnerable self-esteem

Inability to verbalize feelings

Body language: clenched fists, facial expressions, rigid posture, tautness, indicating intense effort to control

Increased motor activity, pacing, excitement, irritability, agitation

Hostile, threatening verbalizations; boasting of prior abuse to others

Provocative behavior: argumentative, dissatisfied, over-reactive, hypersensitive

Overt and aggressive acts; goal-directed destruction of objects in environment

Possession of destructive means: gun, knife, other weapon/substance

Substance abuse or withdrawal

History of violent behavior

CLIENT OUTCOMES/EVALUATION CRITERIA:

Verbalizes understanding of why behavior occurs and precipitating factors. Rechannels hostile feelings into socially acceptable behaviors. Reports anxiety at a manageable level. Demonstrates control of aggressive behaviors.

INTERVENTIONS	RATIONALE

Independent

Convey an attitude of acceptance toward the client. Impart a message that it is not the *client* but the *behavior* that is unacceptable.

An attitude of acceptance promotes feelings of self-worth. These feelings are further enhanced as person and behavior are viewed separately, communicating unconditional positive regard.

Observe client's behavior frequently during routine activities and interactions; avoid appearing watchful and suspicious.

Close observation is required so that intervention can occur if required to ensure the safety of others. Instilling suspicion may provoke aggressive behaviors.

Maintain low level of stimuli in client's environment (low lighting, few people, simple decor, low noise level).

A stimulating environment may increase agitation and provoke aggressive behavior.

Remove dangerous objects from client's environment.

Because client may lack inner control at this time, it is a nursing priority to externally control the environment for the safety of client and others.

Help client identify the true object of hostility (e.g., ''You seem to be upset with . . .'')

Because of weak ego development, client may be using the defense mechanism of displacement. Helping the client to recognize this in a nonthreatening environment may help reveal unresolved issues so that they may be confronted.

Encourage client to gradually begin to verbalize hostile feelings.

May be difficult for client to express negative feelings. Verbalization of these feelings in a nonthreatening environment may help client come to terms with unresolved issues.

Explore with client alternative ways of handling frustration/pent-up anger that channel hostile energy into socially acceptable behavior, e.g., brisk walks, jogging, physical exercises, volleyball, punching bag, exercise bike.

Physically demanding activities help to relieve pent-up tension.

Maintain and convey a calm attitude toward the client.

Anxiety is contagious and can be transferred from staff to client. A calm attitude provides client with a feeling of safety and security.

Have sufficient staff available to convey a show of strength to the client if it becomes necessary.

This display provides reassurance for the client that the staff is in control of the situation and will provide physical security for the client, staff, and others.

Collaborative

Administer medications as indicated, e.g., anti-anxiety or other tranquilizing drugs. (Refer to ND: Violence, potential for: directed at self.)

Tranquilizing medications induce a calming effect on the recipient and may inhibit aggressive behaviors.

NURSING DIAGNOSIS:	ANXIETY (MODERATE TO SEVERE)
MAY BE RELATED TO:	Situational and maturational crises
	Threat to self-concept
	Threat (or perceived threat) to physical integrity

	Unmet needs
	Fear of failure
	Dysfunctional family system
	Unsatisfactory parent/child relationship resulting in feelings of insecurity
	Fixation in earlier level of development
POSSIBLY EVIDENCED BY:	Overexcitement/restlessness
	Fearful affect
	Feelings of inadequacy
	Fear of unspecified consequences
	Insomnia
	Poor eye contact, focus on self
	Continuous attention-seeking behaviors
	Difficulty concentrating; selective inattention
	Increased respiratory and heart rates
	Numerous physical complaints
CLIENT OUTCOMES/EVALUATION CRITERIA:	Identifies behaviors that become evident as anxiety starts to rise. Demonstrates appropriate techniques to interrupt progression of anxiety. Maintains anxiety below the moderate level.

INTERVENTIONS	RATIONALE
Independent	
Establish a trusting relationship with the client. Be honest, consistent in responses, and available. Show genuine positive regard.	Honesty, availability, and unconditional acceptance promote trust, which is necessary for the development of a therapeutic relationship.
Provide activities geared toward reduction of tension	Tension and anxiety can be released safely, and physi-

INTERVENTIONS	RATIONALE

Independent

and decreasing anxiety, e.g., walking or jogging, musical exercises, housekeeping chores, group games/activities.

cal activity may provide emotional benefit to the client through release in the brain of morphinelike substances (endorphins) that promote sense of well-being.

Encourage client to identify true feelings and to acknowledge ownership of those feelings.

Anxious clients often deny a relationship between emotional problems and their anxiety. Use of the defense mechanisms of projection and displacement are exaggerated.

Maintain a calm atmosphere.

Anxiety is contagious and can be transmitted from staff to client.

Assist client to recognize specific events that precede onset of elevation in anxiety. Provide information about signs and symptoms of increasing anxiety and ways to intervene before behaviors become disabling.

Recognition of precipitating stressors and a plan of action to follow should they recur provides client with feelings of security and control over similar situations in the future. This in itself may help to control anxiety response.

Offer support during times of elevated anxiety. Provide physical and psychological safety. (Refer to ND: Violence, potential for, directed at self.)

Presence of a trusted individual may provide needed security/client safety.

Collaborative

Administer medications as necessary, e.g., benzodiazepines, propanediols.

Anti-anxiety medications induce a calming effect and work to maintain anxiety at a manageable level while providing an opportunity for client to develop other ways to manage stress.

NURSING DIAGNOSIS: COPING, INEFFECTIVE, INDIVIDUAL

MAY BE RELATED TO: Situational/maturational crises

Inadequate support systems

Negative role modeling

Unmet dependency needs; low self-esteem

Retarded ego development

Fixation in earlier level of development

Dysfunctional family system

Unresolved grief

POSSIBLY EVIDENCED BY:	Inability to meet role expectations
	Alteration in societal participation
	Inability to problem-solve
	Depressed/anxious mood
	Verbal and physical hostility
	Increased dependency
	Manipulation of others in the environment for purposes of fulfilling own desires
	Refusal to follow rules of the unit
	Substance abuse
	Numerous physical complaints
CLIENT OUTCOMES/EVALUATION CRITERIA:	Verbalizes need for change within dysfunctional system. Identifies, develops, and uses socially acceptable coping skills. Solves problems and fulfills activities of daily living independently. Avoids manipulating others for own gratification.

INTERVENTIONS	RATIONALE
Independent	
Explain rules of the unit and consequences of lack of cooperation. Set limits on manipulative behavior. Be consistent in enforcing the consequences when rules are broken and limits tested.	Negative reinforcement may work to decrease undesirable behaviors. Consistency among all staff members is vital if intervention is to be successful.
Ignore negative behaviors when possible and provide feedback when positive behaviors are noted, encouraging client to give self acknowledgment of success.	Negative behaviors diminish when they provide no reward of attention. When client gives self positive feedback, inner rewards are enhanced.
Encourage client to discuss angry feelings. Help client identify the true object of the hostility. Provide physical outlets for healthy release of the hostile feelings, e.g., punching bags, pounding boards. Involve in outdoor recreation program, if available.	Verbalization of feelings with a trusted individual may help client work through unresolved issues. Physical exercise provides a safe and effective means of releasing pent-up tension, as well as of developing self-confidence and trust in others.
Take care not to reinforce dependent behaviors. Allow client to perform as independently as possible and provide feedback.	Independent accomplishment and positive reinforcement enhance self-esteem and encourage repetition of desirable behaviors.

INTERVENTIONS

Independent

Help client to recognize some aspects of life over which a measure of control is maintained/possible. (Refer to ND: Powerlessness.)

Give minimal attention to the physical condition if client is coping through numerous somatic complaints and organic pathology has been ruled out. Increase attention during times when client is not focusing on physical complaints.

Discuss the negative aspects of substance abuse as a response to stress. Help client recognize difficult life situations that may be contributing to use of substances.

Assist client with problem-solving process. Suggest alternatives, and help to select more adaptive strategies for coping with stress.

Encourage client to learn relaxation techniques, use of imagery.

Collaborative

Refer client to substance rehabilitation program if problem is identified.

RATIONALE

Recognition of personal control, however minimal, diminishes the feeling of powerlessness and decreases the need for manipulation of others.

Organic pathology must always be considered. Failure to do so may place the client in physical jeopardy. Lack of attention to maladaptive behaviors may work to decrease their repetition. Positive reinforcement encourages desirable behaviors.

Denial of problems related to use of substances is common. Client needs to recognize relationship between use of substances and personal problems before rehabilitation can begin.

Because of level of anxiety and delayed development, client may require assistance in determining which methods of coping are most individually appropriate. Increased anxiety interferes with the ability to solve problems.

These skills can be helpful to the development of new coping methods to deal with/reduce anxiety.

A greater likelihood of success can be expected if client seeks professional assistance with this problem.

NURSING DIAGNOSIS:	GRIEVING, DYSFUNCTIONAL
MAY BE RELATED TO:	Real or perceived loss of any concept of value to the individual
	Bereavement overload (cumulative grief from multiple unresolved losses)
	Thwarted grieving response to loss
	Absence of anticipatory grieving
	Feelings of guilt generated by ambivalent relationship with the lost concept/person
POSSIBLY EVIDENCED BY:	Idealization of the lost concept/person
	Denial of loss
	Excessive anger, expressed inappropriately

Developmental regression

Alterations in concentration and/or pursuit of tasks

Difficulty in expressing loss

Labile affect

CLIENT OUTCOMES/EVALUATION CRITERIA:

Verbalizes behaviors associated with the normal stages of grief. Recognizes own position in grief process as progression is made toward resolution. Expresses emotions appropriately. Carries out activities of daily living independently. Expresses feeling of hope for the future.

INTERVENTIONS	RATIONALE
Independent	
Determine stage of grief in which patient is fixed. Identify behaviors associated with this stage. (Most depressed people are fixed in the anger stage, with the anger directed inward on the self.)	Accurate baseline assessment data are necessary to plan effective care.
Develop trusting nurse/client relationship. Show empathy and caring. Be honest and keep all promises.	Trust is the basis for a therapeutic relationship supporting client in dealing with loss/reality.
Convey an accepting attitude; encourage client to express self openly.	An accepting attitude enhances trust and communicates to the client that you believe the client to be a worthwhile person, regardless of what may be expressed.
Encourage client to express anger. Do not become defensive if initial expression of anger is displaced on nurse/therapist. Assist client to explore angry feelings and direct them toward the intended object/person or other loss.	Verbalization of feelings in a nonthreatening environment may help client come to terms with unresolved issues related to the loss.
Assist client to discharge pent-up anger through participation in large motor activities.	Physical activity provides a safe and effective method for discharging pent-up tension.
Provide information about the stages of grief and the behaviors associated with each stage. Help client understand that feelings, such as anger directed toward the loss, are appropriate during the grief process.	Knowledge of the acceptability of the feelings associated with normal grieving may help relieve some of the guilt that these responses generate.
Encourage client to review relationship with loss. With support and sensitivity, point out reality of the situation in areas where misrepresentations are expressed.	Client needs to give up idealized perception and accept both positive and negative aspects about the loss before resolution of grief can occur.
Assist client to determine methods for more adaptive coping with the experienced loss. Provide positive feedback for strategies identified and decisions made.	Feelings of depression may interfere with client's problem-solving ability, resulting in need for assistance. Positive feedback enhances self-esteem and encourages repetition of desirable behaviors.

351

INTERVENTIONS	RATIONALE
Collaborative	
Determine client's perception of spiritual needs as support in the grieving process. Involve chaplain or appropriate spiritual leader as indicated.	Some individuals derive great strength from spiritual support. This strength may be used by the client in the task of grief resolution.

NURSING DIAGNOSIS:	**POWERLESSNESS**
MAY BE RELATED TO:	**Lifestyle of helplessness**
	Health care environment
	Incomplete grief work
	Lack of positive feedback
	Consistent negative feedback
	Numerous real or perceived failures
POSSIBLY EVIDENCED BY:	**Verbal expressions of having no control or influence over situation, outcome, or self-care**
	Nonparticipation in care or decision-making when opportunities are provided
	Expression of doubt regarding role performance
	Reluctance to express true feelings, fearing alienation from caregivers
	Apathy/passivity
	Dependence on others that may result in irritability, resentment, anger, and guilt
CLIENT OUTCOMES/EVALUATION CRITERIA:	**Demonstrates independent problem-solving techniques to take control over life situation. Verbalizes acceptance of life situations over which one does not have control. Verbalizes positive feelings regarding own ability to achieve satisfactory role performance.**

INTERVENTIONS	RATIONALE
Independent	
Encourage client to assume responsibility for own self-care, e.g., setting goals, scheduling activities, making independent decisions.	Providing the client with choices increases feelings of control.
Discuss goals, making sure they are realistic.	Unrealistic goals set the client up for failure and reinforce feelings of powerlessness.
Help client identify areas of life situation that are under own control.	Client's emotional condition may interfere with ability to solve problems. Assistance may be required to perceive the benefits and consequences of available alternatives accurately.
Help client identify areas of life situation that are not within ability to control. Discuss feelings associated with this lack of control.	Client needs to identify and resolve feelings associated with inability to control certain life situations before level of acceptance can be achieved.
Identify use of maladaptive behaviors to gain control. (Refer to NDs: Violence, potential for: directed at self; directed at others.)	Personal attempts to overcome feelings of powerlessness have resulted in ineffective/harmful behaviors.

NURSING DIAGNOSIS:	**SELF-CONCEPT, DISTURBANCE IN: SELF-ESTEEM**
MAY BE RELATED TO:	**Lack of positive feedback**
	Unmet dependency needs
	Retarded ego development
	Repeated negative feedback, diminished self-worth
	Dysfunctional family system
POSSIBLY EVIDENCED BY:	**Difficulty accepting positive reinforcement**
	Nonparticipation in therapy
	Self-destructive ideas/behavior
	Frequent use of derogatory and critical remarks against self
	Hesitancy to undertake new tasks; fear of failure
	Lack of eye contact

353

POSSIBLY EVIDENCED BY—*continued*	Manipulation of one staff member against another in an attempt to gain special privileges
	Inability to form close, personal relationships
	Social isolation
	Degradation of others in an attempt to increase own feelings of self-worth
CLIENT OUTCOMES/EVALUATION CRITERIA:	Verbalizes positive perception of self. Accepts recognition for personal accomplishments. Recognizes and acknowledges the accomplishments of others without degrading own achievements.

INTERVENTIONS	RATIONALE
Independent	
Discuss goals, making sure they are realistic. Plan activities in which success is likely.	Achievement/success enhance self-esteem.
Convey unconditional positive regard for the client. Promote understanding of acceptance for client as a worthwhile human being.	Unconditional acceptance of an individual serves to counteract feelings of worthlessness by reinforcing that they are worthy of another person's respect.
Spend time with client both on a 1:1 basis and in group activities.	Conveys that the nurse sees the client as someone worth spending time with.
Assist client in identifying positive aspects of self and in developing plans for changing the characteristics viewed as negative.	Individuals with low self-esteem often have difficulty recognizing positive attributes. May also lack problem-solving ability and require assistance to formulate a plan for implementing the desired changes.
Encourage and support client in confronting the fear of failure by attending therapy activities and undertaking new tasks. Offer recognition of successful endeavors and positive reinforcement of attempts made.	Recognition and positive reinforcement enhance self-esteem and encourage repetition of desirable behaviors.
Assist client to avoid ruminating about past failures. Withdraw attention if client persists.	Lack of attention to these undesirable behaviors may discourage their repetition. Client needs to focus on positive attributes if self-esteem is to be enhanced.
Minimize negative feedback to client. Enforce limit setting in matter-of-fact manner, imposing previously established consequences for violations.	Negative feedback can be extremely threatening to a person with low self-esteem, possibly aggravating the problem. Consequences need to convey unacceptability of the *behavior,* but not the *person.*
Encourage independence in the performance of personal responsibilities, as well as in decision-making related to own self-care. Offer recognition and praise for accomplishments.	The ability to perform self-care activities independently enhances self-esteem. Positive reinforcement encourages repetition of desirable behaviors.

INTERVENTIONS	RATIONALE

Independent

Support client in critical examination of feelings, attitudes, and behaviors. Help client understand that it is acceptable for attitudes and behaviors to differ from those of others, as long as they do not become intrusive.

The need for judging the behavior of others diminishes as client increases self-esteem through greater self-awareness and the achievement of self-acceptance.

NURSING DIAGNOSIS:	SOCIAL INTERACTION, IMPAIRED
MAY BE RELATED TO:	Unmet dependency needs
	Retarded ego development
	Fixation in earlier level of development
	Negative role modeling
	Low self-esteem
POSSIBLY EVIDENCED BY:	Verbalized or observed discomfort in social situations
	Verbalized or observed inability to receive or communicate a satisfying sense of belonging, caring, interest, or shared history
	Observed use of unsuccessful social interaction behaviors
	Dysfunctional interaction with peers, family, and/or others.
	Exhibits behaviors unacceptable for age, as defined by dominant cultural group
CLIENT OUTCOMES/EVALUATION CRITERIA:	Verbalizes awareness of factors resulting in difficulty in forming satisfactory relationships with others in the past. Identifies feelings that lead to poor social interactions. Interacts with staff and peers with little/no indication of discomfort. Participates in

355

CLIENT OUTCOMES/EVALUATION
CRITERIA—*continued*

group activities appropriately and willingly. Identifies/develops effective social support system.

INTERVENTIONS

Independent

Establish 1:1 relationship with client, which serves as role model for testing new behaviors.

Encourage client to engage in activities out of room. Offer to attend initial group interactions with client. Provide feedback for appropriate interactions.

Confront client and withdraw attention when interactions with others are manipulative or exploitative.

Assist client to understand how unacceptable behaviors have interfered with the ability to form satisfactory relationships in the past.

Act as role model for client through appropriate interactions with client, other clients, and staff members.

Establish schedule of group activities for client.

RATIONALE

Client needs to learn to interact appropriately with nurse, so that behaviors may then be generalized to others.

Decreases opportunity for client to isolate self. Presence of a trusted individual may provide a feeling of security and decrease the anxiety generated by difficult social situation. Positive reinforcement enhances self-esteem and encourages repetition of desirable behaviors.

Attention to the unacceptable behavior may reinforce it.

Client may not realize how others actually perceive actions. Correction of these misperceptions may assist in the improvement of ability to interact with others.

Because of weak ego development, client is inclined to imitate the actions of those individuals admired or trusted.

It is through these group interactions, with positive and negative feedback from peers, that client learns socially acceptable behavior.

NURSING DIAGNOSIS: FAMILY PROCESS, ALTERED

MAY BE RELATED TO: Situational/maturational crises

History of inadequate coping methods

POSSIBLY EVIDENCED BY: Needs of family members not being met

Confusion within family system regarding how needs should be met

Impairment of family decision-making process

Dissonance among family members

Impaired family communication

Family developmental tasks not being fulfilled

Reduced/restricted social involvement

Ill-defined family rules, function, and roles

FAMILY OUTCOMES/EVALUATION CRITERIA:

Develops effective patterns of communication, encouraging honest input from all members. Identifies source(s) of dysfunction and effectively problem-solves to achieve desired resolution. Returns to pattern of functioning improved from premorbid state, having gained knowledge and achieved growth from crisis situation.

INTERVENTIONS	RATIONALE
Independent	
Assess family developmental stage, communication patterns, and extent of dysfunction.	Identifies individual needs and provides direction for care.
Meet with the total family group as often as possible.	The family as a system operates as a single unit. Each member affects, and is affected by, all other members. Therapy is most effective when directed toward the functioning of the family system.
Construct a client/family genogram.	Genograms help to identify emotional closeness among family members over several generations. Family process is clarified, and configuration and dynamics are clearly illustrated.
Assist family to identify true source of conflict. Help them recognize that identified patient's adjustment disorder may be a way to avoid confronting the real problem.	Conflict creates high levels of anxiety within the family system. Common defense mechanisms, such as denial, displacement, projection, and rationalization, are used by the family to decrease anxiety and avoid conflict.
Assist family members to set goals and identify alternatives. Support efforts directed toward positive change. Assist with necessary modifications of original plan.	Life crises interfere with family decision-making and problem-solving ability. Assistance with this process may be required.
Promote separation and individuation and clear, functional boundaries between members.	Emotional connectedness among family members (enmeshment) discourages individual growth and ability to function autonomously.
Assist client-family to identify actions/problem-solve for potential life crises.	Anticipatory guidance/knowing what to expect and having a plan of action for management of situations may help to avert a crisis in the future.

357

INTERVENTIONS	RATIONALE

Collaborative

Involve family in group therapy.	Interacting with others in family/multifamily groups can be helpful to identify dysfunctional patterns and assist in learning new skills and solutions for family problems.
Refer family to other resources, such as support groups, classes, e.g., parenting/assertiveness training.	Sharing with others who have had similar experiences can provide support and assist family members to learn new ways to deal with situation.

CHAPTER 14

PSYCHOLOGICAL FACTORS AFFECTING PHYSICAL CONDITION

Psychophysiologic Disorders

DSM III-R: 316.00 Psychological factors affecting physical condition (specify physical condition on Axis III) These disorders represent a group of ailments in which emotional stress is a contributing factor to physical problems involving an organ system under involuntary control. The organ systems most often affected are respiratory, cardiovascular, gastrointestinal, genitourinary, musculoskeletal, and integumentary.

ETIOLOGIC THEORIES

Although the etiology of psychosomatic disorders is unknown, it is believed that an individual's emotional state and life circumstances significantly affect the onset, form, and course of psychosomatic illness. The interaction of psychological, social, and biologic factors becomes evident as physical symptoms appear and diminish in direct relationship to the amount of stress the person is experiencing. Psychophysiologic disorders do occur without known psychologic components, but generally these disorders have some genetic predisposition in order to respond to stress pathologically.

PSYCHODYNAMICS

Thought to center around issues of unresolved dependency conflicts, undischarged aggressive feelings, repressed anger, hostility, resentment, and anxiety. These conflicts are expressed somatically, with physiologic responses corresponding to unconscious emotional conflict instead of directly through verbalization, indicating inadequate or maladaptive defense mechanisms.

Interpersonal theory proposes that individuals with specific personality traits are predisposed to certain disease processes, e.g., those who are dependent develop asthma; depression, cancer; aggressiveness, coronary artery disease.

BIOLOGIC THEORIES

A new field of psychoneuroimmunology is developing around research of the biologic factors that underlie these illnesses. It has been demonstrated that the immune response can be affected by behavior modification. Skills are being taught to assist people to modify responses which are thought to lead to illness.

In extensive stress studies, it was found that specific physiologic responses under direct control of the pituitary/ adrenal axis occurred in response to stress. When these stress responses are prolonged, psychosomatic disorders can develop. It is postulated that the specific organ system involved and type of psychosomatic disorder the individual develops may be genetically determined.

FAMILY DYNAMICS

Children who grow up observing the attention, increased dependency, or other secondary gain an individual receives because of illness, see these behaviors as a desirable response and subsequently imitate them. The dysfunctional family system uses these psychophysiologic problems to cover up interpersonal conflicts. Anxiety is thus shifted from the conflict to the ailing member. As anxiety decreases, conflict is avoided, and positive reinforcement is given for the symptoms of the sick person.

CLIENT ASSESSMENT DATA BASE

HISTORY

General

In general, these clients do not present a calm, relaxed demeanor but rather a pattern of anxiety and problems of coping with stress that occurs in their lives.

Coronary Artery Disease

Risk factors most frequently reported are cigarette smoking, hypertension, elevated serum cholesterol and triglyceride levels, left ventricular hypertrophy, diabetes, and age.
Males have higher incidence.
May exhibit an abrupt, fast-talking presentation, and are constantly moving, e.g., jiggling knees or tapping fingers.
Measures success by material goods/personal accomplishments.
Usually are "too busy" to notice quiet, beautiful surroundings.

Peptic Ulcer

May report history of stomach complaints, gastritis, hyperacidity, peptic ulcer.
Family history may reveal other affected members.
May express an intense need for perfection and feelings of not having enough control over stressors and environment.

Essential Hypertension

Reports chronic high blood pressure with no known organic origin
More prevalent in black population; onset usually in early adult life (mean age in early thirties).
Increased incidence in urban areas rather than in rural or tropical areas (may be related to a more relaxed lifestyle).
Complains of fatigue, dizziness, nervousness, palpitations, sleep disturbances, and headaches.
May report emotional trauma, presence of stressful situations in daily life.
Predisposing factors include obesity, controlled emotionality, social isolation, sensitivity to salt.

Bronchial Asthma

Can occur at any age (a third are children; two-thirds of these are boys).
The earlier the onset of asthma, the longer it lasts.
Respiratory infections/induced emotionality may trigger/exacerbate attacks.
A strong correlation between asthma attacks and tension in the home/estranged relationships with parents has been demonstrated.

Ulcerative Colitis

Can occur at any age.
May report difficulty in interpersonal relationships/dependency on others.
May express ambivalence/hypersensitivity toward significant others who have been a source of hurt or perceived rejection.

PHYSICAL EXAMINATION

Mental Status:

Psychologic factors linking stress and personality traits include:

Cardiac Type A: Life stressors, ongoing emotional turmoil and overexertion. An intense need to compete and win, even if competing with a child. May be overdutiful to job; hostile, angry and aggressive toward others; feel a need to do everything in a hurry, and become impatient if asked to wait; some cannot tolerate waiting in lines. Driving, idealistic, dominant, compulsive individual, with passive-aggressive tendencies, strict superego, and feelings of insecurity.

Migraine headache: Compulsive/perfectionistic, conscientious, intelligent, neat, inflexible, rigid, resentful, guilt feelings.

Hypertension: Conflicted over expression of hostile and aggressive feelings, struggle with dependency versus achievement needs. Tends to hold anger in and to feel guilty if anger is expressed, and inhibits aggressive wishes. May show greater reactivity to stressful stimuli, even in normal situations.

Asthma: Dependent, meek, sensitive, nervous, compulsive, and perfectionistic. Feelings of insecurity and oppression, insufficient superego, compulsive, overdutiful attitudes, and a tendency to be passive-aggressive are often present. May be shy, irritable, impatient, stubborn, and tyrannical at times. Anxiety, anger, depression, tension, frustration, and anticipation of a pleasurable event can contribute to exacerbation of symptoms.

Ulcerative Colitis: Compulsive, especially regarding punctuality and neatness; difficulty expressing anger/hostility directly, timidity, obstinacy, hyperintellectualism, lack of humor. May perceive even the slightest criticism as rejection and feel a loss of self-esteem, and may respond by using avoidance or by becoming suspicious. Precipitating stressors center around real or feared threats to significant interpersonal relationships or deaths. Other stressors include situations in which the individual feels hurt or humiliated and unable to/not inclined to meet the demands of those on whom they feel dependent.

Peptic Ulcer: Long-standing feelings of anxiety, repressed anger, hostility, resentment, and a sense of helplessness, with difficulty in coping; have a highly developed superego and are conscientious/dutiful; however, may be insecure/nervous.

Common manifestations of psychosomatic disorders (but not limited to) are listed under respective systems:

1. Respiratory: wheezing, shortness of breath, restlessness, cyanosis; hyperventilation, sighing, hiccups.
2. Cardiovascular: elevated blood pressure, migraine headache, tachycardia, palpitations, angina.
3. Gastrointestinal: pain, heartburn, reflux, hyperacidity, diarrhea (with/without blood), weight loss, fatigue, pallor, anemia.
4. Genitourinary: menstrual and urinary disturbances; dyspareunia, impotence.
5. Musculoskeletal: joint stiffness/pain, backache, muscle cramps, tension headaches.
6. Skin: pruritus, cutaneous inflammation (neurodermatitis), excessive sweating (hyperhydrosis).
7. Others: overeating/excessive weight; autoimmune diseases, manifested as rheumatoid arthritis, systemic lupus erythematosus, myasthenia gravis, and pernicious anemia, etc.

DIAGNOSTIC STUDIES

Dependent on specific presenting condition/symptoms.

NURSING PRIORITIES

1. Encourage verbalization of feelings and stressors.
2. Assist client to develop coping skills and assertiveness techniques to reduce/manage anxiety.
3. Promote development of positive self-esteem.
4. Help client to accomplish a sense of autonomy and independence.

DISCHARGE CRITERIA

1. Assertive techniques are used as a more productive, effective means of expression.
2. Demonstrates stress management methods of reducing anxiety.
3. Displays positive self-esteem that satisfies client's needs without compromising self/others.
4. Client/family involved in group therapy/community support programs.

Note: This care plan deals with the psychiatric component of these conditions. The user is referred to a medical-surgical resource (such as *Nursing Care Plans: Nursing Diagnoses in Patient Care,* by Doenges, Jeffries, Moorhouse; 1984) for physiologic considerations.

NURSING DIAGNOSIS:	**ANXIETY (MODERATE TO SEVERE)**
MAY BE RELATED TO:	**Stimulation of the fight or flight reaction**
	Internalized feelings of inadequacy, resentment, frustration, anger
	Inability to obtain relief from stress
	Perceived threat to self-concept
	Unmet needs
	Negative self-talk
POSSIBLY EVIDENCED BY:	**Increase in blood pressure/somatic complaints**
	Denial of relationship between physical symptoms and emotional problems
	Inability to meet role expectations
	Focus on self
CLIENT OUTCOMES/EVALUATION CRITERIA:	**Verbalizes understanding of relationship between feelings of anxiety and physical symptoms. Develops effective methods for decreasing anxiety. Reports anxiety reduced to manageable level. Experiences marked decrease in somatic complaints.**

INTERVENTIONS	RATIONALE
Independent	
Explore situations that lead to feelings of anger, resentment. Discuss possible causes and explore stressors or events that trigger illness. Discuss ways to stop the escalation of anxiety.	Helps client define problem areas and begin to establish goals to work through them. Client reacts to stress psychologically and needs to learn to control emotional responses.
Assist client to learn to be in tune to feelings and recognize situations that cause increase in anxiety.	Client may be out of touch with body and not aware of feelings, therefore does not experience "signal anxi-

INTERVENTIONS	RATIONALE
Independent	
	ety'' which helps to recognize beginning development of anxiety so steps can be taken for control.
Encourage direct expression of feelings. Help client to recognize times when the feelings are internalized.	The client who internalizes feelings is not always aware of doing that and may have trouble even identifying feelings.
Identify the amount of anxiety experienced if not perceiving self as ''perfect'' in job performance and interpersonal relationships.	May put pressure on self to be ''perfect,'' while at the same time not recognizing/accepting feelings and resultant anxiety, which is then expressed in physical illness.
Examine possible cause-effect relationship between ''internalizing'' feelings and somatic symptoms.	Client needs to see the relationship between physical discomfort and turning feelings inward, so steps can be taken to deal more appropriately with them.
Assist client to relate pattern of resurgence of symptoms and stressful life situations.	Reinforces the fact that client does transfer stress to body (GI upset, tension headache, chest pain, respiratory distress, etc.), and needs to learn how to stop this unhealthy reaction.
Ask client to describe difference between assertiveness and aggression, and discuss ways to express feelings assertively.	Assertiveness training is of utmost importance for the client who does not know how to directly express self, in order to defuse inner tension and relieve resulting physiologic effects of anxiety.
Demonstrate/encourage use of relaxation, visualization, imagery techniques, e.g., progressive relaxation, meditation.	Studies show that these techniques decrease anxiety and work to moderate the stimulation of the sympathetic nervous system.
Use gentle, supportive therapeutic approach to develop a positive rapport.	Skill of the therapist is crucial. Care needs to be taken to avoid alienating the client.
Be cautious in using confrontive techniques or making demands for achievement.	Client has low tolerance for stress. It is most critical not to exacerbate onset of symptoms.
Explore possible recreational activities to alleviate and rechannel stress productively (e.g., brisk walks/jogging, volleyball, bowling, swimming).	Physical activity is very effective for relieving stress and providing opportunity to develop new skills to reduce anxiety.

NURSING DIAGNOSIS:	**COPING, INEFFECTIVE, INDIVIDUAL**
MAY BE RELATED TO:	**Personal vulnerability**
	Inadequate repertoire of coping mechanisms
	Difficulty expressing anger/discharging hostile and aggressive feelings
	Use of passive-aggressive maneuvers
	Intolerance and hostility toward others

MAY BE RELATED TO—*continued*	Compelling, intense desire to compete and win
	Feeling pressured to hurry, preoccupation with the urgency of passing time
	Excessive need to achieve success
	Unmet expectations
	Too many deadlines
POSSIBLY EVIDENCED BY:	Failure to obtain relief from and/or not resolving negative feelings
	Inadequate discharge of aggressive feelings/desires
	Internalizing stress/buildup of frustration
	Use of maladaptive coping methods
	Somatic complaints, rise in blood pressure
CLIENT OUTCOMES/EVALUATION CRITERIA:	Develops and implements repertoire of coping strategies based on problem-solving techniques that provide effective relief for conflicts. Uses assertive techniques in place of passive-aggressive, maladaptive behaviors. Demonstrates a more moderate lifestyle. Verbalizes understanding of health risks.

INTERVENTIONS	RATIONALE
Independent	
Assist client to identify present coping patterns and the consequences and evaluate their effectiveness.	A realistic picture of how effective current mechanisms are provides insight and enables client to acknowledge ineffectiveness of these methods and begin to look at healthy alternatives.
Help client identify/understand unmet needs and how present coping patterns relate to relief of anxiety.	Developing a keen sense of self-awareness and how these factors are interrelated provides opportunity for change.
Demonstrate/practice problem-solving techniques. Encourage client to think through problems.	Learning to arrive at thought-out solutions provides base for effective, satisfying coping behaviors.

INTERVENTIONS	RATIONALE
Independent	
Ask client to give examples of situations when resentment and anger were felt but were not expressed. Discuss/role-play alternate ways to handle those situations.	Behavior rehearsal helps client to learn how to handle troublesome situations much more effectively.
Examine how needs are expressed, passively or aggressively.	Client may not be aware of use of passive or aggressive approach. Awareness offers choice to change behavior.
Have client identify and discuss personal dynamics. Are they used to prevent guilt or win approval?	Many interactions may be based on trying to relieve guilt or to please others and ignoring own wishes.
Confront with behaviors that are used to prevent rejection or disapproval by others.	Increases self-awareness of maladaptive pattern(s).
Encourage client to assume control over own reactions to stressful events, even though the circumstances cannot always be controlled.	The client can learn to control how much a stressful event affects feelings, behavior, and becoming upset by changing the way these events are viewed.
Identify competitive behaviors and explore reasons for feeling a compulsion to achieve/win.	Realization that the compulsive drive for achievement can be strong enough to endanger health may provide stimulus for change.
Evaluate the effect these compulsive feelings have had on physical and emotional health.	Heightens awareness of the possible toll on health, longevity.
Explore how these behaviors have affected interpersonal relationships.	Client may be intolerant of others and aggressive in relationships, resulting in problems of interacting with others.
Assist client to identify what needs are really being met by competitive behaviors.	Recognition of own self-esteem needs provides opportunity to meet these needs in a more direct/ successful manner.
Discuss consequences of "driving" oneself and how to moderate lifestyle to reduce stress.	Reinforces the negative effects of continuing an intense lifestyle.
Discuss importance of leisure time and how to develop and use it. Explain how pacing oneself can be a more productive and efficient use of time.	Client has not been used to taking time out to relax, and learning how to relax and enjoy recreation can relieve anxiety and promote effective coping.

NURSING DIAGNOSIS: **POWERLESSNESS**

MAY BE RELATED TO: **Unresolved dependency conflicts**

Feelings of insecurity, resentment

Repression of anger and aggressive feelings

Lacking a sense of control in stressful situations

Sacrificing own wishes for others

MAY BE RELATED TO—*continued*	Retreat from aggression or frustration
POSSIBLY EVIDENCED BY:	**Difficulty expressing self directly and assertively**
	Passive/docile or aggressive behavior
	Internalizing of stress/increased anxiety expressed through somatic complaints, elevated blood pressure
CLIENT OUTCOMES/EVALUATION CRITERIA:	**Recognizes and works through feelings of insecurity, resentment. Uses assertive behaviors to deal with feelings, anxiety-producing situations, and interacting with others. Verbalizes awareness of own control over self and how stress is handled in situations over which client does not have control. Demonstrates fewer physical complaints and episodes of illness.**

INTERVENTIONS	RATIONALE
Independent	
Have client describe events that lead to feeling inadequate or having no control.	Helpful in identifying sources of frustration and defining problem areas so action can be taken
Examine together how client feels when not "perfectly" competent or adequate in performance.	Client may be self-deprecating and believe s/he has failed unless self is perceived as "perfect."
Assess client's attitude toward making mistakes, e.g., able to admit and accept or feels inadequate and worthless.	When client indulges in self-punishment, client needs to learn a rational way of "thinking" regarding mistakes. Failure is seldom a catastrophe and often leads to learning important lessons when the client is open to the opportunity.
Discuss how worry and anxiety prevent dealing with problems efficiently and cause more feelings of incompetency.	Worry and anxiety can prevent objective evaluation of a situation and lead to the use of poor judgment.
Encourage client to do the feared activity to prove that it will not be catastrophic.	Avoiding dreaded events increases unnecessary fears and causes further loss of self-confidence. Confronting the situation can result in an increase in self-confidence.
Discuss behaviors that are self-defeating and explore new, productive behaviors, e.g., looking at problem as a challenge instead of a threat, developing a sense of commitment to something, and gaining a sense of control over own life.	Past solutions to problems may not be relevant at this time, and previous failed experiences are not sufficient reason to discount their reevaluation.
Ask client to describe significant others' behaviors that are perceived as intimidating and how fear of these behaviors can be overcome.	Identifying successful actions to use can improve self-esteem. As self-confidence is gained, the client will be less easily intimidated.

366

INTERVENTIONS

Independent

Explain how a lack of self-confidence in one's own judgment and abilities can result in feeling powerless in stressful situations.

Use role-playing techniques to demonstrate how to assert feelings and help client learn direct self-expression when faced with frustration or aggression.

Have client describe people seen as dynamic or powerful individuals and how they achieved personal power. Explore how client can achieve these desired attributes.

Examine sources of resentment. Identify what has been done to resolve these feelings and whether an effort has been made to get information to justify resentment.

Encourage client to be open and direct in verbal expression. Confront when guarding of feelings is noted.

Assess client's pattern of response to aggression or frustration, and together evaluate the effectiveness of these responses.

Examine situations that produce anger or guilt in client and discuss what triggers these feelings.

Discuss causes of difficulty in making own needs known to others and fears surrounding these issues.

Explore guilt feelings when expressing anger and ways to work through this problem.

Examine causes of hostility and how these feelings can be adequately discharged, e.g., pounding pillows, yelling appropriately, expressing feelings to the other person.

Ask client to verbalize how and why feelings of helplessness and dependency began. Discuss ways to put these feelings into perspective.

Explore with client fears of loss/rejection and evaluate together how realistic these concerns are.

Assist client to think through these concerns and identify ways to deal with them.

Have client identify what will happen if client functions independently. Assist to learn how to use own capabilities.

RATIONALE

Loss of self-confidence serves only to "immobilize"/prevent using effective mechanism in dealing with problems.

Behavior rehearsal is an effective way to practice self-expression/learn to deal with troublesome situations, get the desired need met, and enhance sense of control.

Helps client to clearly define goals and values and look at how these relate to own self.

More information can diffuse an angry or resentful response. Situations are not always as they appear, and individual's perceptions may be distorted. Checking out reality can help the client decide on appropriate follow-up.

Learning new ways of expression is difficult. Reinforcing open/direct expression promotes continuation of activity.

Client first needs to recognize own pattern of maladaptive defense mechanisms in order to learn new adaptive responses.

Unresolved guilt and anger lead to feelings of frustration or powerlessness.

The client does not assert own needs and either passively accepts things as they are or ineffectively tries to assert control, increasing feelings of powerlessness. Discussion and awareness provide opportunity for change.

Client needs to learn that it is acceptable to feel and express anger appropriately.

Client may be harboring undischarged hostility that needs resolution or release instead of allowing these feelings to affect body negatively (e.g., increased blood pressure, tension headache).

Being aware of emotional dependency and how these dynamics originate provides opportunity to change behavior/outcomes.

May tend to exaggerate slight criticism into unrealistic fears.

Client needs to learn to accept the positive and negative aspects of relationships without becoming dysfunctional.

Functioning autonomously and capitalizing on own strengths promote client's sense of control over own life/outcomes.

NURSING DIAGNOSIS:	SELF-CONCEPT, DISTURBANCE IN: SELF-ESTEEM
MAY BE RELATED TO:	Lack of positive feedback
	Unmet dependency needs
	Retarded ego development
	Repeated negative feedback/diminished self-worth
	Dysfunctional family system
POSSIBLY EVIDENCED BY:	Belief that individual should be "perfect"
	Not expressing needs directly, lacking self-confidence, being dependent, not verbalizing negative feelings
	Feelings of worthlessness
	Not working negative feelings through
CLIENT OUTCOMES/EVALUATION CRITERIA:	Verbalizes view of self as a worthwhile, important person who functions well both interpersonally and occupationally. Demonstrates self-confidence by setting realistic goals and active participation in life situations. Experiences a decrease in somatic complaints.

INTERVENTIONS	RATIONALE
Independent	
Assess client's strengths and limitations and compare with client's own assessment of self.	An accurate picture of the client's sense of self-worth is important in developing the plan of care.
Assist client to learn to accept disapproval from others without feeling a sense of failure.	Helps to develop confidence in own abilities and judgment despite what others think.
Discuss client's goals. Are they what the client really wants or are they what the client thinks they "should" or "ought" to be?	Typically tends to ignore own wishes and do what client thinks others expect.
Explain why it is necessary to take risks in order to build self-esteem.	Self-confidence is built on taking risks and learning from success and/or failure.

INTERVENTIONS

Independent

Ask client to discuss feelings about criticism from others. Discuss ways to cope with these feelings.

Identify what needs are being met by preoccupation with neatness and orderliness. Relate these needs to self-esteem needs.

Discuss possible feelings of ambivalence toward significant other(s) who have been a source of disappointment, rejection, or loss.

Explore expectations family and/or significant others hold for client.

Assist to identify realistic needs for change in relation to self, family/significant other(s).

Reinforce client's ability to assume responsibility and reliance on own abilities.

RATIONALE

May have unrealistic feelings when criticized and needs to learn how to apply constructive criticism for personal growth rather than becoming devastated.

Client more than likely experiences a sense of failure if unable to keep environment perfect.

Often experiences ambivalent feelings toward significant others due to inability to deal with negative feelings directly and having a fear of rejection if negative feelings are expressed.

Client may be trying to meet unrealistic expectations, further increasing sense of failure and anxiety.

Without guidance, may misinterpret/block needs, setting self up for failure.

Needs emotional support and encouragement to become self-reliant.

NURSING DIAGNOSIS:	**COPING, INEFFECTIVE, FAMILY: COMPROMISED/DISABLING**
MAY BE RELATED TO:	**Inadequate or incorrect information or understanding by a primary person**
	Client providing little support for primary person
	Prolonged disease progression that exhausts supportive capacity of significant other(s)
	Significant person with chronically unexpressed feelings of guilt, anxiety, hostility, despair
POSSIBLY EVIDENCED BY:	**Client expresses despair regarding family reactions/lack of involvement**
	Intolerance/abandonment
	Psychosomatic tendency
	Taking on illness signs of client
	Distortion of reality regarding the client's health problem

POSSIBLY EVIDENCED BY—*continued*	Significant other(s) display protective behavior disproportionate (too little or too much) to client's abilities or need for autonomy
FAMILY OUTCOMES/EVALUATION CRITERIA:	Identifies/verbalizes resources within themselves to deal with situation. Interacts appropriately with the client and each other, providing support and assistance as indicated. Verbalizes knowledge and understanding of illness. Participating actively in treatment program.

INTERVENTIONS	RATIONALE
Independent	
Explore past relationships and feelings about successes and failures.	May help identify a pattern of interacting that is doomed to failure.
Discuss precipitating stresses regarding real or feared threats to significant personal relationships.	Unrealistic fears may be dictating relationships.
Determine extent of "enabling" behaviors evidenced by family members; explore with family/client.	"Enabling" is doing for the client what s/he needs to do for own self. People want to be helpful and do not want to feel powerless to help their family member to be well. When the family members' "roles" are to "help" the client stay ill, they need to learn new ways of interacting to attain/maintain health for each individual.
Assist to develop communication skills that enable needs to be met by using assertive expressions, e.g., "I-messages."	Using assertive, direct communication can make significant differences in communicating needs and having these needs met in more effective ways.
Explore possible negative feelings or fears caused by feeling compelled to meet demands of others.	May frustrate own wishes to please others due to fear of rejection or loss of the relationship.
Discuss ways of handling troublesome situations by using newly learned coping skills.	Having a plan for handling situations before they arise helps increase successful interactions.
Give positive feedback for efforts toward using constructive new behaviors.	Client may lack self-confidence and require emotional support and assurance of capability.
Collaborative	
Refer to support groups, family therapy, if indicated.	May need additional assistance to promote healthy ways of interacting and assist client to deal effectively with illness/improve quality of life.

370

Late Luteal Phase Dysphoric Disorder (Premenstrual Syndrome)

DSM III-R: Recommended for further systematic clinical study and research

Premenstrual syndrome (PMS) is a group of symptoms occurring during the luteal phase of the menstrual cycle, becoming progressively worse, interfering with familial, social, and work-related activities, and improving after the onset of menses. The symptoms cannot be the sole result of cyclic or environmental stress, but may be enhanced by these stressors. This diagnosis is not used when the person is experiencing a late luteal phase exacerbation of another disorder, such as major depression, panic disorder, or dysthymia.

ETIOLOGIC THEORIES

PSYCHODYNAMICS

Although etiology is not understood, it is believed to be related to the interaction of psychologic, social, and biologic factors. Underlying personality and psychiatric conditions contribute to how any particular individual deals with these physical problems. It has been suggested that an individual's past and present negative attitudes toward menstruation likely influence the symptomatology of PMS. Emotion is the result of complex interactions between hormonal changes and cognitive variables. Hormonal changes during the menstrual cycle are likely to increase the female's susceptibility to negative psychologic experiences rather than to cause such experiences.

BIOLOGIC THEORIES

Although not completely understood, it is believed to be related to the alterations (fluctuations) in estrogen and progesterone and the fluid-retaining action of estrogen during the menstrual cycle. Estrogen excess/deficiency, progesterone deficiency, vitamin deficiency, hypoglycemia, and fluid retention have all been proposed to contribute to PMS. In addition, levels of androgen, adrenal hormones, and prolactin have also been hypothesized to be important in the etiology of this syndrome. An increase in prostaglandins secreted by the uterine musculature has also been implicated in accounting for the pain associated with PMS.

FAMILY DYNAMICS

It is possible that the behaviors associated with PMS are learned through modeling during the socialization process. Children may observe and identify with this behavior in significant adults and incorporate it into their own responses as they grow up. Positive reinforcement in the form of primary or secondary gains for these behaviors may serve to perpetuate the learned patterns of disability.

CLIENT ASSESSMENT DATA BASE

HISTORY

Age of onset may be any time after menarche, but may not be noticeable until the twenties (may not seek treatment until thirties or forties, when the symptoms worsen).

May report a history of personality changes not unlike Jekyll and Hyde (e.g., feeling happy or serene during the follicular phase of the menstrual cycle and tense, irritable, and depressed beginning anytime in the luteal phase but primarily during the last week), occurring during a majority of menstrual cycles and ceasing at the onset of the menstrual period.

Reports interference with the quality of life (home, social, and work)

May have close female relative(s) with similar problems.

May relate intolerance or multiple side effects to birth control pills. (However, a small percentage of women with PMS become better on birth control pills.)

May have history of pregnancy-induced hypertension.

May report poor nutritional habits, lack of exercise, and difficulty maintaining a stable weight.

May complain of nervous tension, mood swings, irritability, anxiety (Type A); headaches, dizziness or fainting, heart pounding, sugar and other specific food cravings/increased appetite, and fatigue (Type C); swelling of extremities, abdominal bloating, overeating/weight gain, breast tenderness and swelling (Type H); depression, forgetfulness, crying, confusion, and insomnia (Type D); as well as cramps, alcohol intolerance, acne, cystitis, oliguria, joint pain/swelling, and backache.

PHYSICAL EXAMINATION

Mental status:
>Changes in body image, sense of depersonalization may be reported.
>Affective changes of dysphoria or depressed mood, irritability, anxiety, and feelings of being unable to cope/ sense of loss of control may be noted.

Multiple symptoms may be present, e.g., tension (including depression), anger, lethargy, and anxiety; sudden mood swings, including hostility, aggressiveness, nagging, irrational thought processes involving suicide and suicidal attempts.

Psychologic symptoms, such as altered sexual drive, restlessness, decreased concentration, confusion, crying spells, fatigue, decreased interest in usual activities, forgetfulness, and altered sleep patterns.

DIAGNOSTIC STUDIES

As indicated by individual situation, dependent on: age, medication therapy, family history, and symptomatology.

In nonmenstruating females who have had a hysterectomy, the timing of luteal and follicular phases may require measurement of circulating reproductive hormones and/or daily self-ratings.

Serum progesterone and estradiol 17 (midluteal phase): To assess an inadequate luteal phase and confirm Type A in client with unexplained infertility.

Serum prolactin and TSH: To rule out pituitary/thyroid abnormalities in Type H and any PMS client with galactor-rhea.

Adrenal suppression test: To locate source of androgen excess and serve as a guide for therapy for Type D clients with hirsutism.

Abraham Menstrual System Questionnaire (MSQ), the Dalton Diagnostic Checklist (or similar PMS worksheet), and PMS calendar of symptoms (minimum 2 months).

Psychologic assessment: Minnesota Multiphasic Personality Inventory (MMPI) twice, once during the follicular phase of the menstrual cycle and again during the luteal phase (preferably the client's most critical day) of the menstrual cycle.

NURSING PRIORITIES

1. Provide emotional support and relief of symptoms.
2. Present information about condition/health care needs/resources available.
3. Encourage client to adopt a lifestyle promoting health and diminishing PMS symptoms.

DISCHARGE CRITERIA

1. Assertive behavior/stress management techniques are used to manage problems.
2. Expresses knowledge about PMS and sources for assistance.
3. Implementing lifestyle changes to promote health/diminish symptoms.
4. Client/family are involved in support group.

NURSING DIAGNOSIS:	COMFORT, ALTERED: PAIN CHRONIC
MAY BE RELATED TO:	Changes in estrogen/progesterone levels
	Vitamin deficiency
	Hypoglycemia

Fluid retention

Increased secretion of prostaglandins

POSSIBLY EVIDENCED BY:

Headache

Breast engorgement

Edema

Lower abdominal pain

Nausea/vomiting

Backache

Nervousness and irritability

CLIENT OUTCOMES/EVALUATION CRITERIA:

Verbalizes relief from discomfort associated with symptoms of PMS. Demonstrates ability to maintain anxiety at manageable level and minimize feelings of discomfort.

INTERVENTIONS	RATIONALE
Independent	
Note and record type, duration, and intensity of pain.	Background assessment data is necessary to formulate an accurate plan of care for the client.
Provide nursing comfort measures with a matter-of-fact approach that does not provide added attention to the pain behavior (e.g., backrub, warm bath, heating pad).	May serve to provide some temporary relief of pain. Secondary gains from solicitous response may provide nontherapeutic reinforcement to the behavior.
Encourage client to get adequate rest and sleep and avoid stressful activity during the premenstrual period.	Fatigue exaggerates symptoms associated with PMS. Stress elicits heightened symptoms of anxiety during this period affecting perception of pain.
Assist client with activities that distract from focus on self and pain. Demonstrate techniques, such as visual or auditory distractions, guided imagery, breathing exercises, massage, application of heat or cold, and relaxation techniques, that may provide symptomatic relief.	Use of techniques described may help to maintain anxiety at manageable level and prevent the discomfort from becoming disabling.
Provide positive reinforcement for times when client is not focusing on self and personal discomfort and is functioning independently.	May encourage repetition of desired independent behaviors while eliminating the secondary gain of dependency for the client.

INTERVENTIONS	RATIONALE
Collaborative	
Administer medication as indicated:	When other measures are insufficient to bring about relief, symptomatic drug therapy may be necessary/useful.
Diuretics, e.g., hydrochlorothiazide (Esidrix, HydroDIURIL), furosemide (Lasix);	Provides relief from discomfort of bloating and edema when fluid retention is extreme and does not respond to other measures, e.g., diet and sodium restriction
Nonsteroidal anti-inflammatory agents, e.g., ibuprofen (Motrin);	For relief of pain due to increased prostaglandin secretion.
Propranolol (Inderal), naproxen (Naprosyn);	May be used for relief of migraine.
Muscle relaxants, diazepam (Valium);	For relief of muscular tension.
Bromocriptine (Parlodel).	May be given for control of pain of mastodynia/symptoms of PMS, although side effects (especially nausea) may preclude use in some clients.

NURSING DIAGNOSIS:	ANXIETY (MODERATE TO PANIC)
MAY BE RELATED TO:	Cyclic changes in female hormones affecting other systems
POSSIBLY EVIDENCED BY:	Feelings of inability to cope/loss of control
	Depersonalization
	Increased tension
	Apprehension, jitteriness
	Somatic complaints
	Impaired functioning
CLIENT OUTCOMES/EVALUATION CRITERIA:	Verbalizes awareness of feelings of anxiety and appropriate ways to deal with them. Demonstrates understanding of illness and problem-solving skills to reduce stress and PMS symptoms. Uses resources effectively.

INTERVENTIONS	RATIONALE
Independent	
Assess level of anxiety and degree of interference with	Degree to which this disorder is affecting life will indi-

INTERVENTIONS

Independent

daily activities/interpersonal relationships.

Review history and have client maintain a PMS calendar, noting occurrence of nervous tension, mood swings, irritability, and feelings of anxiety.

Encourage client to acknowledge and express feelings, accepting client's perception of the situation.

Assist the client to use anxiety to promote understanding and deal with situation.

Assist client to identify precipitating factors and learn new methods of coping with anxiety, e.g., stress reduction techniques, relaxation and visualization skills.

Collaborative

Administer medications, as indicated:

> Anti-anxiety: e.g., alprazolam (Xanax), diazepam (Valium).

Identify helpful resources/people, e.g., physicians, nurse practitioners/clinicians, psychiatrist/psychologist, lay support groups.

RATIONALE

cate need for/type of intervention.

Aids in identification of disorder and type by specific identification of symptoms and their frequency.

Listening to the client promotes feelings of worthwhileness and normalcy, thereby reducing anxiety.

A moderate degree of anxiety can be helpful to heighten awareness and when client learns to use this, problem-solving can be enhanced.

Knowing these factors and ways of handling them reduces anxiety and allows client to feel more in control of situation/self.

May be used for short-term control of anxiety. Dose may be increased as necessary to prevent panic attacks during the luteal phase.

Professionals who specialize in PMS can assist the client to accept self/feelings as reality-based and begin to identify necessary lifestyle changes.

NURSING DIAGNOSIS:	**COPING, INEFFECTIVE, INDIVIDUAL**
MAY BE RELATED TO:	**Pain, threat to self-concept**
	Personal vulnerability
	Poor nutrition
	Work overload
	Multiple stressors (PMS syndrome) repeated over period of time
POSSIBLY EVIDENCED BY:	**Verbalization of difficulty coping or asking for help**
	Muscular tension
	Frequent headaches/neckaches
	Emotional tension

POSSIBLY EVIDENCED BY—*continued*	Lack of appetite
	Chronic fatigue
	Insomnia
	Inability to meet role expectations
	Alteration in societal participation
	High illness rate
	Overeating
CLIENT OUTCOMES/EVALUATION CRITERIA:	Indentifies ineffective coping behaviors and consequences. Meets psychologic needs as evidenced by appropriate expression of feelings, identification of options, and use of resources. Participates in treatment program.

INTERVENTIONS	RATIONALE
Independent	
Assess current functional level/coping ability, noting substance use, smoking habits, eating patterns.	Identifies needs and appropriate interventions for individual situation.
Note understanding of current situation and previous methods of dealing with life problems.	Provides information about how the client views what is happening and provides opportunity for her to look at previous methods of coping that may be helpful now.
Determine effect(s) of problem on client's relationships/family.	Destructive impact of symptoms can seriously undermine family systems, resulting in alienation, divorce.
Identify extent of feelings and situations when loss of control occurs. Discuss/problem-solve behaviors to protect self/others, e.g., call support person, remove self from situation.	Recognition of potential for harm to self/others and development of plan enables client to take effective actions to meet safety needs.
Discuss importance of learning new coping strategies and developing more supportive relationships (based on information from psychologic testing).	Realization that past behaviors have contributed to current situation/lack of support may provide impetus for change.
Encourage client to reduce or shift workload and social activities during the premenstrual period as part of a total stress management program.	By coping realistically with life stresses, the decreased responsibility should relieve stress and therefore help relieve symptoms.
Have client identify most troublesome symptoms, which may persist after initial therapy trials.	If other measures are inadequate/unsuccessful, pharmacologic treatment may be needed to enhance coping abilities.

INTERVENTIONS	RATIONALE

Collaborative

Review psychologic assessments, e.g., Minnesota Multiphasic Personality Inventory (MMPI) and clinical interview. (The first MMPI should be taken during the follicular phase, and a second MMPI during the most critical day of the luteal phase.)

Evaluation of these tests can determine the difference in emotional overlay and psychologic functioning. MMPI results can show very different patterns of emotional and personality functioning between these two phases. Consideration of these results are essential to an accurate picture of an individual's dynamics, coping skills, and stresses, which play such a significant role in this problem.

Provide for counseling at each appointment, reviewing past month's charting, and evaluating symptoms and effects of therapy, as well as client relationship(s).

This opportunity for assessing ongoing problems and making needed changes helps both client and nurse to know whether program is successful.

Administer medications, as indicated, e.g.,

Medications are individually prescribed by type of PMS and severity of symptoms. (Refer to ND: Comfort, altered: Pain, chronic for additional drug therapy.)

Progesterone vaginal suppositories;

Used to relieve symptoms of PMS when nonpharmacologic measures have not relieved symptoms.

Spironolactone (Aldactone);

May reduce fluid retention relieving depression and helping crying spells, abdominal bloating.

Trycyclic antidepressants: amitriptyline (Elavil); monoamine-oxidase inhibitors (Nardil);

Used for depression that does not respond as other symptoms are resolved.

Antiprostaglandins;

Relieves dysmenorrhea.

Lithium carbonate (Eskalith).

May be used in the presence of affective lability when other treatments have not been successful.

Encourage participation in support group, psychotherapy, marital counseling on a regular basis.

May be needed to help client/family members learn effective coping strategies and support lifestyle changes that might be needed.

NURSING DIAGNOSIS:	KNOWLEDGE DEFICIT [LEARNING NEED] (SPECIFY)
MAY BE RELATED TO:	Lack of exposure to information/misinterpretation/unfamiliarity with resources about PMS
	Inaccurate/incomplete information
POSSIBLY EVIDENCED BY:	Verbalization of the problem
	Request for information
	Inappropriate or exaggerated behaviors, e.g., hysterical, hostile, agitated, apathetic

INTERVENTIONS	RATIONALE
Independent	
Determine client's knowledge of PMS and misconceptions about condition.	May have incomplete information and misunderstandings about problem.
Provide information about condition in written/verbal form.	Provides different methods for accessing/reinforcing information and enhances opportunity for learning/understanding.
Have client do a nutritional survey/record entire food and liquid intake for one month.	Assists in interpretation of whether the client's diet is a contributing factor/cause of PMS symptoms. (Commercial computer analysis may be available for interpretation of the survey.)
Encourage client to limit smoking.	Smoking decreases the absorption of vitamins.
Suggest participation in mild exercise five days a week, e.g., walking one mile per day.	Exercise alters the level of certain neurotransmitters in the brain. These neurotransmitters (endorphins) are important in determining mood and anxiety and can reduce PMS symptoms.
Encourage client to do self-exam of breasts regularly. Demonstrate as necessary.	While an important practice for all women, statistics have suggested that PMS-Type A clients have a higher incidence of breast cancer.
Review medication regimen, importance of follow-up visits to health care provider.	Client needs to understand importance of monitoring on a regular basis to be sure program is continuing to be helpful, note necessity for change, and determine client cooperation.
Collaborative	
Review the premenstrual worksheet, confidential personal data sheets, and Life Events Stress scale.	Joint evaluation of all the assessment data, noting the interaction between life stress and PMS symptoms, is essential to making a correct diagnosis and developing an appropriate treatment program.
Refer client who does not respond to treatment regimen within three months for further evaluation for premature menopause, hypoglycemia, diabetes, hypothyroidism, polycystic ovaries, and ovarian failure.	Although one-third of clients seeking treatment respond to an initial multifaceted, nonhormonal treatment, it is important to rule out hormonal abnormalities, as the client will respond best to treatment for specific need.
Establish recommended diet plan, e.g.:	Beginning an early self-help program may relieve clinical symptoms and encourage the client emotionally.

INTERVENTIONS	RATIONALE
Independent	
Limit red meat to 3 oz/day, reduce intake of fats, especially saturated fats;	Decreases arachidonic acid, which helps balance PGE_1 ("good") with PGE_2 ("bad") prostaglandin, improving many PMS symptoms.
Limit intake of dairy products to two servings a day;	Excessive dairy products block the absorption of magnesium.
Increase intake of complex carbohydrates (vegetables, legumes, cereals, and whole grains) and cis-linoleic-acid-containing foods, e.g., safflower oil;	Stimulates insulin release in a less abrupt and more sustained manner. Although the value of cis-linoleic acid has not been proven, some women have found it to be helpful for the relief of PMS symptoms.
Decrease refined and simple sugars;	Increases insulin release rapidly, thus lowering the blood sugar, which initiates the craving for sweets and so completes the vicious cycle. Excess sugar is thought to cause nervous tension, palpitations, headache, dizziness, drowsiness, and excretion of magnesium in the urine, thus preventing the body from breaking down sugar for energy.
Decrease salt intake to 3 gm/day but not less than 0.5 gm/day;	Insulin prevents the kidneys from excreting salt; however, too little salt stimulates norepinephrine and causes sleep disturbances. Salt restriction also prevents edema.
Limit intake of caffeine (coffee, tea, and chocolate) and alcohol (one or two drinks a week);	Increases breast tenderness and pain, negates the effect of vitamins on Type A. Alcohol can cause reactive hypoglycemia and fluid retention, and may be the biggest reason for treatment failure.
Discuss starting an economical, complete vitamin therapy program, such as Optivite.	Women with PMS tend to eat more junk food and be too busy to eat well, and growing and cooking fresh vegetables is rare in today's lifestyle. Therefore, the client may be short of vitamins and minerals, which act as cofactors in a number of chemical reactions in the body that are involved in making, using, and excreting hormones. Abnormal levels of hormones are one cause of PMS symptoms.
Refer to available support groups/research centers.	Provides additional resources to understand and deal with condition.

CHAPTER 15
PERSONALITY DISORDERS

Antisocial Personality Disorder

DSM III-R: 301.70 Antisocial personality disorder (coded on Axis II)

The terms *sociopath* and *psychopath* are often used to describe the individual with antisocial personality. The disorder is extremely difficult to treat. Imprisonment has been society's major method for controlling the most dangerous behaviors.

ETIOLOGIC THEORIES

PSYCHODYNAMICS

Psychodynamically, this individual remains fixed in an earlier level of development. Because of parental rejection or indifference, needs for satisfaction and security remain unmet, and the ego is underdeveloped. Behavior is id directed, due to lack of ego strength, and results in the need for immediate gratification. An immature super-ego allows this individual to pursue gratification, regardless of means and without experiencing feelings of guilt.

BIOLOGIC THEORIES

Genetic involvement has been implicated in studies that showed that individuals with antisocial personality, and their parents, showed excessive EEG abnormalities when these examinations were conducted on both groups. (Despite genetic or environmental factors, sociopaths choose their lifestyle; therefore, it is up to them to *choose* to change it.)

FAMILY DYNAMICS

Family functioning has been implicated as an important factor in determining whether or not an individual develops this disorder. The following circumstances may predispose to the disorder: absence of parental discipline, extreme poverty, removal from the home, growing up without parental figures of both sexes, erratic and inconsistent discipline, being "rescued" each time the person is in trouble (never having to suffer the consequences of own behavior), and maternal deprivation.

CLIENT ASSESSMENT DATA BASE

HISTORY

More prevalent in males than females. Presents in females, often at the onset of puberty; in males, early childhood.

381

These behaviors usually diminish after age 30, when the individual seems to "mellow out"/get tired of the situation.

Occurs most frequently in lower socioeconomic populations.

May be history of violence in the home. Family may be dysfunctional with little positive interaction.

Displays chronic antisocial behavior incompatible with the value system of general society, e.g., excessive drinking, substance abuse, lying, stealing, fighting, frequent conflicts with the law, and early, aggressive, sexual acting-out behaviors. Repeatedly violates the rights of others without guilt or shame (thought to be without any conscience).

Rejects authority, has contempt for morality, does not learn from the past, and does not care about the future.

Lacks motivation for change, often not seeking therapy voluntarily unless client no longer tolerates the mess the client has made of own life/is facing long-term imprisonment.

History often reveals significant impairment in social, marital, and occupational functioning (generally has poor employment history).

PHYSICAL EXAMINATION

Mental status:
  Lacks emotional attachment to others, even parents.
  Personality appears charming, engaging, and is usually intelligent.
  Demeanor is often a pretense intended to deceive others or to facilitate exploitation of others.
  Signs of personal distress may be evident, e.g., tension and poor tolerance for boredom.
  Displays preference for stimulation rather than isolation.
  Manipulation is style of operating. Needs and demands immediate gratification.
  Low tolerance level results in feelings of frustration when desires are not immediately gratified.
  Affect: Emotional reactions may be erratic and extreme, with lack of concern for other people's feelings.
  Mood: Adaptive to individual's intended goal, ranging from charming and pleasant to intense anger.
  Thought processes: Preoccupied with own interests, grandiose expressions of own importance.
  Insight/judgment: poor

Heart rate: Slight increase may be demonstrated when anticipating stress. (This correlates with electrodermal responses indicating little anxiety.)

Experiences low level of autonomic arousal and responds to dangerous or painful stimuli with minimal anxiety.

DIAGNOSTIC STUDIES

EEG: Abnormally higher amounts of slow-wave activity, reflecting a possible deficit in inhibitory mechanisms, which may lessen impact of punishment.

Aversive stimuli: Tend to be slower in learning to avoid shock, associated with a lower than normal level of physiological arousal. Heightened ability to tune out aversive stimuli.

NURSING PRIORITIES

1. Limit aggressive behavior; promote socially acceptable responses.
2. Develop a trusting relationship.
3. Assist client to learn healthy ways to deal with anxiety.
4. Increase sense of self-worth.
5. Promote development of alternate, constructive methods of interacting with others.

DISCHARGE CRITERIA

1. Self-control is maintained.
2. Assertive behaviors are used to gain desired responses.
3. A trusting relationship is beginning to be established.
4. Anxiety is recognized/diminished/managed.
5. Client/family are involved in ongoing therapy/support groups.

NURSING DIAGNOSIS:	**VIOLENCE, POTENTIAL FOR: DIRECTED AT OTHERS**
MAY BE RELATED TO:	**Contempt for authority/rights of others (antisocial character)**
	Frustration; need for immediate gratification
	Easy agitation
	Use of maladjusted coping mechanisms including substance use
	Negative role modeling
POSSIBLE INDICATORS:	**Becoming assaultive when angry**
	Choice of aggression to meet needs
	Overt and aggressive acts
	Hostile, threatening verbalizations; boasting of prior abuse to others
	Possession of destructive means
	Substance abuse
	Vulnerable self-esteem
	Inability to verbalize feelings
CLIENT OUTCOMES/EVALUATION CRITERIA:	**Verbalizes understanding of why behavior occurs, its consequences, and how it affects outcome(s). Demonstrates self-control as evidenced by relaxed posture and manner. Develops and uses assertive/nonaggressive, socially acceptable behaviors to gratify needs and interact with others.**

INTERVENTIONS	RATIONALE
Independent	
Note prior history of violent behavior. Determine seriousness of homicidal tendency, gestures, threats.	Therapist needs to be aware of client's style of acting-out behaviors to provide a safe environment and pro-

INTERVENTIONS	RATIONALE

Independent

(Use scale of 1 to 10 and prioritize according to severity of threat, availability of means.)

	tect client and others.
Be aware of escalating behaviors, e.g., increased psychomotor activity, threats, attempts to intimidate. Isolate if observed to be losing control.	Client can become dangerous very quickly with or without provocation. Early detection provides opportunity to alter behavior before violence occurs.
Note distortions of the truth, manipulation. Confront client with these behaviors in a calm, but firm manner.	Confronting unacceptable behaviors helps to increase client's awareness of own feelings and the effect these feelings and behaviors have on others.
Encourage verbalization of feelings and provide outlet for expression.	Increases client's self-awareness of feelings and stressors.
Set firm limits; follow through with consequences.	Environment needs to be structured to discourage escalation of aggressive behaviors.
Discuss ways to detect potentially provocative/volatile situations before becoming involved.	Sociopaths tend to tune out aversive stimuli and need to increase awareness of environment to avoid becoming involved in volatile situations.
Review with client the benefits of using assertive behaviors and the consequences of aggression. Ask client to identify situations when aggression was used and discuss alternate methods for handling those situations.	Consequences serve as the best motivation for changing behavior. Client needs a plan of action rehearsed to aid in handling situations differently.
Assist client to learn to anticipate situations that usually result in anger and develop a plan to handle anger before losing control.	Restructuring helps to eliminate old behavioral patterns that result in acting out. A plan of action provides client with a feeling of control.
Explore with client how aggressive, destructive behaviors have affected interpersonal relationships, e.g., children, spouse, parents.	Needs to realize own role and responsibility in personal interactions.
Remain calm and nonaggressive in communicating with client. Avoid responding to client's verbal hostility with anger.	Anger is released through others. Not responding to client's anger breaks cycle, providing opportunity for change.
Help client to find healthy outlets for anger, e.g., telling other person in an assertive manner, use of large motor skill activities/relaxation techniques.	Developing new ways of reacting is essential to breaking the maladaptive pattern of responding.

NURSING DIAGNOSIS:	POWERLESSNESS
MAY BE RELATED TO:	**Unsatisfactory interpersonal interaction and unmet needs**
	Experience of severe abuse as a child
	Lifestyle of helplessness
POSSIBLY EVIDENCED BY:	**Antisocial behavior, e.g., repeated violation of rights of others, use of intimidation to get needs met, resorting to**

crime when faced with adversities or for self-gratification.

Overwhelming need to create self-stimulation

Need to increase sense of having control over environment

Nonparticipation in treatment program

Expressions of dissatisfaction and frustration over inability to perform tasks and/or activities

Reluctance to express feelings

Apathy; anger

CLIENT OUTCOMES/EVALUATION CRITERIA:	Verbalizes a sense of control over present situation, future outcomes. Demonstrates increased tolerance for external stress and meets needs with assertive behaviors. Makes healthy choices related to and is involved in own care.

INTERVENTIONS

Independent

Investigate pattern of attempting to control environment through anger and intimidation.

Explore client's need for immediate gratification. Ask client to describe feelings when someone says "no."

Assist client to identify when feelings of loss of control began and events that led to this situation.

Review with client feelings regarding authority and violating rights of others.

Discuss with client thoughts and fantasies present before committing crimes. Ascertain how much planning went into the crimes. Did the client "experience" the crime "mentally" before commission?

RATIONALE

Increases client's awareness of inappropriate mode of interaction and the consequences.

Client needs to understand own feelings in order to work on resolution.

Recognition of these events provides an opportunity for resolution/adaptation of more effective behaviors. (Note: Sociopaths have often been victims of child abuse and need to deal with these feelings.)

Often experiences pleasure through antisocial behaviors and needs to gain insight regarding personal motives.

Fantasizing about crime plays a large role in eventual commission. In order to restructure cognitive processes, client needs to break this pattern.

385

INTERVENTIONS	RATIONALE
Independent	
Ask client to discuss thoughts on family, peers, authority figures, opposite sex, violence, and victims. Give feedback on the "correctness" of thinking process.	Reinforces positive values or attitudes and exposes problem areas in thinking process. This is important for cognitive restructuring.
Be aware of slow progress when working with this client, acknowledge difficulties openly, and avoid becoming discouraged.	Major obstacles in working with the sociopath lie in an inherent inability to form a trusting, open relationship with a therapist.

NURSING DIAGNOSIS:	**ANXIETY (MODERATE TO SEVERE)**
MAY BE RELATED TO:	**Low tolerance for external stress**
	Unconscious conflicts
	Threat to self-concept
	Unmet needs
POSSIBLY EVIDENCED BY:	**Choice of maladaptive/aggressive behaviors (stealing, lying, fighting)**
	Use of alcohol/other drugs to relieve stress
	Feelings of inadequacy
	Concern for unspecified consequences
	Expressed concern regarding changes in life events
	Focus on self
CLIENT OUTCOMES/EVALUATION CRITERIA:	**Verbalizes awareness of feelings of anxiety. Develops and demonstrates socially acceptable and nondestructive ways of reducing anxiety. Reports reduction of anxiety to a manageable level. Uses resources effectively.**

INTERVENTIONS	RATIONALE
Independent	
Maintain structured environment, e.g., consistent schedule, ward rules, expectations of the client for co-operating.	Sociopaths often function better in a controlled setting. Structure facilitates therapeutic intervention by reducing the anxiety caused by ambiguity.

INTERVENTIONS	RATIONALE

Independent

Provide outlet for expression of feelings/concerns.

Assist client to recognize anxiety by describing feeling states.

Help to formulate possible rationales for current anxious feelings.

Explore anxiety-producing situations.

Assist to identify/recognize early warning signs of increased anxiety and to implement effective coping skills before loss of control occurs.

Guide client in choosing constructive behaviors. Give positive feedback when client demonstrates an effort to use constructive behaviors.

Discuss fears or anxieties of others' responses to client's new behaviors and feelings concerning these responses.

Help client recognize behaviors that do not get intended response and discuss possible modifications.

Needs to identify sources of fears and anxieties to work through them.

Increases understanding and self-awareness of feelings to facilitate appropriate actions.

Clarifying basis of anxious feelings may help eliminate unnecessary worry.

Useful in establishing a possible cause-effect relationship, providing opportunity for insight.

Establishing a plan in advance helps client, on becoming aware of feelings, to apply new skills that aid in controlling/reducing anxiety and impulsive actions.

Provides education/knowledge for new behaviors. Reinforces appropriate behaviors and enhances self-esteem.

Gives client a sense of what might be expected from others to help alleviate fears.

Sociopaths have difficulty interpreting others' feelings and need guidance in this area.

NURSING DIAGNOSIS: COPING, INEFFECTIVE, INDIVIDUAL

MAY BE RELATED TO:

Very low tolerance for external stress

Lack of experience of internal anxiety such as guilt or shame

Personal vulnerability

Inadequate support systems

Multiple life changes

Unmet expectations

Conflict

Difficulty delaying gratification

POSSIBLY EVIDENCED BY: Use of maladjusted coping, such as denial, projection (inappropriate use of defense mechanisms)

POSSIBLY EVIDENCED BY—continued	Choice of aggression and manipulation to handle problems and conflicts
	Chronic worry, anxiety, depression
	Poor self-esteem
	Inability to problem-solve
	High rate of accidents
	Substance use/abuse
	Destructive behavior toward self or others
CLIENT OUTCOMES/EVALUATION CRITERIA:	Identifies maladaptive coping behaviors and consequences. Verbalizes awareness of own positive coping abilities. Develops and uses appropriate, constructive, effective coping skills. Verbalizations of feelings are congruent with behavior.

INTERVENTIONS	RATIONALE
Independent	
Discuss present patterns of coping with anxiety and effectiveness of these mechanisms.	Client needs to become aware that present patterns are self-destructive as well as harmful to others.
Assist client to identify sources of anxieties and how they relate to use of denial and projection.	Needs to get in touch with own feelings, own them, and be responsible for them before individual can begin to change behavior.
Provide information about constructive, effective coping strategies, e.g., discussing feelings with staff, running or jogging.	Client has likely not learned effective coping skills and needs information to begin to replace maladaptive skills.
Confront client with manipulative and intimidating behaviors when they occur.	Helps reinforce the need to stop this pattern.
Explore the implications/consequences of continuing antisocial activities.	Needs to be constantly aware of the direction life is taking and the effect these behaviors have on society and self.
Discuss the importance of being responsible for own actions and not blaming others for own behaviors.	Sociopaths tend to externalize blame onto others and do not accept responsibility for own actions.
Give positive feedback when client demonstrates use of constructive alternatives.	Enhances self-esteem and reinforces acceptable behaviors.
Evaluate with client effectiveness of new behaviors and discuss modifications.	If client's new methods of coping are not working, assistance will be needed to reassess and develop new strategies.

INTERVENTIONS	RATIONALE
Independent	
Encourage participation in ward activities, groups, outdoor education program.	Interaction with others provides opportunities for client to begin to experience success, feel good about self, get needs met in positive ways.

NURSING DIAGNOSIS:	**SELF-CONCEPT, DISTURBANCE IN: SELF-ESTEEM**
MAY BE RELATED TO:	**Lack of positive feedback**
	Unmet dependency needs
	Retarded ego development
	Repeated negative feedback
	Dysfunctional family system
	Fixation in earlier level of development
POSSIBLY EVIDENCED BY:	**Acting-out behaviors, such as excessive use of alcohol and other drugs, sexual promiscuity**
	Inability (difficulty) accepting positive reinforcement
	Nonparticipation in therapy
	Feelings of inadequacy/diminished self-worth
CLIENT OUTCOMES/EVALUATION CRITERIA:	**Acknowledges self as an individual who has responsibility for own actions. Verbalizes a sense of worthwhileness. Demonstrates pro-social functioning. Recognizes and incorporates change into self-concept in accurate manner without negating self-esteem.**

INTERVENTIONS	RATIONALE
Independent	
Encourage verbalization of feelings of inadequacy, worthlessness, fear of rejection, and need for acceptance from others.	Client may relate acting-out behaviors to a poor self-concept, and acceptance of reality of own behaviors in relation to others' reactions can assist decision to change.
Assist client to identify positive aspects about self related to social skills, work abilities, education, talents, and appearance.	Helps to build on positive aspects of personality and use them to improve self-concept.
Provide clear, consistent, verbal/nonverbal communication. Be truthful and honest.	Client's perception is keen and can instantly detect insincerity.
Explore the relationship between feelings of inadequacy and aggressive behaviors, use of drugs, sexual promiscuity.	Provides opportunity for client to understand relationship between low self-esteem and ineffective measures taken to "feel" better.
Discuss how companions are chosen. Ask if these people reinforce client's own antisocial activities/values.	Aids client to see how much peers can influence thinking and thereby reinforce antisocial behavior.
Ask client to describe interpersonal relationships, their quality and depth. If relationships are superficial, discuss how this came about.	Sociopaths have great difficulty forming close relationships. Perhaps exploring early relationships with parents or siblings may provide insight into the problem.
Review ways to improve the quality of interaction with others.	Learning to recognize/respect feelings of others in relation to own helps client to develop more satisfactory relationships.

NURSING DIAGNOSIS:	**COPING, INEFFECTIVE FAMILY: COMPROMISED/DISABLING**
MAY BE RELATED TO:	**Temporary family disorganization and role changes**
	Client providing little support in turn for the primary person
	Prolonged disability progression that exhausts the supportive capacity of significant people
	Highly ambivalent family relationships
POSSIBLY EVIDENCED BY:	**Expressions of concern or complaint about significant other(s) response to client's problem**
	Significant person reporting preoccupation with personal reactions regarding illness

390

	Significant person displaying protective behavior disproportionate (too little or too much) to client's abilities or need for autonomy
FAMILY OUTCOMES/EVALUATION CRITERIA:	**Identifies/verbalizes resources within themselves to deal with the situation. Interacts appropriately with the client/each other, providing support and assistance as indicated. Provides opportunity for client to deal with situation in own way. Expressing feelings openly and honestly.**

INTERVENTIONS

Independent

Identify behaviors/interactions of family members. Note factors affecting abilities of family members to provide needed support.

Listen to client/significant others' comments and expressions of concern, noting nonverbal behaviors and/or responses.

Discuss basis for client's behavior(s).

Assist family and client to understand "who owns the problem" and who is responsible for resolution.

Encourage free expression of feelings, including frustration, anger, hostility, and hopelessness.

Assist family members to identify coping skills being used and how these skills are/are not helping them to deal with the situation.

Collaborative

Refer to additional resources as needed, e.g., family therapy, financial counseling, spiritual.

RATIONALE

Provides information about patterns within family and whether they are helpful to resolution of current problems. Personality disorder/mental illness of other family members inhibits coping abilities.

Provides clues to underlying feelings, unconscious motivations/defenses.

Helps family begin to understand and accept/deal with unacceptable actions.

When each individual begins to assume responsibility for own actions, each one can begin to problem-solve without expectation that someone else will take care of them.

Expression of feelings can be the beginning of recognition and resolution of short-/long-term problems.

Identification of what is helpful and what is not will allow for learning new ways to cope with behaviors/situation.

May need further assistance to help with resolution of current/long-term problems.

NURSING DIAGNOSIS:	**SOCIAL INTERACTION, IMPAIRED**
MAY BE RELATED TO:	**Factors contributing to the absence of satisfying personal relationships, e.g., inadequate personal resources (shallow feelings), immature interests, underdeveloped conscience, unaccepted social values**

391

POSSIBLY EVIDENCED BY:	Difficulty meeting expectations of others
	Sense of emptiness/inadequacy covered up by expressions of self-conceit, arrogance, and contempt
	Behavior unaccepted by dominant cultural group
	Lack of belief that rules pertain to them
CLIENT OUTCOMES/EVALUATION CRITERIA:	Identifies causes and actions to correct isolation. Expresses increased sense of self-worth. Participates willingly in activities/programs without use of manipulation. Demonstrates behavior congruent with verbal expressions.

INTERVENTIONS

Independent

Note expressions of hopelessness/worthlessness, e.g., "I'm a loser," "It's fate."

Listen to expressions of feelings and "insight," pointing out discrepancies between what is said versus behaviors.

Confront expressions of powerlessness, inability to control situation/make difference in relationships/commitments.

Encourage client to make requests/ask for what is wanted in a clear, straightforward manner and express feelings clearly to others.

Collaborative

Involve in group activities, e.g., occupational/vocational/therapy, outdoor education program, co-dependency meetings.

RATIONALE

These may be the only genuine emotions this individual feels and may be expressed in subtle ways when failures can no longer be denied. Although these feelings may be dismissed quickly, this may be the time when the client is most accessible to change.

Client may be very good at saying what others want to hear. However, behavior is the ultimate determinant of real change. It is almost impossible for this person to understand the feelings of others.

Consistent confrontation with reality of how client's behavior affects interactions and trust of others may force client to begin to look at own responsibility for problems in these areas. This person's refusal to accept criticism and/or projection of failure as the fault of others make it difficult to change behavior.

As needs are met by direct action, client may begin to see the value of this approach.

Provides opportunity for interaction with others to learn new behaviors, gain support for change.

Borderline Personality Disorder

DMS III-R: 301.83 Borderline personality disorder (coded on Axis 2)

ETIOLOGIC THEORIES

PSYCHODYNAMICS

Unconscious processes that are believed to shape personality are set in motion by drives or instincts that are then influenced by conflicts among them as well as instinctual wishes and demands of reality. Defensive maneuvers are unconsciously developed to protect against anxiety arising from this conflict. This personality is seen as a painstaking but poorly constructed defense.

It is also seen as resulting from a fixation of libido at stages of psychosexual development associated with certain body parts. Although it is difficult to agree on how personality is formed, it is believed that severe personality disorders do begin early in childhood and milder forms are influenced by factors during later development.

BIOLOGIC THEORIES

Personality is believed to have a hereditary basis known as "temperament," biologic dispositions that affect mood and level of activity, e.g., cranky, placid, self-contained, outgoing, impulsive, cautious. There is little agreement about how this affects the development of personality disorders.

FAMILY DYNAMICS

The social environment of the child, particularly the family, is assumed to be the main force that shapes personality.

The theory of object relations provides a basis for personality development and an explanation of the dynamics that manifest the borderline characteristics. It has been suggested that the individual with borderline personality is fixed in the rapprochement phase of development (18–25 months of age). In this phase the child is experiencing increasing autonomy, while still requiring "emotional refueling" from the mothering figure. The mother feels threatened by the child's efforts at independence, so strives to keep the child dependent. Nurturing and emotional support become bargaining tools. They are withheld when the child exhibits independent behaviors and used as rewards for clinging, dependent behaviors. This engenders a deep fear of abandonment in the child that persists into adulthood as the child continues to view objects (people) as parts, either good or bad. This is called splitting, which is the primary dynamic of borderline personality.

CLIENT ASSESSMENT DATA BASE

HISTORY

More prevalent in females.

Higher incidence found in families with history of both chronic schizophrenia and major affective disorders.

History may reveal previous physical violence directed at self and others, including self-mutilation, which is used to "punish the bad self." (This is thought to provide some relief from anxiety and may be an attempt to identify self-boundaries as a form of maladjusted coping.)

May be associated with other personality disorders that have histrionic, narcissistic, schizotypal, or antisocial features.

Reports significantly impaired social, marital, and occupational functioning.

May indulge in unpredictable/impulsive behaviors, e.g., spending, sexual promiscuity, gambling, substance abuse.

Experiences ambivalence toward being independent.

Complains of feelings of emptiness and boredom; does not like to be alone, becoming depressed and sad.

PHYSICAL EXAMINATION

May reveal evidence of self-mutilative acts, e.g., cutting, burning.

Mental status:

May display overall poor reality base with difficulty making decisions.

Lacks insight and does not learn from past experience.

Magical thinking and difficulty in identifying the self may occur; may display severely impaired self-concept.

Displays intense emotions with rapid, unpredictable, and strong mood swings; quick to anger, which may be intense, inappropriate; lacks ability to control; severe anxiety.

Affect may appear genuine but not necessarily appropriate to the situation.

Mood may be anxious and depressed, dysphoric.

Behavior may be erratic, impulsive, intense, clinging.

May use and exploit others; lacks empathy for others and seems unable to gain insight into own behaviors.

Relationships may be transient, shallow and/or demanding, with little flexibility and unstable interpersonal behavior.

Often attempts to provoke guilt in others and makes endless demands

May present a profound disturbance in gender identity and the inability to form long-term goals or values.

May border on neuroses and psychoses, exhibiting transient psychotic symptoms when experiencing extreme stress.

Lying and fabrication become habitual, almost delusional.

Self-centered, often to the point of narcissism, inordinately hypersensitive, and inflexible.

Major defense mechanism used is projection (seeing in others those attitudes one fails to see in self).

DIAGNOSTIC STUDIES

P-300 (a change in brain electrical activity that occurs in most people about 300 milliseconds after they perceive a tone, light, or other signal indicating that they have to perform a task): may be abnormal, smaller than average, and slightly delayed.

Drug screen: To identify substance use.

NURSING PRIORITIES

1. Limit aggressive behavior; promote socially acceptable responses.
2. Encourage assertive behaviors to attain sense of control.
3. Assist client to learn healthy ways of controlling anxiety/developing positive self-concept.
4. Promote development of effective coping skills.
5. Assist client to learn alternate, constructive methods of interacting with others.

DISCHARGE CRITERIA

1. Impulsive behavior(s) recognized and controlled.
2. Establishing goals and asserting control over own life.
3. Problem-solving techniques used constructively to resolve conflicts.
4. Interacting with others in socially appropriate manner.
5. Client/family involved in behavioral therapy/support programs.

NURSING DIAGNOSIS:	VIOLENCE, POTENTIAL FOR: DIRECTED AT SELF/OTHERS
MAY BE RELATED TO:	Use of projection as a major defense mechanism
	Pervasive problem with negative transference
	Feelings of guilt/need to "punish" self

POSSIBLE INDICATORS:	Easily agitated, angry when frustrated, may become assaultive
	Choice of maladjusted ways of getting needs met (e.g., splitting, projection, provocation, depression)
	Use of unprovoked anger, hostility toward others
	Self-mutilative acts
	Vulnerable self-esteem
	Provocative behavior: argumentative, dissatisfied, overreactive, hypersensitive
CLIENT OUTCOMES/EVALUATION CRITERIA:	Verbalizes understanding of why behavior occurs. Recognizes precipitating factors. Demonstrates self-control, using appropriate, assertive coping skills. Clarifies feelings of negative transference and eliminates the use of projection.

INTERVENTIONS	RATIONALE
Independent	
Establish therapeutic nurse/client relationship. Maintain a firm, consistent approach.	Building rapport and trust is imperative, although difficult, for this client.
Assist to identify how much anger is elicited by significant other(s) and how much results from own unresolved feelings.	Becoming aware of the use of projection helps to break this maladjusted pattern.
Intervene immediately in a nondefensive manner when acting out occurs. Set firm, consistent limits.	Intervention is critical to prevent dangerous situation for either client or others. Therapeutic milieu helps client to manage self and develop self-control. Environmental safety provides external control until internal control is regained.
Encourage client to evaluate situations in which client becomes angry. Was the amount of anger appropriate to the actual event?	Needs to learn to recognize/assess inappropriate, unwarranted anger directed at others.
Explore what client expects from others, and self, in interpersonal relationships.	Assists client to learn to define roles and recognize own responsibility in the situation.
Define expectations and rules of the situation clearly and state what the client can/cannot do.	Structure reduces ambiguity and anxiety, providing sense of security and minimizing escalation of violent behavior.

395

INTERVENTIONS	RATIONALE

Independent

Determine negative transference feelings and clarify the actual source of anger, hostility.

Heightens self-awareness of these feelings to assist with resolution.

Provide care for client's wounds, if self-mutilation occurs, in a matter-of-fact manner. Do not offer sympathy or provide additional attention.

Additional attention and sympathy can provide positive reinforcement for the maladaptive behavior and may encourage its repetition. A matter-of-fact attitude can convey empathy/concern.

Make an agreement or contract to discuss angry or hurt feelings when they begin instead of ''internalizing'' and displacing anger, hurt onto others.

Helps client learn to work through feelings as they occur to prevent intensification and promote resolution.

Collaborative

Have client participate in group therapy sessions with feedback given by peers.

Group setting aids in promoting diffusion of anger; provides insight as to how negative, aggressive behaviors affect others, making feedback easier to digest.

NURSING DIAGNOSIS:	THOUGHT PROCESSES: ALTERED
MAY BE RELATED TO:	**Brief psychotic episodes that may include delusional thinking**
	Cognitive distortions
	Increasing anxiety/fear
	Poor reality base
POSSIBLY EVIDENCED BY:	**Persecutory thoughts or statements of ''I am victim''**
	Perception of events as either grossly distorted or ''did not happen at all''
	Interference with ability to think clearly and logically
CLIENT OUTCOMES/EVALUATION CRITERIA:	**Defines methods to validate perceptions before drawing conclusions. Recognizes warning signs of increasing anxiety. Deals with anxieties and fears with more reality-based thinking.**

INTERVENTIONS	RATIONALE
Independent	
Assess escalating anxiety and observe client contact with reality, e.g., presence/development of psychotic symptoms, delusions/hallucinations, disorganized thinking, confusion, altered communication patterns. (Refer to CP: Paranoia.)	Underlying feelings of worthlessness, inadequacy, powerlessness can lead to increasing anxiety with resultant inability to think clearly.
Note rapid changes in behavior, e.g., from cooperative to angry, demanding, argumentative.	Need for immediate gratification can lead to frustration and changes in behavior, which may indicate loss of touch with reality.
Monitor for substance use; note physical symptoms of abuse, e.g., dilated/constricted pupils, abnormal vital signs, needle marks.	May cloud symptomatology, potentiate erratic behavior, and interfere with progress.
Provide information in brief, clear, calm manner.	Specific instructions and expectations about what is happening help client maintain contact with reality.
Maintain calm, quiet, nonstimulating environment.	Auditory and visual stimulation may increase labile affect and potential for acting out.
Correct misinterpretations of environment as expressed by the client.	Confronting misinterpretations honestly, with a caring and accepting attitude, provides a therapeutic orientation to reality and preserves client's feelings of dignity and self-worth.
Encourage client to develop a relationship with more than one person.	Helps client to achieve object constancy. Client may feel abandoned when therapist leaves and have a feeling that the person ceases to exist. Dependency can be avoided and client can begin to develop independent activities in this atmosphere.
Maintain open communication and provide consistency of care.	Provides for accurate information and reduces anxiety.

NURSING DIAGNOSIS:	SELF-CONCEPT, DISTURBANCE IN: SELF-ESTEEM/PERSONAL IDENTITY
MAY BE RELATED TO:	**Lack of positive feedback**
	Unmet dependency needs
	Retarded ego development
	Fixation at an earlier level of development
POSSIBLY EVIDENCED BY:	**Difficulty identifying self or defining self-boundaries**
	Extreme mood changes

POSSIBLY EVIDENCED BY—*continued*	Lack of tolerance of rejection or being alone
	Unhappiness with self, striking out at others
	Performance of ritualistic, self-damaging acts, such as "cutting veins and watching the blood flow to cleanse the soul"
	Belief that punishing self is necessary
CLIENT OUTCOMES/EVALUATION CRITERIA:	Verbalizes a sense of worthwhileness. Demonstrates increased self-worth/respect with reduction in punishing/mutilative behaviors. Uses improved self-image to promote good interpersonal relationships.

INTERVENTIONS	RATIONALE
Independent	
Encourage client to describe and verbalize feelings about self.	Aids in assessing in which areas negative feelings are most intense.
Explore need to punish self. When did this begin and what events precipitated these acts? (Refer to ND: Violence, potential for: directed at self/others.)	May help to establish a cause-effect relationship.
Discuss what stressors usually bring on depression. Explore ways to deal with depression before it becomes overwhelming.	Information can be used to learn and implement effective methods to prevent onset of depression.
Note attitude of superiority, arrogant behaviors, exaggerated sense of self, resentment, and anger.	Indicative of attempt to compensate for feelings of worthlessness, inadequacy, and powerlessness.
Encourage client to verbalize feelings of insecurity and need for constant reassurance from others.	Provides insight into sources of insecurities.
Discuss feelings of worthlessness and how these feelings relate to need for acceptance by others.	Gives client the message that life cannot be spent trying to meet others' expectations.
Identify situations in which client pushed others away because of fear of rejection. Help client to look at reality that rejection will happen.	Needs to learn that some risk-taking is necessary, reaching out to others does not always end in rejection, and when it does, client can use skills to deal with it appropriately.
Identify positive, realistic behaviors the client possesses.	Helps client begin to look at possibility of making desired changes to meet needs in a more satisfying way.
Encourage increased sense of responsibility for own behaviors.	Use of projection has enabled client to blame others for own problems/consequences of behavior.
Define sexual identity and what areas create confusion, fears.	Helps to assess possible knowledge deficit or which direction to take in alleviating anxiety.

INTERVENTIONS

Independent

Assess knowledge of human sexuality and supply needed information.

Give feedback regarding nonverbal behaviors.

RATIONALE

Provides information appropriate to learning needs.

Increases awareness of the possibility of double messages that client may be giving.

NURSING DIAGNOSIS:	**POWERLESSNESS**
MAY BE RELATED TO:	**Lifestyle of helplessness**
	Need for control
POSSIBLY EVIDENCED BY:	**Becoming enraged and hurt**
	Manipulative behavior
	Self-centered and hypersensitive attitude
	Provoking guilt in others
	Making endless demands
	Using and exploiting others
	Ambivalence toward being independent
	Alternating clinging and distancing behaviors
CLIENT OUTCOMES/EVALUATION CRITERIA:	**Expresses sense of control over present situation and future outcome. Develops a sense of being in charge of own life. Interacts with others without abusing or violating their rights. Makes choices related to and is involved in care.**

INTERVENTIONS

Independent

Develop alliance with the client and assist to overcome fear of closeness and intimacy.

RATIONALE

This individual is generally frightened by close relationships; an alliance demonstrates that it is possible to trust.

INTERVENTIONS	RATIONALE

Independent

INTERVENTIONS	RATIONALE
Identify behaviors used to gain control of others, e.g., manipulation, attempts to influence, intimidate.	Increases awareness of modes of interaction that are used to get own way and feel in control of the situation.
Explore areas of life in which client is feeling inadequate or having no control.	Provides insight into feelings that are necessary for learning adaptive behaviors.
Encourage verbalization of how feelings of anger, hurt, and loss of control relate to desire to strike out at others.	Enhances understanding of how the use of projection has become a pervasive pattern.
Confront inconsistencies in statements; discuss what needs these statements serve.	Reinforces that lying and manipulation are maladaptive and lead to feelings of low self-esteem.
Recognize client manipulations and respond differently.	Redirection stops the manipulation, allowing for straight, congruent communication.
Provide opportunities to learn how to get needs met in an acceptable, truthful way.	Promotes inner strength and adaptive functioning.
Ask to discuss feelings about someone in life who seems self-centered. Compare behaviors.	By comparing behaviors, client may understand how others perceive self-centeredness and the feelings about these behaviors.
Assist client to learn to listen to others and consider their feelings by putting self in their place.	Promotes feelings of empathy for others.
Encourage client to participate in developing treatment plan.	Aids in promoting a sense of control over life.
Role-play behaviors, e.g., appropriate anger, admitting mistakes, shared humor.	Avoiding angry confrontations, maintaining sense of humor help client learn new ways of control.

NURSING DIAGNOSIS:	**ANXIETY (SEVERE TO PANIC)**
MAY BE RELATED TO:	**Unconscious conflicts (experience of extreme stress)**
	Perceived threat to self-concept
	Unmet needs
POSSIBLY EVIDENCED BY:	**Transient psychotic symptoms**
	Abuse of alcohol/other drugs
	Easy frustration and feelings of hurt
	Performing self-mutilating acts
CLIENT OUTCOMES/EVALUATION CRITERIA:	**Verbalizes awareness of feelings of anxiety and healthy ways to deal with them. Develops and implements**

effective methods for decreasing anxiety. Reports anxiety reduced to manageable level. Uses resources effectively.

INTERVENTIONS	RATIONALE
Independent	
Encourage client to identify events that precipitate stress/anxious feelings; e.g., real or anticipated anxiety of relationships with others.	Helps to establish a cause-effect relationship, enhancing awareness and promoting change.
Assist in learning to identify early warning signs that anxiety is escalating and request intervention before it becomes overwhelming.	Promotes development of internal control.
Ask client to describe events/feelings preceding cutting or hurting self. Explore ways to relieve anxiety without self-damaging acts. (Refer to ND: Violence, potential for: directed at self/others.)	Provides knowledge for adapting new effective coping skills and breaking the pattern of self-destruction.
Discuss times when substances were taken to relieve tension, anxiety.	Provides an understanding of the relationship between anxiety and drug use.
Discuss fears involving interactions with parents, spouse, children or significant other(s).	Knowledge of specific fear may provide insight into problem areas.
Identify constructive ways of releasing tension, e.g., jogging, talking with nurse/therapist, use of relaxation/imagery techniques, involvement in outdoor education programs.	Client needs to learn constructive methods of coping to replace the maladjusted behaviors that have been used.

NURSING DIAGNOSIS:	**COPING, INEFFECTIVE INDIVIDUAL**
MAY BE RELATED TO:	**Use of maladjusted defense mechanisms such as projection, denial, externalizing**
	Chronic feelings of emptiness and boredom
	Repetitive use of the same patterns of coping, even though they do not work
POSSIBLY EVIDENCED BY:	**Low tolerance for being alone**
	Not learning from previous experiences
	Relief of anxiety through self-destructive acts

POSSIBLY EVIDENCED BY—*continued*	Wanting own way, not coping with slight frustration of wishes
	Sexual promiscuity, impulsive spending, gambling, substance abuse
	Not controlling anger
CLIENT OUTCOMES/EVALUATION CRITERIA:	Identifies ineffective coping behaviors and consequences. Develops and demonstrates use of constructive coping skills. Verbalizations of feelings are congruent with behavior.

INTERVENTIONS	RATIONALE
Independent	
Ask client to describe present coping patterns and their consequences.	Identifies which defenses are maladjusted, ineffective, destructive in order to effect change.
Have client identify problems and perceptions of their cause.	Exposes problem areas in thinking process and possible cognitive distortions.
Promote development of effective ways to deal with stress, anger, frustration.	Client will need help in learning new behaviors, e.g., acceptable expression of anger, "I-messages."
Discuss ways of dismissing feelings of boredom and assist client to understand that these feelings can be controlled.	Client needs to get in touch with own feelings and own/be responsible for them before they can be resolved.
Be aware of attempts to split staff. Avoid manipulative games and be consistent in dealing with the client.	Staff splitting can be a major problem. Client may behave in one way (quiet/cooperative) with some staff and in another way (angry/demanding) with others.
Confront manipulative and other maladaptive behaviors.	Consistent confrontation removes the reward and reinforces need for the client to adopt new behaviors and to stop directing anger at others.
Give feedback on how effectively client is handling situations and discuss suggestions for improvement.	May need assistance and guidance in modifying behaviors that are not working.
Give positive feedback when client demonstrates use of appropriate, constructive behaviors.	Reinforces use of positive techniques
Evaluate antisocial behaviors and resulting problems. (Refer to CP: Antisocial Personality.)	Destructive behaviors may lead to legal involvements and other problems in which client needs to learn new behaviors.

NURSING DIAGNOSIS:	SOCIAL ISOLATION
MAY BE RELATED TO:	Immature interests
	Unaccepted social behavior

POSSIBLY EVIDENCED BY:	Inadequate personal resources Inability to engage in satisfying personal relationships Difficulty meeting expectations of others Experiences feelings of difference from others Expresses interests inappropriate to developmental age Shows behavior unaccepted by dominant cultural group
CLIENT OUTCOMES/EVALUATION CRITERIA:	Identifies causes and actions to correct isolation. Verbalizes willingness to be involved with others. Participates in activities at level of desire. Expresses increased sense of self-worth.

INTERVENTIONS	RATIONALE
Independent	
Determine presence of factors contributing to sense/choice of isolation.	Identification of individual factors allows for developing appropriate plan of care/interventions.
Differentiate isolation from solitude and loneliness.	The latter are acceptable or by choice, and this differentiation helps client to identify which is applicable to self so steps to deal with problem can be taken.
Let client know the nurse will not abandon the client.	Client is often fearful that the therapist will become angry or discouraged and give up.
Ask client to identify significant other(s) with whom client can talk. If there is no one, ascertain how this came about.	Aids in seeing a pattern of interaction that is ineffectual.
Examine guilt feelings involving significant other(s). Discuss how these feelings occurred.	May have unrealistic guilt feelings that need resolution before work on the relationship can begin.
Discuss/define fears about being alone. Develop a schedule to "practice" being alone a few minutes each day, gradually increasing the time.	Provides knowledge for developing adaptive coping skills and desensitizes person to feelings of anxiety.
Identify how fears, anxieties have affected quality and depth of interpersonal relationships.	Reinforces a sense that projection does indeed cripple relationships.
Develop plan of action with client, e.g., look at available resources, support risk-taking behaviors.	Structure of a plan with support of a trusted person helps client to try out new behaviors.
Encourage client to identify positive, realistic behaviors currently being used.	As client recognizes that there are already some positive behaviors to build on, self-confidence will be enhanced and client may be willing to take more risks.

403

INTERVENTIONS	RATIONALE
Collaborative	
Encourage involvement in classes/group therapy, e.g., assertiveness, vocational, sex education; psychotherapy.	Provides opportunity to learn social skills, enhance sense of self-esteem, and promote appropriate social involvement.

Passive-Aggressive Personality Disorder

DSM III-R: 301.84 Passive-aggressive personality disorder (coded on Axis II)

ETIOLOGIC THEORIES

PSYCHODYNAMICS

These clients are unaware that ongoing difficulties are the result of own behaviors. They experience conscious hostility toward authority figures but do not connect own passive-resistant behaviors with hostility or resentment. They do not trust others, are not assertive, are intentionally inefficient, and try to get back at others through aggravation. Anger and hostility are released through others, who become angry and may suffer because of the inefficiencies. This disorder can lead to more serious psychological dysfunctions such as major depression, dysthymic disorder, alcohol, and other drug abuse/dependence.

These behaviors are not disturbing to the individual but are to those in the environment who interact with the client. Therapy is not usually sought, but client is generally referred by family members.

BIOLOGIC THEORIES

Personality disturbance is attributed to constitutional abnormalities. It is suggested that there is a biologic base to behavioral and emotional deviations, and researchers hope to demonstrate a correlation between chromosomal and neuronal abnormalities and a person's behavior.

FAMILY DYNAMICS

Theories of development implicate environmental factors occurring in the very early years of the child's life. Feelings of rejection or inadequate nurturing by the mother figure result in anger that is then turned inward on the self. Depression is common.

CLIENT ASSESSMENT DATA BASE

HISTORY

Demands for adequate performance are met with resistance expressed indirectly, resulting in pervasive social or occupational ineffectiveness, interfering with job performance and leading to difficulty adjusting to close relationships.

Covert aggressive behaviors are chosen over self-assertive behaviors.

Passively resists demands, to increase or maintain certain level of performance, through behaviors such as dawdling, stubbornness, procrastination, and "forgetfulness."

Habitually "forgets" commitments, arrives late for appointments.

PHYSICAL EXAMINATION

Mental Status:

  Behavior: may not appear uncomfortable in social situations but is cold and indifferent, reflecting stiff perfectionism. Interpersonal relationships may be strained because of passive-aggressive behaviors.

  Mood and affect: displays a seriousness with difficulty expressing warm feelings. May sulk and pout, passively acquiesce/conform, but resentment is unspoken.

  Emotion: anxiety and depression, expresses low self-esteem, lacks self-confidence, and may be dependent and passive

  Thought processes: views world in a negativistic manner but fails to connect behavior to others' reactions, feels resentful, and believes others are being unfair. Sees the world as a hostile and unfair environment.

DIAGNOSTIC STUDIES

Drug screen: to identify substance use.

NURSING PRIORITIES

1. Assist client to learn methods to control anxiety and express anger appropriately.
2. Promote effective, satisfying coping strategies.
3. Promote development of positive self-concept.
4. Encourage client/family to become involved in therapy/support programs.

DISCHARGE CRITERIA

1. Resolving feelings of anger, hostility.
2. Assertive techniques are learned and used.
3. Self-esteem is increased.
4. Client/family involved in therapy programs.

NURSING DIAGNOSIS:	ANXIETY (MODERATE TO SEVERE)
MAY BE RELATED TO:	Unconscious conflict
	Unmet needs
	Threat to self-concept
	Difficulty in asserting self directly, trusting others
	Feelings of resentment toward authority figures
POSSIBLY EVIDENCED BY:	Difficulty resolving feelings/trusting others
	Passive resistance to demands made by others
	Extraneous movements: foot-shuffling, hand/arm movements
	Irritability, argumentativeness
CLIENT OUTCOMES/EVALUATION CRITERIA:	Defines and uses effective methods for decreasing anxiety. Demonstrates problem-solving skills. Reports anxiety is reduced to a manageable level. Uses resources effectively.

INTERVENTIONS	RATIONALE
Independent	
Encourage direct expression of feelings. Help client to recognize when open, honest feelings are not being expressed.	Client has established a pattern of expressing feelings indirectly through covert aggression. Needs to learn to express feelings directly as they occur.
Explore situations that lead to feelings of anger, hostility. Discuss possible causes.	Client needs to gain insight into areas that cause resentment and anger in order to plan resolution.
Examine feelings toward authority figures. Discuss how these feelings come about.	Authority figures are a common target for client's aggression. May have started in early childhood, leaving multiple unresolved conflicts.
Assist client to be in tune to own feelings and increasing internal anxiety.	Client is often unaware that responses are consequences of anxiety.
Discuss fears concerning intimate relationships. Does client feel betrayed by significant other(s)?	Inability to trust is a significant problem for this client. Examining situations in past provides opportunity for insight.
Review how the inability to express feelings has resulted in covert acting-out behaviors.	Important for establishing the correlation between hostility and covert maneuvers.
Aid client in establishing a possible cause and effect relationship of "forgetfulness," dawdling, procrastination, etc., to internal resentment toward the person making demands.	Important for heightened awareness of own feelings and behaviors manifested.
Encourage client to recognize need to act out with covert aggression to "get back" at others. Together develop effective methods to alter response.	Client is not always aware of own feelings/needs, and assistance in redirecting aggression can help client to change behaviors.
Support verbalization of feelings in an assertive manner instead of using flight response.	Client needs to learn to face issues directly using assertive techniques.
Discuss client's fears regarding new assertive behaviors. Help define ways to alleviate these fears.	Self-assertion is a new experience for this client. Discussing fears helps diminish them.
Explore with client how often anger is displaced onto others because client believes the target of the anger cannot be approached.	Reinforces need for client to deal directly with target of feelings.
Explain "pressure cooker" effect of "stuffing" feelings.	Has established a lifelong pattern of internalizing feelings, and this eventually leads to exploding inappropriately. Education is necessary to understand relationship of "thoughts—feelings—behavior."
Define methods of expression that effectively control anxiety, e.g., relaxation, use of "I-messages."	This is a new approach for the client who therefore needs guidance in learning effective anxiety control.
Give positive feedback for new behaviors. Discuss any needed modifications.	Provides reassurance and encourages repetition of newly learned skills. This client has difficulty trusting own judgment.

NURSING DIAGNOSIS:	**COPING, INEFFECTIVE INDIVIDUAL**
MAY BE RELATED TO:	**Personal vulnerability**
	Unrealistic perceptions

MAY BE RELATED TO—*continued*	Unmet expectations
	Inadequate coping method (does not use self-assertive behaviors)
	Lack of recognition of relationship between passive-aggressive behaviors and internal anxiety
POSSIBLY EVIDENCED BY:	Use of maladaptive, temporary relief behaviors that do not last or really satisfy
	Real issues remaining unaddressed and unresolved
	Maneuvers such as dawdling, procrastination, stubbornness, forgetfulness, habitual tardiness
	Difficulty meeting basic needs
	Alteration in societal participation
	Lack of assertive behaviors
CLIENT OUTCOMES/EVALUATION CRITERIA:	Identifies ineffective coping behaviors and consequences. Develops and implements repertoire of coping strategies that are based on problem-solving techniques and that provide effective relief of conflicts.

INTERVENTIONS

Independent

Discuss present patterns of coping and evaluate their effectiveness.

Assist client to identify how passive-resistant behaviors are maladaptive relief behaviors.

Confront client with what needs the behaviors are really serving when forgetfulness and procrastination are used.

Review what unmet needs are and why present coping patterns do not afford lasting relief.

Discourage client from justifying current automatic relief behaviors. Point out the inadequacies of these behaviors.

RATIONALE

Client needs to recognize pattern and see that current methods do not bring positive results.

Needs to associate behaviors with an attempt to gain relief from anxiety and hostility.

Confrontation heightens awareness of problem, providing stimulus for change to get needs met in more constructive ways.

Brings to light that client's needs are really not being satisfied.

Client will have difficulty changing old behaviors and has already spent a lifetime justifying them to self.

INTERVENTIONS

Independent

Encourage client to identify examples of situations when the client felt imposed upon or angered but did not speak up. Discuss alternate ways to handle those situations.

Ask client to discuss how it feels when others are habitually forgetful and don't keep commitments. Discuss importance of following through with what is promised.

Give feedback on how passive-resistant behaviors affect others.

Provide information about problem-solving techniques to provide base for effective, satisfying coping behaviors.

Give positive feedback when client demonstrates use of adaptive skills and makes suggestions for improvement.

RATIONALE

Promotes understanding that avoidance of dealing directly with anger often leads to a negative outcome. Realization is crucial to learning new coping skills.

Developing empathy may help break this pattern.

Client needs to realize how destructive the behaviors can be.

Aids client in learning to think through problems and arriving at well-thought-out solutions that are successful.

Aids in reinforcing positive behaviors.

NURSING DIAGNOSIS:	SELF-CONCEPT, DISTURBANCE IN: SELF-ESTEEM
MAY BE RELATED TO:	**Retarded ego development**
	Unmet dependency needs
	Early rejection by significant other(s)
	Lack of positive feedback
POSSIBLY EVIDENCED BY:	**Feelings of inadequacy, fear of asserting self**
	Lack of self-confidence
	Dependency on others
	Directing frustrations toward others by using covert aggressive tactics
	Not accepting own responsibility for what happens as a result of maladaptive behaviors
	Not verbalizing negative feelings and working through them

CLIENT OUTCOMES/EVALUATION CRITERIA:	Verbalizes a sense of worthwhileness. Uses assertive, effective behaviors to interact with others. Actively participating in program(s) to develop positive self-esteem.

INTERVENTIONS

Independent

Encourage client to describe self and perceived inadequacies and how these relate to others. Note whether client compares self to others and in what terms.

Assess client's self-concept. Determine if client is realistic about strengths and limitations.

Encourage client to make adjustments in thinking if expectations of self and others are unrealistic.

Discuss how evaluations by others might have negatively affected the client.

Explore past relationships. Determine if client feels let down or hurt by significant other(s).

Assist client to learn how to express feelings assertively, e.g., "I feel hurt, angry, rejected, discounted, etc." This mode of interaction promotes more comfortable relationships.

Explain that being willing to take some risks by allowing others to get close is necessary, even though getting hurt is a possible outcome.

Discuss specific objectives for self-improvement and enhancing relationships.

Encourage client to learn more about others to gain a clearer perspective of their motives and feelings.

Ask client to describe what is defined as success in others and perceptions of what made them successful, and compare with own life successes.

Explore how the desired attributes can be adopted and put into practice.

Encourage client to accept self with strengths and liabilities and learn to like self.

RATIONALE

Negative self-image often comes from comparing oneself unfavorably to others.

May not have accurate perceptions of own strengths and shortcomings.

Cannot improve self-esteem if expectations are not realistic/achievable.

Often people are hypersensitive to others' comments and allow them to stick as a "label."

Client may be hanging onto old pain that needs to be worked through or let go.

Expressing feelings assertively is self-enhancing.

Taking risks and experiencing success can do much to enhance self-esteem.

Client needs to take action on newly gained knowledge in order to achieve success.

Client uses defense mechanism of projection of own feelings on others. Anger and hostility can be diffused by gaining more information about others and their situations.

May already have qualities for success but has overshadowed them with negative feelings.

Helps client to apply goals to daily life situations.

Self-acceptance is necessary to build self-esteem and improve relationships with others.

NURSING DIAGNOSIS:	POWERLESSNESS
MAY BE RELATED TO:	Interpersonal interaction
	Lifestyle of helplessness

	Difficulty connecting own passive-resistant behaviors with hostility or resentment
	Dependency feelings
POSSIBLY EVIDENCED BY:	Experiencing conscious hostility toward authority figures
	Releasing anger and hostility through others who may become angry or suffer because of their inefficiencies
	Getting back at others through aggravation
CLIENT OUTCOMES/EVALUATION CRITERIA:	Expresses sense of control over present/future outcomes. Verbalizes resolution of hostile feelings. Uses assertive (instead of aggressive) behaviors to deal with feelings, anxiety-producing situations, and interactions with others.

INTERVENTIONS	RATIONALE
Independent	
Examine hostile feelings toward authority figures. Determine when this began and what painful experiences have come about because of those in authority.	A major dynamic for this personality disorder is resentment of authority and the resulting sense of powerlessness. Helps to know what experiences client has had that led to this situation, especially relationship with mother during early years, when client may have felt particularly helpless.
Explore areas of life in which feeling inadequate or having a sense of no control occurs.	Provides insight into feelings necessary for learning adaptive behaviors.
Identify covert aggressive behaviors used to gain control of others.	Increases awareness of mode of interaction used and attempts to maintain sense of own control.
Encourage verbalization of how feelings of anger, hurt, and loss of control relate to desire to strike out at others.	Enhances understanding of how use of covert aggression has become a pervasive pattern.
Provide opportunity to learn how to get needs met in an acceptable, assertive manner.	Promotes inner strength and adaptive functioning, enhancing sense of control.
Assist client to learn to listen to others and consider their feelings by putting self in their place.	Promotes empathy for others and sense of own self-worth.
Have client assist in developing treatment plan.	Aids in promoting a sense of control and involvement in own care/future. This sense of participation enhances cooperation.

411

BIBLIOGRAPHY

General—Books

American Psychiatric Association: Diagnostic and Statistical Manual of Mental Disorders, ed 3, revised. American Psychiatric Association, Washington, DC, 1987.

Beck, CM, Rawlins, RP and Williams, SR: Mental Health-Psychiatric Nursing, ed 2. CV Mosby, St Louis, 1988.

Burgess, AW: Psychiatric Nursing in the Hospital and the Community, ed 4. Prentice-Hall, Englewood Cliffs, NJ, 1985.

Carpenito, LJ: Nursing Diagnosis: Application to Clinical Practice, ed 2. JB Lippincott, Philadelphia, 1987.

Doenges, M, Jeffries, M and Moorhouse, M: Nursing Care Plans: Nursing Diagnoses in Planning Patient Care. FA Davis, Philadelphia, 1984.

Doenges, M and Moorhouse, M: Nurse's Pocket Guide: Nursing Diagnoses with Interventions. FA Davis, Philadelphia, 1988.

Gettrust, KV, Ryan, SC and Engelman, DS (eds): Applied Nursing Diagnosis: Guides for Comprehensive Care Planning. John Wiley, New York, 1985.

Gordon, M: Nursing Diagnosis: Process and Applications, ed 2. McGraw-Hill, New York, 1987.

Kaplan, H and Sadock, B: Modern Synopsis of Comprehensive Textbook of Psychiatry/IV. Baltimore: Williams & Wilkins, 1985.

Kreigh, HZ and Perko, JE: Psychiatric and Mental Health Nursing: A Commitment to Care and Concern, ed 2. Reston Publishing, A Prentice-Hall Company, Reston, VA, 1983.

Haber, J, et al: Comprehensive Psychiatric Nursing, ed 3. McGraw-Hill, New York, 1987.

Hagerty, BK: Psychiatric-Mental Health Assessment. CV Mosby, St Louis, 1984.

Hogan, R: Human Sexuality, ed 2. Appleton-Century-Crofts, Norwalk, CT, 1985.

Janosik, EH and Davies, JL: Psychiatric Mental Health Nursing. Jones and Bartlett, Boston, 1986.

Lego, S (ed): The American Handbook of Psychiatric Nursing. JB Lippincott, St Louis, 1984.

McFarland, G and Wasli, E: Nursing Diagnoses and Process in Psychiatric Mental Health Nursing. JB Lippincott, Philadelphia, 1986.

Neal, MC, et al: Nursing Care Planning Guides for Psychiatric and Mental Health Care, ed 2. Nurseco, Pacific Palisades, CA, 1985.

Pasquali, EA, et al: Mental Health Nursing. CV Mosby, St Louis, 1985.

Schultz, J and Dark, S: Manual of Psychiatric Nursing Care Plans, ed 2. Little, Brown and Co, Boston, 1986.

Stuart, GW and Sundeen, SJ: Principles and Practice of Psychiatric Nursing, ed 3. CV Mosby, St Louis, 1987.

Townsend, M: Nursing Diagnoses in Psychiatric Nursing: A Pocket Guide for Care Plan Construction. FA Davis, Philadelphia, 1988.

General—Articles

Bauer, A: Dual diagnosis patients: The state of the problem. Tie Lines 4(3):1–4, July 1987.

Chapter 1—Books

Goldenberg, I and Goldenberg, H: Family Therapy: An Overview. Brooks/Cole, Monterey, CA, 1980.

Minuchen, S: Families and Family Therapy. Harvard University Press, Cambridge, MA, 1976.

Chapter 1—Articles

Joel, LA: Reshaping nursing practice. AJN 87(6):793–795, June 1987.

McHugh, MK: Has nursing outgrown the nursing process? Nursing87, 17(8):50–51, August 1987.

Lombard, N and Light, N: On-line nursing care plans by nursing diagnosis. Computers in Healthcare, pp 22–23, November 1983.

Chapter 2—Books

Kelly, MA: Nursing Diagnosis Source Book, Appleton-Century-Crofts, Norwalk, CT, 1985.
Kim, MJ, et al: Classification of Nursing Diagnosis, Proceedings of the Fifth National Conference. CV Mosby, St Louis, 1984.

Chapter 2—Articles

American Nurses' Association: Nursing: A social policy statement. Pub Code: NP-63 35M 12/80, Kansas City, 1980.
American Nurses' Association: Standards of nursing practice. Pub Code: NO-41 10M 1:77, Kansas City, 1973.
Baer, C (ed): Nursing diagnosis. Topics in Clinical Nursing 5(4), January 1984.
Carter, EW: Psychiatric nursing: 1986. J Psychosocial Nursing 24(6):26–30, June 1986.
Fadden, TC, et al: Nursing diagnosis: A matter of form. AJN 84(4):470–472, April 1984.
Jacoby, MK: The dilemma of physiological problems: Eliminating the double standard. AJN 85(3):281, 285, March 1985.
Kim, MJ: Without collaboration, what's left? AJN, 85(3):281, 284. March 1985.
Tartaglia, MJ: Nursing diagnosis: Keystone of your care plan. Nursing85, 15:34–37, March 1985.

Chapter 3—Books

Adams, CG and Macione, A: Handbook of Psychiatric Mental Health Nursing. John Wiley, New York, 1983.
Arieti, S: Interpretation of Schizophrenia. Basic Books, New York, 1974.
Campbell, C: Nursing Diagnosis and Intervention in Nursing Practice. John Wiley, New York, 1984.
Critchley, DL and Maurin, JT (eds): The Clinical Specialist in Psychiatric Mental Health Nursing. John Wiley, New York, 1985.
Freedman, AM, Kaplan, HI and Sadock, B: Modern Synopsis of Comprehensive Textbook of Psychiatry/III, ed 3. Williams & Wilkins, Baltimore, 1981.
Johnson, BS: Psychiatric-Mental Health Nursing Adaptation and Growth. JB Lippincott, Philadelphia, 1986.
Kalkman, ME and Davis, AJ: New Dimensions in Mental Health-Psychiatric Nursing. McGraw-Hill, New York, 1980.
Kyes, J and Hofling, CK: Basic Psychiatric Concepts in Nursing, ed 4. JB Lippincott, Philadelphia, 1980.
Manfreda, ML and Krampitz, SD: Psychiatric Nursing, ed 10. FA Davis, Philadelphia, 1977.
Murray, RB and Huelskoetter, MW: Psychiatric/Mental Health Nursing: Giving Emotional Care. Prentice-Hall, Englewood Cliffs, NJ, 1983.
Stewart, MA and Gath, A: Psychological Disorders of Children. Williams & Wilkins, Baltimore, 1978.
Slaby, AE, Lieb, J and Tancredi, LP: Handbook of Psychiatric Emergencies. Medical Examination, Inc, New York, 1975.
Taylor, CM: Mereness' Essentials of Psychiatric Nursing, ed 12. CV Mosby, St Louis, 1986.
Wilson, HS and Kneisl, CR: Psychiatric Nursing, ed 2. Addison-Wesley, Menlo Park, CA, 1983.

Chapter 3—Articles

Baird, SF: Helping the family through a crisis. Nursing87, 17:66–67, June 1987.
Marks, RG: Anorexia and bulimia: Eating habits that can kill. RN, pp 44–47, January 1984.
Ornitz, EM and Ritvo, ER: The syndrome of autism: A critical review. American Journal of Psychiatry 133:6, June 1976.

Chapter 4—Books

Burnside, IM: Nursing and the Aged. McGraw-Hill, New York, 1981.
Maci, N and Rabins, RV: The 36-Hour Day (A Family Guide to Caring for Persons With Alzheimer's Disease, Dementing Illnesses, and Memory Loss in Later Life). The John Hopkins University Press, Baltimore, 1981.
Powell, LS (ed): Alzheimer's Disease: A Guide for Families. Addison-Wesley, Reading, MA, 1983.
Reisberg, B, MD Editor: Alzheimer's Disease: The Standard Reference. The Free Press, New York, 1983.

Chapter 4—Articles

"Whole Series, Alzheimer's Disease", AJN 84(2):216–232, February 1984.
Bartol, MA: Non-verbal communication in patients with Alzheimer's disease. Journal of Gerontological Nursing 5(4):21–31, July/August 1979.
Beam, IM: Alzheimer's disease: Helping families survive. AJN 84(2)229–232, February 1984.
Busteed, EL and Johnstone, C: The development of suicide precautions for an inpatient psychiatric unit. Journal of Psychosocial Nursing and Mental Health Services. 21(5):15–19, May 1983.
Cutler, NR and Preom, KN: Drug therapies. Geriatric Nursing, 6(3), May/June 1985:160–163.
Farberow, NL: Suicide prevention in the hospital. Hospital and Community Psychiatry 32(2):99–104.
Kiely, MA: Alzheimer's disease: Making the most of the time that's left. RN, March 1985, pp 34–41.
Ninos, M and Makohon, R: Functional Assessment of the Patient. Geriatric Nursing May/June 1985, pp 139–142.
Reisberg, B: Stages of Cognitive Decline. AJN 84(2):225–228, 1984.

Chapter 5—Books

Asnis, S and Smith, R: Amphetamine abuse and violence. Amphetamine Use, Misuse, and Abuse: Proceedings of the National Amphetamine Conference. Hall, Boston, pp 189–204, 1978.

Bernstein, J: Handbook of Drug Therapy in Psychiatry. PSG, Boston, 1983.

Black, C: It Will Never Happen to Me. MAC, Denver, 1982.

Blum, K: Handbook of Abusable Drugs. Gardner Press, New York, 1984.

Burkhalter, P: Nursing care of the Alcoholic and the Drug Abuser. McGraw-Hill, New York, 1975.

Buxton, M, Jessup, M and Landry, M: Treatment of the chemically dependent health professional. In: The addictions: Multidisciplinary Perspectives and Treatments. Heath, Lexington, MA, pp 131–143, 1984.

Cohen, S, et al: Frequently Prescribed and Abused Drugs. Haworth, New York, 1982.

Cohen, S: The Substance Abuse Problems. Haworth, New York, 1981.

Dubin, W and Stolberg, R: Emergency Psychiatry for the House Officer. SP Medical and Scientific, New York, 1981.

Dubovsky, S, Feiger, A and Eiseman, B: Psychiatric Decision Making. BC Decker, Philadelphia, 1984.

Estes, NJ, Heinemann, ME: Alcoholism: Development, Consequences and Interventions. CV Mosby, St Louis, 1982.

Fauman, B and Fauman, M: Emergency Psychiatry for the House Officer. Williams & Wilkins, Baltimore, 1981.

Goth, A: Medical Pharmacology: Principles and Concepts. CV Mosby, St Louis, 1978.

Greist, J, Jefferson, J and Spitzer, R (eds): Treatment of Mental Disorders. Oxford University Press, New York, 1982.

Mannik, M and Gilliland, B: Vasculitis. In: Isselbacher, et al (eds): Harrison's Principles of Internal Medicine, ed 9. McGraw-Hill, New York, pp 351–355, 1980.

Milan, JR and Ketchum, K: Under the Influence. Bantam Books, New York, 1981.

OBrien, R and Cohen S: The Encyclopedia of Drug Abuse. Facts on File, New York, 1984.

Robinson, L: Psychiatric Nursing as a Human Experience, ed 3. WB Saunders, Philadelphia, 1983.

Rund, D and Hutzler, J: Emergency Psychiatry. CV Mosby, St Louis, 1983.

Slaby, A, Lieb, J and Tancredi, L: Handbook of Psychiatric Emergencies. Medical Examination, New York, 1975.

Smith, D: Substance use disorders: Drugs and alcohol. In: Review of General Psychiatry. Lange Medical Publishers, Los Altos, CA, pp 287–289, 1984.

Smith, D, Milkman, H and Sunderwirth, S: Addictive disease: Concept and controversy. In: The Addictions: Multidisciplinary Perspectives and Treatments. Heath, Lexington, MA, pp 145–158, 1984.

Snyder, S: A "model schizophrenia" mediated by catecholamines. Amphetamine Use, Misuse, and Abuse: Proceedings of the National Amphetamine Conference. GK Hall, Boston, pp 189–204, 1978.

Stimmel, B: Cardiovascular effects of mood-altering drugs. Raven Press, New York, 1979.

Youcha, G: A Dangerous Pleasure. Hawthorn Books, New York, 1981.

Chapter 5—Articles

Acee, AM and Smith, D: Crack. AJN 87(5):614–617, May 1987.

Betemps, E: Management of the withdrawal syndrome of barbiturates and other central nervous system depressants. Journal of Psychosocial Nursing and Mental Health Services. 19(19):31–34, September 1981.

Davis, W: LSD or DOB. American Journal of Psychiatry 139(12):1649, December, 1982.

Ehrlich, P and McGeehan, M: Cocaine recovery support groups and the language of recovery. Journal of Psychoactive Drugs, 17(1):11–17, 1985.

Gary, NE and Tresznewsky, O: Barbiturates and a potpourri of other sedatives, hypnotics and tranquilizers. Heart and Lung 12(2):122–127, March 1983.

Goldfrank, L, Bresnitz, E and Weismore, R: Opisids and opiates. Heart and Lung 12(2):114–122, March 1983.

Greenberg, F, et al: A safe psychiatric unit. Hospital Topics, pp 34–36, May/June, 1980.

Grinspoon, L (ed): Treatment of alcoholism—Part I. Harvard Medical School Mental Health Letter 3(12):1–4, June 1987.

Grinspoon, L (ed): Treatment of alcoholism—Part II. Harvard Medical School Mental Health Letter 4(1):1–3, July 1987.

Harris, E: Sedative-hypnotic drugs. AJN 81(7):1329–1334, July 1981.

Heng, MCY: Question and Answers Column. Medical Aspects of Human Sexuality, p 15, November 1987.

Johnsen, CD, Reeves, KO and Jackson, D: Alcohol and sex. Heart and lung 12(1):93–96, January 1983.

King, RCK: Dealing with drug abusers. RN, pp 37–39, April 1985.

Leporati, NC & Chychula, LH: How you can really help the drug-abusing patient. Nursing82, pp 46–49, June 1982.

Lydiard, R and Gelenberg, A: Psychiatric emergencies: Treating substance abuse. Part II. Drug therapy hospital, pp 55–56, April 1982.

McCarthy, J: The concept of addictive disease. Treating the cocaine abuser, pp 21–31, USA, Hazelden, 1985.

McCarthy, J: The medical complications of cocaine abuse. Treating the cocaine abuser, pp 31–49, USA, Hazelden, 1985.

McCoy, S, et al: PCP intoxication: Psychiatric issues of nursing care. Journal of Psychiatric Nursing and Mental Health Services 19:17–23, July 1981.

National Polydrug Collaborative Project: Treatment manual 1: Medical treatment for complications of polydrug abuse. US Dept of Health, Education, and Welfare, 1976.

Nelson, C: The styles of enabling behavior. Treating the cocaine abuser, pp 49–73, USA, Hazelden, 1985.

Olsen, E, McEarue, J and Greenbavor, DM: Recognition, general considerations, and techniques in the management of drug intoxication. Heart and Lung 12(2):110–114, March 1983.

Rector, CS and Foster, ME: Assessment and care of the patient experiencing alcohol withdrawal syndrome. Nursing care plan. Critical Care Nursing, pp 64–68, July/August 1984.

Russ, HA: Nightmare Drug. RN, pp 33–35, October 1979.

Schloemer, NF and Skidmore, JW: Opiate withdrawal with clonidive. Journal of Psychosocial Nursing and Mental Health Services 21(10):8–14, October 1983.

Siegel, R: Treatment of cocaine abuse: Historical and contemporary perspectives. Journal of Psychoactive Drugs 17(1):1–19, 1985.

Silberner, J: Cocaine cardiology: Problems, mysteries. Science News, pp 69, January 31, 1987.

Smith, DE and Wesson, D: Cocaine abuse and treatment: An overview. Treating the Cocaine Abuser. Hazelden, Center City, MN, 1985.

Smith, D, et al: A clinical guide to the diagnosis and treatment of heroin-related sexual dysfunction. Journal of Psychoactive Drugs 14(1–2):91–99, 1982.

Solursh, L and Clement, W: Use of diazepam in hallucinogenic drug crises. Journal of the American Medical Association, 205(9):98–99, 26 August, 1968.

Strassman, R: Adverse reactions to psychedelic drugs: A review of the literature. Journal of Nervous and Mental Disease 172(10):577–594, October 1984.

Washton, AM: Clinical guidelines for cocaine-abusing patients. Medical Aspects of Human Sexuality, pp 138–146, November 1987.

Chapter 6—Books

Paul, GL and Lentz, RJ: Psychosocial Treatment of Chronic Mental Patients: Milieu vs Social-Learning Programs. Harvard University Press, Cambridge, 1978.

Chapter 6—Articles

Braden, W: Vulnerability and schizoaffective psychosis: A two-factor model. Schizophrenia Bulletin 10(1):30–45, 1984.

Clayton, P: Schizoaffective disorders. Journal of Nervous and Mental Diseases, November 1982, pp 646–650.

Goodnick, PJ, Grossman, M and Herbertr, Y: Treatment of schizoaffective disorders. Schizophrenia Bulletin 10(1):30–45, 1984.

Grinspoon, L (ed): Care and treatment of schizophrenia—Part I. Harvard Medical School Mental Health Letter 2(12):1–4, June 1986.

Grinspoon, L (ed): Care and treatment of schizophrenia—Part II. Harvard Medical School Mental Health Letter 3(1):1–4, July 1986.

Grinspoon, L (ed): Schizoaffective disorder. Harvard Medical School Mental Health Letter 4(2):1–4, August 1987.

Harrow, M and Grossman, LS: Outcome in schizoaffective disorders: A critical review and reevaluation of the literature. Schizophrenia Bulletin 10(1):87–105, 1984.

Himmelhock, JM, et al: When a schizoaffective diagnosis has meaning. Journal of Nervous and Mental Diseases, May 1981, pp 277–282.

Meltzer, HY: Schizoaffective disorder: Is the news of its nonexistence premature? Editors' Introduction. Schizophrenia Bulletin 10(1):11–13, 1984.

Pope, HG, Jr, et al: Schizoaffective disorder: An invalid diagnosis? A comparison of Schizoaffective disorder, schizophrenia and affective disorder. American Journal of Psychiatry, August 1980, pp 921–927.

Pope, HG, Jr, and Keck, PE: What is neuroleptic malignant syndrome? Harvard Medical School Mental Health Newsletter 4(4):8, October 1987.

Tsuang, MT and Simpson, JC: Schizoaffective disorder: Concept and reality. Schizophrenia Bulletin 10(1):14–23, 1984.

Tsuang, MT, Dempsey, GM and Fleming, JA: Can ECT prevent premature death and suicide in schizoaffective patients? Journal of Affective Disorders, September 1979, pp 167–171.

Wicklund, S and Devroye, M: Recognizing neuroleptic-induced movement disorders. Nurses' drug alert. AJN 87(12):1651, December 1987.

Chapter 7—Articles

Grinspoon, L (ed): Paranoia and paranoid disorders. Harvard Medical School Mental Health Newsletter 3(12):1–4, June 1987.

Chapter 8—Books

Kolb, LC: Modern Clinical Psychiatry, ed 9. WB Saunders, Philadelphia, 1977.

Chapter 8—Articles

Bower, B: What's in the cards for manic depression? Science News 131(18):410, May 2, 1987.

Harris, E: The dexamethasone suppression test. AJN 82(5):784–785, May 1982.

Jacobsen, FM, et al: Morning versus midday phototherapy of seasonal affective disorder. Am J Psychiatry 144(10):1301–1305, October 1987.

Silver, M: Using restraint. AJN 87(11):1414–1415, November 1987.

The dexamethasone suppression test: An overview of its current status in psychiatry. Am J Psychiatry 144(10):1253–1259, October 1987.

Wilson, JS: Unmasking depression. NursingLife 7(6):58–63, November/December 1987.

Chapter 9—Books

Dollard, J and Miller, N: Personality and Psychotherapy. McGraw-Hill, New York, 1950.

Freud, S: Problem of Anxiety. WW Norton, New York, 1936.

Peplau, H: Process and concept of learning. In Burd, S and Marshall, M (eds): Clinical Approaches to Psychiatric Nursing. Macmillan, New York, 1963.

Rimm, D and Masters, J: Behavior Therapy. Academic Press, New York, 1974.

Smitherman, C: Nursing Actions for Health Promotion. FA Davis, Philadelphia, 1981.

Sullivan, HS: The Interpersonal Theory of Psychiatry. WW Norton, New York, 1953.

Chapter 9—Articles

Keltner, NL, Doggnett, R and Johnson, R: For the Vietnam veteran, the war goes on. Perspectives in Psychiatric Care 21(3):108–113, 1983.

Krupnick, J: The stress response: Recurrent themes. Archives in General Psychiatry 38:428–435, 1981.

Lindy, J: Survivors: Outreach to a reluctant population. American Journal of Orthopsychiatry 51:468–478, 1981.

Mullis, M: The human fallout. Journal of Psychiatric Nursing and Mental Health Services 22(2):27–31, 1984.

Scrignar, CB: Posttraumatic stress disorder and sexual dysfunction. Medical Aspects of Human Sexuality, pp 102–112, February 1987.

Terr, L: Effects of psychic trauma four years after a schoolbus kidnapping. American Journal of Psychiatry 140:1543–1550, 1983.

Chapter 10—Articles

Menenberg, SR: Somatopsychology and AIDS victims. J Psychosocial Nursing 25(5):18–22, May 1987.

Chapter 11—Books

Braun, BG (ed): Symposium on Multiple Personality Psychiatric Clinics of North America, 7/1. WB Saunders, Philadelphia, 1984.

Chapter 11—Articles

Coons, PM: Treatment progress in 20 patients with multiple personality disorder. Journal of Nervous and Mental Disease 144(12):717–719, 1986.

Putnam, FW, et al: The clinical phenomenon of multiple personality disorder: Review of 100 recent cases. Journal of Clinical Psychiatry, pp 285–293, 47(6), June 1986.

Chapter 12—Books

Coleman, E (ed): Integrated Identity for Gay Men and Lesbians. Harrington Park Press, New York, 1988.

Bozett, FW (ed): Holistic Nursing Practice, 1/4. Aspen, Hagerstown, MD, August 1987.

Chapter 12—Articles

Grinspoon, L (ed): Paraphilias. Harvard Medical School Mental Health Newsletter 3(6):1–5, December 1986.

Journal of Homosexuality 14(1/2), 1987.

Chapter 14—Books

Bakal, D: Psychology and Medicine: Psychobiological Dimensions of Health and Illness. Springer, New York, 1979.

Dalton, K: The Premenstrual Syndrome and Progesterone Therapy. Year Book Medical, Chicago, 1977.

Lark, S: Premenstrual Syndrome Self-Help Book. Forman, Los Angeles, 1984.

Taylor, R: PMS answers at last. Optimed, Inc.

Thompson, J, et al: Clinical Nursing. CV Mosby, St Louis, 1986.

Chapter 14—Articles

Abraham, GE: Nutritional factors in the etiology of the premenstrual tension syndrome. Journal of Reproductive Medicine 28(7), July 1983.

Fischman, J: Getting tough: Can people learn to have disease-resistant personalities? Psychology Today, pp 26–28, December 1987.

Havens, C: Premenstrual syndrome: Tactics for intervention. Postgraduate Medicine 77(7), May 15, 1985.

Reale, J: Life Changes: Can they cause disease? Nursing87, 17(7):52–55, July 1987.

Symposium: Helping your patients cope with PMS. Contemporary OB/GYN, April 1984.

Premenstrual Syndrome: The Nutritional Viewpoint. Infection Reporter 1(5):, May 1984.

Chapter 15—Articles

Braverman, BG and Shook, J: Spotting the borderline personality. AJN 87(2):200–203, February 1987.

Grinspoon, L: Borderline personality. The Harvard Medical School Mental Health Newsletter 2(1), July 1985.

Howard, PZ: Dealing with the "difficult person": The borderline personality disorder. Unpublished paper, 1987.

Chapter 15—Books

Mahler, M, et al: Psychological Birth of the Human Infant: Symbiosis and Individuation. Basic Books, New York, 1975.

APPENDIX

TAXONOMY 1

Conceptual base for identifying and classifying nursing diagnoses. (Approved by NANDA General Assembly 1986.)

1. **EXCHANGING:** A human response pattern involving mutual giving and receiving.
   - 1.1. ALTERATIONS IN NUTRITION
     - 1.1.1. (Cellular)*
     - 1.1.2. (Systemic)*
       - 1.1.2.1. More than body requirements
       - 1.1.2.2. Less than body requirements
       - 1.1.2.3. Potential for more than body requirements
   - 1.2. (ALTERATIONS IN PHYSICAL REGULATION)*
     - 1.2.1. (Immune)*
       - 1.2.1.1. Potential for Infection
     - 1.2.2. Alteration in Body Temperature
       - 1.2.2.1. Potential
       - 1.2.2.2. Hypothermia
       - 1.2.2.3. Hyperthermia
       - 1.2.2.4. Ineffective Thermoregulation

   - 1.3. ALTERATIONS IN ELIMINATION
     - 1.3.1. Bowel
       - 1.3.1.1. Constipation
       - 1.3.1.2. Diarrhea
       - 1.3.1.3. Incontinence
     - 1.3.2. Urinary Patterns
       - 1.3.2.1. Incontinence
         - 1.3.2.1.1. Stress
         - 1.3.2.1.2. Reflex
         - 1.3.2.1.3. Urge
         - 1.3.2.1.4. Functional
         - 1.3.2.1.5. Total
       - 1.3.2.2. Retention [Acute/Chronic]
     - 1.3.3. (Skin)*
   - 1.4. (ALTERATIONS IN CIRCULATION)*
     - 1.4.1. (Vascular)*
       - 1.4.1.1. Tissue Perfusion
         - 1.4.1.1.1. Renal
         - 1.4.1.1.2. Cerebral
         - 1.4.1.1.3. Cardiopulmonary
         - 1.4.1.1.4. Gastrointestinal
         - 1.4.1.1.5. Peripheral
       - 1.4.1.2. Fluid Volume
         - 1.4.1.2.1. Excess
         - 1.4.1.2.2. Deficit
           - 1.4.1.2.2.1. Actual
           - 1.4.1.2.2.2. Potential

---

*Recommended by Taxonomy Committee but not yet approved by NANDA.

1.4.2. (Cardiac)*
    1.4.2.1. Decreased Cardiac Output
1.5. (ALTERATIONS IN OXYGENATION)*
  1.5.1. (Respiration)*
    1.5.1.1. Impaired Gas Exchange
    1.5.1.2. Ineffective Airway Clearance
    1.5.1.3. Ineffective Breathing Pattern
1.6. (ALTERATIONS IN PHYSICAL INTEGRITY)*
  1.6.1. Potential for Injury
    1.6.1.1. Potential for Suffocating
    1.6.1.2. Potential for Poisoning
    1.6.1.3. Potential for Trauma
  1.6.2. Impairment
    1.6.2.1. Skin Integrity
      1.6.2.1.1. Actual
      1.6.2.1.2. Potential
    1.6.2.2. Tissue Integrity
      1.6.2.2.1. Oral Mucous
            Membrane

2. COMMUNICATING: A human response pattern involving sending messages.
2.1. ALTERATIONS IN COMMUNICATION
  2.1.1. Verbal
    2.1.2.1. Impaired
  2.1.2. (Nonverbal)*

3. RELATING: A human response pattern involving establishing bonds.
3.1. (ALTERATIONS IN SOCIALIZATION)*
  3.1.1. Impaired Social Interaction
  3.1.2. Social Isolation
3.2. (ALTERATIONS IN ROLE)*
  3.2.1. Role Performance
    3.2.1.1. Parenting
      3.2.1.1.1. Actual
      3.2.1.1.2. Potential
    3.2.1.2. Sexual
      3.2.1.2.1. Dysfunction
    3.2.1.3. (Work)*
  3.2.2. Family Processes
3.3. Altered Sexuality Patterns

4. VALUING: A human response pattern involving the assigning of relative worth.
4.1. ALTERATIONS IN SPIRITUAL STATE
  4.1.1. Distress

5. CHOOSING: A human response pattern involving the selection of alternatives.
5.1. ALTERATIONS IN COPING
  5.1.1. Individual
    5.1.1.1. Ineffective
      5.1.1.1.1. Impaired
            Adjustment
  5.1.2. Family
    5.1.2.1. Ineffective
      5.1.2.1.1. Disabled
      5.1.2.1.2. Compromised
    5.1.2.2. Potential for Growth
  5.1.3. (Community)*

5.2. (ALTERATIONS IN PARTICIPATION)*
  5.2.1. (Individual)*
    5.2.1.1. Noncompliance
  5.2.2. (Family)*
  5.2.3. (Community)*

6. MOVING: A human response pattern involving activity.
6.1. (ALTERATIONS IN ACTIVITY)*
  6.1.1. Physical Mobility
    6.1.1.1. Impaired
    6.1.1.2. Activity Intolerance
    6.1.1.3. Potential Activity Intolerance
  6.1.2. (Social Mobility)*
6.2. (ALTERATIONS IN REST)*
  6.2.1. Sleep Pattern Disturbance
6.3. (ALTERATIONS IN RECREATION)*
  6.3.1. Diversional Activity
    6.3.1.1. Deficit
6.4. (ALTERATIONS IN ACTIVITIES OF DAILY LIVING)*
  6.4.1. Home Maintenance Management
    6.4.1.1. Impaired
  6.4.2. Health Maintenance
6.5. ALTERATIONS IN SELF CARE
  6.5.1. Feeding
    6.5.1.1. Impaired Swallowing
  6.5.2. Bathing/Hygiene
  6.5.3. Dressing/Grooming
  6.5.4. Toileting
6.6. ALTERED GROWTH AND DEVELOPMENT

7. PERCEIVING: A human response pattern involving the reception of information.
7.1. ALTERATIONS IN SELF CONCEPT
  7.1.1. Disturbance in Body Image
  7.1.2. Disturbance in Self Esteem
  7.1.3. Disturbance in Personal Identity
7.2. SENSORY/PERCEPTUAL ALTERATION
  7.2.1. Visual
    7.2.1.1. Unilateral Neglect
  7.2.2. Auditory
  7.2.3. Kinesthetic
  7.2.4. Gustatory
  7.2.5. Tactile
  7.2.6. Olfactory
7.3. (ALTERATIONS IN MEANINGFULNESS)*
  7.3.1. Hopelessness
  7.3.2. Powerlessness

8. KNOWING: A human response pattern involving the meaning associated with information.
8.1. ALTERATIONS IN KNOWLEDGE
  8.1.1. Deficit
8.2. (ALTERATIONS IN LEARNING)*
8.3. ALTERATIONS IN THOUGHT PROCESSES
  8.3.1. (Confusion)*

9. FEELING: A human response pattern involving the subjective awareness of information.
9.1. ALTERATIONS IN COMFORT

9.1.1. Pain
    9.1.1.1. Chronic
    9.1.1.2. Acute
9.1.2. (Discomfort)*
9.2. (ALTERATIONS IN EMOTIONAL INTEGRITY)*
9.2.1. Anxiety
9.2.2. Grieving
    9.2.2.1. Dysfunctional

9.2.2.2. Anticipatory
9.2.3. Potential for Violence
9.2.4. Fear
9.2.5. Post Trauma Response
    9.2.5.1. Rape Trauma Syndrome
        9.2.5.1.1. Rape Trauma
        9.2.5.1.2. Compound Reaction
        9.2.5.1.3. Silent Reaction

INDEX OF NURSING DIAGNOSES

424

The Worlds Great

CLOCKS
&
WATCHES

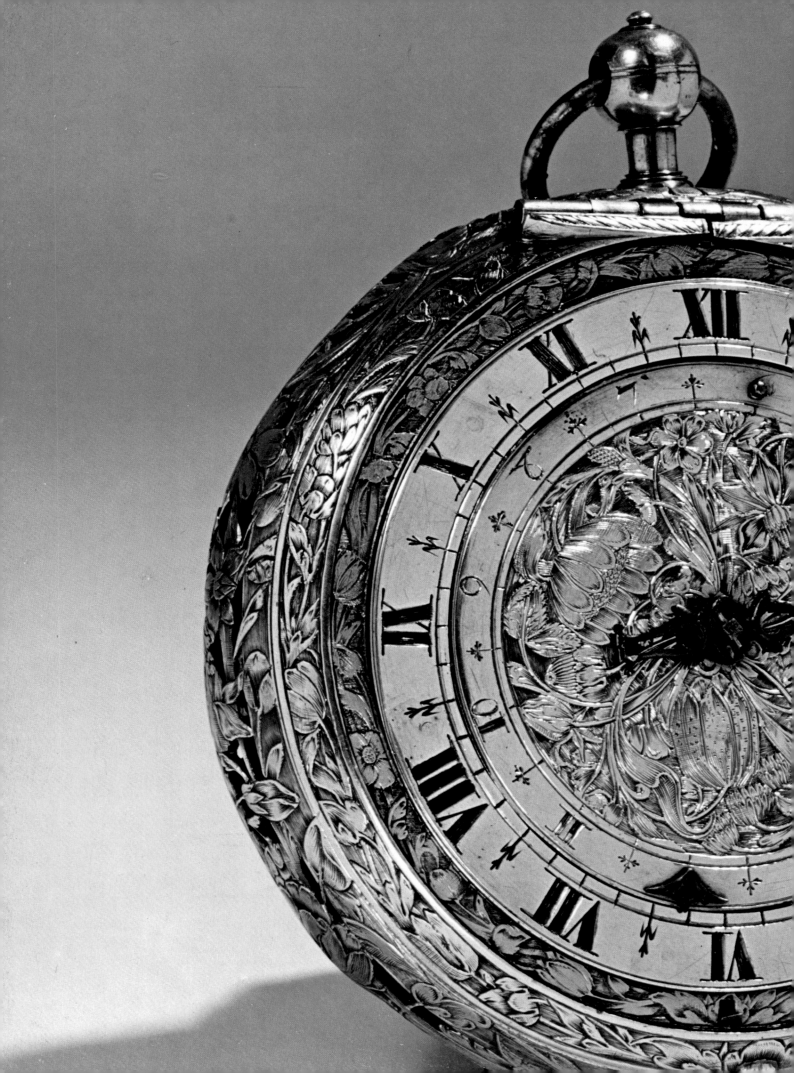

The Worlds Great

CLOCKS & WATCHES

Cedric Jagger

Galley Press

To my wife
CHRISTINE
with my love and gratitude for her skilled
and unstinting help with the preparation of this
book

endpapers
A London dealer's workshop. It is not easy to find a dealer with such expert facilities of his own. Aubrey Brocklehurst, London.

title page
See page 106.

Copyright © 1977 Hamlyn Publishing,
a division of The Hamlyn Publishing Group Limited

Published in this edition 1986
by Hamlyn Publishing for Galley Press,
an imprint of W.H. Smith and Son Limited
Registered No. 237811 England.
Trading as WHS Distributors, St John's House,
East Street, Leicester, LE1 6NE

ISBN 086136 6859

Printed in Spain

Acknowledgments

A.C.L., Brussels 21 top and bottom; Antique Collectors' Club, Woodbridge 241; Ashmolean Museum, Oxford 89 top, 96 top and bottom, 97 right; Bayerisches Museum, Munich 92 top, 159 top and bottom; Bibliotheque Nationale, Paris 16; British Museum, London 14, 31, 41, 50, 52, 53, 54, 58, 59, 68, 70, 71, 73, 74, 76 left and right, 78 left, 79 top and bottom, 80 top and bottom, 81, 82, 83, 84 left, 86, 88, 89 bottom, 91, 101 left and right, 105 top and bottom, 110, 119, 121, 122, 124, left, 125, 127, 132, 143 right, 147 right, 158 left, 162 left and right, 173, 175, 182, 186 left, 202, 203, 215, 216 left and right, 217, 218, 219 left and right, 220 top and bottom, 221, 222 top and bottom, 223 left and right, 224, 225, 227, 230; Eric Bruton, Widmer End 8, 30, 236 bottom; J. Allan Cash, London 17; Copenhagen Town Hall 49 top and bottom; Glasgow Herald and Evening Times 69; Clockmakers' Company Museum, Guildhall, London 34 right, 65 left, 72 left and right, 75 left and right, 98 bottom, 144 top and bottom, 170, 171 left and right, 193 top; Hamlyn Group Picture Library endpapers, 2–3, 102 left, 226, 228 left and right; Hamlyn Group – John R. Freeman & Co, 13 right, 29 left and right, 46, 57 bottom, 78 right, 93 left and right, 95, 97 left, 98 top, 102 right, 103 bottom, 104 top, 108 left and right, 109 left and right, 111 top and bottom, 112 bottom, 113 top and bottom, 114 left and right, 115, 116 left, 117 left and right, 120, 123 left, 126, 128 bottom, 129, 120, 131, 147 left, 150 left, 155 bottom, 160, 163, 164 right, 165, 178 top and bottom, 179 top and bottom, 180 top, 181 left and right, 183 right, 184, 185, 187 top and bottom, 188, 189 left and right, 190 top, centre and bottom, 191, 194, 197 left, 199 bottom, 201 top, 205, 209, 210 top, 211, 212 top, 213 left and right, 231 bottom, 235 top, bottom left and bottom right, 242 right, 248 right, 249 left, 250 bottom; Hamlyn Group – Hypsos 135 left, 143 left; Hamlyn Group – Marcus Taylor 195; Herzog Anton Ulrich-Museum, Brunswick 92 bottom; Hessisches Landesmuseum, Kassel 84 right, 85 left and right, 87 left, 90 top; Historisches Uhren-Museum, Wuppertal 12 right; Cedric Jagger 34 left, 37, 51, 55 left and right, 56 top, 100, 124 right, 183 left, 233 bottom; Jurg Stuker Gallery, Berne 208; A. F. Kersting, London 67; Kunsthistorisches Museum, Vienna 90 bottom; Edward Leigh, Cambridge 198; Merseyside County Museums, Liverpool 150 right, 152; Museen der Stadt Vienna 142 left; Museum of Fine Arts, Boston 10; Museum of the History of Science, Oxford 25 left, 155 top; National Maritime Museum, London 172 top and bottom, 174 left, 177; Nederlands Goud, Zilver en Klokkenmuseum, Utrecht 60; Partridge, London 156, 157 left and right; Derek de Solla Price Yale University, Newhaven, 26; Rapho, Paris 25 right; Richmond Reference Library, London 234; Rijksmuseum voor de Geschiedenis der Natuurwetenschappen, Leiden 136; T. R. Robinson, Bristol 66 top; Science Museum, London 11, 12 left, 13 left, 22 left and right, 23 top, 62 right, 63 left, 66 bottom, 135 right, 138, 145, 176; Ronald Sheridan, London 64 left and right, 65 right; Smithsonian Institution, Washington 62 left; Spectrum, London 23 bottom, 233 top; Strike One, London 142 right, 199 top, 201 bottom; Victoria Art Gallery, Bath 149 right, Vienna Clock Museum 161 top left and top right; Wallace Collection, London 137, 139, 140 top and bottom, 141, 146; Zwinger Museum, Dresden 87 right.

The photographs on pages 123 right, 148, 158 right, 168 top and bottom are reproduced by Gracious Permission of Her Majesty the Queen.

The remaining photographs were taken for the Hamlyn Group by John Webb.

Contents

Preface

While naturally I hope that the specialist in antiquarian horology may find one or two features, at least, to interest him in this book, I have nevertheless assumed that the majority of its readers will be contemplating the subject, if not for the very first time, then certainly at a very early stage in their developing interest in it. Twenty-five years ago I found myself in precisely that situation and, by the sheerest good fortune, able for a time to indulge my taste for antique timepieces – thanks to the exceptional kindness of its original owner – with the Ilbert Collection. It seemed to me then, and I still hold to the belief, that it is supremely important to start with a solid diet of the best horological practice, both technically and artistically, and thoroughly to assimilate this before coming to grips with second or third rate work, of which there will always be an abundance in any era. It is of first importance, in other words, not to risk letting the inferior cloud one's judgement before proper standards have been established with which it can be compared.

I have therefore made no attempt – as seems customary in books of this nature – to 'spread' the illustrations over as wide a spectrum of different artisans' work as possible. On the contrary, I have deliberately allotted anything up to half a dozen illustrations to the work of one craftsman, if he happens to be a member of that select group of master horologists of the past who are household names to the initiates of the present day. From David Ramsay, first Master of the Worshipful Company of Clockmakers early in the seventeenth century, to Abraham-Louis Breguet, the French genius almost two centuries later, there are certain illustrious names that will become important to the aspiring antiquarian horologist, whether he shops for his specimens in the world's great auction rooms or its street markets, and whether or not he ever owns an example by any of them.

There is a precedent of a kind for this somewhat arbitrary approach, in that the Master, Wardens and Court of Assistants of the Worshipful Company have, by the terms of their Royal Charter, a traditional power – albeit nowadays no longer exercised – to make periodic inspections of the horological workshops within the geographical limits of the Company's responsibility, for the sole purpose of seeking out and destroying any work not attaining those standards of quality and craftsmanship which the Charter requires it to uphold. Side by side with such harsh discipline, however, the Company for almost the last two hundred years has made a practice of acquiring the best examples of the work of the craft that have come within its reach, whether these were bequeathed, donated, loaned or purchased. It has also assembled the best library that it could find over the years, and this by no means restricted to works in the English language. The original purpose both of the collection and the library was to educate members of the craft and show them, by example as well as by theoretical exposition, exactly how the practice of the very best of their contemporaries was developing. That both the collection and the library have been continuously available, except in times of national emergency, for the aesthetic and intellectual enjoyment of a much wider audience for more than a century now is due to the public-spirited attitude of the Company and the generosity of the Corporation of London, who have consistently provided suitable accommodation for the purpose adjacent to Guildhall Library; and it is a bonus without which London would be appreciably the poorer.

I have a personal debt of gratitude to the Clockmakers' Company, and this seems an appropriate place to voice it. Although I have been fascinated by old clocks and watches for many years, my formal career, all thirty-odd years of it,

6

centred upon the chemical industry. I could not believe my good fortune when, in 1972, I was offered the option of terminating that career on preferential terms and ten years in advance of normal retirement. Privately I had long held the view that a career which throughout followed the same direction was unduly restrictive of human versatility.

Two years later the Clockmakers' Company invited me to take up a part-time consultancy appointment as its Assistant Curator, specifically to look after the collection and to deal with enquiries, requests for photography, the displays, conservation and so forth. I shall always be grateful to the Company for placing such a very fulfilling occupation in my hands. It is partly as a result of having worked with the collection for more than two years now that has led me to the conclusion that it has been under-illustrated in horological books by comparison with other well-known specialist collections in the same field. To some extent I have tried to rectify this omission here.

As a result of this same appointment I have had both the pleasure and the privilege of working closely with a library staff who must rank among the most expert in the world. Guildhall Library specialises, as one would expect, in London – its history, topography, business life, inhabitants and so on. It also has custody of a number of unrelated specialist collections which have been deposited with it over the years and which are, in themselves, of substantial value and interest. The Clockmakers' Company library is but one among many. It follows that there is among the library staff a fund of knowledge on a wide spectrum of subjects, all of which they will willingly share with the multitude of researchers using the Reading Room each day. They are quite unstinting in dealing with questions ranging from the trivial to the most erudite, unfailing in their good humour and, in my own experience, quite without parallel anywhere else in the world of books. To them all, from the Librarian – who is, incidentally, my nominal Curator since he is responsible for the building, services and general staffing – to the most junior attendant, I offer my thanks for all the help I have so consistently received at their hands, and especially while compiling this book.

Although professionally engaged in the museum field for such a short time, I have for years past admired the competence and enjoyed the help, and often enough the friendship, of those in our national museums concerned with the collections relating to timekeeping. In preparing this book I have had inevitably to rely upon their close cooperation over photographs, and they have been meticulous in double-checking whenever there has been any doubt as to exactly what was required. I would particularly thank, in this connection, the staff concerned at the British Museum, the National Maritime Museum, the Science Museum, and the Victoria and Albert Museum, as well as the many helpful people in the overseas museums from which I have also drawn material for the book.

The Antiquarian Horological Society, which is devoted to the needs of students and collectors of old timekeepers, is mentioned elsewhere in this book. Here I would simply express my thanks for its permission to make use, quite freely, of its large photographic library, known as the Lloyd Collection after the late H. Alan Lloyd who assembled it. This is a wonderful horological archive.

I have tried to avoid identifying individuals by name when expressing my thanks because it is so easy to omit someone by mistake, thereby quite inadvertently giving offence. That I omit the names of private collectors is for the additional reason of security. There is a sprinkling of treasures from such sources in these pages, and I am duly grateful that I have been permitted to include them.

Finally, however, there is one person whom I can and will identify. My wife's secretarial and editorial skills, intelligently, devotedly and unstintingly applied to the manuscript of this book over a period of months have been of incalculable worth. I wish I could find words to express my gratitude.

In the Beginning

Evolution is generally associated with living creatures, and though it is not usually thought of in connection with such familiar everyday objects as clocks and watches, it is by no means a new concept. As far back as 1931 the collector and enthusiast J. Drummond Robertson wrote what has come to be regarded as a classic work, *The Evolution of Clockwork*. It broke much new ground at the time, including revelations about the principles and practice of time-measurement in Japan which underlined how very much they differed from those current in the West.

Just as evolution in nature affects not only the animals themselves but also their habitat, so in the human world it touches man's most sophisticated possessions. But while natural evolution is infinitely, laboriously, imperceptibly slow, where machines are concerned change is often almost instantaneous. It was Ralph Waldo Emerson who remarked that 'if a man . . . make a better mousetrap than his neighbour, though he build his house in the woods, the world will make a beaten path to his door.' In the case of time-measurement, certainly, innovation has usually led to fairly rapid change.

It is as well to recognise that time-measurement is both an art and a science, and for a proper understanding, it is best to appreciate them side by side. They seem so far to have passed through two main phases of development, and there are clear signs that they may be on the verge of entering a third. The first and earliest phase is still only imperfectly understood; it might be said to extend from the dimmest recesses of ancient history almost to the end of the Middle Ages. During this period, the time-measuring instruments in use were wholly non-mechanical although at some point within the same span of time some unknown genius conceived the fundamental elements of the mechanical clock. This, when it appeared, seems

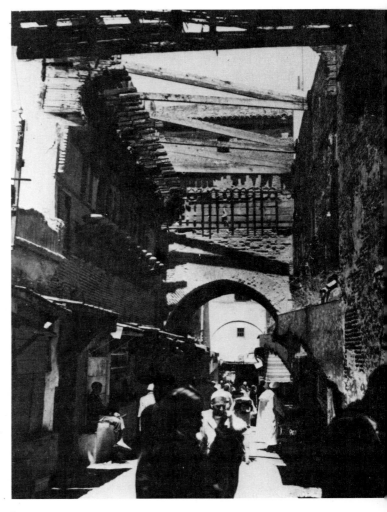

This monumental Arab water clock dates from 1357, when it was built by the Emir Abou Inane at Fez in Morocco. All that remains are the thirteen great bronze bells resting on carved wood brackets below the twelve windows through which formerly automata would have appeared. Of the mechanism nothing but part of the transmission has survived.

8

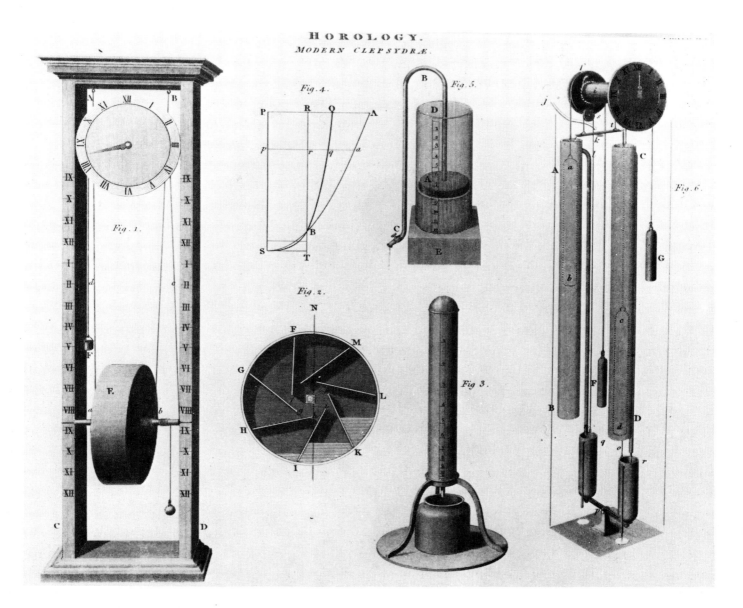

Rees's *Cyclopaedia* published in 1819–20 was the finest reference work to early nineteenth-century technology ever produced in English. This Plate from it demonstrates the continuing preoccupation up to quite recent times with the concept of the clepsydra.

to have burst upon the scene suddenly; but whether this is indeed what happened, or whether some links in the chain of events have not yet been uncovered, is still not certain.

For at least the ensuing six centuries the continuing process of invention, stimulated by evolving human needs, refined and improved the techniques of mechanical timekeeping. Most of the basic inventions in the field had been made by the end of the eighteenth century; and the peak of precision craftsmanship was certainly reached in Victorian times. As early as 1800 it was possible to acquire a pocket watch with a far greater built-in accuracy than the average modern wristwatch, and the principles of self-winding had been used in the pedometer. The ordinary domestic clock had been all but perfected a century earlier.

It may be argued that electrical horology, springing from the inventions of Alexander Bain in the 1840s, really constitutes a third phase of evolution. On the other hand, however, while electrical systems have run alongside mechanical ones for decades now, they have never superseded them. Again, in many cases electricity has been used simply as a power source to drive a pendulum or a balance, and the main transmission remains mechanical. Finally, of course, it would have been little short of miraculous if the Industrial Revolution, affecting virtually every aspect of people's lives, had not produced at least one viable alternative to the mechanical methods for regulating their day-to-day activities which had existed for so long.

The development of time-measuring methods has broadly paralleled man's own evolution. Coarser, non-mechanical means coincided with a life-style largely governed by natural phenomena – the rotation of crops and seasons, day and night, and so forth – where there can have been no particular sense of urgency or immediacy and where errors of an hour or more in twenty-four were of no

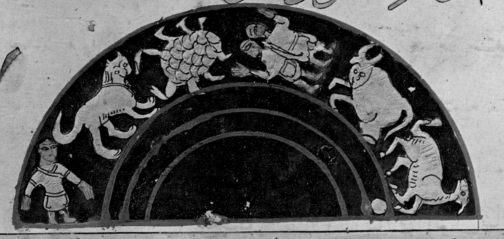

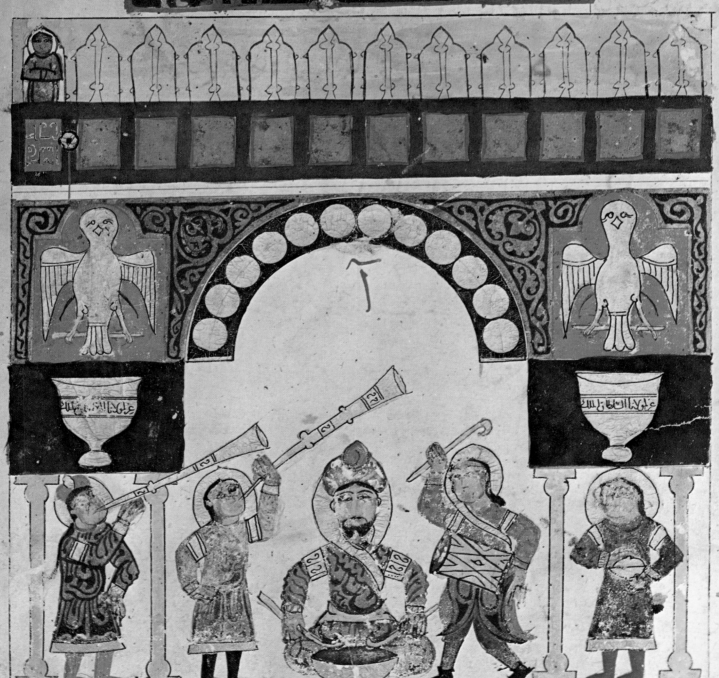

great moment. Even when mechanical systems were at last introduced, to aid the proper observance of religious offices, their initial accuracy, which was subject to then unknown forces such as friction, was not at all impressive, even though it was far better than anything that had gone before.

Necessity, it is said, is the mother of invention. As the process of civilisation gathered momentum so also did the efficiency of man's time-measuring. Two examples of this will illustrate the principle. By the beginning of the eighteenth century, losses at sea from shipwreck and other natural hazards, not to mention avoidable diseases such as scurvy, had become so great that the British Parliament was stung into offering a considerable cash prize for a solution to the problem of exact navigation. In essence the difficulty was that, to calculate with any precision a ship's position when out of sight of land, the captain had to have at his disposal a timekeeper which would function not only despite the motion of the vessel – and technically this was not then possible – but also with predictable accuracy, maintaining its performance throughout what, in those days, might well be a lengthy voyage. It took half a century to find answers to the complex questions this provoked; but it gave Britain a lead in chronometry which, when based on mechanical systems, has never been surpassed.

For a second example, it is only necessary to turn, once again, to the Industrial Revolution. The advent of railways in Britain rendered obsolete, almost overnight, the grid of local times throughout the country which had sufficed during the coaching era. Occupancy of the permanent way in accordance with pre-published timetables, and the absolute necessity of avoiding accidents caused by misplaced trains, enforced upon the country a universal time system, as well as the means to measure it accurately. Also, the industrialisation of a hitherto agricultural work-force, more or less at the farmer's beck and call at any hour and governed only by the needs of crop or livestock, brought in its wake the concept of hours of work at the office or factory, and the need to arrive and depart to time. There was also, of course, a resulting rise in the wealth and independence of the worker, and this certainly provided much of the impetus towards mass-production, not least of clocks and watches. Where previously it was necessary to be fairly well-to-do to possess a clock, let alone a watch, such gradually became essentials and within the reach of all.

So we come to the present century, now in its final quarter. Mechanical time-measurement is still generally preferred, but for how much longer?

Arabian water clocks, like this medieval example by Al-Jazari, not only told the time but were entertaining on account of their theatrical complications and complex automata. Museum of Fine Arts, Boston.

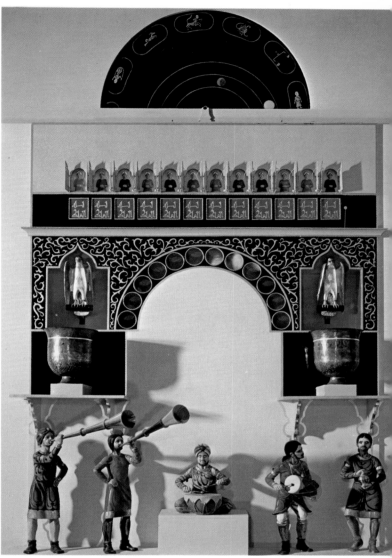

This working reconstruction by P. N. Haward, D. R. Hill and C. Melling demonstrates clearly that complicated feats of hydraulic engineering – of which usually only remnants of the originals survive – were nonetheless thoroughly feasible. Science Museum, London.

The system is by no means perfect – not, certainly, in its everyday manifestations – so that error is still measured in seconds per day for the average clock or watch. Yet the techniques involved have probably reached their peak of perfection, certainly in economic terms. To make further demonstrable improvements in mechanical time-measurement would be so costly as to nullify the effort involved, since any resulting instruments would certainly be beyond the reach of the great mass of consumers. What happens next?

The twentieth-century equivalent of the earlier Industrial Revolution may well appear, when assessed by future historians, to be the enormous investment, mainly by the United States and the Soviet Union but also, in a smaller way, by many other nations, in aerospace research and exploration. Present indications are that, in the course of

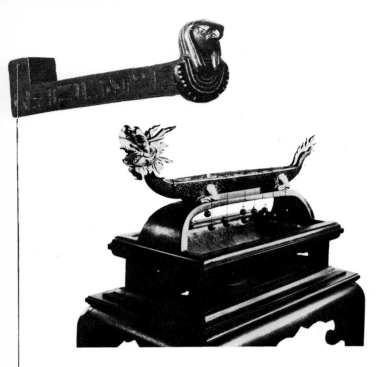

The 'merkhet' (*top*) enabled early Egyptians to tell the time at night, and was also used in surveying. This example has an inscription attributing its ownership to Bes, who was an astronomer priest in Upper Egypt about 600 BC. It is of bronze inlaid with a gold-silver alloy. Science Museum, London.

above
'Destructive' timekeepers depending on the consumption of one or another commodity are found in a number of countries, and this Chinese dragon vessel measures the time passing by burning incense. The Japanese had a timekeeper working on the same principle but of different design. Historisches Uhren-Museum, Wuppertal.

time, it will bring as many beneficial changes in its wake, as a direct 'spin-off' from the highly specialised technologies developed over a wide range of fields, as did its predecessor. One of these, and invaluable in its original context, has been the extremely accurate guidance systems springing from succeeding generations of ever more sophisticated computers and, of course, from the ancillary time-measuring equipment. In all of these the basis has been electronics.

Electronic timekeepers for domestic use have been on the market for about a decade now, and manufacturers continue to develop newer and more attractive modules as each year passes. Consumers are rapidly becoming accustomed to the very functional illuminated display which is a recent feature of such equipment – the same applies to the pocket calculator, for instance – and there is much to be said for the direct readings thus obtained, by contrast with the need to interpret two hands against a dial whose legibility can vary greatly from one style to another, not to mention the problem of reading it in the dark.

But possibly the principal factor to be taken into consideration, as always, is the economic one. The manufacture of mechanical timekeepers is a labour-intensive industry; that of electronic timekeepers is not, or at least not to anything like the same extent. While there may remain, for a very few with both the money and the inclination, a top-price market for the best in mechanical timekeepers, it would be strange indeed if we were not at this moment witnessing the start of a third phase in the evolution of time-measuring systems, based on electronics, and a true system in the sense that it will completely supplant its predecessors.

The old adage that 'beauty is in the eye of the beholder' is nowhere more clearly demonstrated than among those enthusiasts who collect the instruments of time-measurement – and especially among those who have narrowed their enthusiasm to some small corner of what is indeed a wide field. It probably was not always so. While it was still possible, three or four decades ago, to acquire a fine seventeenth-century longcase clock for a modest outlay, it is inconceivable that anyone could have preferred, say, one of the early manifestations of mass-production. Now, of course, the most beautiful pieces judged by any conventional standard have priced themselves out of reach of any but the really rich; and today's enthusiasts have perforce to confer the accolade of beauty on what are often some of the ugliest machines imaginable. They do it with great gusto!

This is just one of the considerations that needs to be taken into account in trying to arrive at a definition of what constitutes a 'great' clock or watch. There are all sorts of standards which may be applied. Domestic clocks, for example, have always tended to follow, or at least to merge happily with, contemporary furniture design which in its turn, often enough, has clear associations with the architectural fashions of the period. It must follow then that the finest architectural periods have inevitably given rise to the best clocks; but is the reverse also true? The reader may contemplate, perhaps, the present-day enthusiasm for Art Nouveau and Art Deco in arriving at a conclusion.

Again there are those who insist that beauty and greatness together can be found in mechanical design – for example, in the relationships of the numbers of teeth on wheels and the leaves of pinions with which they engage; in the way wheels are 'crossed out', i.e. the care with which the spokes have been cut as well as their number; in the symmetry with which a clock or watch movement has been laid out and its various elements 'planted', i.e. positioned. There are many criteria which can be brought into play when judging clocks and watches from this viewpoint; the enthusiast-mechanic will extol the 'proportions' of, say, an escapement with all the verve and spirit of an admirer of classical sculpture.

So it is probably important for anybody taking an active acquisitive interest in time-measuring paraphernalia to decide for themselves, before get-

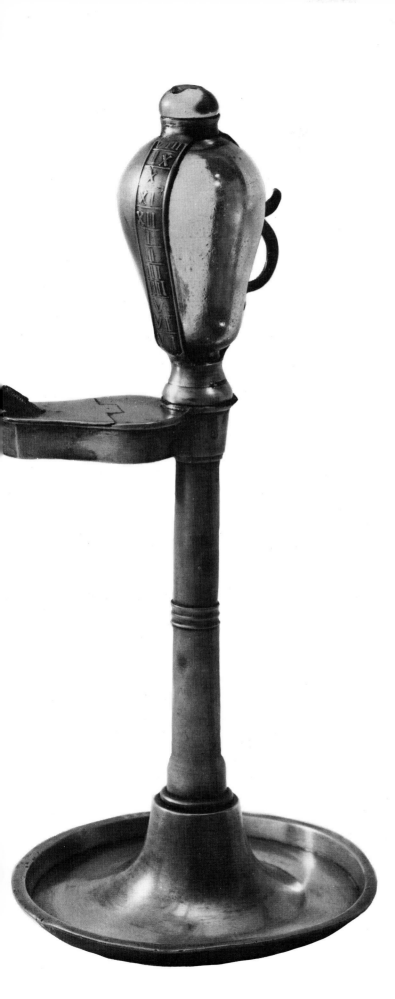

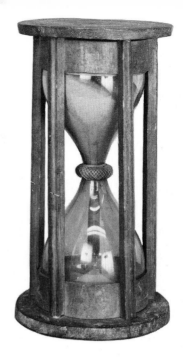

Sand glasses came in all sizes. Standing over thirteen inches high, this one measures a period of four hours, and was probably made in France before 1750 for use at sea. The frame is oak. Museum of the Worshipful Company of Clockmakers, Guildhall, London.

Another form of 'destructive' timekeeper, this eighteenth-century pewter oil clock from north Germany incorporates a glass reservoir equally graduated in hours from 8 p.m. to 7 a.m., the level of unburnt oil indicating the time. Such clocks, useful though they may have been at night, could hardly have been other than inaccurate, in view of the irregular shape of the reservoir. Science Museum, London.

ting too immersed in the study, the particular keystone of taste with which they are in sympathy, always accepting, of course, that their tastes will change over the years. This is inevitable since there are no hard-and-fast standards; but at least it is not without purpose to decide upon some such propositions as 'the Vienna Regulator of the late nineteenth century is the finest clock ever made' – or not, as the case may be – if only in order to set one's personal parameters, against which those objects that will be encountered in the course of pursuing the subject may be measured.

Earlier, the concept of evolution was considered in relation to living things and to the inanimate objects associated with them. There are also, of course, evolutionary tendencies in ideas, and, not least, in ideas about taste. The definition of the word 'great' as it appears in the title of this book, therefore, may be taken to be more relative to those particular developments in practical horology that have influenced subsequent mechanical and stylistic trends than to any catalogue of individual masterpieces which might, under one heading or another, qualify for that same overworked adjective. If in so doing, the book helps the reader to arrive at a personal, as well as satisfying,

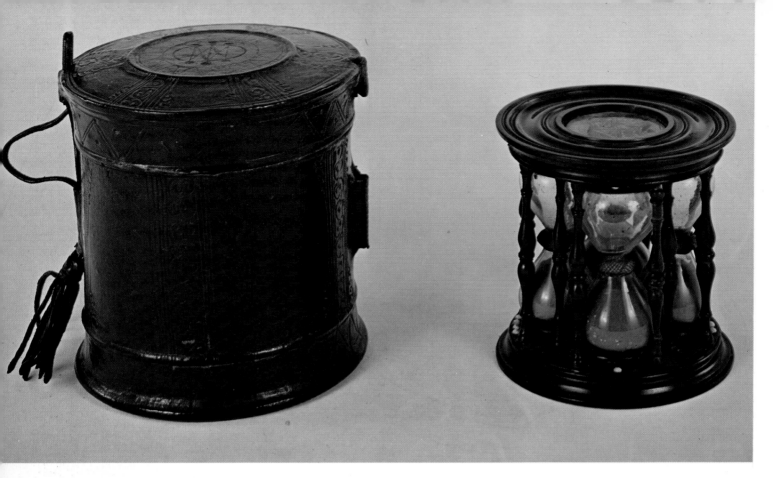

determination of the meaning of 'great' in the context of horology, then its principal purpose will have been fulfilled.

There can be little doubt that the pace of modern civilisation continues to accelerate. As good an example of this as one could wish for is to be found in the realisation that, until not much more than two centuries ago, the clock was by far the most sophisticated machine invented by man. His achievements in technology during that period have been immense and, if you broaden the perspective – simply in the field of time-measurement – to encompass the dawn of civilisation, little short of miraculous.

But how did it all start? Life on this planet has always revolved round repetitive sequences of events based entirely upon natural phenomena by which, in a rough and ready manner, time can be measured. Admittedly the units were large: twelve hours (and subject to considerable variation) in the case of day and night, much longer if you consider the passage of the seasons (as well as much more liable to inaccuracy on the grand scale). The human stomach requires to be fuelled at relatively shorter intervals and must certainly have been used by primitive man as a rough and ready guide; it is in any case a more feasible, not to say reliable, method.

Nevertheless all this is reasoned supposition; supporting evidence is hard to find. The situation does not greatly improve when we move on from the earliest manifestations of civilisation – when, apart from the needs of agriculture and the

impulse of superstition, there was really little necessity to mark events in time anyway – to some point, probably centuries later, when man's innate intelligence enabled him to conceive of more artificial but, at the same time, more consistent methods of measuring off time. There is no clear-cut starting-point for the introduction of such techniques and certainly no finishing point; indeed, in some cases – for example, sundials and sand glasses – it is easy to find examples of their usage right to the present time, if only, in the latter instance, to boil the breakfast egg. This blurring of the edges between one style and another, between any particular type of time-measuring instrument and another, in general between the entry and exit of any stylistic or technical innovation, is typical of the whole history of horology. Thus at a much later period it is not uncommon to find an interval of several decades before the best usage of a metropolitan centre of clockmaking drawing upon a rich clientèle or substantial patronage, filtered down to the individual craftsmen working in the provinces of the same country. Certainly so far as man's first attempts to construct and use time-measuring apparatus are concerned, it is well-nigh impossible to encompass them within any chronological parameters.

If man was capable of utilising the regular recurrence of sunrise and sunset as a makeshift clock, then it can only have been a matter of course before he refined, by observation, his employment of the motions of heavenly bodies for timekeeping. The single most important instrument originating

left
Mary Queen of Scots' sand glass is probably the most famous instrument of its kind in the world. It is described on page 18. British Museum, London.

right
Portable sundials come in a variety of attractive designs, one of the less common being a cube with faces on all five exposed sides. National Maritime Museum, Greenwich.

below right
Michael Butterfield, who worked in Paris during the last quarter of the seventeenth century, designed a form of pocket dial which was much copied by other makers and is always described by his name. The adjustable gnomon carries a scale which is read against the bird's beak and must be set to the latitude of the place where the dial is being used. The back of a Butterfield dial always carries a list of principal cities with their relevant latitudes. National Maritime Museum, Greenwich.

below
Back of the Butterfield dial.

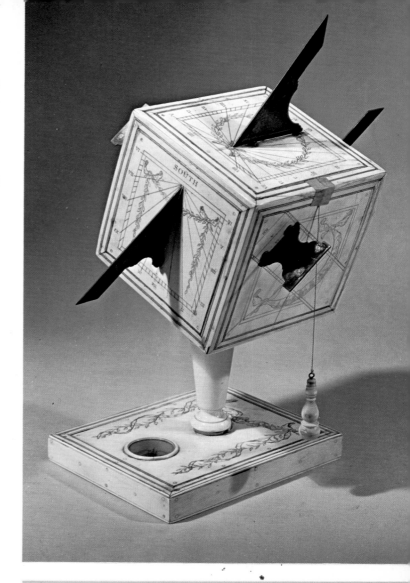

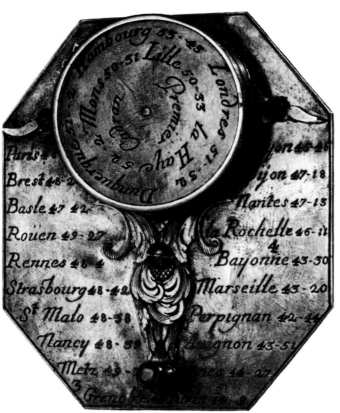

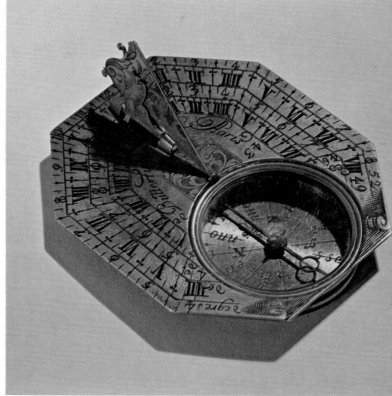

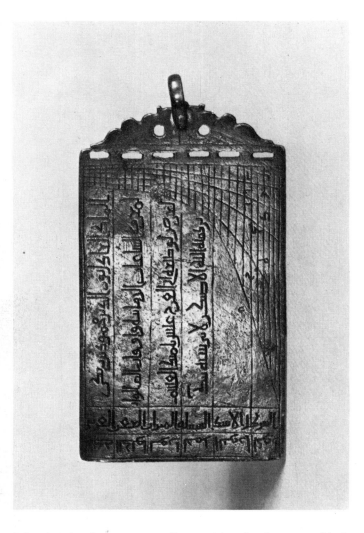

Islamic scientists are generally considered to have provided the link in scholarship between the classical and medieval worlds. In Islam, the sundial aided Muslims not only in determining times for prayer, but also in finding the direction of the Holy City of Mecca which must be faced at such times. This earliest known portable Islamic sundial is dated 1159 AD. Bibliothèque Nationale, Paris.

from this development was, of course, the sundial; but it may be helpful first to mention other forms of apparatus for marking the passage of time which were neither so long-lasting nor so scientifically well founded, even though they were still in use long after the introduction of this most important of the non-mechanical timekeepers.

The rate at which a flame will burn down a candle or smoulder along a knotted rope can obviously be related to the passage of time. Techniques like this – so called 'destructive' timekeepers – certainly existed in the orient, and there are quite elaborate examples from China, often based on the rate of consumption of joss sticks or incense. In one arrangement, the Chinese 'dragon boat', this system can even be made to sound an alarm at predetermined intervals. At a later period, lamps burning oil from a graduated glass reservoir became fashionable.

Equally ingenious was man's utilisation of fire's opposing element – water. The water clock – called by the Greeks the clepsydra, and sometimes known by this name in other countries – occurs in several versions based either on the concept that water can escape at a predetermined rate from a perforated container, or that a similar container, placed upon the surface of a body of water, will fill up at a predetermined rate and eventually sink. Elaborated versions of these principles, enabling time to be read off by a moving pointer against a dial, or by such means as the sounding of gongs, are also on record. Water clocks probably first appeared in Egypt, from where they were introduced into Greece and used extensively during the times of the Greek and Roman Empires; and there are quite a number of references to them in classical literature.

In considering clepsydrae, however, a few cautionary words are not out of context. Nobody would be so foolish as to dispute their existence in antiquity, but no less an authority than Courtenay Ilbert – the world's leading collector of clocks, watches and the like until his death in 1956, when his enormous collection was acquired by the British Museum – used to say that, throughout a lifetime of collecting his treasures all over the world, he was never offered a water clock of whose genuineness he was convinced. It is also a fact that for years a firm in Birmingham was quite openly manufacturing 'water clocks', each bearing a spurious date, and catalogued by the maker as reproductions, but that subsequently these have not infrequently been passed off as genuine by unscrupulous antique dealers. Even if a genuine clepsydra was encountered, it might not be recognised by the uninitiated. There is, for example, one in the collection belonging to the Worshipful Company of Clockmakers, of London, which is simply an unmarked copper bowl with a small hole in the base. The all-revealing detail is that this tiny hole is bushed in gold, to prevent the water acting upon the copper so as eventually to restrict the inflow. The bowl comes from Ceylon, and in use was certainly floated upon a surface of water, into which it sinks after about twenty-five minutes. It is impossible to date on the basis of presentday knowledge.

Another 'elemental' device which measured flow – in this case, of sand – probably arrived on the scene rather later than the water clock, but survives in use to this day. Sand glasses – sometimes called hour glasses, but incorrectly, because they can be constructed to measure any interval of time – were used in the Royal Navy to time the duty watch right up to 1839, as well as in the House of Commons to time divisions. The 'sermon glass' in church was used by preachers in the sixteenth century and later, and there still exist sets of glasses – usually four in number, all in one frame –

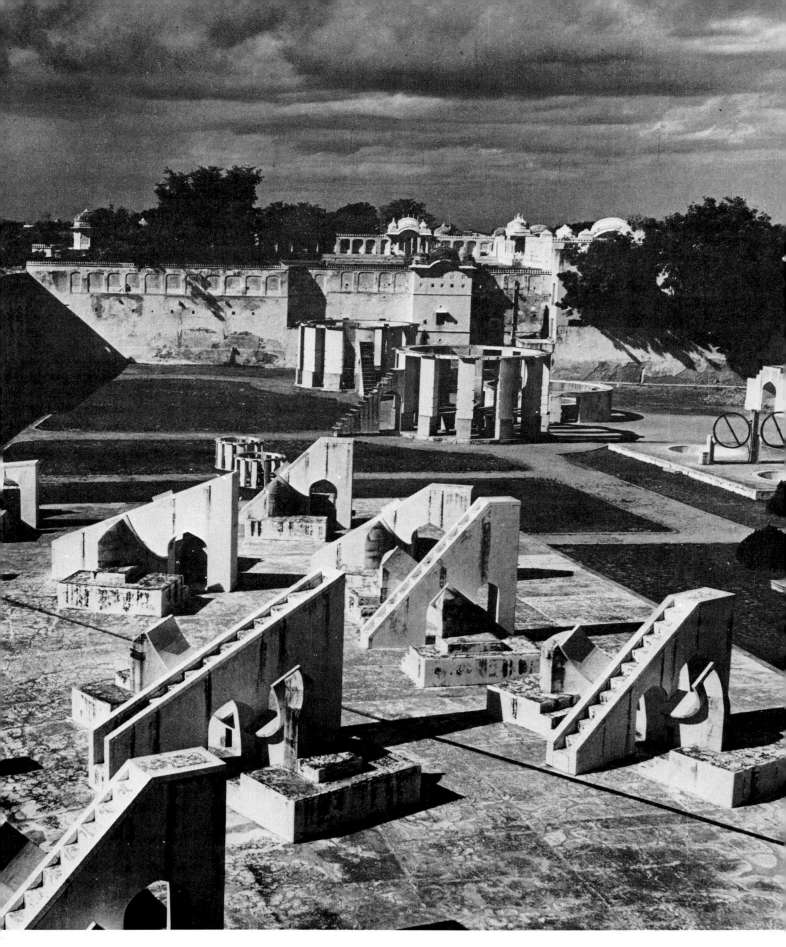

A general view of the astronomical observatory at Jaipur
constructed by the Maharaja Sawai Jai Singh II
(1686–1743).

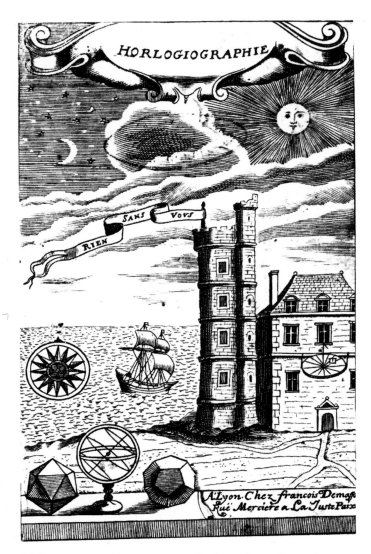

This seventeenth-century treatise by a French monk went through five editions between 1641 and 1701, and treated the subject of dialling with considerable erudition.

each measuring a different interval, sometimes compounds of fifteen minutes, which must have had numerous domestic uses.

Of this latter version there exists a particularly elegant example in the same Ilbert Collection in the British Museum to which reference has already been made. The four glasses are arranged between circular ebony plates with moulded borders, separated by turned baluster pillars, the whole contained within a cylindrical leather case with cover. The top and base have recessed panels painted with the arms of Scotland and France. Ilbert purchased this beautiful object unseen: it had been hidden for years in a jeweller's safe that was bombed during the Second World War, and for the contents of which he offered a lump sum. At the time, the significance of the very individual monogram – 'M' for Mary entwined with the Greek 'φ' or 'phi', representing King Francis II of France, the Queen's first husband – escaped him, and it was not until some months later that he woke in the early hours of the morning, suddenly

recollecting where he had seen the same monogram previously. Waiting only to put on his dressing gown, it is said, he stumbled out of his house, found a taxi and drove straight to the private home of a very celebrated museum director, whom he unceremoniously awoke. They both then, taking the waiting taxi, drove to the museum, to which they managed to obtain access. Their researches there, at about 3 a.m., are said to have confirmed the provenance of the sand glass. The monogram, in fact, appears on a small cannon, reputedly the property of the Scottish Queen.

The contrivances which have so far been described, at least in their most sophisticated forms, appear to have been current in those parts of the world which we now call the Near and Middle East, and in China. The Egyptians certainly were most advanced in such matters – there is even a hieroglyph which is believed to represent a water clock – while the Christian world was largely starved of such useful appliances except in their most simple form. They were reputedly current during a total span of some two thousand years – excluding freak survivals to the present time such as the sand glass egg-timer, of course!

Of the more scientifically based non-mechanical timekeepers, however, rather more information is available. It is reasonable to suppose that, certainly in all those areas mentioned above where sunshine is a fairly continuous feature of the climate, it cannot have been long after the dawn of civilisation that the movement of cast shadows – of trees, perhaps – was noticed. Trees, however, were not always sited in the most convenient locations, so that it was probably necessary at first to erect poles in public places, where the movements of their shadows across the ground could indicate to all concerned the passage of the daylight hours. These in turn were replaced by large stone 'needles' or obelisks, of which plenty of examples remain. There are something like twenty of these in Rome, carried there by the early Emperors; one in Paris, which came originally from Luxor; and the famous Cleopatra's Needle, which was first erected at Heliopolis, outside Cairo, in 1500 BC, removed to Alexandria in 23 BC, and finally brought to London in 1878. It weighs 166 tons, stands 70 feet high, and is otherwise celebrated for the great variety of its Egyptian inscriptions, in one of which, for the first known time, is found the phrase 'King of Kings'. It was, incidentally, one of a pair of such obelisks, of which the other was erected in Central Park, New York, in 1881.

The first documentary reference to a sundial would appear to be in chapter twenty of the Second Book of Kings, where Isaiah the prophet miraculously retarded the shadow of the sun by ten degrees or steps. This particular dial belonged to King Ahaz and may well have been of the monumental kind; fine examples of this sort from the

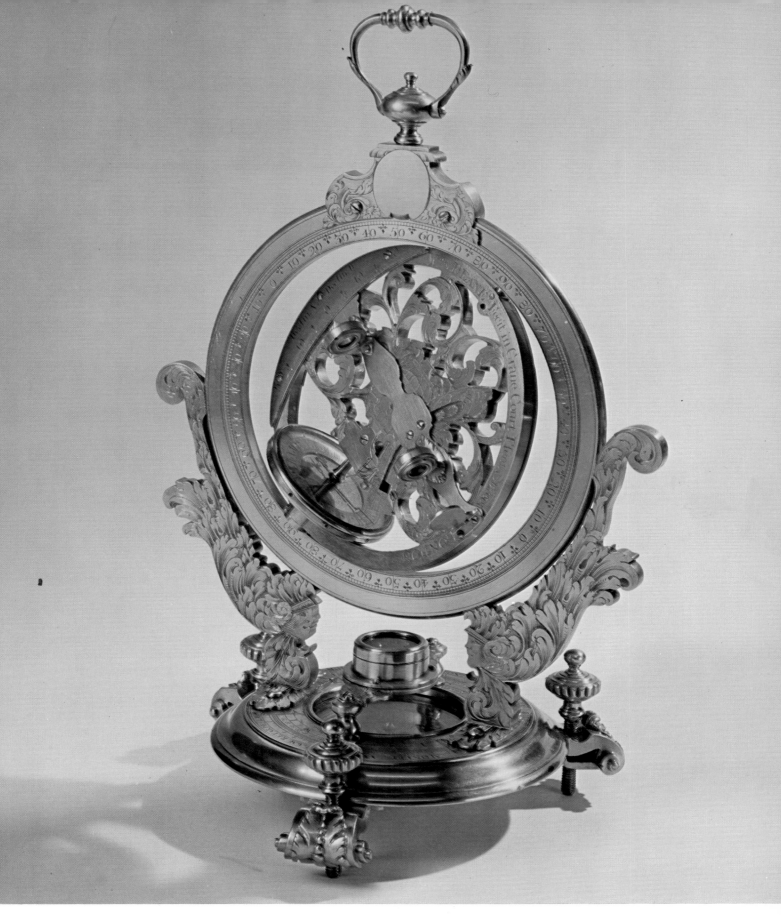

This magnificent equinoctial ('equal hours') dial was made by William Dean of London about 1690. A number of different craft skills have been combined to make this both a scientific instrument and a work of art. National Maritime Museum, Greenwich.

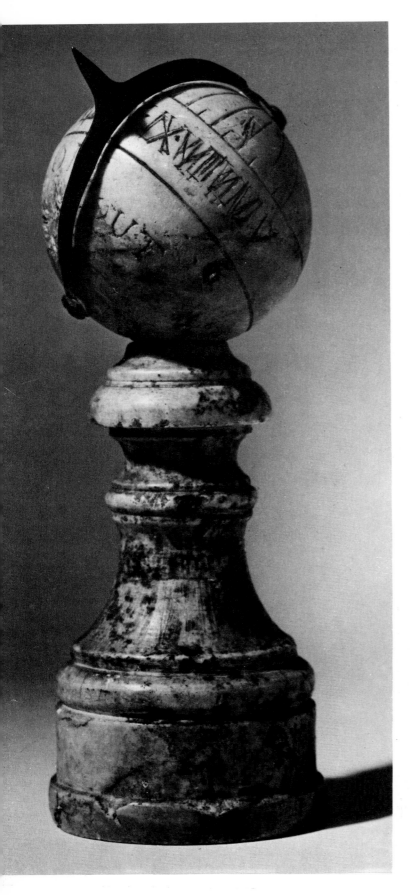

The seventeenth and eighteenth centuries saw the design of sundials reach a peak. This spherical dial of French origin was made in 1767. National Maritime Museum, Greenwich.

early Islamic observatories in Persia still exist, in which the shadow of a wall or similar projecting object falls upon an ascending flight of steps.

Ruins of other massive sundials are scattered throughout a number of countries. In Britain, the rings of megalithic stones on Salisbury Plain, known as Stonehenge, fall into this category; estimates of their age suggest about 2000 BC. At Jaipur, in India, some vast curved stones serve a similar purpose; the Aztecs in Peru constructed rock pillars as their sun clocks. Such instruments were, of course, the equivalent of public clocks or for the use of astronomers; personal sundials, as used in India and Tibet, were in the form of a simple time-stick with a peg inserted in it at right-angles. The side of the stick was calibrated, and the shadow of the peg falling upon these gradations gave a reading of the time.

Clearly the sundial could only be used by day, but other systems, particularly the clepsydra, were available for night use. In addition, however, the Egyptians had the merkhet, which was in essence a plumb-line; its use was to observe the transit of known fixed stars across the meridian. At later periods various types of 'nocturnals' were designed, often being built into a compendium with a conventional sundial, for portable use.

Sundials come in an enormous variety of designs: cubes on a carved stand, with each of the five available faces showing a different time system; so-called diptych or tablet dials, which open like books; dials with built-in compasses to ensure that they were set up on the correct bearing, facing south, and plumb-bobs to verify their level. There were also, of course, horizontal dials on baluster pillars for public use, as well as vertical dials often set upon church walls.

In use, the only snag with such a seemingly simple and efficient tool as the sundial, is that day and night are not the same length all the year round, certainly in northern Europe where winter nights can be twice as long as those in summer. In the Mediterranean basin, though, the variation is very much smaller, so that for the early civilisations in that region such an instrument was certainly a practical proposition.

The problem, whether it be more or less acute, can be resolved into two parts: how to divide into convenient quantities the periods of day and night, remembering that except at the equinoxes (Lat., 'equal nights') these vary in length; and, having done that, how to compensate for such variables on a sundial.

A lunar month of thirty days, adapted to a solar year of 365 days to suit their religious celebrations, was in use more than 3,000 years ago by the Egyptians, although probably not originated by them. An even older system, adopted by the ancient Sumerians, divided the period between one sunset and the next into twelve, and each of these 'hours'

Another common form of sundial in the eighteenth century was the folding ring dial. In addition to finding solar time, such dials generally had a subsidiary use of obtaining the altitude of the sun. Musées Royaux d'Art et d'Histoire, Brussels.

below
The nocturnal dial was intended to show the hours during the night by observing the position of the Pole star in relation to certain other stars. This fine specimen, although unsigned, can be dated from other evidence as about 1582, and is possibly French. Musées Royaux d'Art et d'Histoire, Brussels.

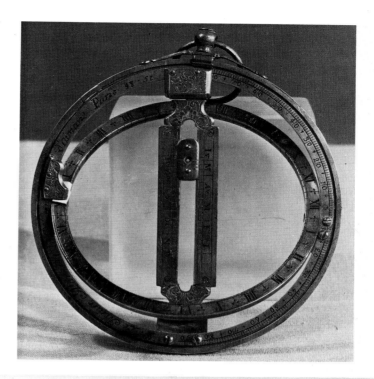

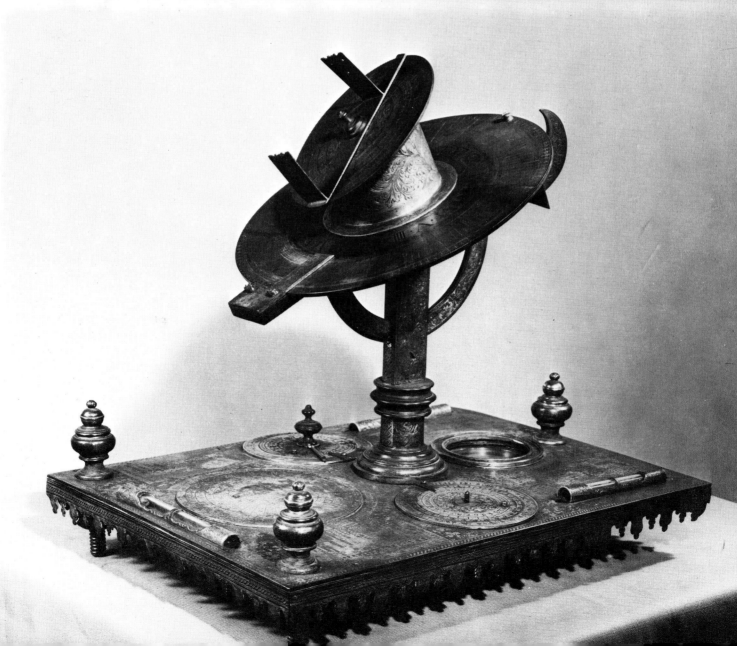

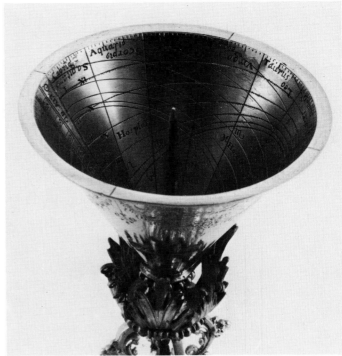

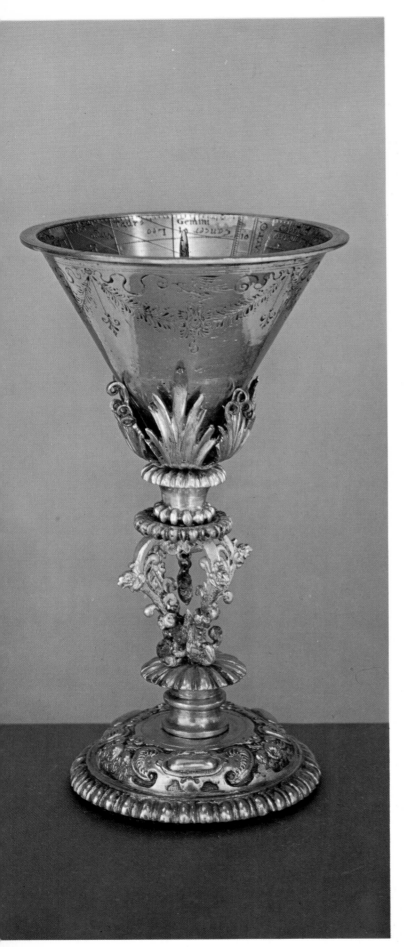

left and above
A beautiful silver gilt chalice sundial dated 1596, this
example was probably made either in Italy or southern
Germany. It is designed for use on the latitude of Rome and
shows the time in Italian hours. The gnomon extends
vertically from the bottom of the cup around which are
engraved appropriate time scales. It is upon these that the
shadow of the gnomon is cast by the sun. Science Museum,
London.

was subdivided into thirty. This system seems to
have found its way across to China and thence to
Japan, where time was reckoned on a similar basis.
Why it should have been determined to assign
twelve 'hours' to a day is not known, although it
has been suggested that there was thought to be a
magical significance in that number. The concept
of twenty-four equal hours – i.e. two periods of
twelve, for day and night – did not enter into
common use until the beginning of the fourteenth
century; and it is interesting to note that there is no
exact term in the English language to differentiate
a daylight from a night-time hour, nor any separate term to denote a complete twenty-four hour
period. It also is simply a 'day'.

Before leaving the pre-mechanical era, there is
one other scientific instrument that should be mentioned – the astrolabe. In its simplest form it was
an altitude dial, consisting of a round engraved
plate with a sighting bar pivoted at the centre to
measure the sun's altitude and thus calculate the
time. As such, its provenance dates back to Greece,

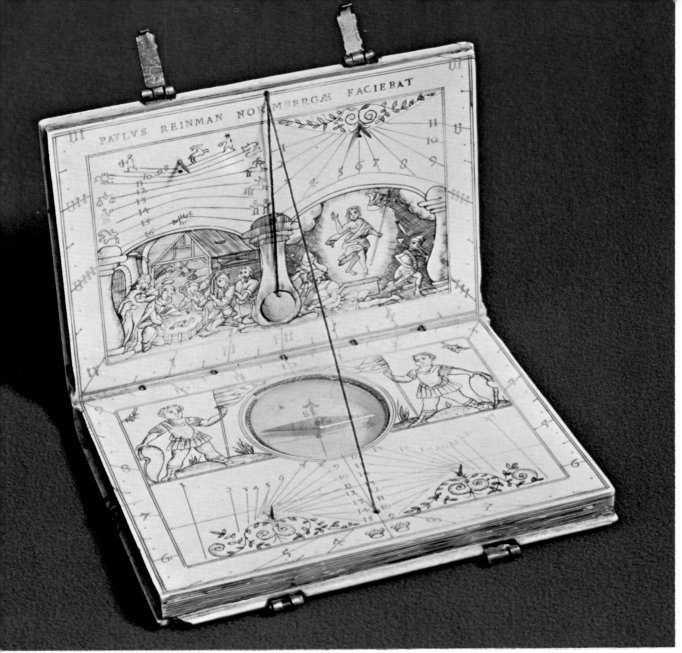

Diptych or tablet sundials were generally made of ivory although examples are known in gilt brass and other materials. This one by Paul Reinman of Nuremberg was made in 1599 and, when closed, is in the form of a book. Tablet dials were a particularly popular design over a long period in the sixteenth and seventeenth centuries. Science Museum, London.

The commonest type of astrolabe – a scientific compendium used for determining the time by day or night, for fixing the times when Muslims must pray, for elementary surveying and navigation and for teaching astronomy – is called 'planispheric' because it functions on a flat surface as opposed to a spherical one.

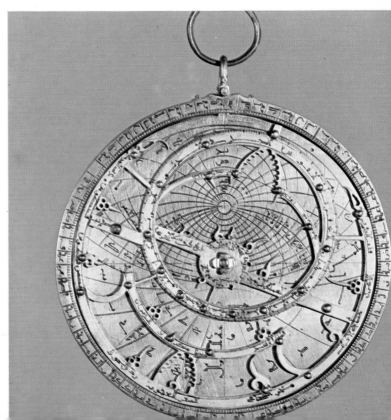

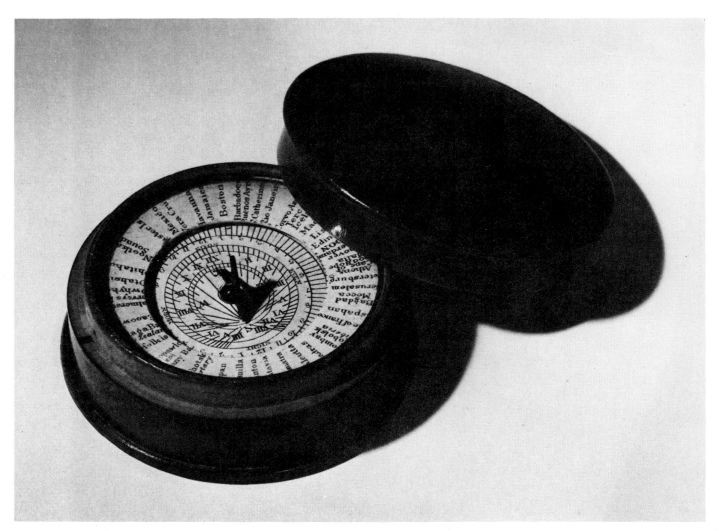

Sundials have remained sources of fascination and interest into modern times. A so-called 'Patent Pantochronometer', this pocket device, according to instructions printed on the bottom, gives a reading of the time, not only where it is used, but also in a range of principal cities throughout the world, and can also be used as a compass. Internal evidence points to its having been made for use in Australia, probably at the turn of the nineteenth century.

somewhere about 150 BC. Also pivoting upon the disc was a star map which, when rotated, reproduced the appearance of the sky at any moment, past, present or future. From this could be deduced the rising or setting of a star, the length of day or night, the time of ritual prayers, as in Islamic practice, and it even performed certain functions related to predictions by astrology, to which, formerly, so many cultures subscribed. The astrolabe has been described as combining all other astronomical instruments in one; certainly it has had a long history, for the earliest surviving specimens are Islamic, of the late ninth century. It first came to Christian Europe about two centuries later. In the seventeenth century it was improved for more accurate navigational use at sea. Astrolabes were in use in the mosques of Morocco within the last fifty years; and to this day there is still one workshop in Isfahan which manufactures them.

The sundial also, of course, survived as a very functional tool long after the appearance of the mechanical timekeeper. The earliest mechanisms were so very haphazard in their performance that the easiest – indeed the only – means of keeping a check on them was to compare their readings with those obtained with a sundial. The latter, of course, only displayed solar time, and a conversion factor had to be applied to such readings in order to calculate mean time such as should be shown on a clock or watch. The calculation was described as the Equation of Time, and tables giving the appropriate conversion according to the time of year were produced, in particular in the seventeenth and eighteenth centuries when pocket sundials in a variety of attractive designs, and principally intended for checking clocks and watches, were produced in quantity. Several of the makers of these became famous in their own right, notably such French craftsmen as Michael Butterfield and Nicholas Bion in Paris, and Charles Bloud in Dieppe, while in Germany there was Johann Willebrand of Augsburg and a number of others. Such dials were often sufficiently sophisticated as to have a gnomon – the projection whose shadow falls on the calibrated dial plate – that could be adjusted, so that the angle it formed with the plate could be made to conform with the latitude of the locality where the dial was being used; they also had several concentric time scales, each relating to a different span of latitudes. This was essential in order to obtain a correct reading, and the reverse of such dials often is inscribed with a list of capital cities and their latitudes. Where a sundial is fitted with a fixed gnomon, it can only be used in places on the one latitude to which it is matched.

The Islamic concept of the astrolabe requires it to be both a scientific instrument and a work of art. Although in Western eyes this remarkable combination instrument – really a form of early computer – has long since been superseded, a few astrolabists continue to this day to pursue their ancient craft.

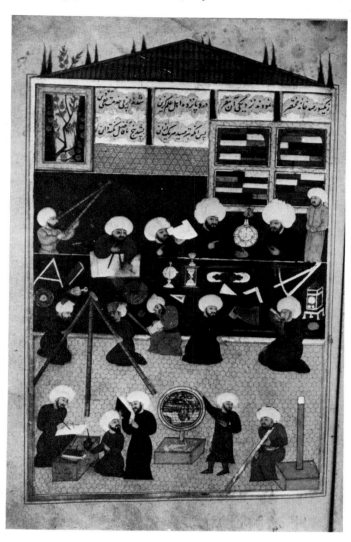

Made of brass with damascening and laminated silver, this Eastern Islamic spherical astrolabe, a great rarity, is signed 'Work of Musa, year 885'. This corresponds to AD 1480. Museum of the History of Science, Oxford.

25

The Rudiments of Clockwork

For the amateur, even if only a dilettante, some knowledge and appreciation of the mechanics of clocks and watches is necessary, not only because it helps to round out data obtained about, say, the historical and decorative aspects but, even more essentially, because it will enable him to communicate much more fully with others of like tastes. Nobody who is active in this field can afford to be so narrowly specialised as to ignore completely any of the complementary disciplines of which it is comprised.

Having said that, the importance which he attaches to his technical knowledge and the extent to which he cultivates it are matters entirely for his own judgement and will largely result from his particular tastes, inclinations and experience. Let it be said straight away that there is nothing so obscure and abstruse about the subject as to render it impossible for even the most unmechanically minded to grasp sufficient of the essentials for all ordinary purposes. The purpose of this chapter will therefore be to explain, in simple terms and avoiding as far as possible the 'private language' of the technologist, the systems of clock- and watch-work which are most likely to be encountered and the salient features by which they can be recognised. The most important developments and inventions over the centuries will be pointed out, and fundamental principles explained. Anything more than this, however, is clearly beyond the scope of this book, and if the reader intends, for instance, to practise as a restorer of antique mechanisms he will need very much more practical information. He is therefore referred to the 'Further Reading' list (page 254); and he is also advised to seek first-hand practical training either by apprenticeship or, if this is inappropriate, by means of a course of instruction. Some information in this regard will be found on page 254, where organisations that cater for both modern industry and the antiquarian horologist are described.

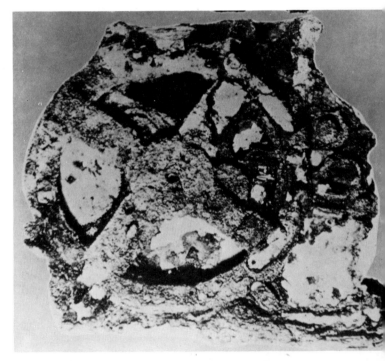

The corroded, almost fossilised, fragments of what is believed to have been some kind of planetary machine were found among the remnants of a treasure ship which sank off the coast of Antikythera in AD 250 (see page 27).

opposite page, left
This plate from Rees's *Cyclopaedia* of 1820 illustrates the principle of the thirty-hour 'endless line' weight-driven clock. Winding the large driving weight is accomplished by pulling on the loop carrying the small counterpoise ring.

opposite page, right
Rees's *Cyclopaedia* contains an admirable diagram of the layout of a common two-train spring-driven clock. The left-hand (striking) train shows the spring coiled in its spring barrel – the cover being momentarily removed – while the assembled driving gear can be seen on the right-hand (going) train.

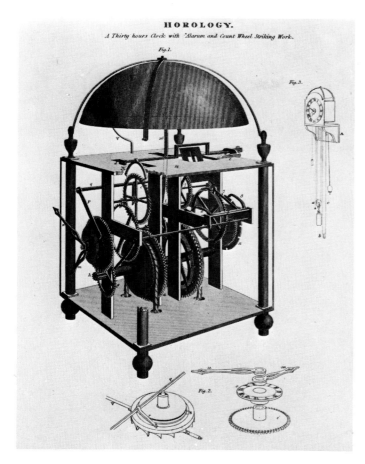

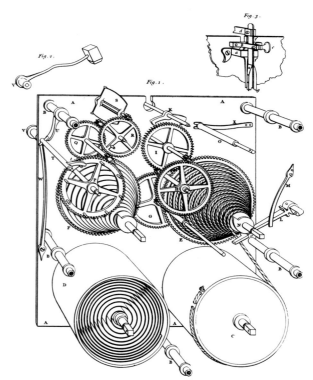

The next chapter describes what little is known – and it is very little indeed – about the birth of the clock, and here it is simply necessary to point out that primitive machinery involving the meshing together of toothed wheels existed long before the clock came upon the scene. Hero of Alexandria, who lived during the first century AD although his exact dates have not been ascertained, describes two examples of the use of wooden wheels with widely spaced teeth, but in a context which suggests that even in his lifetime this was nothing new; so it is quite conceivable that such devices extended back to the birth of Christ. There is also some material evidence of much more recent discovery. Seventy-five years ago there was salvaged from a Greek treasure-ship, thought to have sunk off the island of Antikythera about 250 AD, the remains of a machine which consisted of metal wheels having finely cut teeth which meshed with one another to form a kind of gearing. From considerations of the mechanics of the machine, so far as the remaining fragments reveal them, and also of the inscriptions, of which there are some traces, it seems most probable that in its original state the device was some kind of manually operated planetarium which was used to illustrate the motions of certain heavenly bodies.

When one is examining such archaeological remains, how can one be so certain that they were not once part of a clock? The answer is that early clock mechanisms have one element peculiar to themselves alone, which does not figure in any kind of machinery that is not devoted wholly or partially to measuring intervals of time. This single element is the escapement, which is dealt with in some detail on page 34; suffice it to say at this point that unless there is clear evidence of the existence of an escapement, even if no longer *in situ*, then there is a strong presumption that a machine is not a clock.

Like any other machine, a clock or watch needs stored up energy – a power source – to drive it, and when we wind up our longcase clock once a week or our wristwatch every day, we are simply regenerating this supply. The use of a particular power source is governed by the type and size of timekeeper concerned, its age, the purpose for which it was designed and similar considerations.

Everybody has encountered a clock driven by a falling weight which is periodically hauled up again, either as a result of being wound up with a key fitting on to a winding 'square' which can be seen through a hole in the clock dial, or, especially with clocks of thirty-hours 'duration of going', by pulling directly upon the 'line' hanging down inside the clock case. In the latter instance, the clock weight is simply threaded on an endless rope or chain, a loop, in fact; this loop passes through the clock movement and hangs down below it on either side, the driving side containing the main weight on its pulley, the slack side simply held reasonably taut with a small counterpoise, either

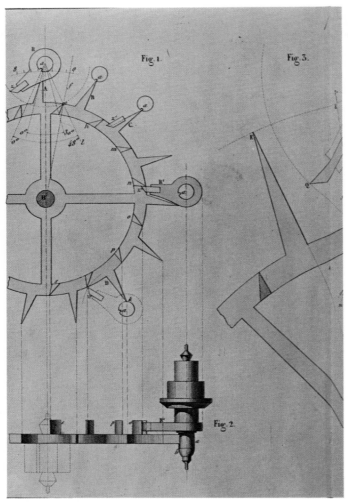

One of the best-known nineteenth-century French horological textbooks is Claude Saunier's *Treatise on Modern Horology* which first appeared in 1869 in Paris. The best English edition which has the technical drawings in colour to demonstrate the use of the two principal metals, brass and steel, and ruby jewelling, appeared in 1880. This is part of Plate 2 which shows the duplex escapement with its characteristic escape wheel employing two sets of teeth cut in planes at right angles to one another.

just a ring of lead like a weight for a fishing line, or sometimes a smaller version of the driving weight and also on a pulley. Pulling down the counterpoised side of the line pulls up the main driving weight and thus winds up the clock. In either case, the weight is pulling upon a line wound round a drum, called a 'barrel', with which is associated the main driving wheel of the machine – the 'great' wheel, as it is called.

The falling-weight type of power source is probably the most efficient that could have been contrived, since the weight is acting under the force of gravity, which is constant; thus, at whatever height the weight may be in its passage from fully wound up to fully 'run out', the driving force it applies to the clock remains the same. Its only disadvantage as a system is that, while the weight is being wound up, the power supply to drive the

clock is interrupted, since the two motions cannot coexist except in the case of the loop-drive of thirty-hour clocks, where it does not apply. To overcome this, especially in the finest clocks, 'maintaining power' is provided. This takes the form of a small ancillary spring, so arranged that the clock cannot be wound at all without activating it; this gives sufficient additional power to keep the clock running while the winding-up procedure takes place. When a clock has the type known as 'bolt and shutter' maintaining power, it is necessary first to operate a lever, sometimes projecting through the dial but on other clocks at the side of the movement, in order to lift shutters that normally obstruct access to the winding squares in the dial. Not only weight-driven but also the finest quality spring-driven clocks, as well as many watches, are fitted with maintaining power, on much the same principle.

The falling weight was the earliest source of power, apart from the very rare, almost freak, use of hydraulics in clocks that were anyway only partially mechanical; these will be considered in the next chapter. The other main mechanical power source was the coiled spring, contained within a cylindrical drum also called a 'barrel'. It was a long time after the first use of falling weights to drive a clock that iron and steel technology became sufficiently advanced to allow a spring to be made successfully. The metal had first to be beaten into a ribbon by hand; and it must have been extremely difficult to obtain uniformity in all dimensions throughout its whole length. Then it had to be heat-treated to obtain the correct 'temper'. It seems likely that when, probably in Italy during the fifteenth century, the first springs were made – possibly by a swordsmith or locksmith rather than a clockmaker – the reject rate must have been inordinately high.

The disadvantages of the coiled spring as a power source are, first, its liability to break without warning, and second the uneven 'pull' which it exerts to drive the timekeeper. The first of these has been largely overcome – but only in the present century – by the perfection of various alloys that are nearly, if not completely, unbreakable. The second has required a great deal more mechanical ingenuity to cure.

When a spring is fully wound up, it exerts a much stronger force – in its efforts to unwind – than when it is partially or nearly run down. Clearly this inconsistency of energy supply must affect the going of the clock, so that it would run fast when fully wound up, its rate falling away as the spring uncoils. Among early attempts to correct this fault was a device called the stackfreed. Developed in Germany, it was a far from satisfactory remedy and did not survive long into the seventeenth century. In essence, it used a cam to turn with the mainspring, its rotation being helped

When used with the fusee, the central arbor is held fast and the barrel revolved by pulling upon a fine chain or, in the case of spring clocks, a gut or wire line, coiled around the outside of the barrel and fixed at the far end to it. The other end of this line is attached to the fusee, which is a cone-shaped pulley around which is cut a spiral groove in which the line runs.

To wind up the spring, a key is placed on the squared end of the fusee arbor and turned. This action pulls the line on to the fusee and off the spring barrel, thus rotating it; and since the barrel arbor is held tight, the spring is thereby coiled up. The reverse of this action – that is, as the spring runs down – sees the coiled spring rotating the barrel, and pulling the line back off the fusee again. But the fusee is essentially a cone, and the arrangement provides that when the spring is fully wound it is pulling, via the line to the fusee, against the smallest diameter of the latter, which will therefore be exercising the least leverage – called 'torque' – to the system. Maximum torque, on the other hand, comes into play when the mainspring is nearly run out, by which time the line is then pulling upon the largest diameter of the fusee. The

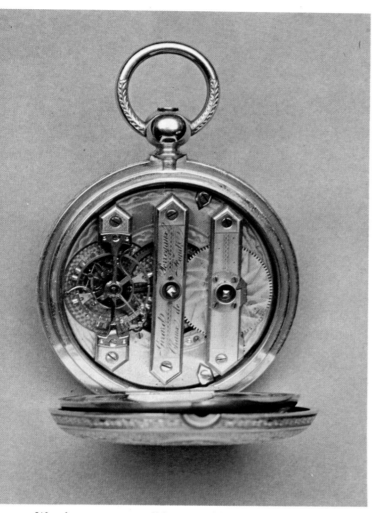

Watches are susceptible to positional error, and this is mainly felt in the escapement. To compensate for this, two similar devices, called respectively the tourbillon and the karrusel, have been used. The former was invented by Breguet, and the latter by Bonniksen. Both involve mounting the escapement in a slowly rotating carriage – the average time for one revolution can be about forty minutes. This illustration shows the tourbillon of a watch by Girard Perregaux. Museum of the Worshipful Company of Clockmakers, Guildhall, London.

or impeded by a spring-loaded roller acting along its edge, the intention being thus to cancel out the natural irregularity of the mainspring's action.

The first and still the commonest device to correct this fault, both on clocks and watches of any quality, is called the fusee. It provides a most elegant solution, not only practical as well as satisfactory in operation, but also theoretically perfect. In essentials, the ends of the mainspring coiled in its barrel are both fixed, the outer end hooked on to the inside of the barrel wall, and the inner to a spindle´ – or 'arbor' – which passes through the centre of the barrel. To wind up the mainspring – that is, to coil it up under maximum tension – clearly either the central spindle can be held static and the barrel revolved, or the barrel held static and the central arbor revolved.

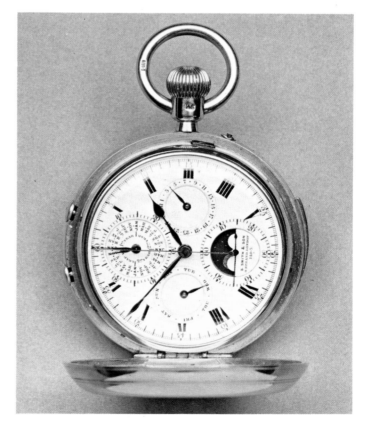

So called 'triple-complicated' watches are well illustrated by this example made by S. Smith & Son in 1899. The dial shows not only the time, but also the phases of the moon, and has a perpetual calendar. Apart from this, the watch is a minute repeater and has split-seconds chronograph action. Museum of the Worshipful Company of Clockmakers, Guildhall, London.

29

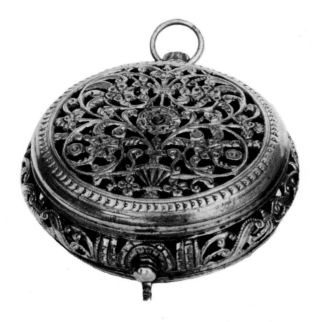

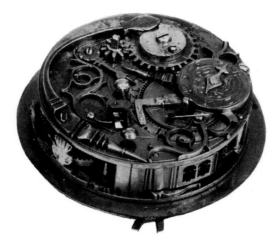

arrangement completely compensates, therefore, for the innate defects of the spring; and since the main driving wheel to the mechanism, the great wheel, shares the same arbor as the fusee but is connected with it only by a ratchet arrangement – so that, in one direction only, the fusee can be rotated separately from the great wheel, this being necessary when winding up – the source of power must be delivered evenly to the mechanism throughout the duration of its going, and right at the start of the transmission.

With the fusee, it will be remembered that the barrel arbor is fixed tight and the barrel itself turned to wind up the spring. There is, however, another arrangement – of rather more modern usage and, to some extent, associated with the decline in the market for the finest quality clocks and watches – which goes by the name of a 'going barrel'. In this, the fusee is dispensed with altogether, and the concept depends upon eliminating the worst effects of uneven drive from the mainspring by utilising only a certain portion – effectively the middle coils of the spring – as a power source. It is true that the worst manifestations of unevenness occur when the spring is either fully wound or almost run out; so if you can ensure – by a device called 'stop work' – that even when the spring stops driving the clock it is still under some residual tension in the barrel, and similarly that when it is effectively wound it would still coil up further, were it not for the stop work, then you are principally using the middle coils of the spring, which in practice give a fairly even pull throughout their length. In a going barrel, the great wheel is integral with it; and the system requires that the spring be wound by turning the barrel arbor itself, the barrel being unable to rotate except as it drives the mechanism through the great wheel.

A short-lived device for equalising the pull of the mainspring was tried out in Germany during the last half of the sixteenth century. Called the stackfreed (see page 28), this consisted essentially of a spring-loaded roller abutting against a snail-shaped cam both of which can be clearly seen in this picture. Also visible is the dumb-bell foliot and hog's bristle which regulated it. Basingstoke Museum.

right
One of the finest examples of a clock showing the equation of time, this one by George Graham is dated about 1740. In addition to the equation dial in the break-arch, there is a gilt minute hand which always points to solar time, while the steel hand points to mean time. See also page 162. British Museum, London.

Before leaving the question of residual tension, it is just worth mentioning that, whereas in the going barrel the residual tension is achieved by using stop work, with the fusee also some residual tension must remain in the spring even when the system is effectively run out, in order that the device shall operate most efficiently and so as to keep the line from barrel to fusee taut. To achieve this, the mainspring has to be 'set up', and this is normally done by a ratchet and click applied to the end of the barrel arbor, or by an endless screw. There is a special tool, called a fusee testing rod, by which watch- and clockmakers have to test such pretensioning of the mainspring to ensure that it is compatible with the proportions of the barrel and fusee actually in use, and thus that the system provides an even power supply throughout its cycle of operation.

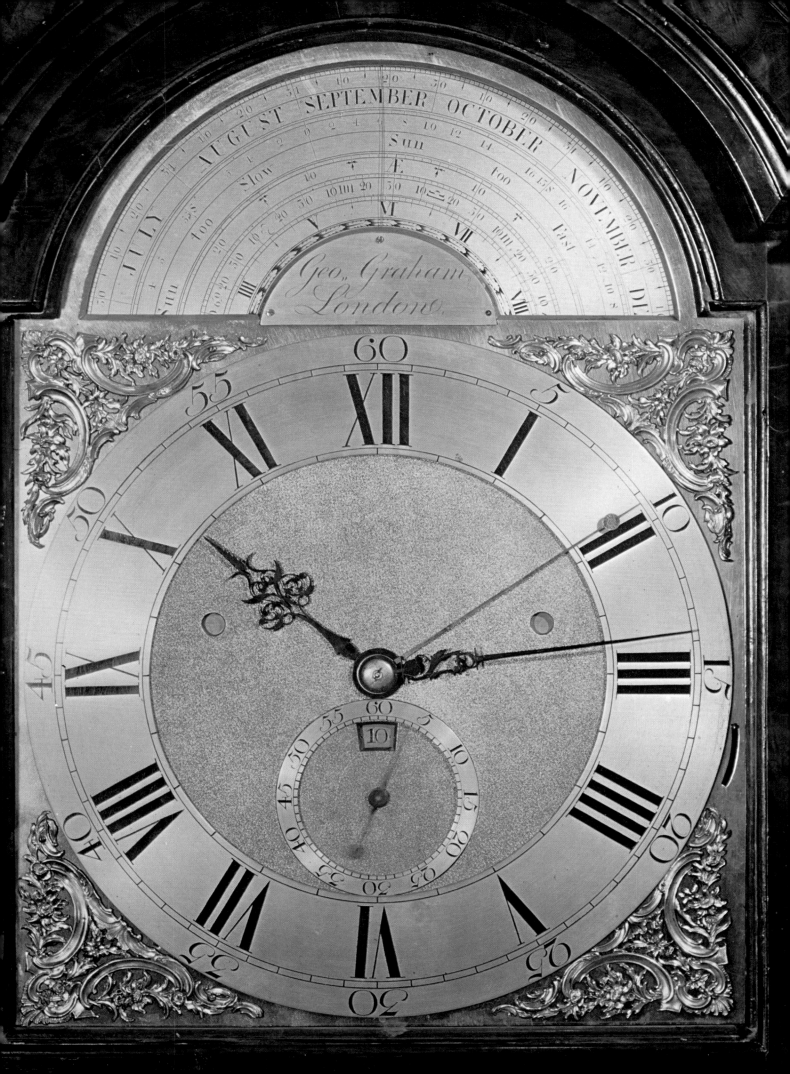

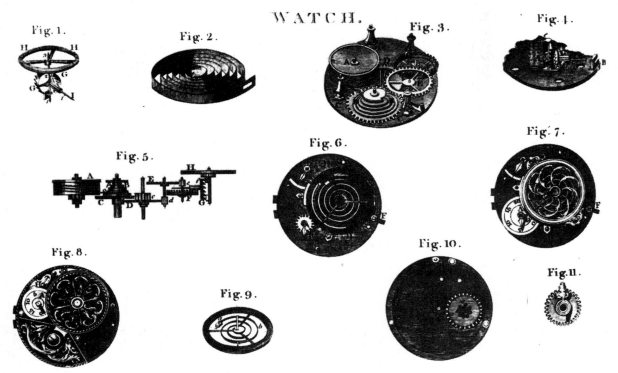

Fig. 1. Fig. 2. Fig. 3. Fig. 4. Fig. 5. Fig. 6. Fig. 7. Fig. 8. Fig. 9. Fig. 10. Fig. 11.

The nineteenth century was remarkable for the plethora of well-produced technical encyclopedias that appeared, and this is the plate dealing with 'watch' taken from *The English Encyclopaedia* of 1802. Self-evident among the various figures can be seen the verge escapement as applied to a watch, an unhoused mainspring and the layout of spring barrel, fusee and train in a watch whose back plate has not yet been placed in position. Figure 5 shows the relationship of wheels and pinions in the same train, starting from the spring barrel at left and extending to the escapement – a verge – at right. Figures 7 and 8 show the typical continental and English watch movements of the period as seen from the back.

Once given an efficient power source, it is clearly necessary to have some means of passing it through the machine, dividing it up into the right proportions to fit the eventual needs of each particular part to which it travels. This is done by a 'train' of engaging gears; and any clock or watch may have more than one train. Thus, a big clock is likely to have a going train, a striking train (to strike the required number of times at each hour) and a chiming train (to chime at each quarter), the two last-named being interdependent and triggered off by the going train, which, of necessity, provides the basic control of the machine.

A train of gears consists of a sequence of wheels meshing with pinions; usually the wheels are of brass, mounted upon steel arbors out of which are also formed the pinions, and it is customary to speak of the wheels as having teeth but pinions as having leaves. In early clockwork, wheels were made of iron by smithing techniques, and the teeth were cut out by hand; at that time, too, lantern pinions were the usual design, that is, instead of being formed from solid metal, they were in the form of a cage, made up of two end-discs separated by pins which constituted the leaves. For some centuries past, however, it has been possible to produce wheels on a wheel-cutting 'engine', which utilises a 'dividing plate' to direct the cutter, somewhat in the manner of a pantograph.

In most going trains – that is, the gear train that leads from the power source eventually to show the time by hands on a dial – the starting point, as has been shown, is the great wheel. Except where the train has an unusually long duration of going – more than eight days, at any rate – the usual arrangement is for the great wheel to drive the pinion of the centre wheel; that wheel drives the third wheel pinion, the third wheel drives the fourth wheel pinion and so on. The fourth or fifth wheel is generally the escape wheel – an integral part of the escapement, which will be described shortly.

Arbors carrying wheels and pinions are shaped at their ends into 'pivots' running in pivot holes in the main frame of the clock or watch. Such a frame will usually consist of front and back 'plates' separated by turned or otherwise ornamental 'pillars', and between which the movement is supported. These pivot holes may simply be drilled in the metal, or they may be 'jewel holes', that is to say, bushed with hardstone to make a hard-wearing bearing. While nowadays synthetic stones are used, formerly ruby, sapphire or garnet were the customary material. Jewelled surfaces were also used elsewhere in both clocks and watches where much wear was likely as, for instance, on the bearing faces of the pallets in the escapement.

The centre wheel arbor extends through the dial, in most arrangements, the projecting part

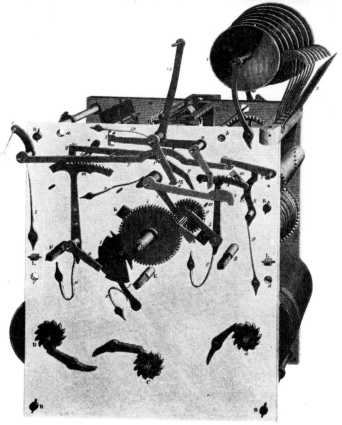

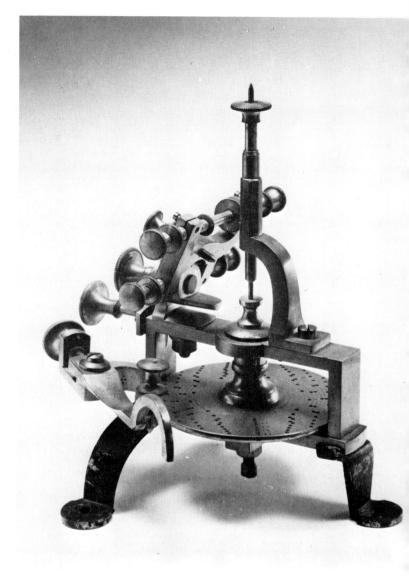

being called the centre post. Friction tight upon this post is carried the 'cannon pinion', which drives the 'motion work', as it is called. Its sole purpose is to divide the rotation of the centre post between the requirements of the hour and minute hands – the latter, of course, rotating twelve times as fast as the former. The motion work is a mini-train all of its own, consisting of the cannon pinion which drives the minute wheel, which rides free upon a stud fixed to the main frame of the clock or watch. The minute wheel pinion drives the hour wheel, which is mounted upon a pipe that fits freely over the cannon pinion. On this pipe is mounted the hour hand. The end of the cannon pinion is squared off and projects through and beyond the pipe of the hour wheel carrying the hour hand; and upon this squared end is mounted the minute hand. If there is a 'supplementary' seconds hand – frequently sited just above six on the dial – it is usually carried upon the extended arbor of the fourth wheel, or, in the case of the conventional seconds-beating pendulum clock, upon the escape wheel arbor.

If the mechanism, as it has been described so far, were wound up and allowed free rein, it would race to unwind itself in a totally uncontrolled way and most probably cause itself irretrievable damage in so doing: teeth would be stripped from wheels, and the whole machine might even disintegrate. Clearly this would serve no useful purpose whatever.

The element that is lacking is that single device which, as we said earlier, is peculiar to early time-measuring instruments and features in no other sort of machinery – the escapement. This is, in effect, the governor that slows down the rate at

above left
A beautifully engraved plate from Rees's *Cyclopaedia* shows a conventional three-train spring-driven rack striking and chiming clock, the chime being on eight bells.

above
The principle of a wheel-cutting engine is based on the precise graduating of a circular plate – called the dividing plate – so that a range of concentric circles engraved thereon are each marked out in a different number of equal arcs. It is necessary then only to select that circle which is divided into the same number of sections as a wheel-blank is to have teeth cut into it, and then to line up the cutter point by point around that circle on a system something like a pantograph. This small wheel-cutting engine, which is Swiss, of about 1850, is specially designed to cut the teeth of verge escape wheels which, because of their shape, are usually called crown wheels. The number of teeth in such a wheel is limited, and the dividing plate of this engine ranges from seven to twenty-one teeth only.

33

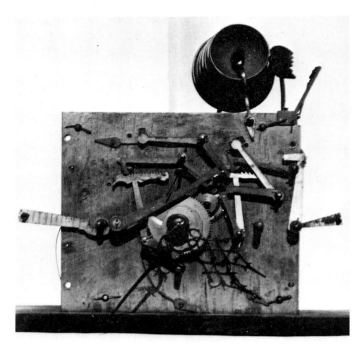

which the power supply is used up to one that is commensurate with the passage of time; in other words, it allows power to 'escape' at carefully controlled intervals which, within limits, can be slowed down or speeded up to make the clock run 'to time'.

In understanding the fundamentals of an escapement, it is necessary to bear in mind, firstly, that the escape wheel is always the last wheel in the going train – right at the end of the line, as it were – and secondly that its natural inclination is to rotate freely under the influence of the power being applied to it through the rest of the train, starting from the power source. It is necessary, therefore, to impede that natural motion, but this can only be done to a wheel that is not meshing with yet another pinion – hence the need for it to be the last one in the train.

The wheel can be impeded from rotating freely by first locking, and then releasing it, one tooth at a time; and if some kind of regularly swinging or vibrating component be used for the purpose, the wheel can be made to give that component 'impulse' – that is, give it a push – each time it is frustrated in its endeavour to run free. Imagine, therefore, a pendulum on a free suspension with, attached to it, a pair of jaws designed to embrace a number of teeth of the escape wheel; set the pendulum swinging, so that at each extreme of its swing it locks – or intercepts – a tooth on one side of the wheel but releases one on the other, and there is the simplest form of escapement. Providing the shape of the escape wheel teeth and the 'pallets' – the contacting surfaces of the jaws – are properly designed, the pendulum, once set in motion, will continue swinging until the spring or weight runs out, obtaining all the impulse it needs through the system.

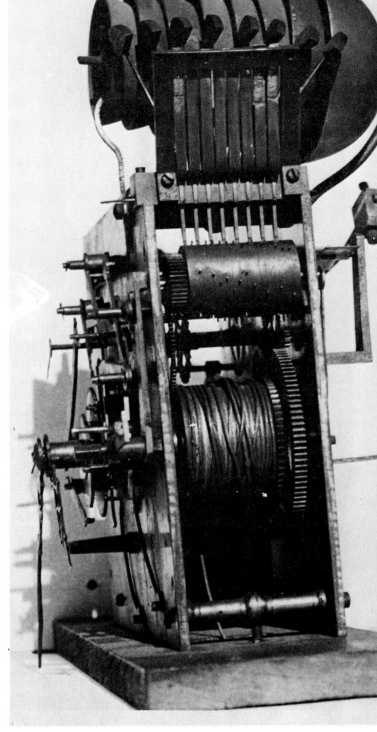

above left
Although this three-train clock is weight-driven, there are clear points of resemblance with the plate from Rees's *Cyclopaedia*. The hands – including seconds hand above centre – have been replaced to aid orientation, and the system of striking and chiming by rack and snail is clearly demonstrated.

above
This end-on view of the same clock shows the chiming barrel, pinned as in a musical box, and in this case it can be altered at will to chime on four or eight bells. The change is effected by raising or lowering the lever in the foreground which shifts the pin-barrel slightly sideways to bring a different set of pins into action.

The theory of pendulums is complex. An ideal length exists for pendulums 'beating' certain intervals of time, and probably that most commonly encountered is the seconds pendulum, the theoretically perfect length of which is approximately one metre. This is the pendulum used in most longcase – familiarly called grandfather – clocks. To obtain a perfect pendulum that will beat longer intervals than one second, however, it is not enough simply to multiply up – a two-seconds pendulum, for instance, should measure four metres in length, and these are sometimes found on church clocks. Short 'bob' pendulums are also found on small domestic clocks, and one beating three times per second has a length of only 10.6cm.

This extraordinary clock movement – how it was originally cased is now not known – is a short-period timer which might possibly have been used for horseracing. It was made at the end of the eighteenth century by Justin Vulliamy, and its nine dials can be activated by levers to work in various combinations. The escapement, unusually for a clock, is a very large cylinder of which it seems to be the only known weight-driven example.

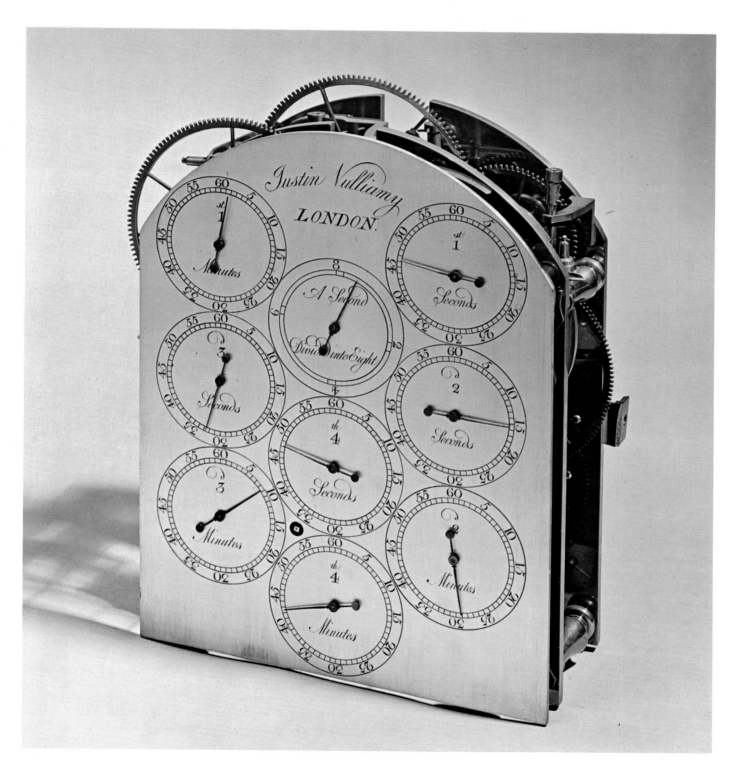

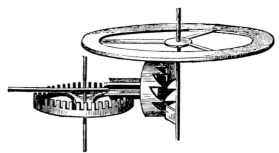

right

The verge escapement, when applied to watches, is arranged as in this illustration, also from *Clocks and Watches and Bells*. The wheel in a horizontal plane with teeth sticking upwards is usually called the contrate wheel, and this drives the pinion of the escape – or crown – wheel. The pallets, which look like two small flags on the upright arbor of the balance wheel, are clearly visible.

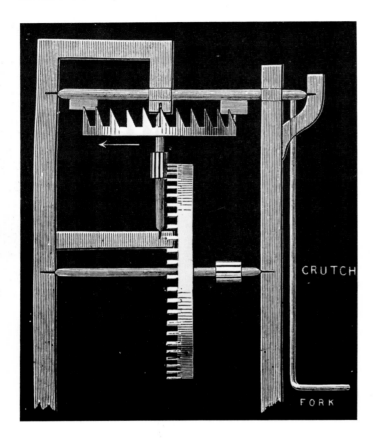

CRUTCH

FORK

This illustration – which shows the verge escapement as applied to a clock – comes from the seventh edition which appeared in 1883 of a celebrated nineteenth-century treatise on horology entitled *Clocks and Watches and Bells* by Sir Edmund Beckett, Q.C. The author of this book, afterwards Lord Grimthorpe, designed the mechanism for 'Big Ben'. In the illustration, the pendulum hangs on the right, passing between the right-angled forked end of the crutch.

A fine drawing, again from Sir Edmund Beckett, of the action of the cylinder or horizontal escapement. Identifying features of this assembly include the curiously shaped escape wheel teeth with their small platforms on top, so formed in order to pass through the cylinder seen in action with the escape wheel, and also, on extreme left, by itself. The swinging balance wheel would be attached to the latter.

For any timekeeper that is going to remain reasonably static, a pendulum is probably the best form of controller for the escapement that can be devised; it is also true, that the longer the pendulum the more perfectly it will perform in a clock, since it is desirable that, whatever type of controlling device is used, the interval between the impulses it receives from the escape wheel should be as long as possible, to allow it to remain 'detached' from the machine and able to 'vibrate' – or swing – freely for as much of the time as can be contrived.

But for smaller clocks as well as for portable timekeepers, especially watches, the alternative to the pendulum is the balance wheel; and the balance spring was invented to recreate, often in a horizontal rather than a vertical plane, the backwards and forwards effect which, in the pendulum, is a combination of impulse from the mainspring pushing it outwards and gravity bringing it back to the zero point again.

To put this in correct historical perspective, the very first type of controller, on the earliest monastic clocks, was a flat bar, pivoting at the centre and oscillating in a horizontal plane. Called a 'foliot', this had movable weights suspended from each half of the bar by which some adjustment could be effected. It can be argued that the balance wheel, which simply added a rim to the foliot to turn it into a kind of flywheel, was a logical progression from it rather than a separate invention; in any event, neither can be attributed to any particular person in the present state of our knowledge. The pendulum, however, was certainly recognised by Leonardo da Vinci even though he never applied it to a clock, so far as is known. Galileo wrote about the pendulum as a philosophical instrument; and it was left to Christiaan Huygens, the eminent

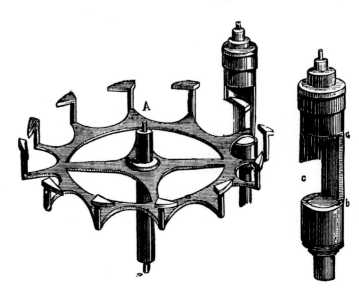

Dutch physicist, to apply the pendulum to a timekeeper. As for that other component, the balance spring – often called the hairspring, although such is not a correct horological term – this was originated by Robert Hooke for application to watches, and later perfected and marketed by Huygens.

It is probably not an exaggeration to say that dozens upon dozens, if not indeed several hundred, designs of escapement have been drawn up over the centuries – although far fewer than that were ever actually made; and it is possible to say with certainty that many of those which exist only as figments on paper could never have worked anyway. There are perhaps nearly a dozen types of escapement with which anybody taking an interest in horology should familiarise themselves, and these can be summarised as follows.

The verge is the oldest of all escapements. Found in the first clocks, where it was controlled by a foliot, it was quickly adapted for watches, when the technology permitted of these being made. Provincial craftsmen in Britain were still using it as late as 1900. It is robust and relatively trouble-free in use, and will run for long periods with minimal attention, but its timekeeping properties are not remarkable.

The cylinder, which was perfected by Thomas Tompion's partner George Graham and used in virtually all his watches after 1725, became the preferred escapement for the well-to-do, although it never completely supplanted the verge. The escape wheel works in a horizontal plane, hence it is sometimes called the 'horizontal' escapement. The cylinder is an extremely difficult escapement to make, and – except in that variant known as the ruby cylinder, in which the acting surfaces are made of precious hardstone – subject to wear. It is also much more fragile than the verge, and these disadvantages tend to cancel out any slight timekeeping edge it may possess over the best verge watches.

Incidentally, the cylinder was reincarnated by the Swiss in the latter half of the last century, in the enormous quantities of fairly low-grade export watches which they manufactured, and also as a platform escapement in the poorer carriage clocks'.

The duplex was originally invented and perfected in Paris during the first half of the eighteenth century by J. B. Dutertre and Pierre Le Roy. It appeared in England in 1782 under a patent taken out by Thomas Tyrer, and became the heart of the English high-quality watch – apart from the pocket chronometer – for at least the first three decades of the nineteenth century. It was still being made until at least 1845. The individual characteristic of the duplex is that its escape wheel

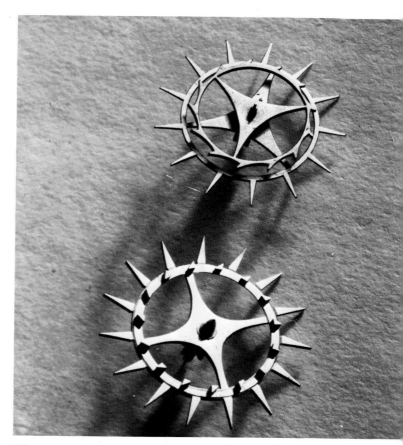

These two escape wheels, both for use with the duplex escapement, show the difference between English and continental practice. The English preferred to cut their two sets of teeth on the same wheel, whereas elsewhere it was commonplace to cut two separate wheels and mount them on the same arbor.

requires two sets of teeth in planes at right angles to one another. In the English version, this is usually accomplished by cutting the two sets of teeth on the same wheel, but on the Continent the preferred arrangement is usually to have two separate wheels mounted upon the same common arbor.

Like the cylinder, the duplex was also resuscitated, but this time in cheap machine-made American watches towards the end of the nineteenth century. Its inherent disadvantage is difficulty of lubrication.

The detent or chronometer escapement existed in several designs, based mainly upon the inventions of John Arnold and Thomas Earnshaw in this country, and of Pierre Le Roy and Ferdinand Berthoud in France, during the second half of the eighteenth and the earliest years of the nineteenth centuries. The two forms most usually encountered are the spring detent and the pivoted detent, with sub-forms of the former according to Arnold's or Earnshaw's patterns. This escapement is the one most suitable for marine chronometers and deck watches – that is to say, for navigational use – and might be thought a little too fragile for everyday wear, although plenty of examples were carried on the person.

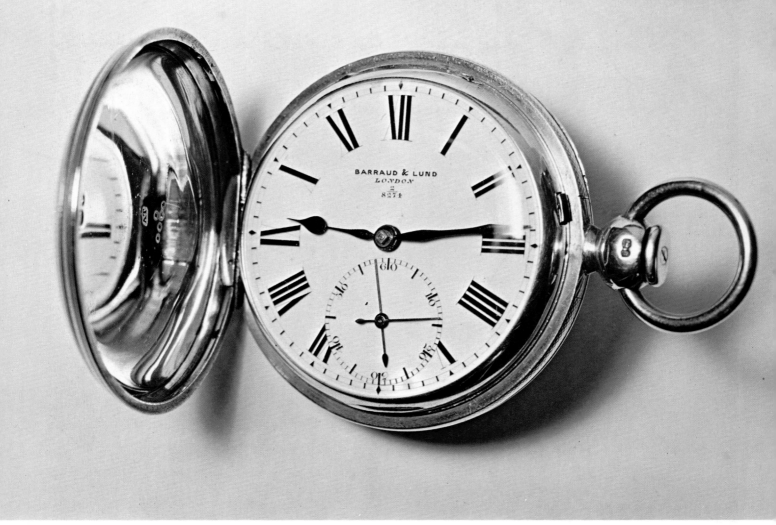

The split-second chronograph is so named because in its original form it consisted of two seconds hands, one above the other, which normally rotated together. By pressing a push-piece, it was possible to halt one of the seconds hands while the other continued. When the end of the interval to be measured was reached – and for convenience it had to be less than a minute – the difference between the two seconds hands could be read off. A further pressure on the push-piece caused the hand that was stationary to catch up with the other one. This particular specimen by Barraud & Lund of London was made in 1859.

In this simplified sketch of the English lever escapement, which is also taken from Sir Edmund Beckett's book, the plain flat balance wheel swings backwards and forwards taking with it the pin P. This engages and disengages with the notch at the end of the lever which is pivoted at C, causing this to rock backwards and forwards, alternately engaging with and releasing a tooth of the escape wheel.

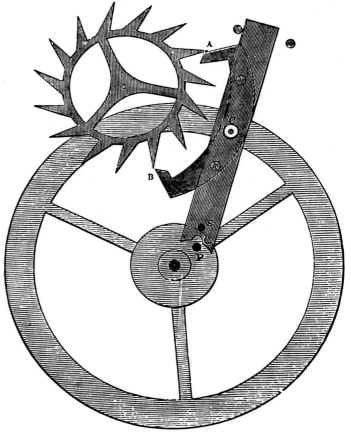

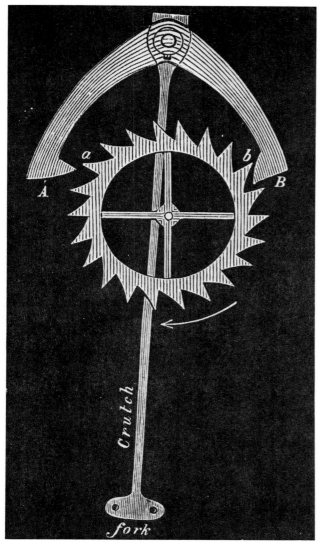

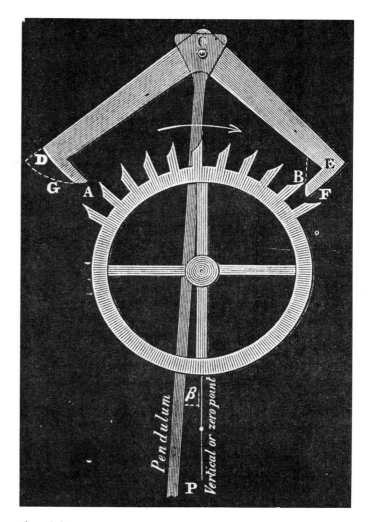

The lever, the principal escapement used today in mechanical wristwatches and in many small clocks, was invented in its original form by Thomas Mudge in the mid eighteenth century, but discarded by him as too complicated for ordinary purposes. Towards the end of the same century a handful of the finest craftsmen made a few special watches incorporating versions of this escapement, which are numbered among the great rarities by collectors today. The lever escapement then died a second death, only to re-emerge eventually, in a simplified form known as the table-roller lever, about 1825. There were intermediate developments, examples of which are still to be found: these include Peter Litherland's rack lever, patented in 1791, Edward Massey's crank-roller lever of 1814, and George Savage's two-pin lever of only two or three years later. Quite independently, one or two French craftsmen had tried their hand at a similar device; both the great A.-L. Breguet and Robert Robin, for instance, made some interesting lever watches in the last decade of the eighteenth century. By about 1860, the lever watch had swept all before it; gone were the duplex and chronometer watches and, apart from the cheap Swiss version, the cylinder had long since disappeared.

above left
The recoil anchor escapement in its application to clockwork, in an illustration from *Clocks and Watches and Bells*. As with the verge illustrated earlier (see page 36), the pendulum is suspended at a point above the crutch and passes between the pins on the fork. As it swings backwards and forwards, it takes the crutch with it and, of necessity, the anchor to which the latter is attached.

above
The deadbeat anchor escapement, while operating in the same manner as the recoil anchor, will be seen from this illustration from Beckett's book to have escape wheel teeth of a different profile and also differently shaped pallets.

With the exception of the verge, nearly all the escapements listed so far have had their main application in watches – and there were a number of others, too, which are more rarely encountered even among advanced circles of collectors today. Such were the virgule – and that exceptional rarity, the double virgule – and the Debaufre-type escapements, of which no two ever seem to be quite the same. The chance of the average collector coming face to face with one of these is becoming increasingly less likely as each year succeeds the last.

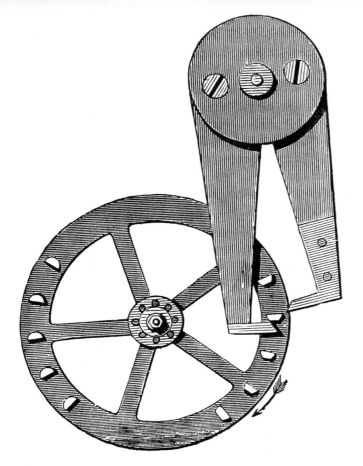

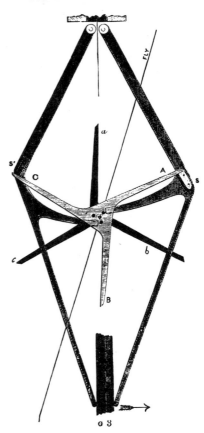

But what about clock escapements? Apart from the solid long-lasting verge, the commonest antique clock escapement is:

The anchor or recoil escapement. Variously attributed to Robert Hooke and William Clement, it seems to have appeared about 1671 and for the first time made really accurate clocks possible. It supplanted the verge escapement in clocks, and many originally fitted with verges were subsequently converted to this more accurate form. When, on page 34, a basic escapement was described as a swinging pendulum fitted with jaws that embraced a number of teeth of the escape wheel, this was an oversimplified description of the anchor escapement.

The dead-beat escapement is a recoilless version of the anchor, invented in 1715 by George Graham and especially used in regulator clocks, that is to say, clocks built to observatory standards of accuracy. Such clocks are frequently fitted with the most sophisticated means of improving and maintaining performance, so that it is not unusual to find bearings running in jewels – in the same manner as so many watches boast of nowadays, although not all their jewelling is necessarily quite what it may appear to be. The pallets, too, may be surfaced in the same material.

There are other forms of clock escapement – the pin-pallet, for example, much loved by the Victorians, and not to be confused with the pin-wheel escapement found in many good-quality French

clocks – including, from the collector's point of view, several great rarities. The grasshopper is one of these. The invention of John Harrison for his great wooden regulator clocks, its great advantage is that it needs no oil. It was modified and used later by Vulliamy and rarely by one or two other makers.

The gravity escapement will be the last one to be mentioned here, and this because, in one or another version, it is to be found on some of the finest turret clocks. Towards the end of the third

above left
There are several versions of the pin-wheel escapement for clocks, even though the principle is the same. This example is Sir Edmund Beckett's design, the difference being that for technical reasons he has flattened the underside of the pins on the escape wheel, which are generally left rounded, as shown on the left of the illustration.

above
Sir Edmund Beckett's greatest contribution to horology was probably his design of the double three-legged gravity escapement for large public clocks. It was originally intended for the Westminster clock 'Big Ben' and the performance of that timekeeper is world-famous.

right
Automata in clocks have a very long history. This example of the Heralds and Electors paying homage to the Emperor is a detail from the ship-clock or *nef* attributed to Hans Schlottheim, and which was made for Emperor Rudolf II, probably in Prague about 1580. British Museum, London.

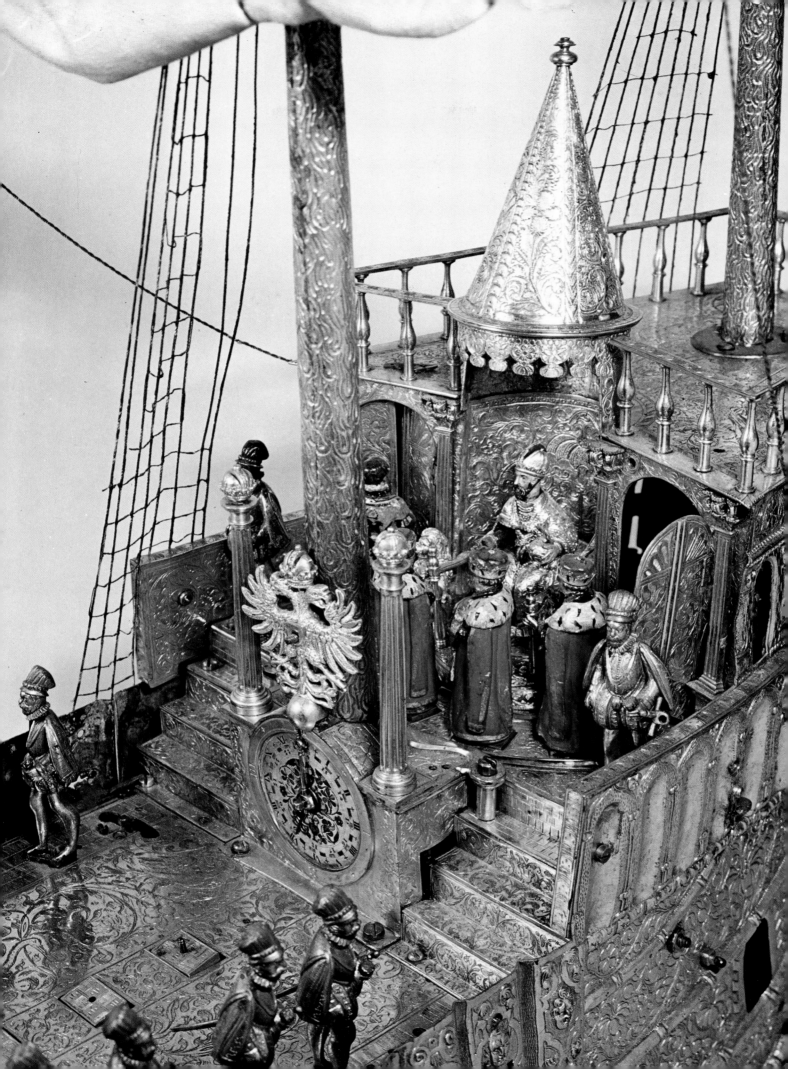

quarter of the eighteenth century, two famous London makers, Thomas Mudge and Alexander Cumming seem independently of one another to have devised escapements of this kind. The essential principle of them is that impulse is imparted by the mainspring not directly to the pendulum or balance but through an intermediary system which the mainspring activates. Thus the pendulum is never in direct contact with the power source, and variations in power will not affect it, providing there is always sufficient energy to activate the intermediary system. This principle is usually called a remontoire. One of the most spectacular gravity escapements to be found in turret clocks – and especially in its prototype, London's 'Big Ben' on the Houses of Parliament – is the double three-legged gravity escapement especially invented by Lord Grimthorpe as part of his design for this famous clock.

The final word on escapements should perhaps be to reiterate something implied earlier on, in postulating the amateur's approach to clockwork. The technical complexities of escapements, studied in depth, are immense. Proponents of the early forms of lever, for example, will argue for hours on whether they incorporate 'draw', which is a stage in the cycle of operation of this escapement. Arguments will embrace mathematical and mechanical concepts calling for specialised knowledge, not to say aptitude. Yet, for the amateur, an escapement need not really mean any more than a system that twists or swings, back and forth, letting the escape wheel revolve one tooth at a time in a manner compatible with its main function which is to measure time!

Any clockwork mechanism is a comedy – or perhaps tragedy would be more appropriate – of errors; and at least part of the art of persuading it to run to time is to find means of getting these errors to compensate for one another, or cancel each other out. Some of the errors are due to friction which, for example, acts differently upon such parts as the pivots, depending upon the position of the timekeeper; that is to say, whether it is upright, upon its back, front or whatever. This applies only to watches, and their position is designated 'dial up' or 'down', 'pendant up', 'down', 'left' or 'right' when they are tested 'in positions'.

Yet other errors are due to changes in the temperature of the timekeeper's surroundings. It is a well-known phenomenon that metals tend to expand in heat and contract in cold, and obviously any compensation for this effect needs to act automatically upon the regulating component, adjusting it to make the machine run fast when the temperature change would cause it to slow down, and vice versa.

A number of devices have been tried, in attempts to correct for positional error in watches. The most successful have been directed towards

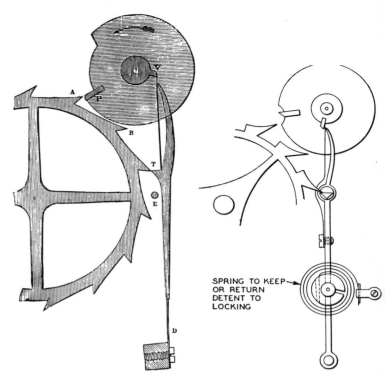

SPRING TO KEEP
OR RETURN
DETENT TO
LOCKING

mounting the entire escapement in a revolving carriage. Of two similar designs of this kind, the best-known is probably the tourbillon, one of Breguet's brilliant inventions and dating from 1801. Generally, in his arrangement, the carriage revolves once a minute. The other one, called a karrusel and originated by Aarne Bonniksen of Coventry in 1894, revolves in 52½ minutes.

While of course temperature error acts on all metal parts, its most serious effects are upon the pendulum rod of a clock, and, separately, upon the balance wheel and balance spring of a watch.

There are several well-established temperature compensation systems for metal pendulum rods. In the mercurial pendulum, which was designed by George Graham in 1721 and applied by him to his regulator clocks, the pendulum bob takes the form of a reservoir of mercury. As the pendulum rod lengthens in heat, the mercury expands upwards, thus keeping the effective length the same.

In Harrison's gridiron pendulum, of 1726, the same objective – maintaining the effective length constant – is achieved by using a grid of brass and steel rods, their ends fixed to cross-members alternately top and bottom so that the expansion upwards of the one metal cancels out the corresponding expansion downwards of the other. Yet again, in 1752, John Ellicott published details of a device he had perfected twenty years before, by which the downward expansion of a pendulum rod pressed upon levers located inside the pendulum bob, raising it and thus preserving its effective length.

Temperature compensation devices for watches and chronometers mostly depend upon the principle that a bi-metallic strip of brass and steel, riveted together, bends under the influence of heat

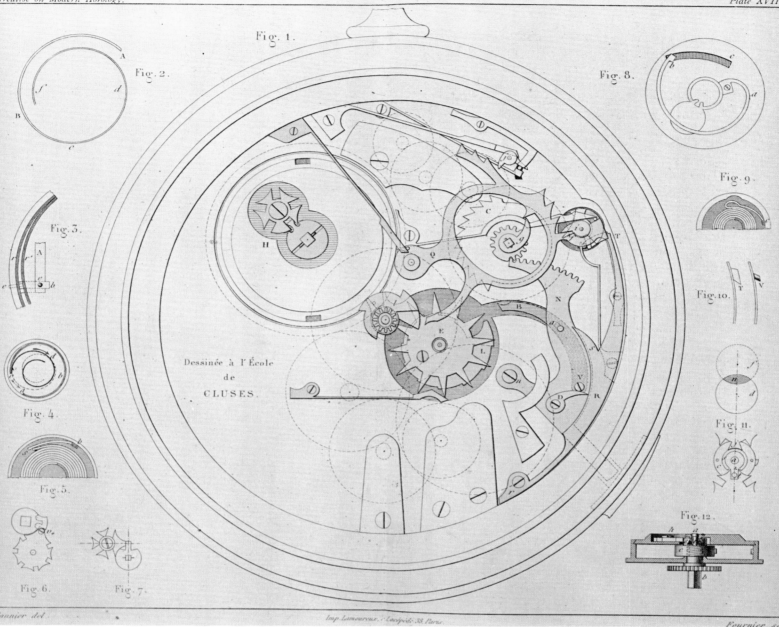

Fig. 1.

Fig. 2.

Fig. 3.

Fig. 4.

Fig. 5.

Fig. 6.

Fig. 7.

Fig. 8.

Fig. 9.

Fig.10.

Fig. 11.

Fig. 12.

Dessinée à l'École de CLUSES.

Saunier del.   *Imp. Lemourvux. Lacipite 33. Paris.*   *Fournier sc.*

opposite page, left

After the initial pioneering efforts of John Harrison, complemented by experimental work from a small number of makers such as Thomas Mudge and Josiah Emery, the final form of marine chronometer escapement followed two superficially similar patterns devised respectively by John Arnold and Thomas Earnshaw. Modern chronometers have settled upon the latter arrangement, and this is shown in this drawing from *Clocks and Watches and Bells*. The most significant feature is the tooth V which, when it is moving anti-clockwise – it being on the same arbor as the balance wheel – displaces the detent DTV. When, however, it returns in the opposite direction, it simply pushes aside a weak spring TV, set on the end of the detent, which is called the passing spring.

opposite page, right

Another form of chronometer escapement defined as the pivoted detent was originally developed in France and has been favoured by continental manufacturers. The main difference between this form and the spring detent previously described is the necessity to incorporate a spiral spring similar to a balance spring.

above

Plate 17 from Saunier's *Treatise on Modern Horology* of 1880 (see also page 28) illustrates very well the high standard of technical drawing reached in the late nineteenth century. This particular diagram represents a typical continental design for a quarter-repeating watch.

43

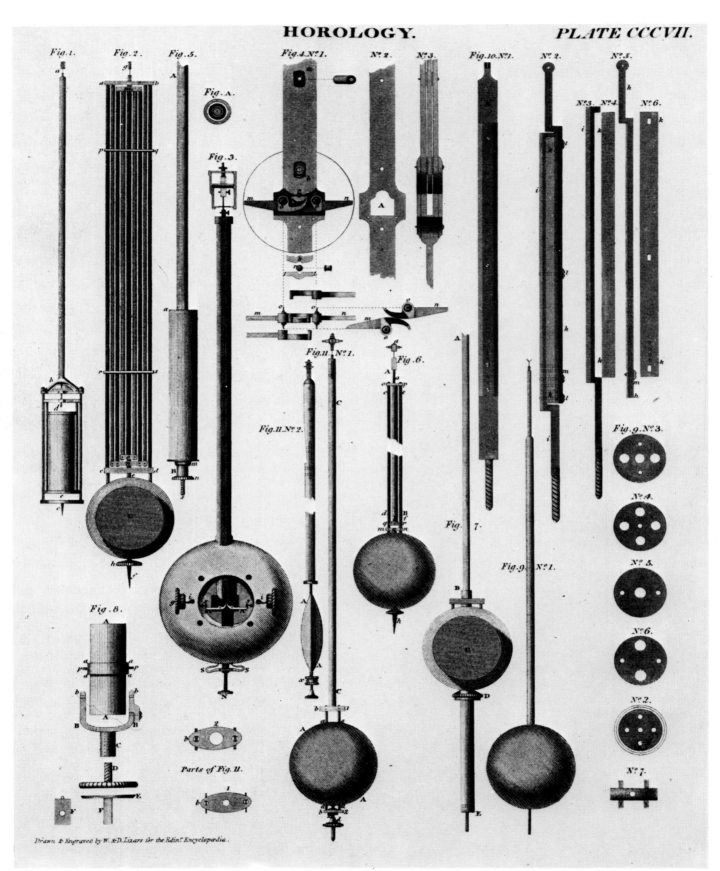

Once the necessity of temperature compensation for both clocks and watches had been accepted, a great deal of experimentation was applied to the problem as this plate taken from *The Edinburgh Encyclopaedia* shows. This work, which was edited by David Brewster LL.D., F.R.S.,

appeared in 1816, and some of the designs include: Figure 1, Graham's mercury pendulum as improved by Thomas Reid; Figure 2, Harrison's gridiron pendulum; Figure 3, Ellicott's pendulum.

or cold. The compensation curb, usually a U-shaped bi-metallic strip, is so arranged that the ends of the 'U' close up in heat; if one of these is fixed and the other grasps the outermost coil of the balance spring, it will, under these conditions, pull on the spring, effectively shortening it and thus causing the watch to gain when it would otherwise lose. This system has certain defects and was eventually abandoned in British watches, although elsewhere in Europe it survived in use even on the more expensive products providing that no exceptional degree of accuracy was required.

A better system was possible once the laminating of the brass and steel strips had been perfected; riveting was insufficiently rigid, so that soldering, and eventually fusing, the strips together was infinitely preferable. The improved arrangement, which survives in use today, depended upon forming the rim of the balance wheel out of two semi-circular bi-metallic strips, one end of each being fixed to the arm of the balance wheel, the other, unattached end carrying a small weight. The free ends of the strips move towards or away from the the centre of the balance with changes in temperature. Balances of this kind are sometimes called 'cut balances', to distinguish them from those with a solid rim. For most practical uses they give an adequate performance, but they do introduce an added complexity called 'middle temperature error' which, when affecting marine chronometers used in navigation, can be significant. To correct this, many different methods of so called 'auxiliary compensation' have been tried.

There are other factors – barometric pressure, for instance – that can affect the accuracy of timekeeping of a clock, but none of such significance as those mentioned at length. Positional errors nowadays are averaged out; that is to say, a good wristwatch is tried in the six principal positions and the best average performance obtained in each. An inexpensive wristwatch will only be tried in two positions, while in a pocket watch positional errors have a relatively small effect anyway. As for temperature compensation, the situation was revolutionised by the inventions earlier this century of the alloys 'Invar' and 'Elinvar'. The inventor, Dr Guillaume of Paris, won the Nobel Prize in 1920 for these improved alloys, which undergo negligible change as a result of differences in temperature. 'Invar' was used for pendulum rods, while 'Elinvar', used for balance springs, eliminated middle temperature error as well as rendering both balance wheel and spring non-magnetic.

'Complications', as applied to clocks and watches, is almost a self-explanatory term. A 'complicated' clock or watch is, at least in theory, any that does more than simply tell the time. Nowadays many so-called complications have become so commonplace as to make the term inapprop-

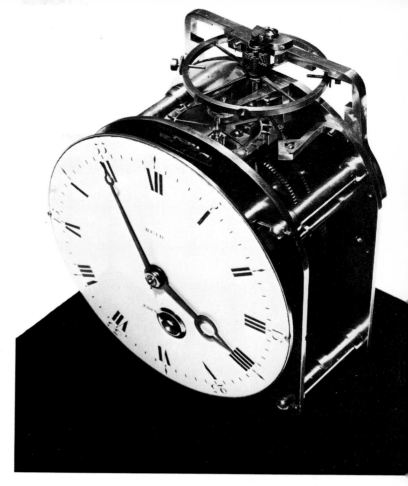

Edinburgh was the home not only of the *Encyclopaedia*, but also of a very fine early nineteenth-century horologist and technical writer, Thomas Reid. This clock of his presents some curious contradictions. Its massive chronometer escapement, beating two seconds, and therefore essentially a precision controller, is nevertheless allied to a solid uncompensated balance wheel. The back plate of the movement is signed 'Thos. Reid, Edinburgh. 1803', and it is possible that it was intended mainly for demonstration purposes.

riate. Nevertheless, for the sake of completeness, it may be convenient to review the various kinds of 'attachments', as they are also sometimes called, which may be superimposed upon the basic 'going' train, that is, the mechanism that just tells the time.

The indicators of any clock or watch are, of course, the dial and hands; the first is usually fixed, with the second moving against it. There is a whole range of complications that extend these visible indications, of which a number derive from the calendar. A simple calendar mechanism, which is just pushed forward once every twenty-four hours by the going train, can still give both day of the week and day of the month indications, as well as the month itself and sometimes the year. Such a mechanism has, of course, to be adjusted manually for leap years, as well as for months of less than thirty-one days. In the most complicated clocks and watches, however, it is possible for this to be done automatically, and then the mechanism is described as a 'perpetual calendar'.

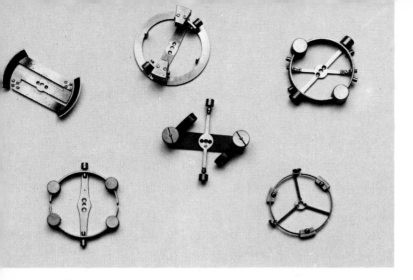

The need to compensate a balance wheel against temperature changes is most marked when it is applied to chronometers, and many chronometermakers of the eighteenth and nineteenth centuries designed special balances to this end. A selection of these is shown. Museum of the Worshipful Company of Clockmakers, Guildhall, London.

An extension of simple calendarwork is the moon dial. The lunar cycle is 29½ days, and 'age of the moon' or 'moon phases', as it is variously called, was a popular adjunct in both clocks and watches, even until quite recent times. Essentially it consists of a disc with, usually, two representations of the moon thereon; this disc revolves behind a cut-away aperture in the dial. Generally the moon disc has fifty-nine teeth cut upon its outer edge – twice 29½, that is – and these are nudged forward one at a time every twelve or twenty-four hours, depending upon the particular arrangement. Before the time when street lighting became universal, it was quite important to know whether or not the moon would be up; and lunar work on clocks is a well-recognised feature from about 1750.

Associated with a moon dial is, rather more rarely, a tidal dial which purports to give an approximation of high tide at a designated place. Found on some eighteenth-century longcase and spring clocks, they must have been useful in tidal waters where the river or coast provided a means of transport.

Another visible indication of value in earlier times, but even then rarely provided, was an 'equation' dial. The equation referred to is the so-called equation of time, that is to say, the relationship between mean time and solar time. Given this relationship, it is possible, whenever the sun shines, to check one's clock or watch by a sundial; and before the advent of the time signal by telephone or radio, and unless one lived within easy reach either of an observatory or of a watch- or clockmaker possessing a regulator clock, this was the only way to do it, except by setting up a telescope and carrying out an observation of 'a transit of a specified star across a meridian' – which no layman in his right mind would be inclined to undertake! Having said this, tables setting out the equation of time were printed year by year – they will sometimes be discovered fixed inside the longcase clocks – so that a separate equation dial was something of a luxury. Technically, too, it was not without its difficulties of accomplishment. Mean time and solar time only agree on four days during any year, and at other times the difference between them varies between extremes of about +16½ minutes and −14½. The principal component of the motion work by which this reading is given continuously on a clock is an ingeniously designed cam, which, because of its shape, is called the 'kidney piece'.

Remembering that mechanical clocks can be designed to go for as long as a year at one winding, any information at all which is based on time-measurement, whether the interval concerned be long or short, can be shown on a clock dial – and probably has been, at some time or another. Thus times of sunrise and sunset for the farmer, Saints' days for the religious community, or just a ship rocking on painted waves to show that time passes – or that the clock is still going – are all to be found in varying degrees of rarity. In some early clocks, certainly in the monumental astronomical clocks of the sixteenth century, much more information was provided, since these catered not only for the astronomer but for the astrologer as well. To appreciate that there was formerly a most intimate relationship between astronomy and astrology, it is only necessary to know that, in the latter, it was firmly held that the five planets which had up to that time been located, together with the sun and the moon, influenced the lives of all on earth, successively each hour according to their distances from it, starting with the most distant and working inwards. Hence the appearance on such clocks of the Zodiac, which was thought to be a belt, about 18° wide, in the heavens, outside which the sun, moon and planets do not pass. There was also a certain amount of other miscellaneous information, probably of use both to laity and to clergy, such as the Dominical Letter, from which was ascertained the date of Easter Sunday; the Golden Number, which is related to the nineteen-year cycle regulating the repetition of the days of the full moon; the Epact, which is the age of the moon on each 1st January; and the Solar Cycle, a period of twenty-eight years after which the days of the month fall on the same days of the week once again. It is really not too long a step from clocks of this kind, to those much more modern ones with a multiplicity of dials, which each show the time in some stated capital city of the world. Anyone who may wish to see a modern example of a hyper-complicated clock, embracing a number of those indications listed above as well as many more, has only to visit the Jens Olsen World Clock in Copenhagen, completed as recently as 1945.

46

Another whole class of visible complications, of which mention must be made, is that which would nowadays be called 'timers'. These are devices drawing upon the main timekeeping property of the clock or watch mechanism to measure off smaller intervals for special purposes. The 'stop watch' is, strictly speaking, simply a watch with a seconds hand and a means of halting the escapement – that is to say, the entire watch – usually by the simple expedient of a lever that pushes a pin in between the teeth of the escape wheel. Many watches were so equipped during the nineteenth century and earlier, and they are sometimes called 'doctor's watches' although whether they served any useful purpose when measuring the pulse it is hard to say. The chronograph, in horology, is associated with the kind of watch that has a separate seconds hand, capable of being stopped, started and returned to zero, although its literal meaning – a writer of time – does have some foundation in the so-called 'inking chronograph', patented by F. L. Fatton in 1822. In his design, there was a dial on both sides of the watch. That on the back revolved, but there was a fixed arm terminating in an ink reservoir and nib which, by pressing a button on the outside of the case, could be brought momentarily in contact with it, leaving a tiny mark. At the end of the

below left
This under-dial view shows a particularly complicated Swiss watch by Nicholas Monnier, of the early nineteenth century. Not only does it strike the hours – properly, it is called a clock-watch – but it repeats the quarters; furthermore, by operating a slide on the band, Grande Sonnerie is obtainable. If that was not enough, this clock-watch possesses the rare virgule escapement.

The most common form of musical watch movement is that introduced by the Swiss, early in the nineteenth century in which a disc, pinned on both sides, revolves between individually tuned steel teeth. This example by Piguet et Meylan illustrates the arrangement. Such watches are generally based on the cylinder escapement and often also have a quarter-repeating motion.

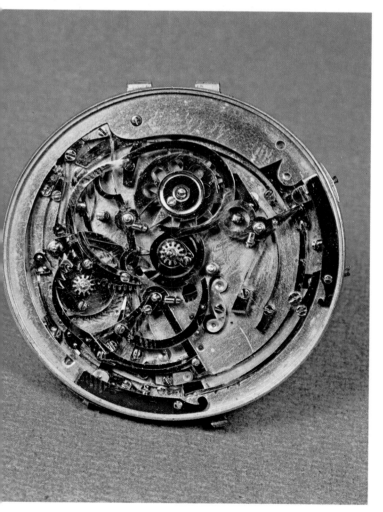

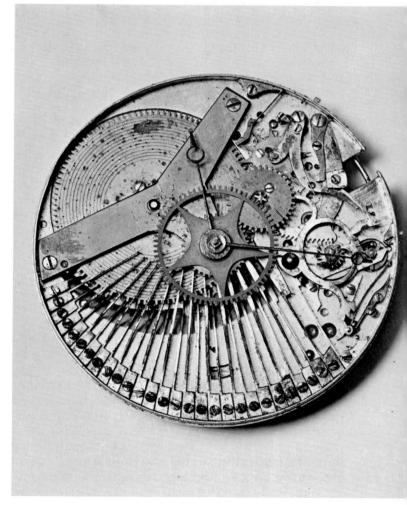

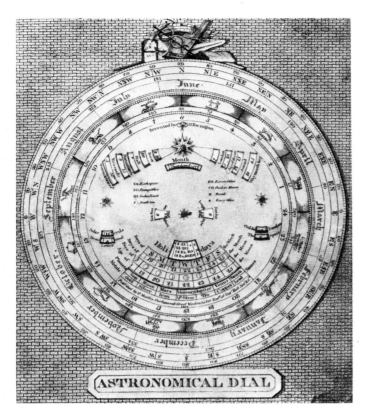

ASTRONOMICAL DIAL

The ordinary man's continuing interest in astronomical – and, in view of the inclusion of the zodiac, presumably also astrological – phenomena is well demonstrated by this cardboard 'Astronomical Dial'. Apparently 'invented by H. Ewington' and 'Published by G. Medley, Parliament Street, Westminster, entered at Stationers' Hall, November 25th, 1802', it consists essentially of a printed dial with a number of cut-out sectors behind which volvelles can be moved by hand to give a variety of interrelated information.

interval being timed, a second mark could be made upon the dial and the time between the two marks computed. Afterwards, the marks were simply erased and the procedure could start again. Another form of this type of instrument is called a 'split seconds chronograph'. In this, two seconds hands, mounted on the same axis one above the other, revolve together continuously in normal use. However, one of them can be stopped at will, for instance at the start of a period to be timed, the end of the period being noted on the other hand as it continues to revolve. The stopped hand can then be zeroed back to the revolving hand. In yet another form, of long usage throughout the eighteenth and nineteenth centuries, subsidiary hands, often driven by an independent train with its own mainspring, 'jumped' various fractions of a second, usually fifths or quarters, and could be stopped and started by a lever or push-piece. It is difficult, at this distance of time, to say with certainty what some of them may have been used for; they are generally beautifully made, yet their actions sometimes have an air of novelty about them. Present-day chronographs, of course, not only measure

seconds, but also have dials recording minutes and even hours.

So far we have been concerned with visible complications, and before we leave them to deal with audible ones mention should be made of another sort of visual effect, which, although generally not intended to be of an informative nature, occurs in various forms at virtually all horological periods. This is the automation, defined as 'a machine which moves by concealed machinery'. In clocks and watches, the word is applied to any image of man or beast of which part, or the whole, moves.

There were certainly some simple automata incorporated in various early water clocks, but the first application to a mechanical clock was probably the monumental cock which surmounted the first Strasbourg cathedral clock, constructed about 1355. This remarkable automaton is dealt with at length in the next chapter.

Other automata were regularly associated with huge astronomical clocks of similar type. Usually these took the form of processions – either of religious figures or of royal ones – which passed through a cycle of movements at set times, returning to their original state at the end in readiness for their next appearance. The sixteenth and early seventeenth centuries were renowned for the great heights to which the finest mechanics had developed clockwork, and many examples of their skill remain. The great gilt ship-clock or *nef* attributed to Hans Schlottheim, and made for Emperor Rudolph II about 1580, almost incidentally incorporates a clock; far more spectacular was its capacity to run up and down the banqueting table under its own power, swaying to imaginary waves and firing its guns as it went, while an organ played and the Heralds and Electors processed past the enthroned Emperor. Then again, the clocks of Isaac Habrecht – who made the second Strasbourg cathedral clock between about 1571 and 1574 – tend to combine a fine show of astronomical information with automata. The lineal descendants of such clocks as these are to be seen in the succession of Guinness exhibition clocks which were such a feature of life in Britain in quite recent years, and also the Liberty's clock, set above the entrance to that department store just off Regent Street in London.

So far, examples given have been on the grand scale – public clocks, in the main. This prolific early period surprisingly also provided many examples of domestic clocks incorporating automata, the great majority coming from centres such as Augsburg, renowned for its highly skilled mechanics. There is such a huge variety of these clocks that it is only possible to summarise them briefly. Their themes were either religious – the Crucifix clock is a well-known type – or else animals were the basis of the design, and in these cases it was customary for their eyes to roll in time with the escapement, wings to flap or beaks to open at the hour, and so on.

There was, from earliest times, a much simpler automaton than any of the rather sophisticated mechanisms so far described. This was the clock 'jack' – contracted by the English from '*jaquemart*', which is said to mean 'Jack o' the clock' in reference to the fourteenth-century clock in Dijon, in France. A 'jack' is simply a figure holding a hammer, with which it strikes the hour on a bell. One of the best-known examples is Jack Blandifer, the figure that performs this duty in Wells cathedral; he also kicks the quarters with his heels on two other bells.

Watches were not without their automata, too, although generally this was a much later development than in clocks, and often somewhat less reputable. The Swiss, by the beginning of the nineteenth century, had perfected watches which, on depressing the pendant, set in motion complete scenes of moving people and animals – stonemasons or woodcutters at work, smithy work of all kinds, often accompanied by swans feeding on a millpond, goats browsing and so forth. In another version, *jaquemart* figures were placed either side of a dial made smaller to accommodate them; these appeared to strike the hours on tiny bells when activated by the pendant, although such striking was actually carried out inside the watch, upon curved tuned wire gongs sited around the edge of the case. It was not long, however, before this penchant for mechanical invention degenerated, resulting in a spate of so-called erotic watches, often incorporating secret panels above the dial or in the back of the case which had first to be opened before the scene could be viewed. Some of these were well executed, but the great majority were of coarse workmanship, and have been correctly compared to that other phenomenon, of more recent provenance, which is so aptly summed up in the opening gambit of the trader in such objects: 'Filthy postcards for nice English gentleman?' Such products do not bear comparison, either, with another type of erotic watch, usually of the late eighteenth century, in which a static scene is painted in enamels behind a secret double back of the case. Many watches of this variety are of genuinely high quality, incorporating painting of exceptional standard so that despite their content, they will frequently be acceptable as works of art in their own right.

The final variant, as well as the commonest, in this catalogue of the complications that can be associated with simple time-measurement is the audible effect. The first device to sound the time was the alarm; it preceded any arrangement for striking the hours or even for showing the time. Indeed, the first clocks in monastic usage were nothing other than what nowadays would be called 'timers'. They simply sounded a bell at pre-

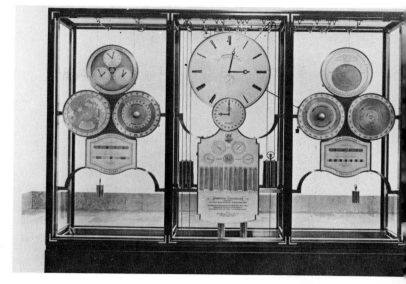

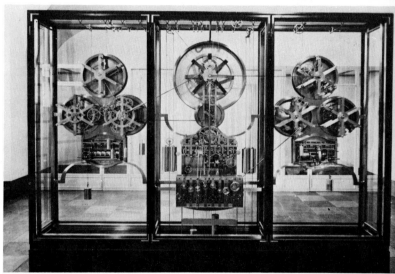

The Jens Olsen World Clock, housed in Copenhagen City Hall, was completed in 1945 and is probably the most complicated modern mechanical clock in existence. It is a worthy successor to the tradition of great complicated clocks elsewhere in Europe.

determined intervals, to warn the clock-keeper that some particular office was due. In effect, the going train unlocked the alarm train when the correct point in time was reached, and the latter continued ringing until it ran down. Alarms have been commonplace ever since those early days, in both clocks and watches, with no great variation in the principle involved, except perhaps that the alarm action can usually be curtailed at will.

The ability to strike hours upon a bell has been known from very early times, and the first, and simplest, method of doing it, which was applied to both clocks and watches, is known as 'count wheel' or 'locking plate' striking. The count wheel, which effectually 'counts' the strokes of the hour being struck, is a toothless wheel, the edge of which has been divided into unequal sections, running

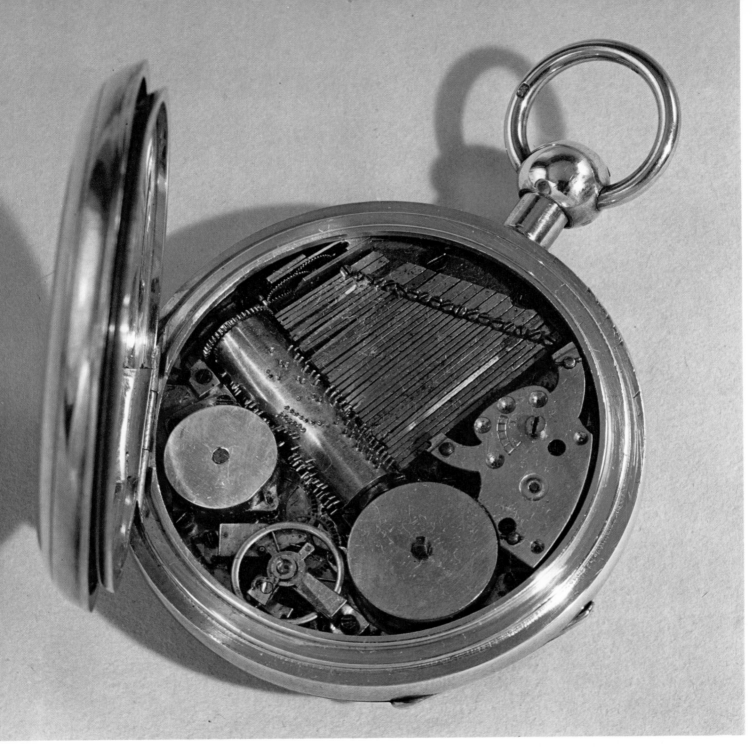

Another variant of the musical watch exactly copies the principle of a musical box in that the tunes are pinned out – the horological term is 'pricked' – on to a revolving cylinder which abuts upon the ends of the tuned teeth of a steel comb. This model also generally dates from the early nineteenth century. British Museum, London.

from the shortest to the longest in relation to striking the hours of one through to twelve. A notch divides each section from its neighbour, and, at rest, the striking detent, which is a kind of lever used for locking and unlocking parts of a machine, lies in one of the notches. When the going train reaches the hour, it lifts the detent out of its notch, and the count wheel starts to rotate, at the same time as the hammer sounds the hour at a controlled rate on the hour-bell. The detent rides over the slowly turning edge of the count wheel until the hour corresponding to that segment of the wheel has been struck, when it reaches the next notch along the edge, into which it drops, locking up the striking train until the next time.

The system works quite well although it is more susceptible to derangement than the one which succeeded it; but its major drawback is its capacity for getting out of synchronisation with the going train, more often than not due to resetting the hands without allowing the striking train to strike in full every intervening hour between the old setting and the new, a time-consuming operation. It is quite easy to correct this fault if it arises: it is simply necessary to leave the clock hands as they are, but keep on releasing the striking train by hand until eventually it strikes the hour shown on the dial; but the system is not foolproof, and misuse can possibly damage it. Even so, in some countries and in clocks where there were no complications, locking plate striking found considerable popularity; it appears in many French and American clocks throughout the nineteenth century.

A better system, invented by the Rev. Edward Barlow in 1676, is called 'rack and snail' striking. A rack, in horological parlance, is a segment of a toothed wheel, while a snail is a cam cut in steps. At the hour, the rack drops, its tail resting against the snail. This component revolves with the hour hand, exhibiting to the tail of the rack a different step for each hour, and leaving to be gathered up only the related number of teeth on the rack. When the train is released, a 'gathering pallet' rotates, collecting up the rack one tooth at a time until the hour striking is completed. The train is then locked up once more. The great advantage of this system is that, since the hour snail is directly connected to the hour hand, the two can never get out of synchronisation, and the hands can always be reset in a continuous manoeuvre, without any need to strike out each intervening hour in full. The system catches up by itself.

In passing, it is worth noting that there have been other forms of striking than that with which most of us today are familiar. Joseph Knibb, a celebrated seventeenth-century clockmaker, devised 'Roman striking', in which two bells of different pitch were used, the one representing the Roman 'I', the other the Roman 'V'. Using this method, and regarding 'X' as twice 'V', no more than four strokes need ever be heard, whatever the hour; and this was particularly important at a time when most domestic clocks went for eight days, throughout which duration it would require an inordinately long spring to drive the striking train, with only one winding. Another method of striking, known as Dutch striking, was directed towards clarifying the half-hour stroke of a clock which, if heard from so far away that the hands could not be read against the dial, was of little practical use. In this system, again, two bells were used. The hour was struck on the larger, deeper bell; but when the half-hour arrived, the next succeeding hour was struck on the smaller, higher-pitched bell. This system eventually led to that

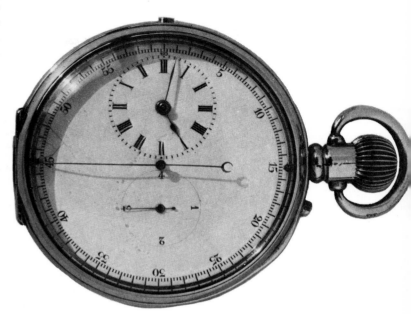

Although this particular watch, which is unsigned, dates from about 1860 and is apparently of Swiss manufacture, it is not clear, as with so many early timers, what it was intended to do. The escapement beats quarter-seconds, and both the large hand and the small hand below the centre of the dial, measure off quarters. The small hand was probably intended to confirm to the nearest quarter second the movement of the larger second hand, and it is possible that the watch was associated with gunnery. This type of watch – although previously key wound, rather than keyless – was made from the end of the eighteenth century onwards, beating either quarters or fifths of a second, and usually based on a cylinder escapement.

known as full Grande Sonnerie striking, during the last quarter of the seventeenth century. In this latter arrangement, after each quarter is sounded, it is followed by the last preceding hour.

It was a simple step from hour striking by rack and snail to chiming the quarters by a similar system. Dr Barlow further modified his system to produce the first 'repeater', that is to say, a clock or watch that one can cause to sound the time at will, either by pulling a cord at the side of the case or, for a watch, depressing the pendant or pushing a sliding piece set into the band of the case. His application for a patent for this invention was opposed by the celebrated London clockmaker Daniel Quare, supported by the Worshipful Company of Clockmakers. In the end, the matter was referred to the monarch, who gave preference to Quare only because in his arrangement one process activated both hours and quarters, whereas in Barlow's two actions were necessary to achieve the same result.

In case it may be thought that hour-striking has always been a facility confined to clocks, it may perhaps be mentioned at this point that hour-

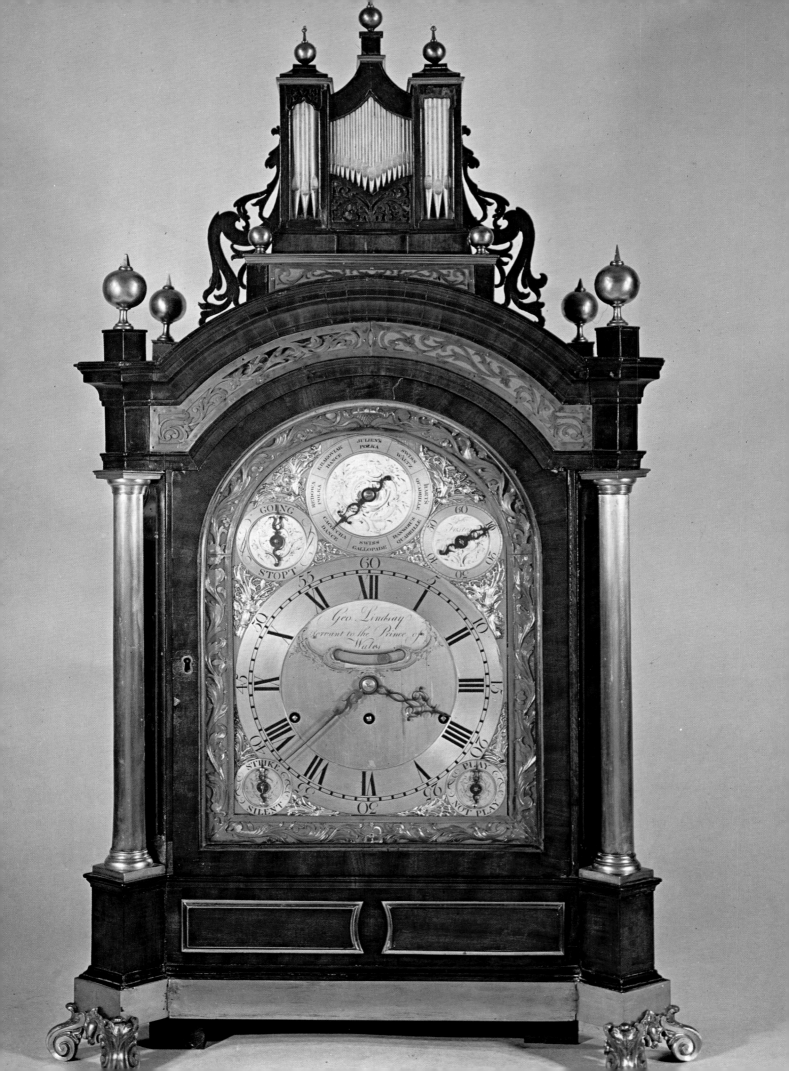

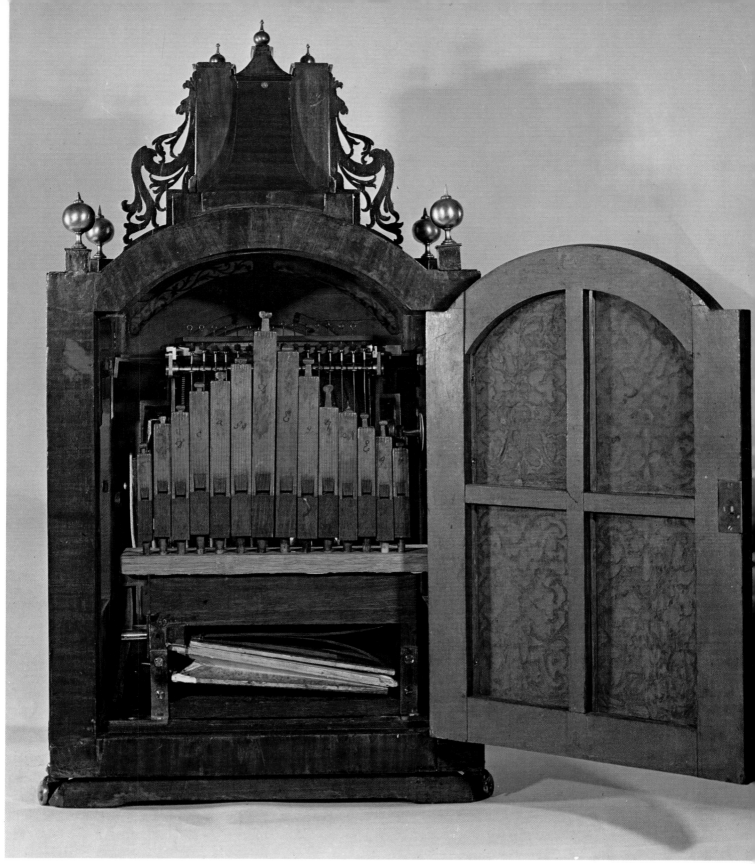

This large clock by George Lindsay was a favourite of the late Courtenay Ilbert when it was in his collection. Lindsay, who frequently signed himself 'Servant to the Prince of Wales' or 'Watchmaker to His Majesty', enjoyed a Royal Warrant from George III and seems to have specialised in elaborate musical clocks; both organ clocks and clocks incorporating a musical train on bells are recorded. British Museum, London.

This rear view of the previous illustration shows the small organ operating automatically. It plays a choice of eight tunes every three hours. British Museum, London.

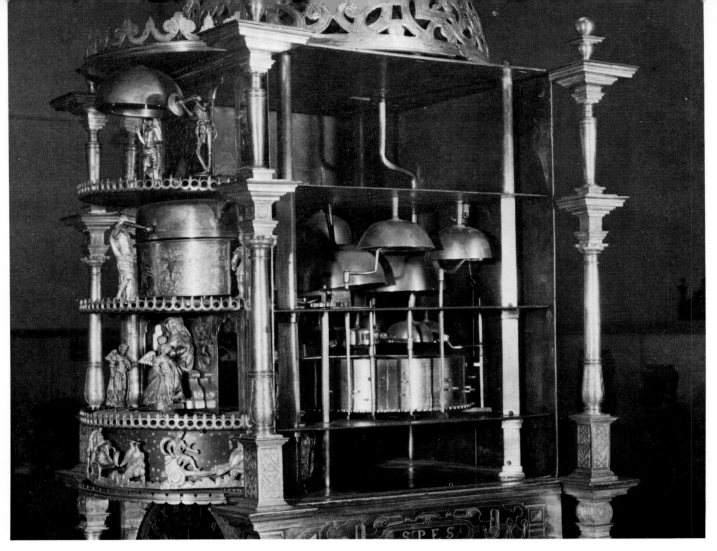

Isaac Habrecht's famous clock of 1589 has four levels of automata above the clock mechanism proper. These show, starting from the bottom, the planetary deities representing the days of the week, next a seated Madonna and Child in silver accepting the homage of angels. The third floor up has four silver figures representing the four Ages of Man, and on the topmost floor is the figure of Death who strikes the hours, whilst from the left and through a door the figure of the resurrected Christ appears. British Museum, London.

striking watches have been known for centuries, certainly from early in the seventeenth century to the present time. Correctly, they are called 'clock-watches' – or, a more recent usage, 'striking watches' – and some of the finest early watches combined striking and alarm facilities.

Repetition work, in general, utilises the rack and snail system used for hour striking and quarter chiming, but allows them to be activated at will. The first repeating systems gave the time only to the nearest quarter, usually on two bells – 'ting-tang quarters', as they were sometimes called – the usual arrangement being first to sound the last hour struck, followed by double strokes, one on each of two bells, for each quarter-hour completed since that last full hour. Thus, say, at a quarter to ten, the repeater would sound nine strokes for the last full hour, followed by three double strokes, one for each subsequent quarter.

During the eighteenth century, repetition work was greatly refined, so that the hour became divided by half-quarters – that is, eight periods of seven and a half minutes each – and then into twelve periods of five minutes. Half-quarter and five-minute repeaters operate upon the same system as quarter repeaters, only that, after the last complete quarter sounded, there may be a further 'tang' if more than seven and a half minutes of the

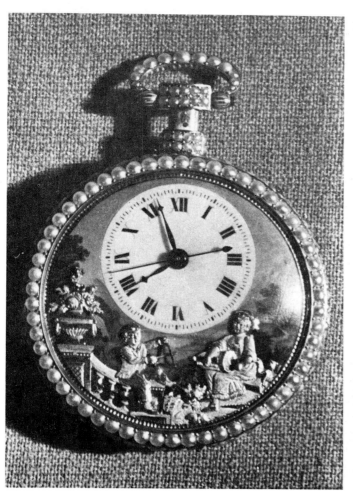

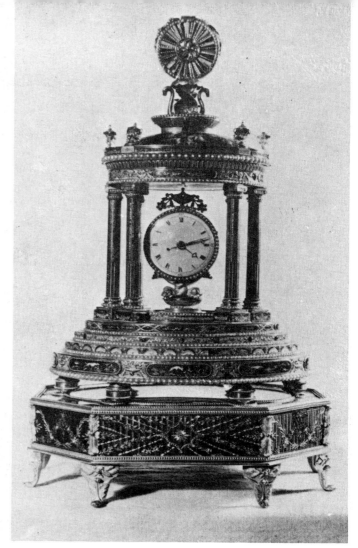

The Swiss have been supreme in devising automata for watches, and this particular example by Piguet et Meylan and dating from the early nineteenth century was formerly in the collection of King Farouk of Egypt which was sold up in 1954. Not only has the watch a musical train, but below the dial is a figure of a boy playing a triangle and a girl playing a hurdygurdy, both in vari-coloured gold.

above right
In this remarkable creation, the automaton is not in the image of a human being, but in the coloured revolving spiral supported by swans which surmounts the whole. In the base is a carillon musical movement, while the timekeeping is by Staplin of London and dates from the late eighteenth century. Formerly the property of King Farouk of Egypt.

succeeding quarter has passed; or, if it is a five-minute repeater, conceivably up to two 'tangs' indicating ten minutes of the next quarter has been measured off. Inevitably, of course, the final refinement, the minute repeater, appeared upon the scene; there are eighteenth-century examples of this, although it was not until the nineteenth century that it was made in any quantity, particularly in the case of watches. In the minute repeater, the last hour is struck upon the lower-pitched of two bells or gongs; the last quarter is represented as double strokes, exactly as previously; then the number of minutes completed after the last quarter struck is sounded with single strokes upon the higher-pitched bell.

Although not frequently encountered, it might make a fitting finish to this examination of the rudiments of clockwork to mention the part played in it by music of various kinds. It has always been only a short step, technically, from a clock that chimes quarters upon eight bells to one that plays a selection from several different tunes on, perhaps, fourteen. The principle is simply that of the commonplace musical box, but with the rotating barrel and the strategically placed pins protruding from it actuating the tails of bell hammers, rather than the steel teeth of the tuned musical 'comb' with which everyone is familiar.

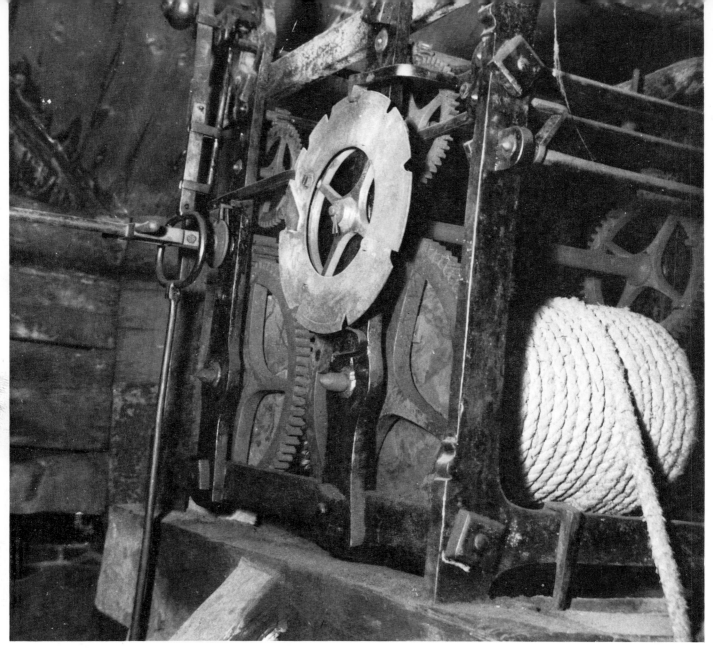

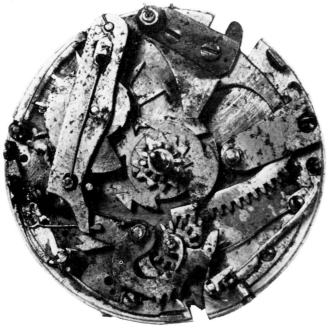

Of the two methods of controlling the striking used on both clocks and watches, the later and more efficient was that known as the rack and snail, which can be seen on page 33. The earlier system was known as count wheel striking and depended upon dividing the circumference of a wheel into sectors proportional to the number of hours to be struck from 1 to 12. This photograph shows the count wheel of a tower clock on a large country house: the clock dates from Queen Anne's time and has recently been thoroughly restored.

It was not long after quarter-repeating work had been perfected that this was further refined to give half quarters – i.e. seven and a half minutes – and then five-minute repeaters. This early eighteenth-century movement by John Bushman is an example of the latter.

The ultimate refinement of a repeating watch had to be striking the time to the nearest minute. It is possible that this was perfected before the end of the eighteenth century, but it did not come into common usage until the nineteenth. This example is by Dent, watchmakers to the Queen and the firm that built Big Ben. The unique characteristic of a minute repeating mechanism is clearly visible: this is the four-armed snail, each arm having fourteen teeth cut into it, which can be seen in the centre of the movement.

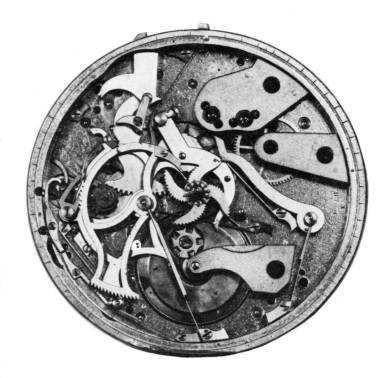

Carillons of bells operating upon this system have been associated with quite early church clocks, as well as with rather smaller creations. There is in the British Museum, for instance, a carillon clock by Nicholas Vallin dated 1598, which, with an overall height of only 23 inches, cannot have been intended for public use. This clock, the earliest known clock with a carillon to be made in England, albeit by a Flemish craftsman, plays a tune on thirteen bells just before each hour, a short phrase at the quarters and a slightly longer fragment at the half-hour. As for carillons in larger clocks, it is known that the original Strasbourg cathedral clock, built in the fourteenth century, incorporated such a mechanism. The oldest surviving one, however, is probably the clock said to date from 1542, which was taken from the church of St Jacob, in The Hague, and which is now preserved in the Clock Museum in Utrecht.

Musical watches were being made in London by a certain John Archambo early in the eighteenth century, the tunes being played upon sets of hemispherical bells set upon a common stem and concealed in the back of the watch case. Inevitably, however, such watches were large, and musical watches did not really enjoy much of a vogue until the early nineteenth century, when the tuned comb was adapted from the musical box. Two types of musical watch, both made principally in Switzerland, are known from this period. In the first, the action exactly replicates that of a musical box, with a small pin-barrel revolving against tuned steel teeth set parallel to one another. The other version, which is the more common, as well as enabling the watch to be made thinner, utilises instead of a pin-barrel a revolving disc, in which pins are inserted upon both sides. The separate teeth of the comb have their feet planted around the outer circumference of the movement, where they are out of the way of the mechanism proper; the effect, however, is to form a wedge of steel rods pointed at the disc, which would be quite incapable of operation were it not for the fact that alternate ones pass above and below it.

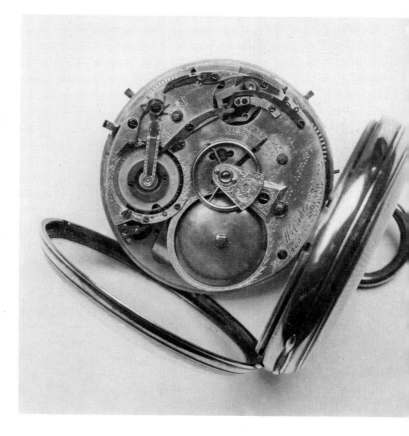

This musical watch by James McCabe which dates from about 1800, is a throw back to an earlier era when makers such as John Archambo, in the first half of the eighteenth century, were making large watches which played tunes on bells. This very much smaller watch nevertheless employs five hammers striking on four bells. Museum of the Worshipful, Company of Clockmakers, Guildhall, London.

57

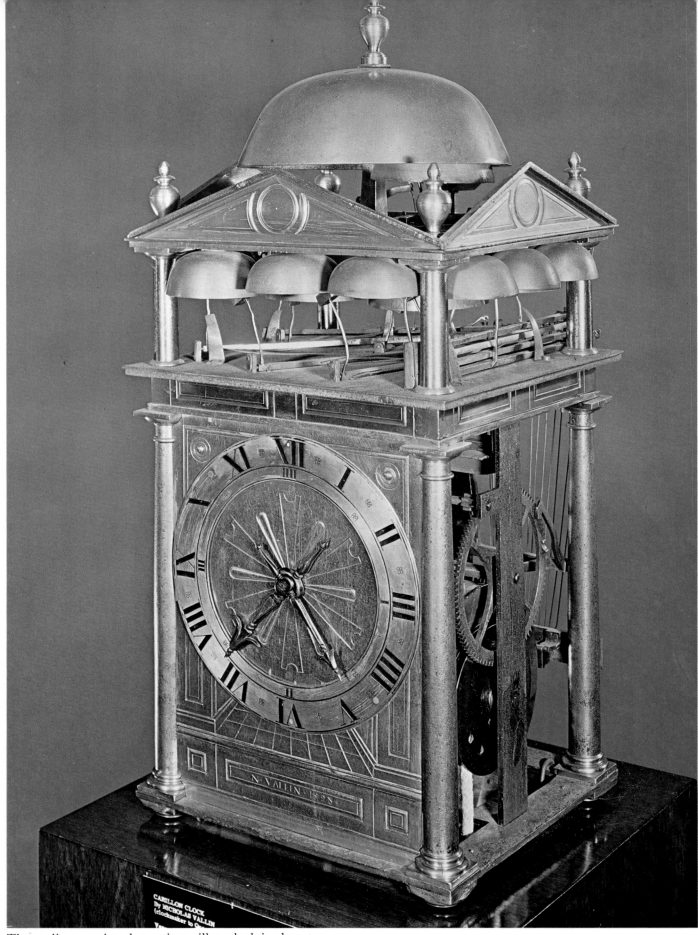

The earliest surviving domestic carillon clock is almost certainly this one by Nicholas Vallin which is dated 1598. The carillon consists of thirteen bells. British Museum, London.

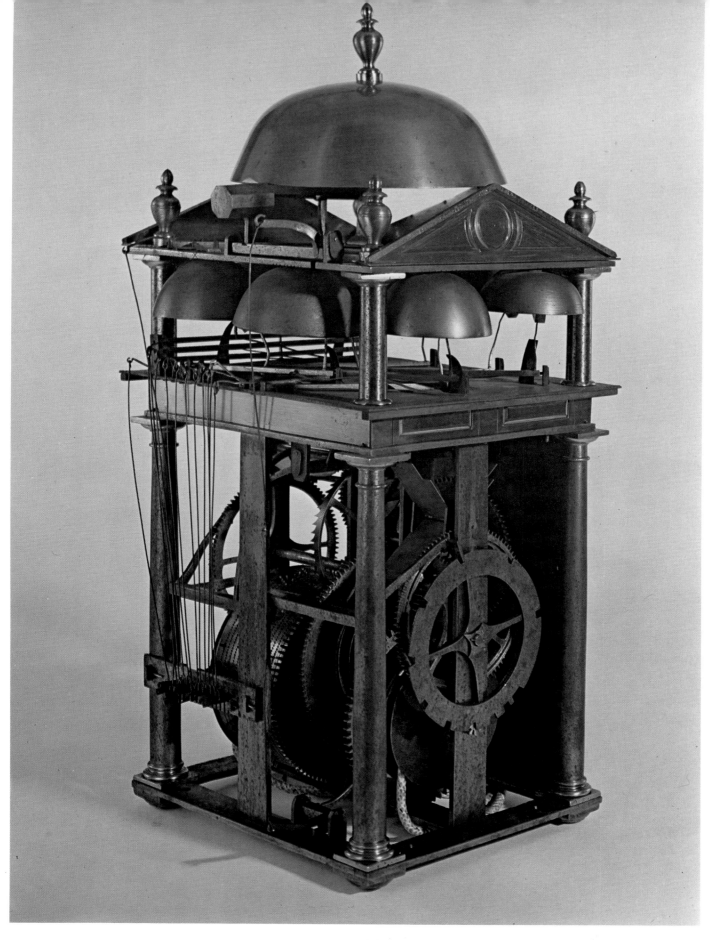

This view shows more clearly the operation of the carillon with its vertically mounted pin-barrel. Visible in the centre foreground is the striking count wheel. British Museum, London.

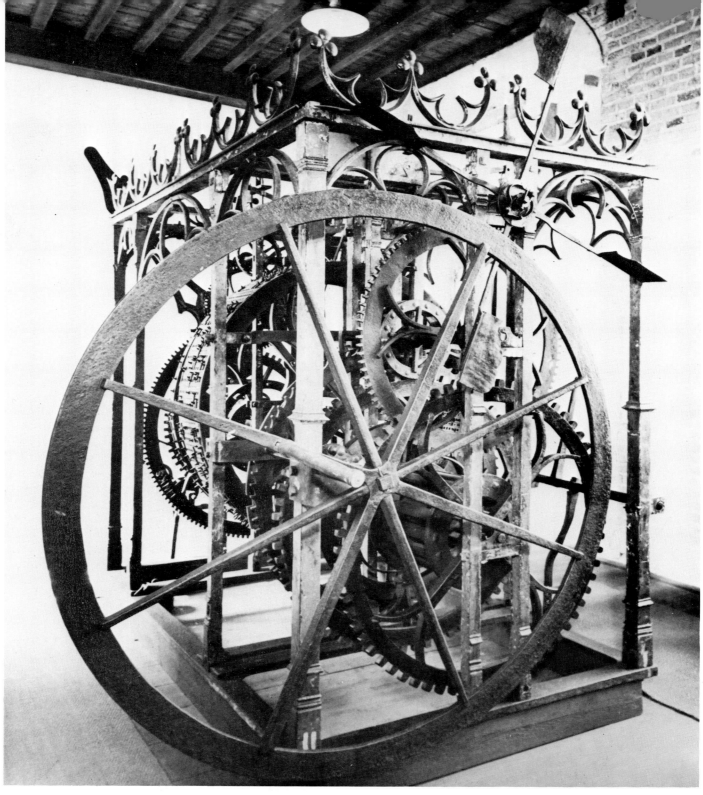

The church of St Jacob in The Hague originally possessed a clock with what is believed to be the earliest surviving carillon mechanism, which is attributed to the year 1542. The pinned drum which operated the carillon is visible towards the end of the mechanism. It is five feet in diameter and fifteen inches wide.

Other musical forms incorporated into clocks and watches at various times have included organs, singing birds and even a barking dog, if that can be classified under this heading! Almost any combination of complications is possible – and has probably been made, at some time or another –

so that it is understandable that terms like 'triple-complicated watch', which means a watch incorporating chronograph mechanism, repeatingwork and a calendar, should come into use, ugly though it may sound. There must be some slight sense of loss, however, that such objects are unobtainable new and, as antiques, are prohibitively expensive. They added some quality, springing from pure craftsmanship and the pride taken in its practice, to daily life which nowadays is totally absent, and which is certainly missed by discriminating people.

Great Clocks of the 'Iron' Age

As has been mentioned before, the precise – or even the approximate – moment of breakthrough which gave birth to the mechanical clock has so far escaped the historians of science. There are a few established milestones which it will be helpful to review, even though any final conclusion is likely to be elusive.

The single feature of a mechanical clock which must identify it beyond any shadow of doubt is the escapement. When, in the previous chapter, allusion was made briefly to a hydro-mechanical timekeeper of exceptionally early provenance, the clock in question was Su Sung's great astronomical clock of about 1090, although it is apparent that there were other mammoth Chinese clocks in existence and such technology clearly preceded anything that had, up to that time, come into use in either the Arab or European world.

The evidence upon which our knowledge of Su Sung's clock is based is contained in an early Chinese book, of about the date above-mentioned, the significance of which was first discovered by Drs Joseph Needham, Derek Price and Wang Ling in the 1950s. They published their evidence in 1960 (see the Further Reading list on page 254).

Su Sung constructed his clock in the Palace at Kaifeng; it is certain that it was actually built, and that it operated satisfactorily for a number of years. In essentials it was a great astronomical clock-tower, over thirty feet high and surmounted by a bronze power-driven armillary sphere which would have been used for astronomical observation. Below this was a rotating celestial globe – also powered to work automatically – with which comparison could be made from the observations carried out above it. Beneath this again was a five-storeyed pagoda-like structure, each stage of this carrying a procession of automata, ringing bells and gongs and otherwise indicating the hours and special times of the day and night.

Needless to say, all this action required a not inconsiderable power source to drive it. Therefore, also contained within the tower was a great water-wheel, the vanes incorporating scoops to contain the liquid, and this was sufficient to drive all the shafts actuating the various devices. However, from the horological viewpoint, the significant component was the checking mechanism which prevented a scoop descending under the weight of the water it contained until it was full. This device utilised a kind of weighbridge, together with a trip-lever and parallel linkage system, the first to ensure uniformity in filling the scoops, the remainder to stop the wheel at another point so as to bring the next scoop into position on the weighbridge.

This procedure, cumbersome and noisy though it probably was, took place each quarter of an hour; and, although the clock was driven hydraulically, it nevertheless provided for the release and locking of a wheel for the eventual purpose of nudging forward the time-indicating contrivances, step by step, in precisely the manner of any other mechanical escapement. It is a quite remarkable piece of advanced technology, considering its early date; but whether there is any tangible link between it and the clocks of conventional wholly mechanical construction with which we are all familiar, or whether it is a single isolated and individual example of that great genius which typified the Chinese culture at that period, remains to be seen.

Turning now to other considerations regarding the advent of the mechanical clock, it has often been held that, because the first mechanical clocks of which we have any real knowledge are associated with religious institutions, it is reasonable to suppose that it was in such cloistered surroundings, where the tender bloom of philosophical invention might be best expected to flourish, that one should look for the particular spark of

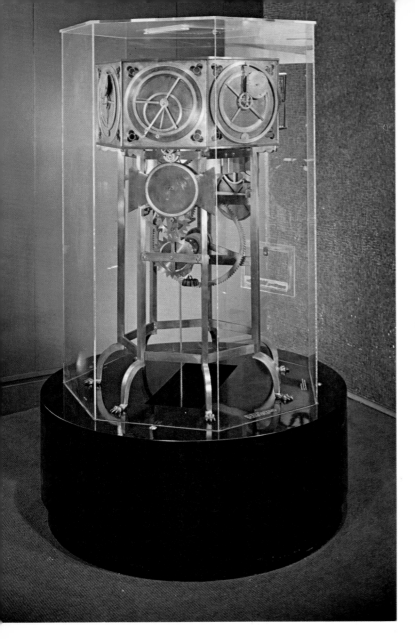

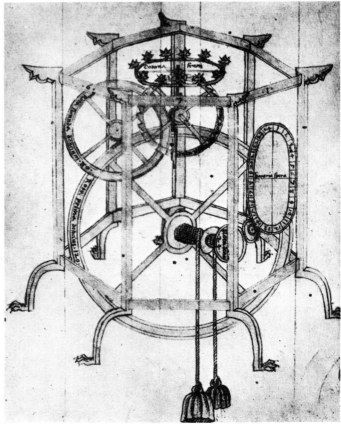

This modern reconstruction of da Dondi's clock, which followed his manuscript in the minutest detail, was carried out under the supervision of the great English horologist, the late H. Alan Lloyd, and was made by Thwaites & Reed of London. The clock itself is now in the Smithsonian Institution, Washington, D.C.

above right
This schematic representation of da Dondi's clock is the earliest known illustration of a weight-driven clock.

creative brilliance that added an escapement to the sum total of mechanical knowledge as it then existed. There are, indeed, in monastic records from very early times innumerable references to 'clocks' described by various linguistic derivatives of the Latin word *horologium*, but what sort of clocks these were is but rarely made clear from the context. Where it is made clear, the reference is invariably to a sundial, a clepsydra or some other kind of non-mechanical timekeeper.

Another school of thought inclines to the belief that clocks somehow arrived in Europe from closer Oriental cultures. The Arabs in the Near East, who were doubtless descended from the Biblical astronomers of Babylon and Chaldea, themselves studied and mapped the heavens and were certainly supreme in designing and manufacturing such essential scientific time-calculating instruments as astrolabes and nocturnals. But so far evidence is lacking as to their mechanical prowess.

What other evidence, of any substance, is left to be considered? There is some documentary evidence that the mechanical escapement had not been discovered by 1277, in which year a remarkable work entitled *Libros del Saber de Astronomia* appeared under the patronage of Alfonso the Wise, King of Castile. Essentially a set of astronomical tables, this work also included an account of past and present inventions for time-measurement, and it is very unlikely that the mechanical clock would have been omitted, had it then been in existence. Yet by 1350 the documentary evidence is of such familiarity with mechanical clocks as to suggest that they had been in common use for some time. It is quite possible that very early clock mechanisms have gone unrecognised since they would have had no dial: indeed only the telltale escapement would reveal to the knowledgeable that they were dealing with a clock.

As to early records, there is a tradition that a clock was erected at Westminster as early as 1288 while in 1286 a record exists of the payment of beer and bread to the 'Orologius' of St Paul's cathedral. There is also a record that a big clock was set up in Canterbury cathedral in 1292. Until comparatively recently it was believed that this series of records, deriving from the twenty years between 1280 and 1300 – in all of which the term for timekeeper remains *horologium* – must have been referring to clepsydrae rather than any mechanical device; but there has recently been a complete reappraisal by experts in this field, as a result of which it is now thought more likely that the mechanical clock first appeared in Europe some time between 1277 and 1300, and that many of these records refer to it. Furthermore, it has long been thought most likely that the clock made its first appearance in Italy or elsewhere in Central Europe. This opinion is also now being revised, since it seems on sound evidence that England may well have been in the van of this technological advance, and that she was certainly no less well informed than other countries at the relevant time. Even so, the first clockmakers were probably so thin on the ground as to make it necessary for them to travel widely in order to pursue their craft, and it is a clear possibility that those working in Britain may have come there from elsewhere in Europe.

The first clocks, therefore, seem certainly to have been used in religious institutions; they may only have been forms of alarm, perhaps with no dial as such, but just a simple means of ringing a bell after a certain period had elapsed; they warned the sacristan of his duties, and they were probably on the ground, rather than hoisted in a tower, as we nowadays expect to find church clocks.

It was not long, however, before true public clocks started to make their appearance in Italy, France and Germany, even though these took the form of belltowers under the control of a bellringer, whose actions in turn were controlled by the sort of mechanical alarm that was used in the monas-

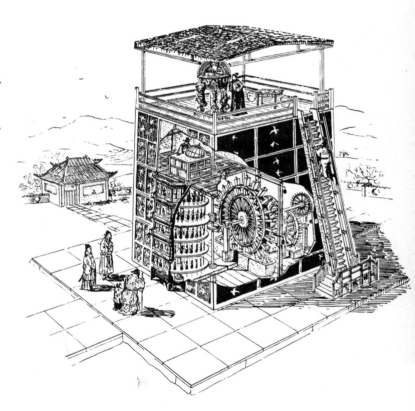

This reconstruction of Su Sung's astronomical clock tower of AD 1090 shows the large water wheel used to drive the various motions including a rotating armillary sphere on the top level and a celestial globe immediately below.

left
In order to test the feasibility of the hydromechanical escapement of Su Sung's clock, this scale model was made in 1962 by Mr J. H. Combridge, an engineer. It proved conclusively that the escapement not only worked, but worked very efficiently. Science Museum, London.

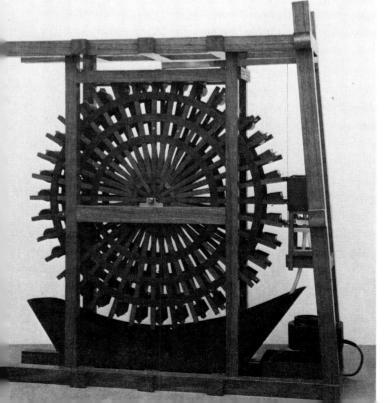

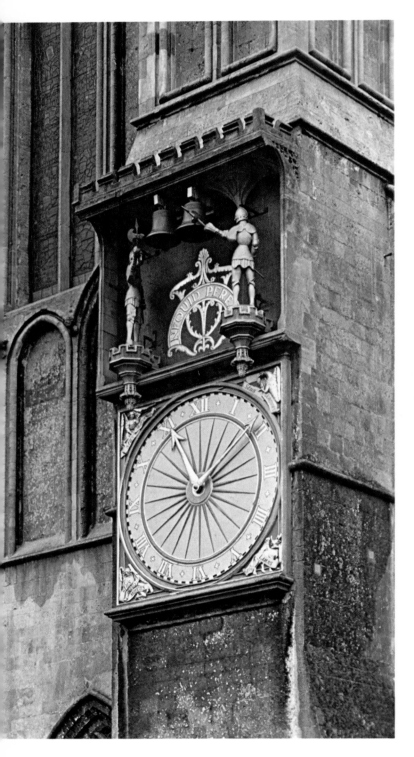

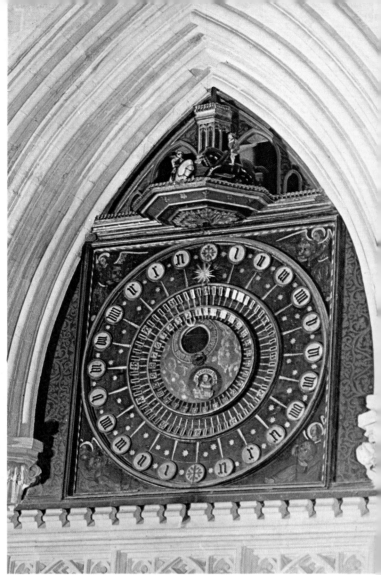

The famous clock at Wells cathedral originally had no dials but now possesses one outside the church and one inside. This is the outside one.

above right
The twenty-four hour astronomical dial – graduated in two periods of twelve hours – at Wells cathedral, is one of the finest medieval dials of its kind in the world. Added to the clock about a century after this was built in 1392, it shows hours, days, dates and moon phases. It also incorporates automata, having four jousting knights above it as well as the oldest *jaquemart* known as Jack Blandifer.

teries. He was required to ring the curfew each night, as well as such other warnings as might become necessary from time to time.

Soon after this, it became possible to substitute a machine for the man ringing the bell – perhaps one of the first instances of automation – and by making it and the bell on a big enough scale and hoisting them up in the air, to provide a time service for the surrounding countryside.

At some quite early moment in the history of mechanical clocks, the mainstream of development split into three separate, even though related, directions. We have so far been following the simplest line – the primitive monastic alarm leading to the eventually somewhat more sophisticated turret clock, which, it might be argued, reached its peak of perfection during the nineteenth century in such masterpieces as the great clock at Westminster. During the period covered by the present chapter, however, such mechanisms were produced in wrought iron by techniques substantially based upon the blacksmith's craft in which hot metal was roughly shaped with the hammer, and files were used for finishing and rounding up. These clocks would have had two trains of gears – at first, perhaps, going and alarm, but soon changing to going and striking – and these were placed end to end; not until several centuries had passed and pendulum control had been introduced were they to be planted side by side. The earliest extant examples of these relatively simple mechanisms include a so-called 'belfry alarm' – of the type, that is, used to alert a bellringer – which is in the Mainfränkisches Museum in Würzburg and is said to date from about 1380; and the original clock of Salisbury cathedral, which can be reliably dated at 1386. This clock, which was most carefully restored in 1954, and then installed on the floor of the cathedral where it can be inspected by visitors, strikes the hours yet has no dial. It is controlled by a large foliot, with a period of oscillation of about four seconds.

In order to follow another subdivision of the mainstream, that of the monumental medieval astronomical clocks, of which, happily, a number of examples still exist albeit in varying states of their original condition, we must revert to the years between 1348 and 1362. During this time a quite remarkable clock was designed and made; and the inventor's description, which has come

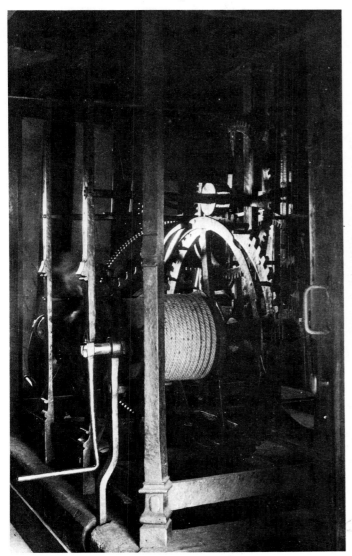

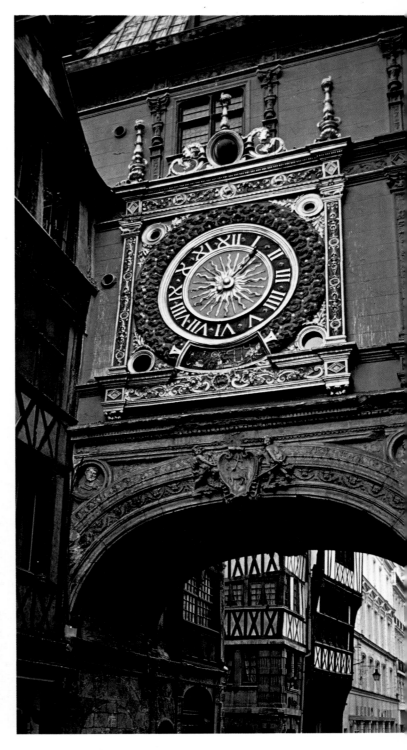

The astronomical clock of 1389 at Rouen possesses the earliest surviving quarter-striking work. It is also very much larger than the clocks of either Salisbury or Wells. Considered to have been built originally by Jehan de Felains, the clock was modified at some unrecorded time, being converted to a verge with pendulum as well as being given some new wheelwork.

The quarter striking train of the Rouen clock of 1389.

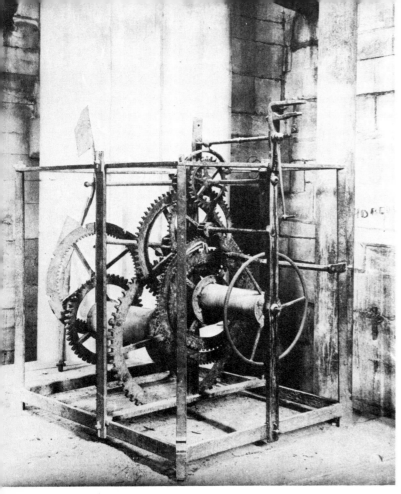

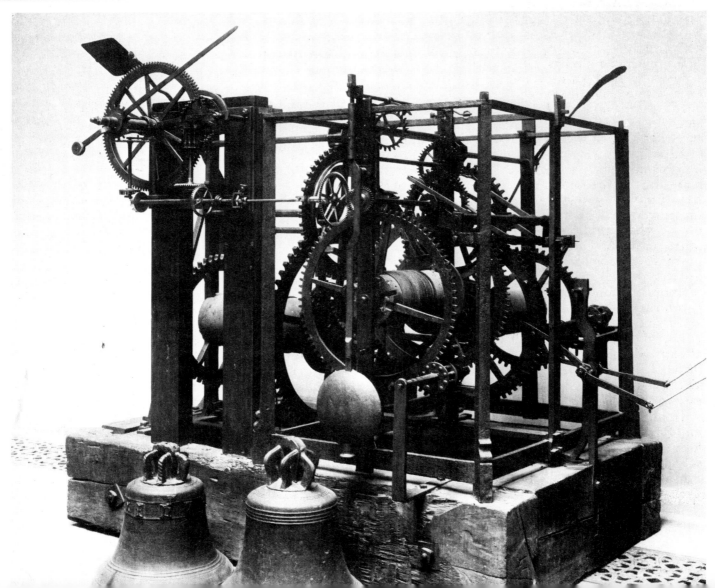

opposite page
At Holy Trinity church, in the Suffolk village of Blythborough, stands this bearded warrior in mid sixteenth-century armour, nowadays disconnected from the clock so that he strikes the bell only when a cord is pulled. Jaquemarts of this kind were once commonplace.

left
Salisbury cathedral possesses one of the two earliest extant church clocks in England, dating from 1386 (see page 65).

below
The other famous early church clock in England at Wells cathedral dates from 1392. Unlike Salisbury, it possesses a quarter striking train which is thought to be contemporary (see page 67). Science Museum, London (on loan from the Dean and Chapter of Wells cathedral).

down to us intact, enters into such fine detail that it has proved possible within recent years to construct a facsimile of the clock with complete confidence that it is indeed a faithful replica. This work was carried out in 1960 under the direction of Mr H. Alan Lloyd, by the specialist firm of Thwaites & Reed of London; the clock itself is now in the Smithsonian Institution in the U.S.A.

The inventor of this clock was Giovanni da Dondi, who was born in 1318. The son of a doctor, he became a doctor himself, being appointed personal physician to Emperor Charles IV in 1349. He lectured in astronomy at Padua university, and in medicine at Florence; and he died at Genoa in 1389. In what was clearly a very full life, he yet found time to design and record in detail a clock the complexity of which was such as had never been seen before his time and which, indeed, was not to be attempted again for two centuries.

Two aspects of this clock are of importance in considering the historical development of clockwork. First, the complexity: the movements of the heavenly bodies, and especially the astrological and religious significance of such motions, were matters of enormous interest to God-fearing peoples – and it is arguable whether astrology necessarily deserves the reputation for absolute charlatanism that it enjoys today. Secondly, the technology employed: it will be remembered that iron was the customary material used for clocks at this early period – yet da Dondi's clock was made from brass, with some parts cast in bronze, and at no point in the manuscript is there any mention whatever of ferrous metal being used.

In the century from 1350 to 1450, very many big clocks were built in the cities of western Europe; there is some record, even if only documentary, of at least sixty. Many of these were simply timekeeping and time-sounding. Clocks striking the hours were more or less commonplace, and of the two English clocks included on the abovementioned list from this period, both that at Salisbury – which has already been described – and the other, at Wells cathedral and dating from 1392, possessed this facility. The latter, in addition, has a quarter-striking train which is thought to be contemporary; and this extra facility compares, chronologically, with a similar feature in the clock at Rouen, which predates Wells by a handful of years, there being clear evidence that it was already completed and working by 1389. So, by the turn of the fourteenth century, public clocks already possessed the basic attributes which we expect of them today.

In addition, however, the clocks at both Wells and Rouen were fitted with astronomical dials, the former being one of the finest medieval dials in the world. Above this dial which was probably fitted a century or so after the clock was first built, since Wells – like Salisbury – originally had no dial,

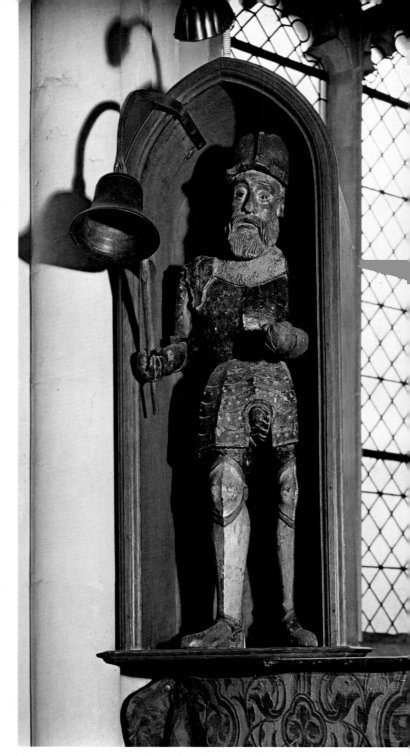

there is a scene with automata, of four knights mounted on horseback who, at each hour, indulge in a joust during which one knight gets knocked off his steed. Other examples of very early clocks with astronomical dials in Britain include those at Exeter cathedral, Ottery St Mary, and Wimbourne Minster. Some of these fine machines, too, have automata figures, often called 'Jacks' (jaquemarts), which strike the hours and quarters, the one at Wells being known as 'Jack Blandifer'.

Perhaps the best-known large astronomical clock in the world is the one in Strasbourg cathedral; perhaps not so well known is that it is the third of its kind. The series started with a clock made about 1350, of which virtually nothing is known

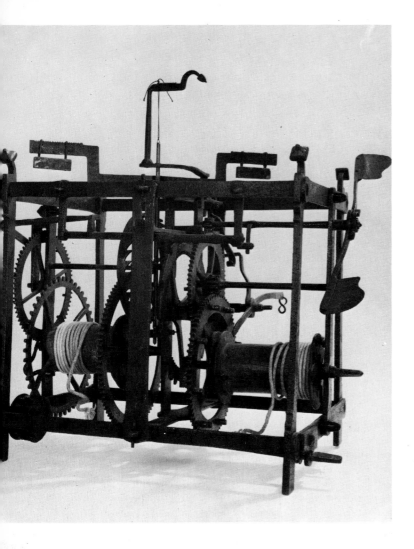

This massive church clock from Cassiobury Park was almost certainly made in the fourteenth century and possibly for the abbey of St Albans; and there is even a possibility that it once belonged to Richard of Wallingford (see page 75). British Museum, London.

save that it was enormous – at least thirty-eight feet high, with a width at the base of about thirteen and a half feet. The only feature of this clock that is still extant is the great cock which crowned it and which, every day at midday, opened its beak, put out its tongue and crowed, simultaneously flapping its wings. One of the engineering miracles of this bird, which, together with the train and bellows operating it, is in Strasbourg Museum, is that each separate one of the primary feathers splayed out when its mechanism was working.

When the first clock was replaced after more than two centuries, the cock was found to be in such excellent condition that it was incorporated into the new design, as were also three pinned drums used to operate the carillon, although the tunes were changed. This second clock was built by Isaac Habrecht (1544–1620), a fine maker of complicated clocks, who took three years to construct it, finishing in 1574. He worked to the technical designs of the then Professor of Mathematics at Strasbourg university, one Conrad Hasenfratz,

sometimes called by the latinised version 'Dasypodius' – his name literally means 'Hare's Foot'. Habrecht, who came from a great clockmaking family – there are said to have been twelve such exponents of the craft within the compass of three generations – may well have been helped by his younger brother Josias and he subsequently made two smaller versions of the Strasbourg clock, both of them still surviving. One of these is in the British Museum and the other in Rosenborg Castle, Copenhagen, while all that remains of his cathedral clock is in Strasbourg museum.

Eventually, the second Strasbourg clock fell into disrepair in its turn – and it seems extraordinary to learn that, two hundred years after it was built, it proved impossible to find anybody to repair it, but that is said to have been the case. It remained out of action for many years, until J. B.-S. Schwilgué, sometime Professor of Mathematics at the College of Silestat as well as in business with a partner making portable scales, balances and turret clocks, was invited by the Mayor of Strasbourg to submit proposals to rectify the situation. He prepared three alternative solutions, starting with an estimate for repairing the old clock, which would, however, never be other than inaccurate and unreliable. Secondly, he proposed the replacement of certain parts of the old clock with new and more functional components; and finally, he offered to build a new clock. Eventually, his third proposition was accepted, then shelved because of the cost; but at long last, in 1832, it was revived although the contract was not finally signed until 1838. Schwilgué started work on 24th June in that year. He was compelled to fit his clock into the old clock case, already *in situ*, which did not please him as it left him no latitude to display his new machinery. His clock was set going for the first time on 2nd October 1842, simultaneously with the opening of the tenth Scientific Congress in France.

Before leaving early turret clocks, either on churches or on other public buildings, mention might be made of one other feature that is often a source of fascination to laymen. This is the very long pendulum. There are a number of churches in Britain where the pendulum can be seen swinging below the ceiling under the tower. Nearly always these will be found to have been a late eighteenth-century modification, except for the pendulum beating 1¼ seconds and corresponding to a length of five feet, which was first tried in longcase clocks at the end of the seventeenth century. The longest pendulum at present working in a turret clock in Britain is probably the one with a period of oscillation of 4 seconds, corresponding to a length of nearly 65 feet. This is installed in a clock dating from 1912, in St Stephen's church, Stockbridge, Edinburgh.

Finally, there is a third subdivision of the mainstream, the first appearance of the domestic clock.

As we have seen, the earliest public clocks were made of iron, and the first domestic clocks were, in essentials, small-scale versions of these, housed in rectangular frames that were reminiscent of those of their bigger brethren. These clocks are called 'Gothic' clocks or 'chamber' clocks, or just iron clocks, and they are usually associated with southern Germany, Switzerland, France and Italy. Technically, it became necessary to extend the gear train, in order to reduce the distance that the weight had to drop in order to drive the clock for a reasonable duration; the alternative would have required that it be hung so high up as to be not clearly visible to those wishing to read the time. These fine iron clocks were controlled by a foliot or a wheel-balance, and they were made over a considerable period, really only dying out after the pendulum had risen to prominence in clockwork.

The longest pendulum on a church clock in Britain measures 65ft and forms part of the clock built in 1912 at St Stephen's church, Stockbridge, Edinburgh. It has a period of 4 seconds.

They continued to be made of iron long after the introduction of brass as a common material in clockmaking; and it is generally believed that they were made by smiths who were accustomed to working on smaller scale objects – probably locksmiths and gunsmiths – than the blacksmiths who made the turret clocks. Gothic clocks generally have an iron dial, with a painted hour circle – more usually called a 'chapter ring', after the chapters or offices to which the monks were summoned by the very first clocks in monasteries – and springing from the tops of the four-posted frame a skeletonised superstructure containing one or more bells, surmounted, often enough, by a spire. Time is shown by a single hand, which may rotate in the normal manner, or remain stationary against a moving dial; the bells are used to strike the hour and sometimes to provide an alarm.

Weight-driven clocks were restricted anyway in their portability, and were quite unsuitable for use on the person, so that the obvious prerequisite for further development was a substitute power source

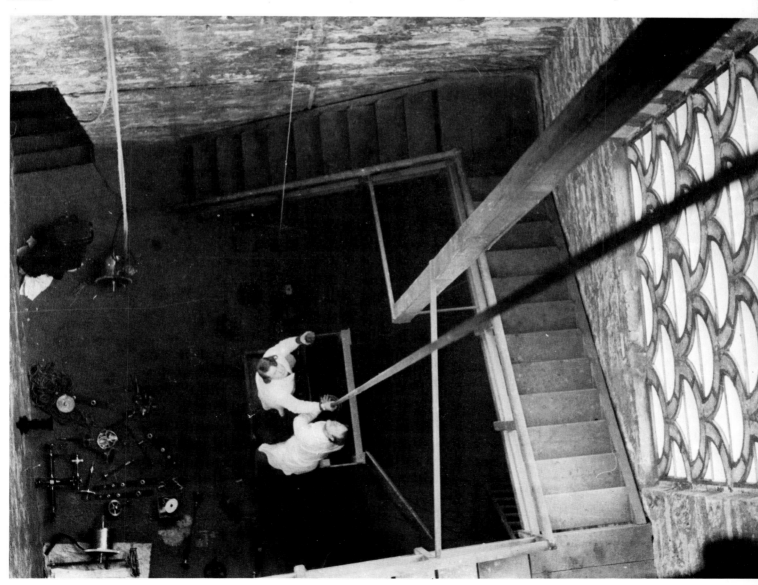

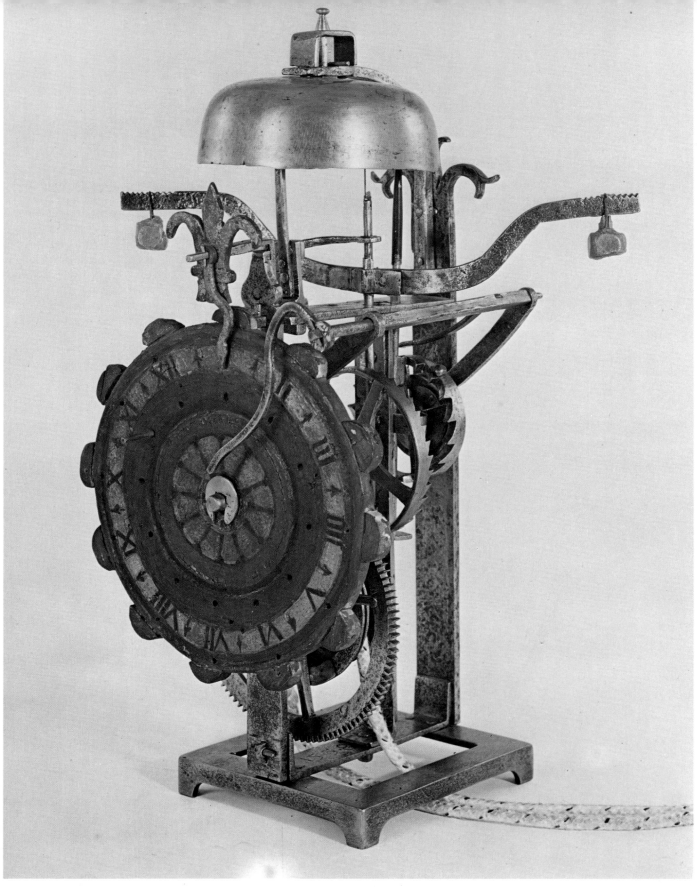

This small domestic clock of the late Middle Ages is simply an alarm clock. Weight-driven, it probably required winding every twelve hours, and the dial revolved against a fixed hand. The alarm is set by putting a peg in the appropriate hole in the dial which, in the course of its revolution, eventually lifts the arm which releases the alarm mechanism. British Museum, London.

opposite
Of much the same period as the previous example, this domestic iron clock is remarkable for its castellated superstructure and for its painted dial incorporating, at the bottom, a bird on a leafy branch. Attribution of this clock is difficult, although it is almost certainly northern European. British Museum, London.

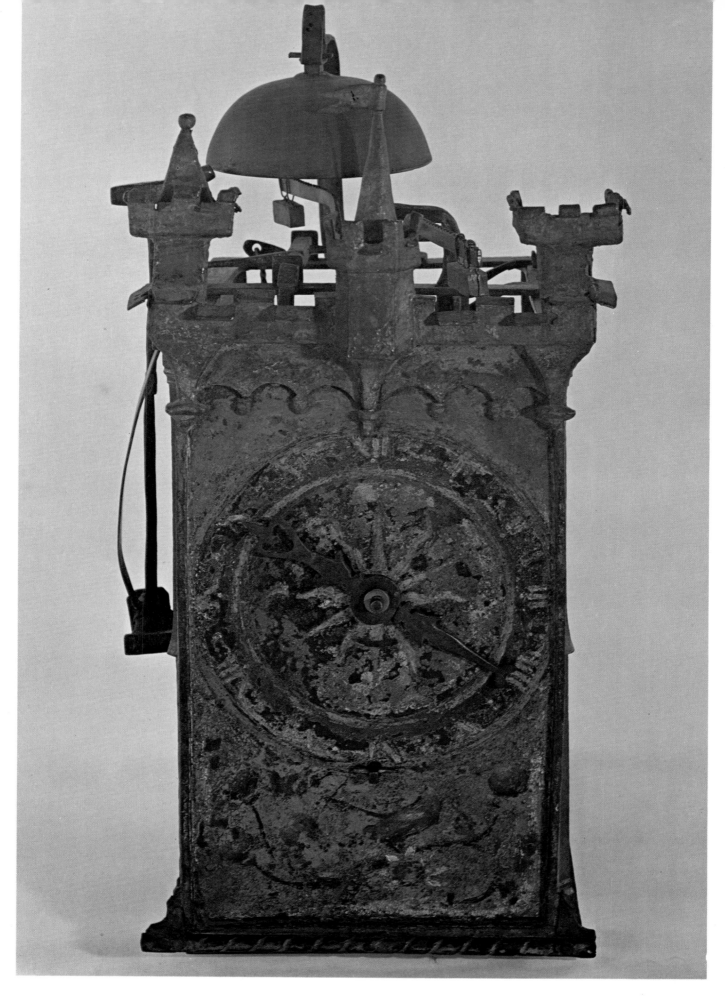

below
The construction of this late fifteenth-century clock clearly follows that of larger public clocks of the time, with its posted frame and curved corner posts carrying rosettes. The primitive dial is a pierced iron plate with painted hour figures. The whole is surmounted by quite an elaborate canopy supporting a bell. Museum of the Worshipful Company of Clockmakers, Guildhall, London.

right
Of similar attribution to the previous illustration and of similar construction, this clock is nevertheless somewhat simpler. It incorporates a dial wheel with twenty-four holes and a pointer, and an alarm could probably be set off by inserting a pin in the appropriate hole. Museum of the Worshipful Company of Clockmakers, Guildhall, London.

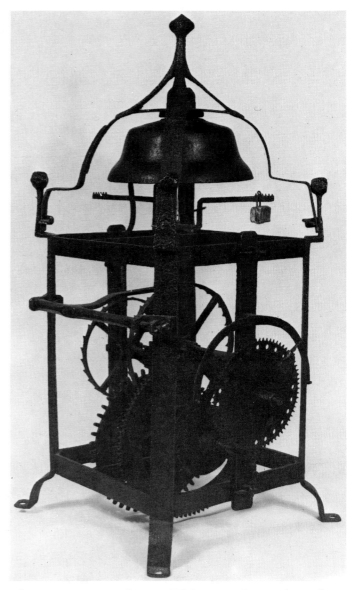

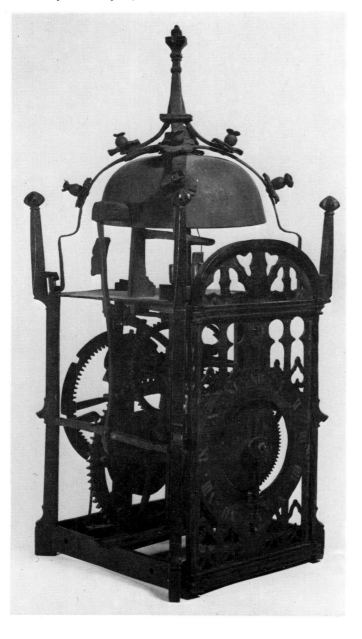

of greater convenience. This was the mainspring, probably developed somewhat earlier, but first applied only during the last half of the fifteenth century. It is possible that the earliest springs may have been beaten out of brass, although steel was always the preferred material; but a major difficulty must have been to make it. Iron has to be made to absorb extra carbon to become steel, and this is done essentially by hammering and reheating. Then there was the associated problem of beating out a ribbon of steel that remained constant in width and thickness throughout its length. Inevitably the reject rate must have been inordinately high.

From evidence in contemporary paintings, the earliest spring clocks may well have looked like their forerunners, the Gothic wall clocks. However, they were soon to diverge into a variety of clearly recognisable types, from one of which it seems likely that the watch was evolved.

Although it has proved impossible up to the present time to pinpoint the invention of the

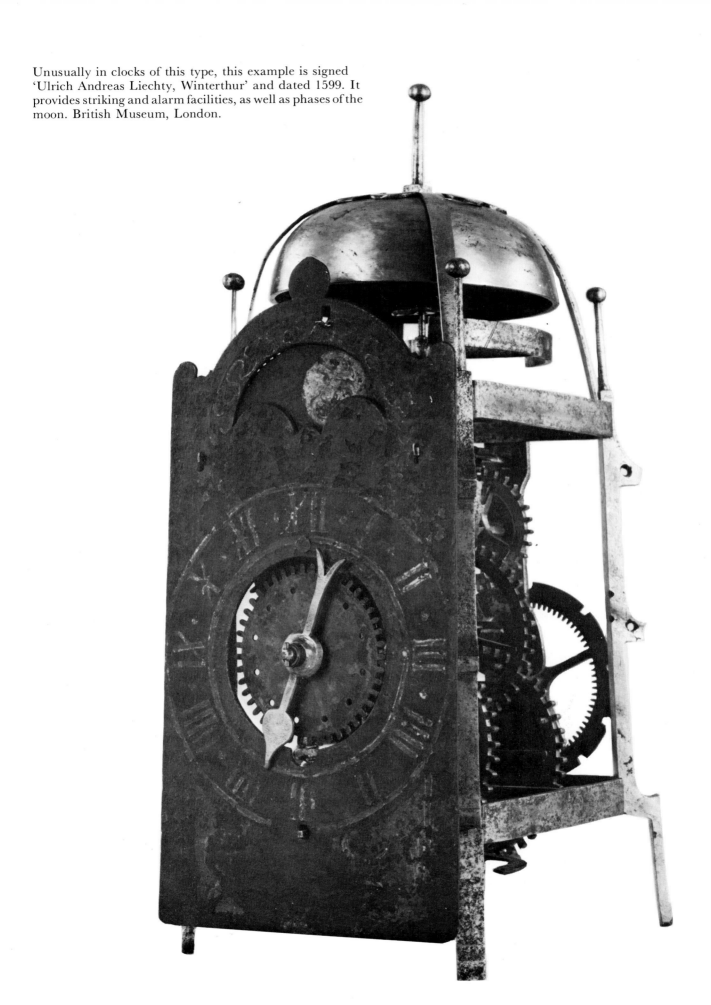

Unusually in clocks of this type, this example is signed
'Ulrich Andreas Liechty, Winterthur' and dated 1599. It
provides striking and alarm facilities, as well as phases of the
moon. British Museum, London.

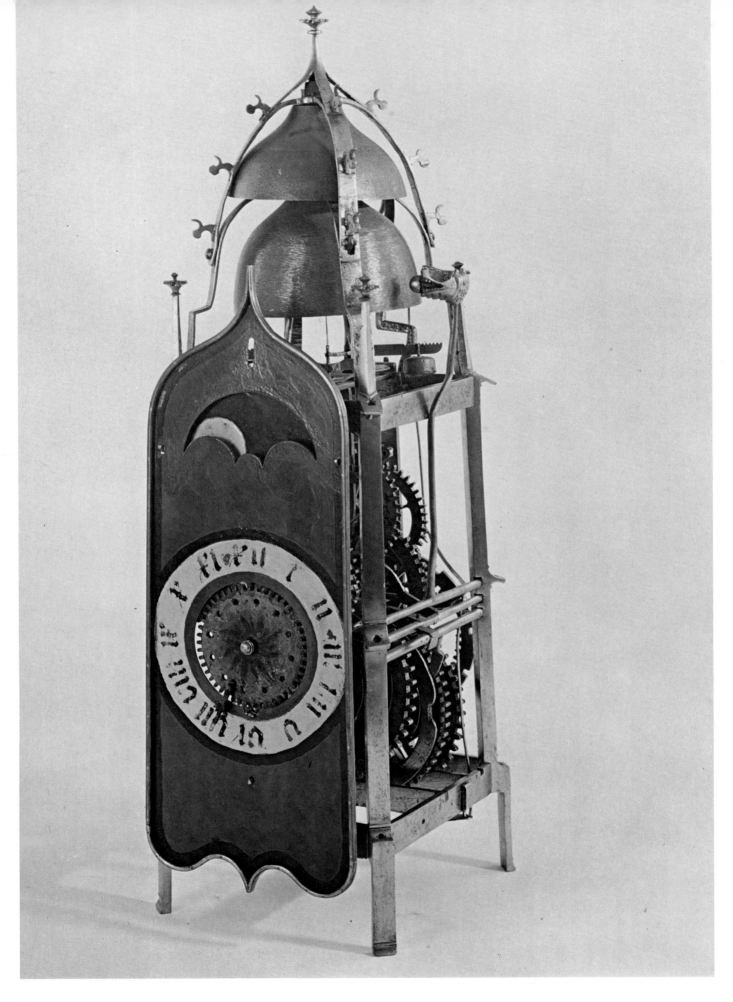

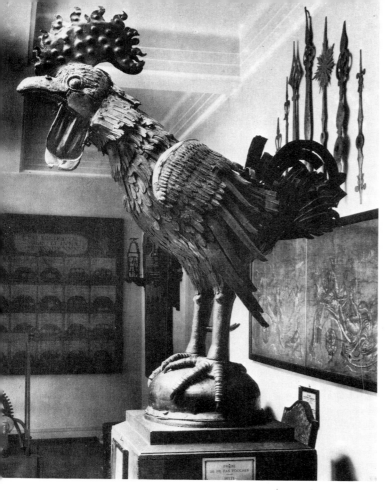

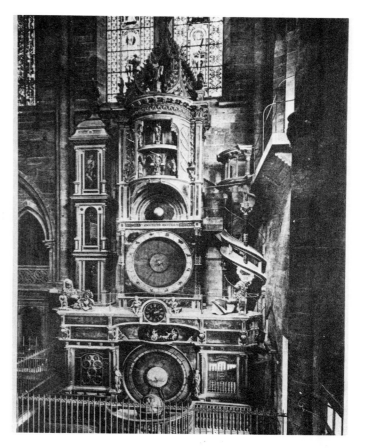

left
This Gothic clock is remarkable for having two bells in its steeple, and the clock in fact has four trains giving going, striking, chiming and alarm motions. There are also phases of the moon visible in an aperture above the painted dial. British Museum, London.

above left
The only substantial surviving part of the original fourteenth-century Strasbourg cathedral clock is the crowing cock which surmounted it. The clock was made about 1350 (see page 67).

above
Schwilgué's clock for Strasbourg cathedral, the third in the series, was completed in 1842 (see page 68).

mechanical clock with great accuracy, some clues can be gained from consideration of the times and conditions of the society in which it appeared. As Professor Cippola remarks in his book *Clocks and Culture 1300–1700*: 'It was not entirely by chance that the mechanical clock and the cannon appeared at approximately the same time. Both were the product of a remarkable growth in the number and quality of metalworkers and . . . many of the early clockmakers were also gunfounders'. In those times there was neither sufficient demand for clocks nor sufficient craftsmen skilled in their making to allow for the formation of guilds of specialists in this field. Furthermore, there can be no doubt that making any kind of clock was a very expensive operation, so that only rich individuals or corporations could afford it; and, in countries where metalworkers with mechanical knowledge were rare, it quite often happened that foreigners with the necessary expertise were imported to undertake the work. Thus it seems quite likely that both the Salisbury and Wells cathedral clocks were made by craftsmen brought to England specifically for the purpose by Bishop

Ralph Erghum, who himself came from Bruges, but who was Bishop of Salisbury from 1375 to 1388, in which year he was translated to Wells. At that particular point in time, large clocks were certainly more common on the continent of Europe than in Britain.

Before that time, though, there had been without doubt mechanical expertise of a high order in England, mainly among the monks. A certain Friar Richard of Wallingford is said to have constructed a complicated astronomical clock about 1320 which, when viewed by an experienced traveller two hundred years later, was not only still going, but was still remarkable enough to draw forth the comment that its like was not to be seen anywhere in Europe. Probably the observer who made this remark had not seen da Dondi's clock, but there can be no doubt that Wallingford's was earlier in the field. So Britain can no longer be lightly dismissed from consideration as a pioneer among European countries in experiments with clocks.

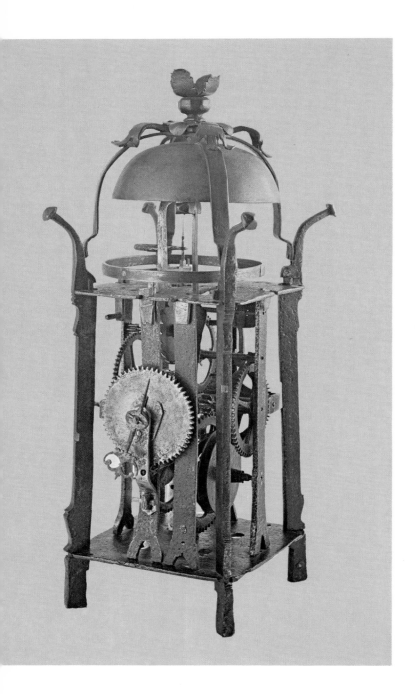

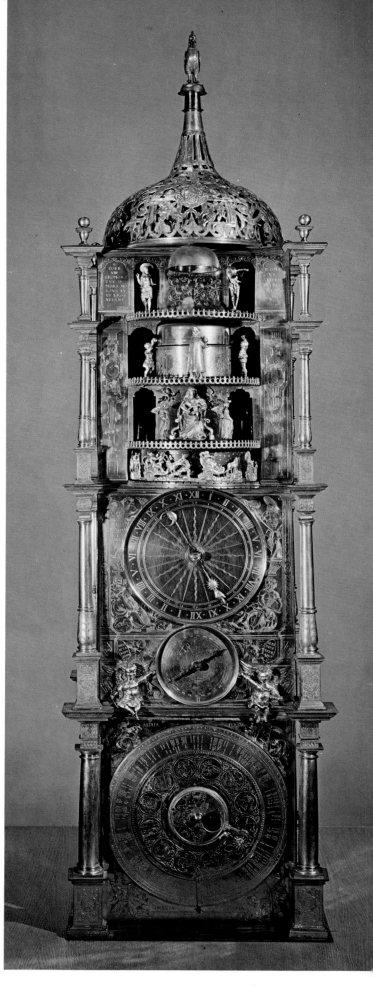

Iron chamber clock with right-handed train and large balance. Possibly Flemish, about 1570. British Museum, London.

right
Apart from his *magnum opus* in Strasbourg cathedral, Isaac Habrecht is particularly known for two smaller astronomical clocks. This one is in the British Museum, London (see also page 54).

The Age of Brass and the Birth of the Watch

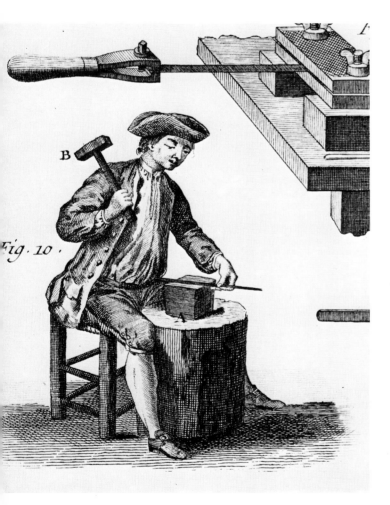

A detail from this plate, which appears in the celebrated eighteenth-century work *La Grande Encyclopédie* of Diderot and D'Alembert, shows one of the first stages in early springmaking with the metal being hammered out by hand.

The appearance upon the horological scene of the spring as a principal power source is of prime importance; but it will be realised by now that, when reviewing the early history of horology, one takes it almost for granted that, whatever else may have survived, inventors' names have not been passed down to us. Thus, most of what we know about the early history of the mainspring is based upon two paintings, both of which unmistakably show spring-driven clocks among the furnishings. The first, depicting a gentleman of the Burgundian Court, is to be found in the Museum of Fine Arts in Antwerp. The portrait dates from 1440 or thereabouts, and there is a spring-driven clock in the background. Another portrait, this time of Louis XI of France and dating from about 1475, includes among the detail a small hexagonal spring-driven table clock.

The first spring-driven clocks seem to have continued the fashion of previous styles, being designed to hang on the wall like weight-driven chamber clocks. It was not long, however, before they gave rise to a change of fashion since they were inherently so much more adaptable than those with weights. The styles that eventually developed, however, were recognisably national, so that designs can be fairly readily identified as originating from particular clockmaking 'schools'.

The two pre-eminent centres of early clock- and watchmaking in Europe were the south German towns of Augsburg and Nuremberg. England, prior to about 1600, had virtually no native industry, relying entirely upon foreign imports or foreign workmen brought into the country to pursue their craft. Thus, its domestic clocks at this period were generally imported iron chamber clocks, copied occasionally by English craftsmen in the smithing tradition, who sometimes also added a sheet metal casing to exclude dust. Apart from Germany, however, there was also, at this

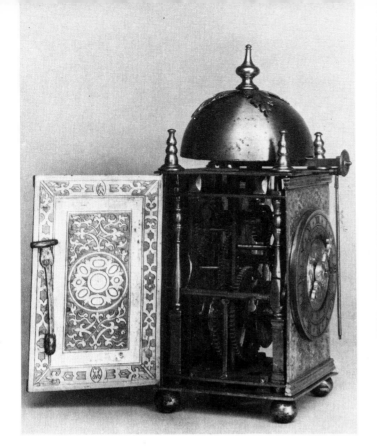

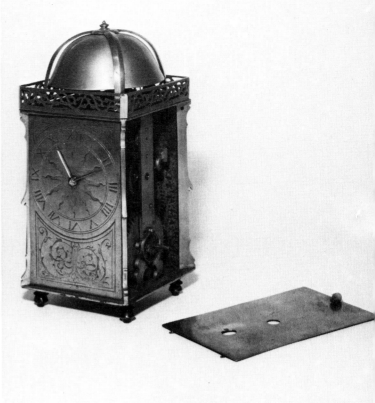

time, a substantial interest in spring-clocks among French and Flemish craftsmen, and in Italy; each developed individual styles.

Although apparently first applied many decades before, the mainspring does not appear in quantity production, so far as can be judged, much before 1500. At quite an early date – perhaps somewhere in the second quarter of the sixteenth century – the watch 'stream' must have split away from that devoted to clocks; but this was anyway a period during which enormous creative effort was being applied to the design of timekeepers in general. It is likely that the new latitude provided by the compact spring drive gave impetus to this effort.

Of the two principal German centres of the craft, Augsburg enjoyed an unrivalled reputation for the enormous variety and superb craftsmanship of its spring-driven clocks, while Nuremberg concentrated mainly upon watches. The Augsburg makers had an insatiable appetite – and presumably also a bottomless market – for clocks incorporating automata which they produced in seemingly endless variety and with the greatest imaginable ingenuity. The fabulous *nef* described in chapter 2 and made by Hans Schlottheim for Emperor Rudolf II – or so it is intelligently surmised, since this magnificent object bears no signature of any kind – is, of course, an outstanding yet not a unique example; there is, for instance, an almost identical *nef*, only perhaps a little later in date because its mechanism is slightly more sophisticated, in the Conservatoire des Arts et Métiers, in Paris. Excluding such extreme examples of the craft, even the average specimen of the output of the Augsburg 'school' was more likely to involve some fabulous

above left
The weight-driven wall clock (this example was made in Germany about 1550) demonstrates the next stage in posted frame design incorporating top and bottom plates. This clock has clear similarities with the English so-called lantern clock, even to the pivoted sides, although this example is very much smaller. British Museum, London.

above
A late sixteenth-century chamber clock, almost certainly of German origin, this example, while preserving the posted frame construction that was normal at the time, has sheet steel sides with the front containing an engraved hour circle and central wavy-rayed sun. The steel arrow hand tells the hours, while the plain hand operates an alarm. The pierced steel balustrade is an interesting feature. The original verge and balance escapement has been replaced by a pendulum. Museum of the Worshipful Company of Clockmakers, Guildhall, London.

above right
The construction of this clock is interesting in that the movement and dial slot into the case. The latter, of gilt metal, is engraved with arabesques, in the manner of Hans Holbein the Younger, and surmounting the whole are 'Jacks' which strike the bell at the hour. The clock was made either in Germany or possibly in England about 1540. British Museum, London.

right
Early Italian clocks are by no means common, and this sixteenth-century example is steel throughout apart from the brass dial; it is controlled by a foliot. British Museum, London.

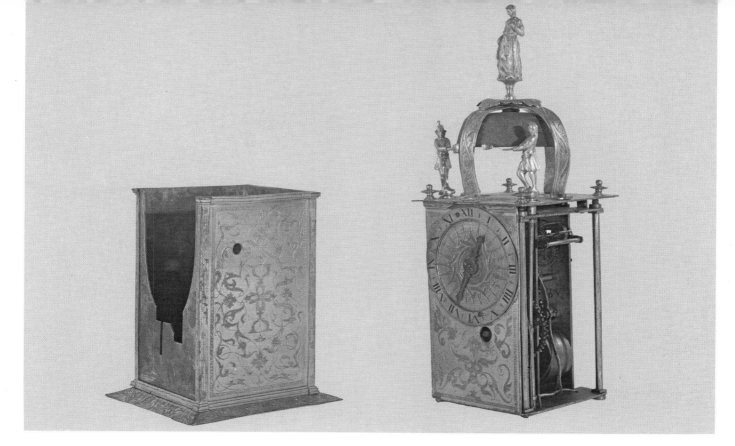

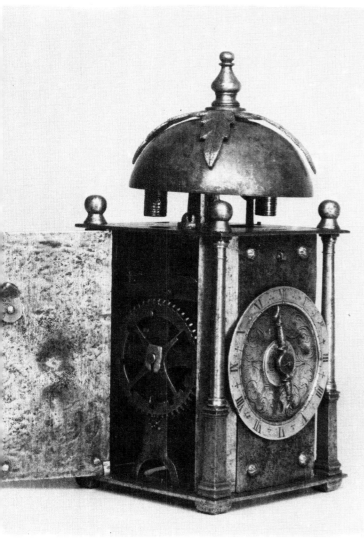

or actual beast which performed one or more functions automatically; or perhaps a little scene involving several people, such as the milkmaid milking the cow under the friendly eye of the farmer – the diversity of these clocks is endless. They also used religious motifs, such as the well-known types called crucifix, monstrance and tabernacle clocks; clocks of the two last-named types are often multi-dialled and extra complicated, with astrolabes and similar accessories incorporated.

Mention of Hans Schlottheim and his connection with the *nefs* – which, incidentally is based upon written evidence that he did supply such an object to the Emperor in 1581, while three years later he was certainly in Prague and actually working for him – brings to mind another celebrated clock with which he was associated. This is usually described as the Tower of Babel clock; it was and presumably still is in the Grünes Gewölbe in Dresden. This clock must have represented one of the earliest attempts to use a rolling ball as a time standard, a principle which was to be further exploited in succeeding centuries. In Schlottheim's arrangement, the mechanism was contained within an octagonal tower some four feet high. Above a base which contained the dial and main part of the machinery were two galleries surmounted by a lantern. The galleries were connected by a track spiralling through sixteen complete turns between one level and the other, and each minute a crystal ball rolled the whole length of this track, taking a minute to do so. On reaching the bottom the ball was raised by the clock mechanism once again to the upper level; but in the meantime another ball had started its down-

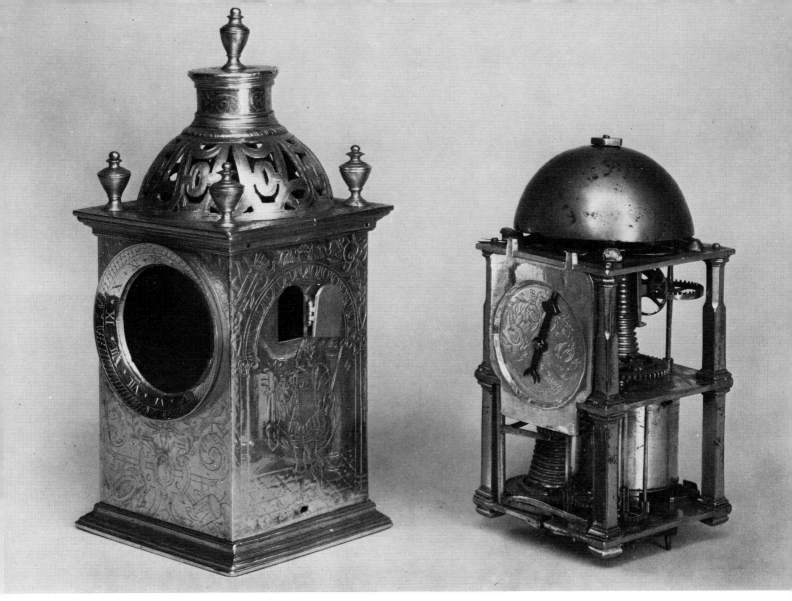

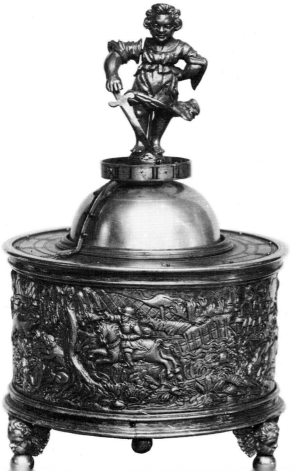

The preference of French makers for the two-tier table clock movement has already been demonstrated, but at least two London makers shared their views. This square table clock signed by Bartholomew Newsam was made about 1580–90. The dial-plate is a modern replacement. British Museum, London.

above right
A complicated version of another early clock style, this drum clock is attributed to Paulus Grimm of Nuremberg and is dated 1576. The dial is made up of eight concentric bands giving a variety of astronomical information. British Museum, London.

left
This elaboration of the cylindrical or drum-shape style of clock, which was made by Hans Gutbub of Strasbourg about 1590, incorporates an automaton figure on top of the bell which moves its arm at the hour. The case is decorated with hunting scenes in relief. British Museum, London.

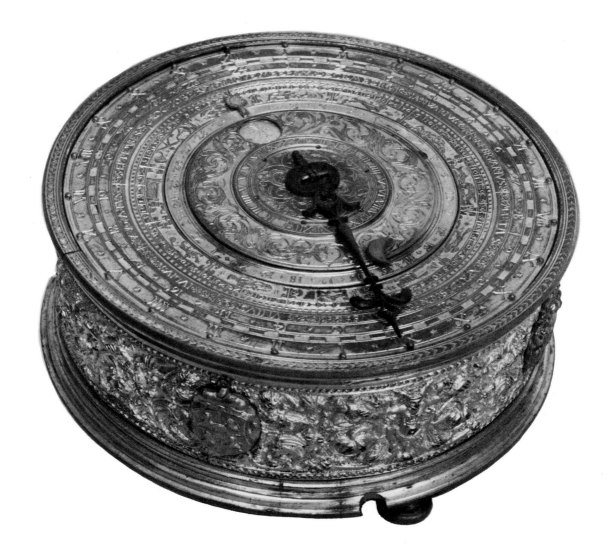

ward journey. As if this were not enough of a novelty in itself – and the continual rolling of balls must have made a noise reminiscent of the early tramways, making it easy to see how the clock acquired its popular name – there were automaton figures of musicians simulating the sounds of an organ which was incorporated into the mechanism, and other figures were also deployed elsewhere upon the structure. Schlottheim started this clock in Dresden in 1592, and it is said to have taken ten years in the building; and unlike the *nefs*, where the actual clock forms but a tiny part of the whole and incorporates no new principles of design or craftsmanship, the Dresden clock is a milestone in horological terms.

Schlottheim was not the only clockmaker towards the end of the sixteenth century to appreciate the possibilities in a rolling ball, which was anyway based upon a fundamental concept of Galileo. Another maker interested in this device was a Viennese, Christof Margraf, who went so far as to take out a patent in 1595. Then, a few years later, Christolph Rohr of Leipzig made a most elaborate rolling ball clock, now in the Herzog Anton Ulrich Museum in Brunswick. Dated 1601, there is a variation of the original principle in this

clock, in that there is only one ball, its periodicity being taken to include not only the length of time it takes to roll down the inclined track – not a spiral this time, but running around the four sides of a flat-topped pyramid – but also the time taken to restore the same ball to its starting point again by lifting it in a cup on an endless chain. Once again, this total period is one minute. As an added attraction, the platform surmounting the runway contains, under a cupola, a carrousel of figures which is set in motion every three hours. Incidentally, the rolling ball as a time standard is not to be confused with the rolling ball as a power source, to which reference will be made in another chapter.

No survey of the great clocks of the sixteenth century, however brief, would be complete without some reference to the work of two other makers. Schlottheim and his contemporaries, by building so much novelty into their masterpieces, may be said to some extent to have equated time-measurement with entertainment, for this is what the adoption of automata on the grand scale must signify. Two centuries earlier – even though a considerable advance on its time – there had been one monumental scientific clock, made for the most serious of purposes between 1348 and 1362, the

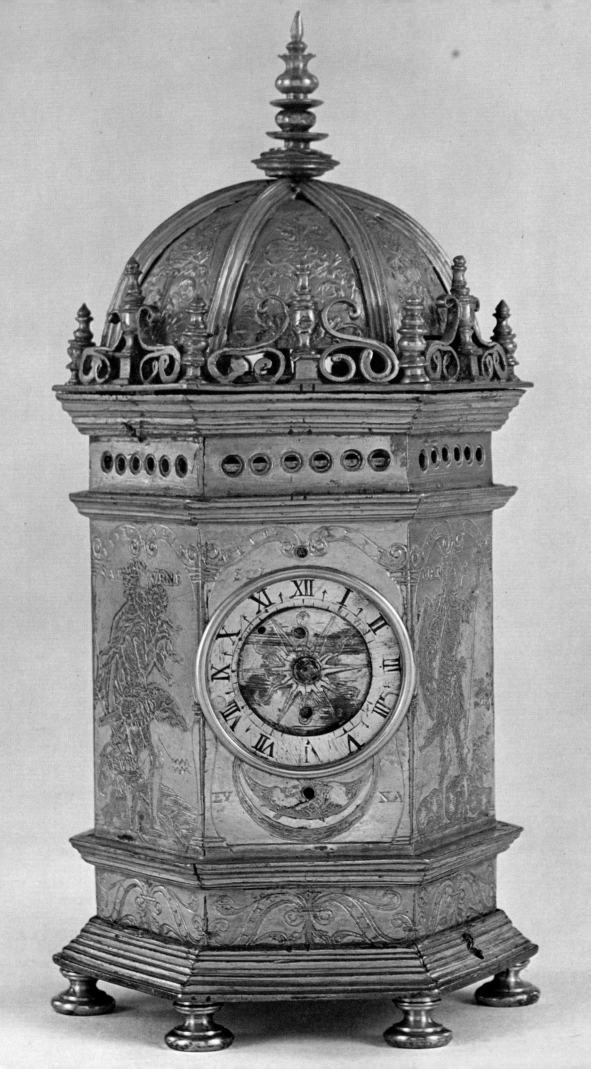

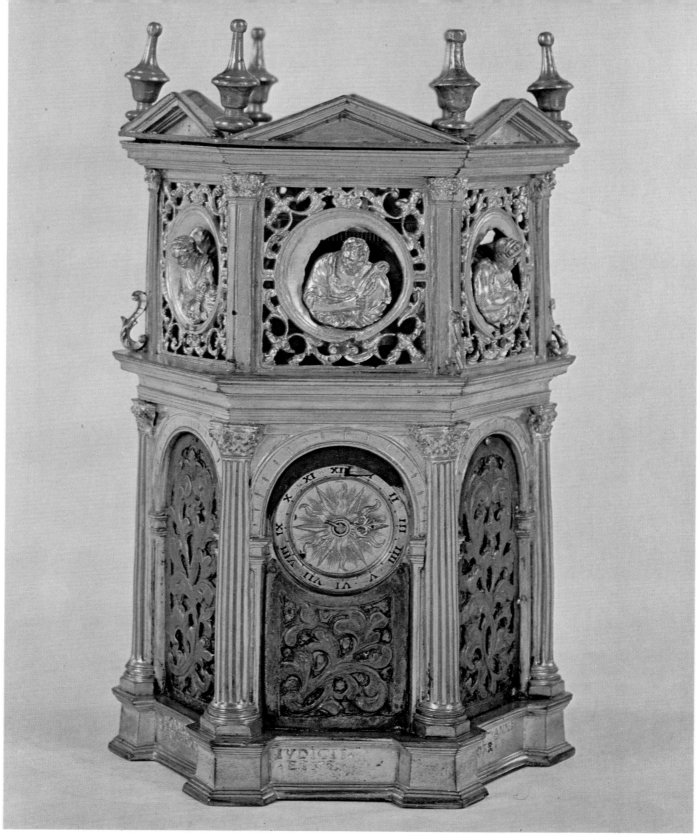

left
The designs engraved on this hexagonal copper gilt French table clock are scrupulously copied from those made in the year 1528 by an engraver who signs himself 'I.B.' The clock, therefore, probably dates from 1530–40 and bears the signature on its base 'LOIS F'. This maker has not been identified. British Museum, London.

above
A very much more elaborate hexagonal table clock, this French product is dated 1545. Aside from the sculptured quality of the case with its figures in the roundels on the upper level, the clock has three dials, one below the hour dial showing the day of the week, and a third dial, shown in the photograph, for setting the alarm. There was originally a fourth dial, above the bell, which recorded certain astronomical data, but this is now missing. British Museum, London.

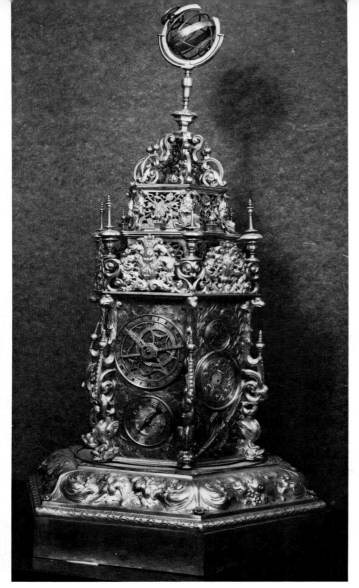

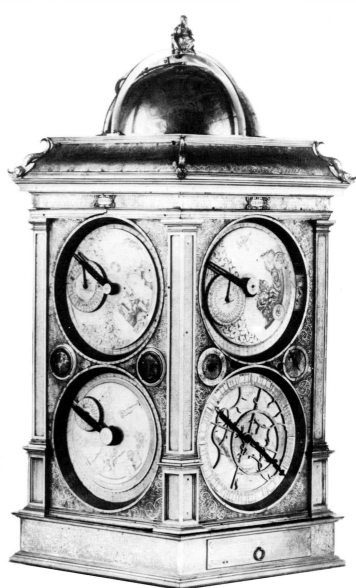

work of Giovanni da Dondi. Was there no comparable equivalent, even by this later period?

The answer to this is to be found in the work of Eberhart Baldewin, who was court clockmaker to Landgraf William IV of Hesse about the middle of the sixteenth century. He made two large astronomical clocks, the first between 1559 and 1561, and the second somewhat later, as well as, in 1575 or thereabouts, a mechanically operating celestial globe. His earlier astronomical clock as well as the globe are now in the Hessisches Landesmuseum in Kassel, while his second clock, which Landgraf William IV subsequently presented to the King of Saxony, is now in the Staatliche Physicalisches und Mathematisches Salon in Dresden. The background to his astronomical masterpieces is to be found in a work entitled *Astronomicum Caesarium*, published in 1540 by Petrus Apianus in Ingolstadt, which incorporated devices called volvelles. These are neither more nor less than rotatable paper discs, from which the position of the planets at any time can be simulated. Landgraf William not only conceived the idea of a clock which should provide this same information mechanically – the project with which

Baldewin was entrusted – but, together with his chief astronomer Andreas Schoener, he himself made fresh calculations of the positions of the chief stars. The decorative work on Baldewin's clock – that is to say, the case and all the associated engraving – was executed by Hermann Diepel of Giessen.

The second important sixteenth-century clockmaker of whom mention must be made is Jobst Burgi (1552–1632). Although born in Switzerland – in Lichtensteig, which is in Toggenburgh – he also entered the service of Landgraf William IV of Hesse, in 1578. There he remained until the Landgraf's death in 1592; and in 1604 he was appointed Imperial Clockmaker to Emperor Rudolf II in Prague.

Burgi's reputation as an outstanding craftsman in the making of globes has been recognised for generations; rather more recently he has come to the fore as a master clockmaker, and this only as a result of research by Professor Dr Hans von Bertele of Vienna. Again Landgraf William IV seems to have been the motivator; his dedication to astronomy necessitated ever more accurate timekeepers, which it was Jobst Burgi's pleasure to

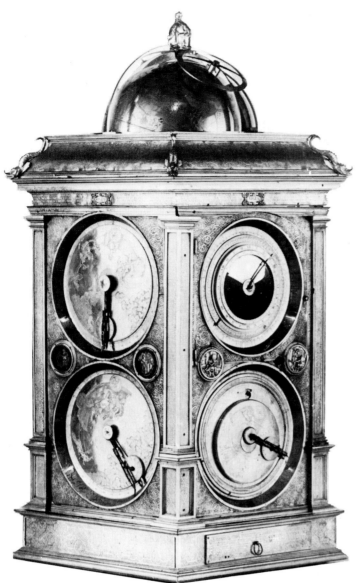

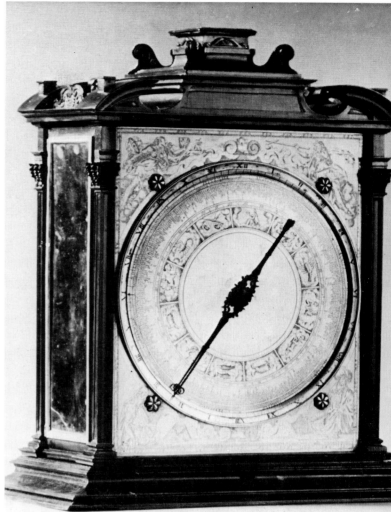

strive to provide for him.

Professor von Bertele discovered three clocks – two in Kassel and one in Dresden – which, although unsigned, are on a number of technical grounds the forerunners of a fourth clock, which is signed. The numerous innovations directed to improved timekeeping performance to be found in this series of clocks include not only long duration – one clock goes for three months at each winding – but also the use of a form of remontoire. This is a device, of which any number of designs have been postulated over the centuries, which is directed towards ironing out idiosyncracies and inconsistencies in the power drive to a clock by converting it into a constant force, usually by using it to rewind a small ancillary spring, which then acts as the direct power source to the clock. This small spring, being frequently returned to maximum tension, exerts a well-nigh constant pull upon the mechanism.

Burgi's principal claim to horological fame, however, rests upon his remarkable development of what is now called the cross-beat escapement. In the third quarter of the seventeenth century the famous astronomer Hevelius mentions an escape-

opposite page, left
One of the more elaborate constructions to emanate from Augsburg, this hexagonal astronomical clock has a case made from gilt metal and silver. It is doubtful if the relatively simple clock mechanism, unfortunately missing, could possibly have lived up to the ambitions exhibited in the profusion of dials. British Museum, London.

opposite page, right
Eberhart Baldewin, clockmaker to the Landgraf William IV of Hesse, made this remarkable astronomical clock, completing it in 1651. The clock has three trains and a thirty-hour movement with quarter striking; it has dials on all four sides.

above left
The other side of Baldewin's clock.

above
Like Baldewin, Jobst Burgi also worked for Landgraf William IV of Hesse. A celebrated craftsman in the making of globes, he also made some outstanding clocks. This one is known as his experimental clock no. 1 and dates from about 1595.

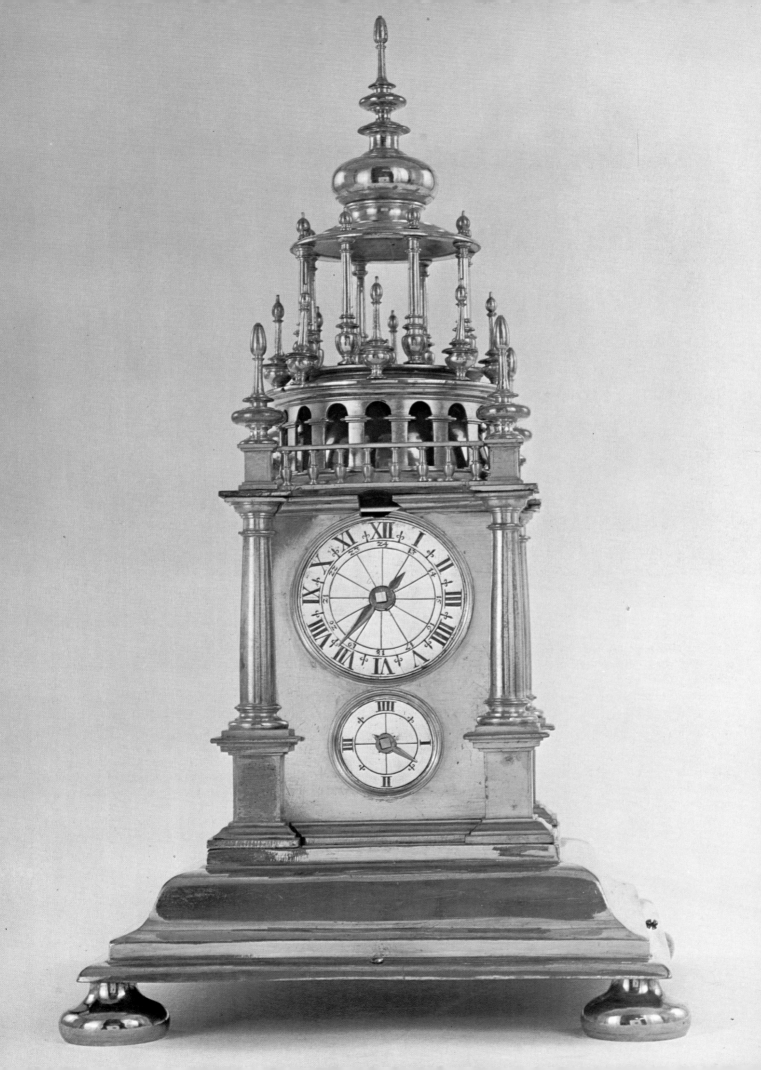

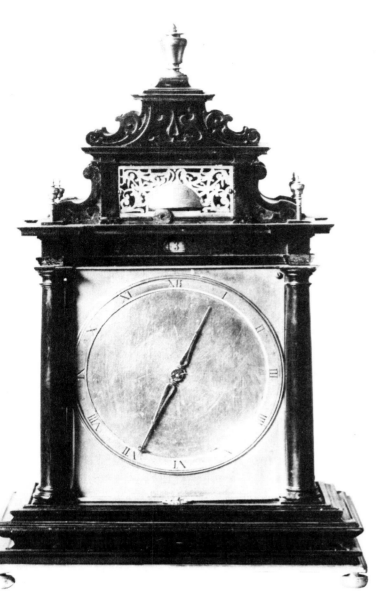

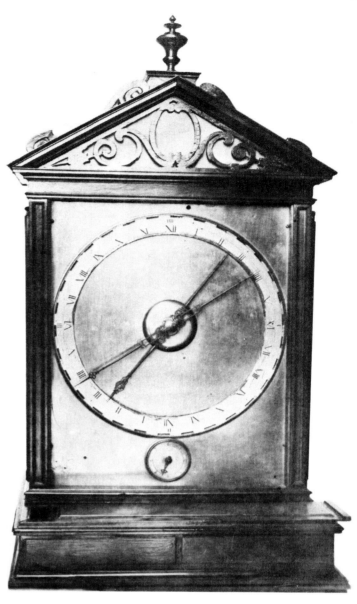

left
This style of clock is generally described as a tabernacle clock, and it was probably made about 1600, in Germany, by makers who signed themselves 'SA.HA'. British Museum, London.

above
Burgi's second experimental clock predates 1600. His outstanding horological invention was the cross-beat escapement.

above right
Burgi's third experimental clock was made about 1605. For more details on this series of clocks see page 89 *et seq*.

ment for which he claims the greatest accuracy then attainable, referring to it as '*libramentum duplice*'. The ordinary escapement of that time – which can only have been the verge – is described simply as '*libramentum*'. Until Professor von Bertele's discoveries, nobody had unravelled this mystery, but it is now quite clear that it is to the Burgi cross-beat escapement that Hevelius was referring. The term '*duplice*' encompasses the two independently pivoted arms, geared together and each having one pallet, which take into an escape wheel having a large number of finely cut teeth. The arrangement permits of much closer adjustment of the escapement than in the case of the simple verge, which thus operates with increased efficiency.

Apart from the appearance of the mainspring, there were two other technical developments around this time of which it is necessary to take account. The first was the gradual assimilation of brass into the craft, as a suitable material for certain components in clock- and watchmaking. Brass is an alloy of copper and zinc, and it seems first to have been used for clocks on the continent of Europe about the middle of the sixteenth century;

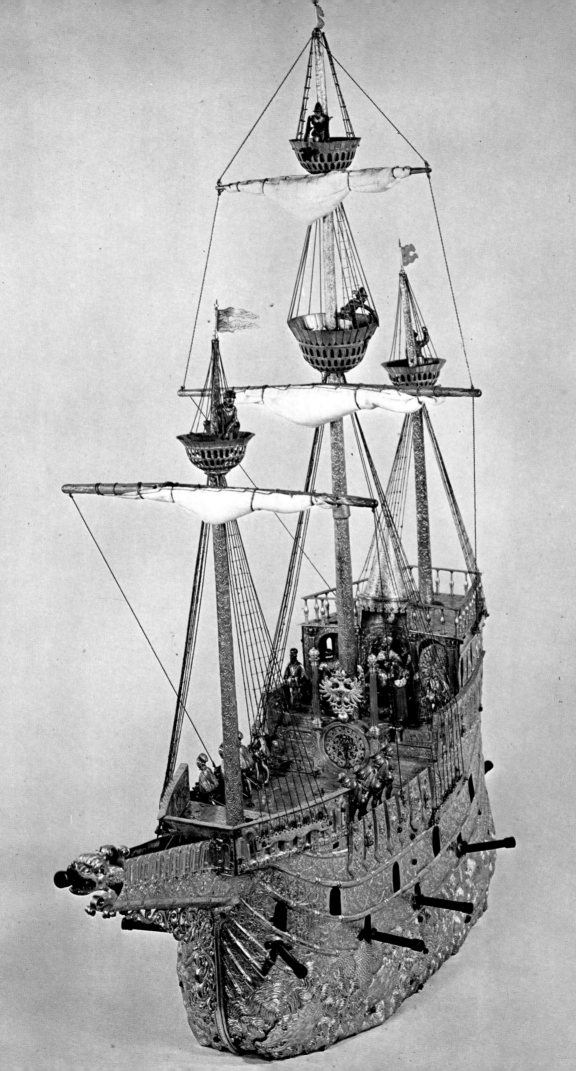

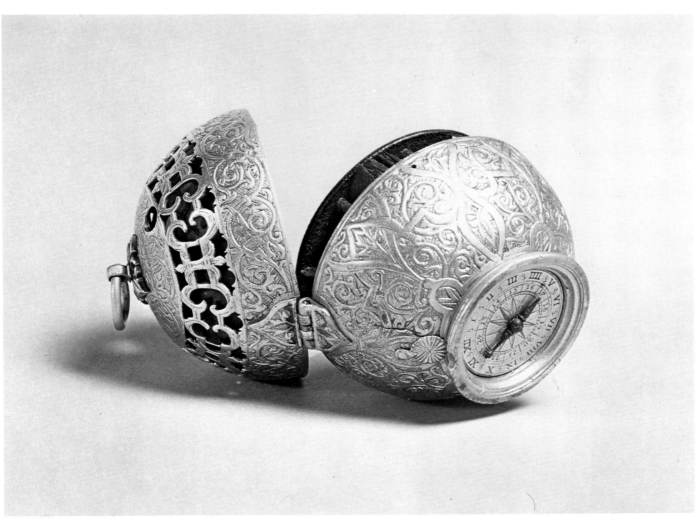

Spherical and tambour-cased watches seem to have originated at about the same time and are the earliest forms of watch known. This German clock-watch, about 1550, has the striking and going trains one above the other, and the movement is fitted with a stackfreed. Ashmolean Museum, Oxford.

left
Dating from about 1600, this exquisite silver gilt enamelled table clock stands only 3¼ in high: a rare and fine example of court craftsmanship, it probably emanated from Augsburg. It incorporates both striking and alarm facilities. British Museum, London.

opposite page
The diminutive clock built by Schlottheim into this elaborate dinner table entertainment piece or *nef* is represented by the small silver and enamelled dial which can be seen at the foot of the mainmast (see page 41). British Museum, London.

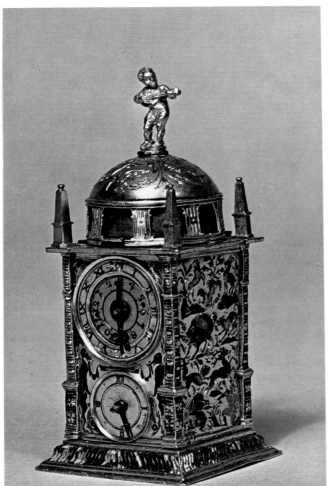

89

but it did not spread to England for some little while thereafter, probably because there was no native brass industry and, even with government aid, it took many years to establish one. Thus it is not usually found in English practice until the beginning of the seventeenth century.

As clock materials go, brass is softer than iron or steel and worked differently. It cannot be hardened, like steel, by heating and then quenching, but only by hammering, or, where appropriate, drawing it into wire or rolling it. The early clockmaker probably cast his own brass; and, although it was at first used mainly for cases and dials, while the movements remained principally of steel, it was not long before brass became accepted as the material of choice first for the framework of the mechanism and subsequently for the wheels. Eventually, brass was adopted as standard for wheels, while steel remained the material for the pinions with which they are meshed. This usage is based upon the proven concept that two surfaces in contact suffer less friction from rubbing against one another if they are made from different metals than if they are the same. The pinions have to withstand more potential wear than the wheels, hence they are made from the harder substance; but the danger is always that dirt, and especially particles of metallic grit, can embed themselves in the softer substance that comprises, *inter alia*, the teeth of the wheels. This can then act as a cutting medium upon the steel pinion leaves, which start to show wear even though the teeth that are doing the damage appear completely unaffected.

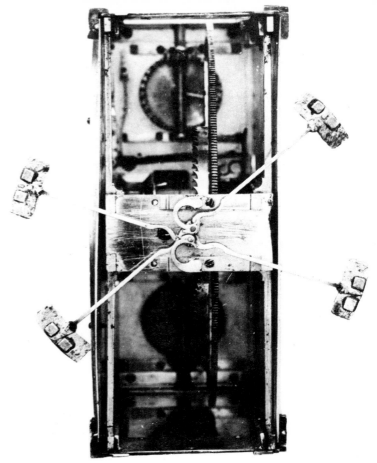

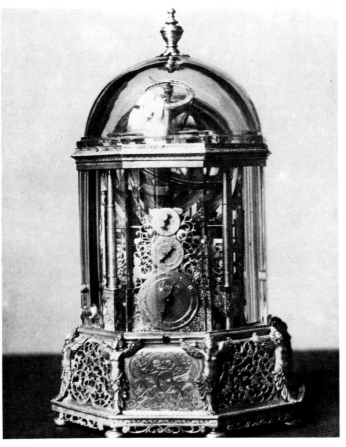

The second technical development which should be noted was the appearance of what is generally called the 'plated' movement. The earliest clocks – and the design persisted for several centuries – were of that type which is commonly described as 'posted' or 'framed'; that is to say, the movements were deployed between metal strips containing the pivot holes for the arbors, and themselves supported within frames of, usually, rectangular open construction top and bottom, separated by four vertical posts, one at each corner. This arrangement had the advantage of great simplicity, both of original construction and when put into operation; the whole movement was so accessible that every part could be observed and adjustments were easy. Furthermore, when cleaning and overhaul were necessary, the main frame could generally be left intact; it served no purpose other than to hold the mechanism together and, as such, needed no maintenance.

In an illuminated manuscript of Flemish or Burgundian origin, of about 1470, there appears for the first time an illustration of a small clock without its outer casing, so that there can be no doubt about the unorthodox manner of its construction. In this new style, the mechanism is contained between two solid metal plates, which are maintained at the correct distance from one another by four pillars. The plates, however, are fundamental to the mechanism because the arbors carrying the wheels and pinions pivot in them — except for the balance wheel, that is. It follows, of course, that when this type of clock requires cleaning, the plates themselves, with their integral pivot holes, have also to be cleaned. The great importance of the movement contained between plates is that, once they were made sufficiently small, they became to all intents and purposes watches and could be carried conveniently on the person.

Every century, certainly up to the end of the nineteenth, has seen great strides in the development of mechanical horology, and the sixteenth was no exception. Reference has already been made, when dealing with the rudiments of clockwork, to two inventions – one only short-lived, but the other both theoretically and practically perfect and surviving for centuries – designed to correct the uneven pull exerted by a mainspring. The stackfreed probably only remained in use for fifty years or so, and was employed almost solely by south German makers. The origin of the word itself is unknown; but it is said to have come into use, being probably a corruption of Low German or Dutch, only in the mid eighteenth century, some two hundred years after the device itself had been abandoned.

The antecedents of the fusee, however, are somewhat better established, as befits the invention that provided both the first and best solution to the problem. The term itself is said to derive from the Latin *fusus*, a spindle, a definition that is not wholly irrelevant in its horological application. It was believed for many years that the first indication of the existence of this device was contained in certain drawings of Leonardo da Vinci that can be dated to about 1485–90. However, this date has been superseded as a result of the discovery of an illuminated manuscript in the Bibliothèque Royale in Brussels which can be dated, on various other grounds, around 1450–60, and which includes, among several clocks, sundials and other associated items, a table clock which unquestionably incorporates a fusee; thoughtfully, its outer case has been removed by the artist, so that the movement can be inspected in some detail. No example survives, of course, that approaches within even reasonable reach of that date. Until comparatively recently it was held that the earliest surviving spring clock with fusee was by Jacob the Zech (the last word means 'miner') of Prague, which is dated 1525, and is owned by the Society of Antiquaries in London; until three decades or so ago, this same craftsman was even credited with its invention, an interesting indication of how horological research has progressed of late. Now, however, pride of place goes to the fragmentary remains of a clock in the Bavarian National Museum in Munich, of which little more than the plates, spring barrel and fusee remain. This clock is signed with four initials and the date '1509'. Apart from this, there is a drum-shaped clock in the Musée des Arts Décoratifs in Paris which purports to date from 1504; but the third digit of this

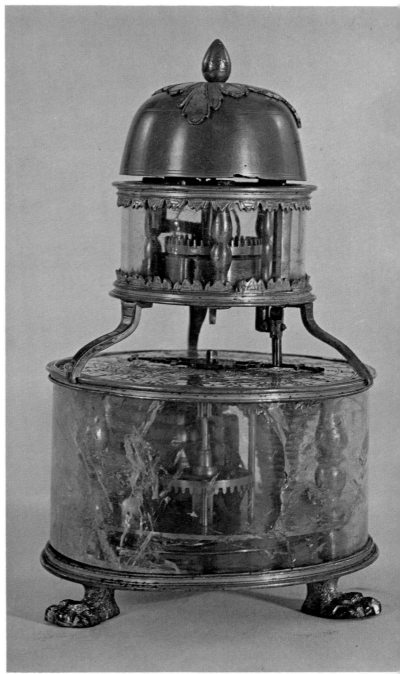

This delightful drum-shaped clock in its rock crystal case is probably French and of late sixteenth-century provenance. It has an attachable alarm, which is positioned above the dial when in use and incorporates a lever projecting downwards in such a manner that it will be tripped by the hour hand when the latter reaches the appropriate time. British Museum, London.

opposite page, left
Burgi's greatest masterpiece is known as the Vienna Crystal Clock and was made about 1615.

opposite page, right
This view of a Burgi cross-beat escapement is taken from his second experimental clock illustrated on page 87.

91

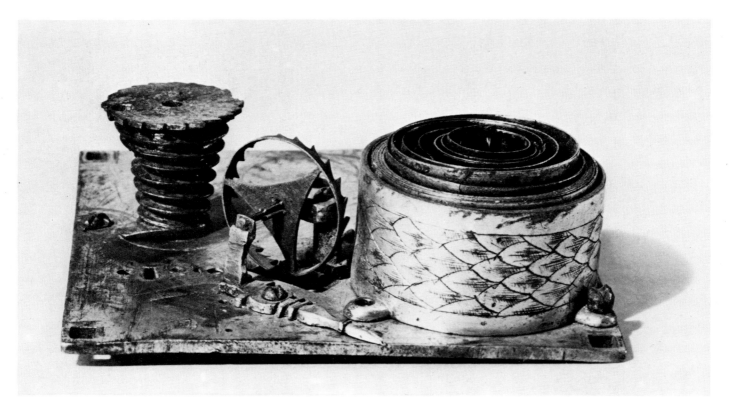

In the Bavarian National Museum in Munich, these fragmentary remains of a clock dated 1509 represent probably the earliest surviving example of the fusee.

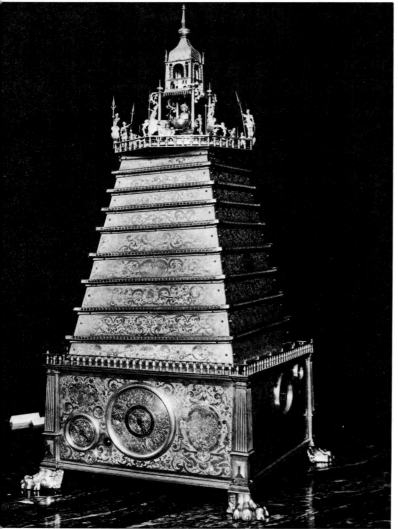

left
The rolling ball as a time standard has been used at various times in horological history. This elaborate example by Christolph Rohr of Leipzig is dated 1601. Only one ball is used, and the time it takes to descend the long track and reach the top again is one minute. Herzog Anton Ulrich-Museum, Brunswick.

opposite page, left
It is possible that portable watches were developed from small clocks in circular canister cases, such as this one of German origin, dating from the second quarter of the sixteenth century. Each of the hours on the dial is fitted with a touch-pin so that the time can be told at night. Museum of the Worshipful Company of Clockmakers, Guildhall, London.

opposite page, right
The movement of the canister clock previously illustrated is mainly of steel, and the only two brass wheels are almost certainly replacements. Museum of the Worshipful Company of Clockmakers, Guildhall, London.

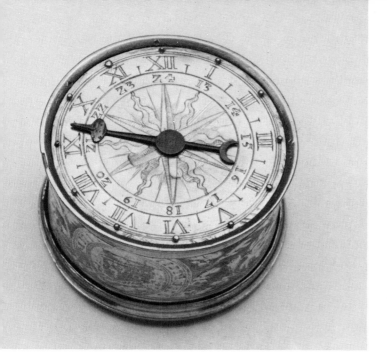

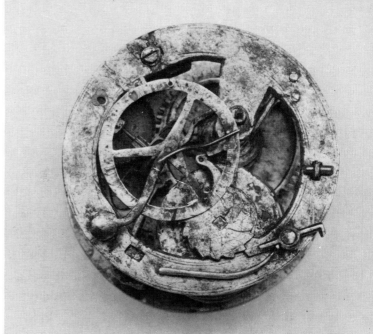

date is suspect, and it would not be safe to rely upon it. The Jacob the Zech clock remains the earliest surviving complete example. The early form of fusee tends to be much too sharply tapered, as presumably the theory had not then been completely worked out; and not until the seventeenth century, when the scientific aspects of horology became more predominant, did the outer curve of the grooved cone become shallower and more flattened out.

The question of regulation – making the clock run faster or slower – was not dealt with at length as part of the rudiments of clockwork, since, in its simplest form, the method must be self-evident. It is necessary only to vary the force of the driving power, for example by increasing or reducing the weight, to obtain what is certainly fairly coarse, rough and ready, regulation of a simple clock; and this is indeed what was done in the earliest times. In addition, of course, the arms of the foliot were supplied with small movable weights, which could be brought nearer to, or removed further from, the centre of oscillation, providing a somewhat finer degree of control. Another method is known as hog's-bristle regulation, of which a clock of about 1500 in the Germanisches Museum in Nuremberg has the earliest surviving example. The method, subsequently applied to early watches as well as to clocks, caused the extent of the swing in either direction – or the amplitude, as it is usually called – of the balance to be limited by interposing in its path two bristles, to catch in turn either side of the balance arm or crossbar. The hog's-bristle was often used in conjunction with that type of balance in which a flat rim had been added to the simple crossbar, to make it a sort of flywheel; this type, and the true foliot, with or without adjusting weights (in the latter case the arms are terminated by rounded bobs which have led to its sometimes being called a 'dumb-bell' balance), seem to have

been used indiscriminately from earliest times, and there is no evidence to show that one superseded the other. It can be appreciated that the bristles possessed their own in-built resilience, so that when limiting the amplitude of the balance, they exerted quite a gentle restraint, much to be preferred to any system which brought the balance to a sudden jarring stop when it had swung as far as it was deemed necessary that it should do. Furthermore, there had of necessity to be provision for the bristles to be adjustable in their proximity to the balance bar at the limits of its swing, otherwise there would be no latitude for regulation. There is, incidentally, another interesting feature in the Nuremberg clock referred to above, and that is the use of screws and nuts, a very early example of this facility being used in horology, and only postdating by about fifteen years Leonardo da Vinci's sketches of a tap and die for making metallic screws.

Over the years, there has been much speculation about the origins of the watch. Two technical requirements were necessary before it could become a practical proposition – the development of a successful spring-drive to power it, and some better arrangement for framing the movement than the open-work, posted method used in the earliest static forms of timekeeper. Both these developments eventually came to pass, and, amongst the plethora of clock-types and shapes that must have poured out of centres like Augsburg, there gradually evolved two basic designs. One of these provided for a movement that was essentially deployed in a vertical plane with a dial likewise, and the other, which is often called the drum or canister type, has the dial and movement arranged horizontally. It is further held that the next stages in clock design sprang from the first, vertical system, while the drum clocks – many of which, from the middle of the sixteenth century

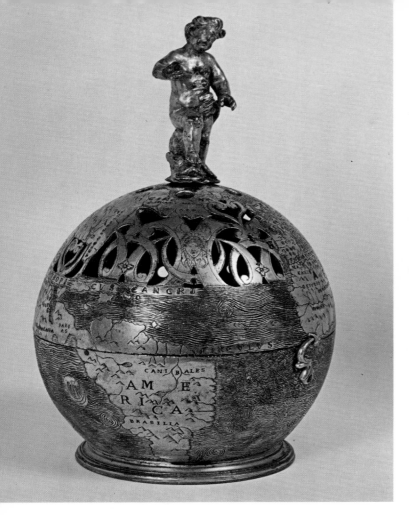

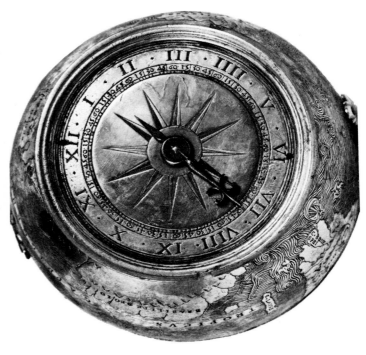

This spherical French clock-watch is by Jacques de la Garde, and, like the rather smaller German clock-watch shown on page 89, dates from about 1550. Unlike the German example, this incorporates a fusee. National Maritime Museum, Greenwich.

opposite page
A good example of the second form of tambour case, in which the outer surfaces are curved. The protective cover over the dial is pierced to allow the time to be read, a fashion which preceded that of fitting a glass cover. Museum of the Worshipful Company of Clockmakers, Guildhall, London.

right
The stackfreed, as a means of evening out the pull of the mainspring, was an interesting, albeit ineffective, device used almost exclusively on watches and on a few horizontal table clocks, all of German provenance. It is almost unknown in small vertical clocks such as this one, which is dated 1612 although thought to be actually somewhat earlier.

94

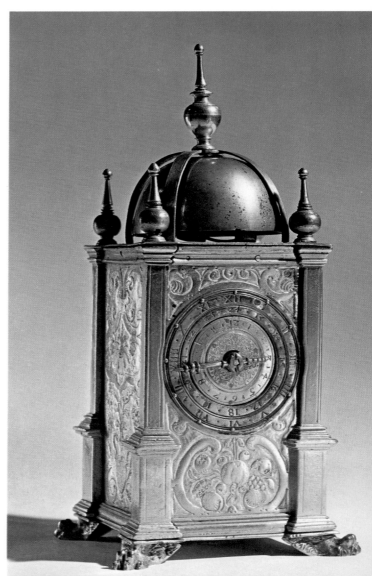

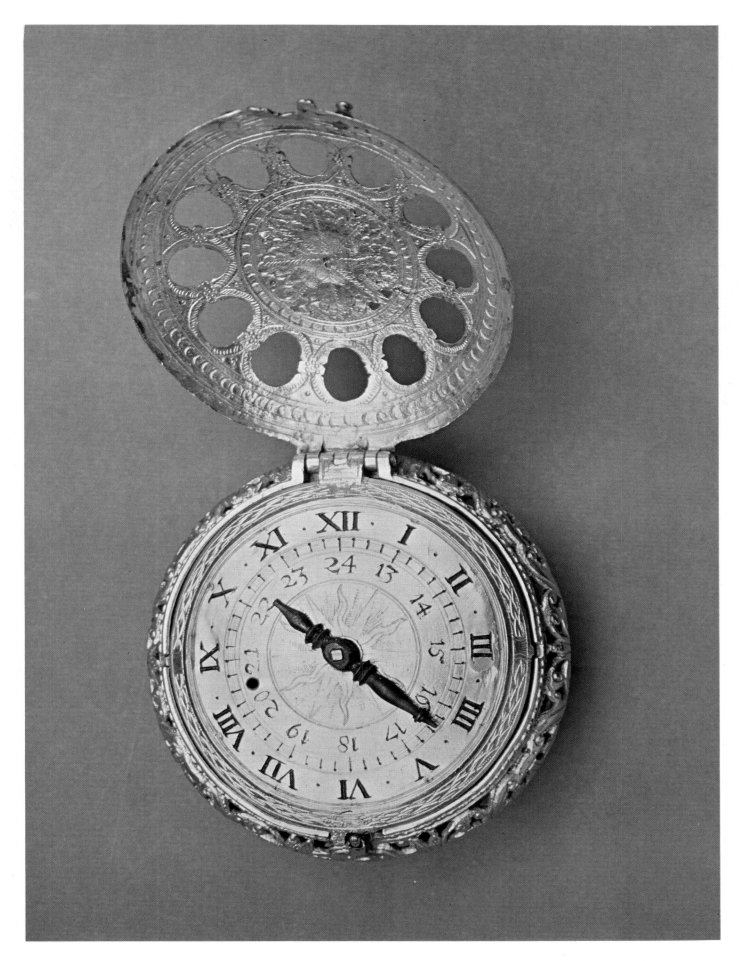

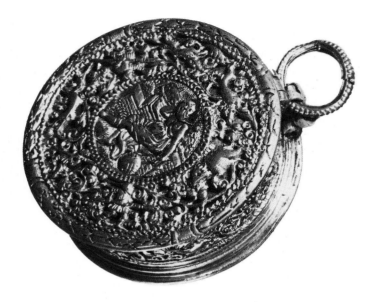

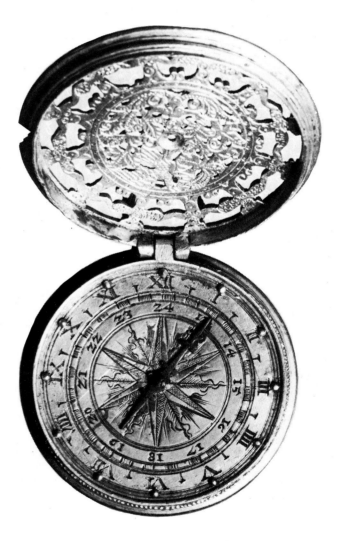

The earliest type of tambour watch-case had a flat top and bottom and a flat band, a fashion which continued till about the end of the third quarter of the sixteenth century. This German clock-watch, an example of this earlier style, also incorporates an alarm. Ashmolean Museum, Oxford.

if not earlier, were already being made quite small enough to be carried on the person – were the progenitors of the watch.

However this may be, the earliest watches seem to fall into two groups. One was indeed a modified form of the drum clock described above: it was flatter in contour, often a little larger in diameter, with hinged covers to either side which were engraved and pierced, as was the band of the case, to allow the sound of the hours being struck to issue forth. Nearly all such watches had an added attachment, usually either alarm or hour-striking – the latter, in other words, were clock-watches. The band of the case – that is, the part separating the back and front covers – might be flat or curved in profile, and the covers flat and overlapping the band or domed and butting with it. Cases with flat bands and overlapping flat lids are usually called tambour cases, preceding the other variety which did not appear until the last quarter of the sixteenth century.

The second style of early watch is spherical. It is extremely rare – probably no more than half a dozen examples survive in the world – but it is clear even from these few specimens that this type of watch was made both in Germany and France. The earliest of all dates from the second quarter of the sixteenth century, while the earliest French model is dated 1551. The latter is by Jacques de la Garde, and is in the Louvre in Paris. A similar, but larger, version by this same maker, dated the following year, is to be found in the National Maritime Museum at Greenwich.

Once upon a time it was unanimously held that the spherical watch was the prototype although recent research tends to suggest that both early types of watch arrived more or less simultaneously. The basis of the earlier belief derives from one Peter Henlein of Nuremberg, a locksmith who was clearly rather more of an artist than his trade description might imply. He first figures in a published reference dated 1511; he is later credited with making 'the small watch works which he was one of the first to make in the form of musk-balls . . .' Since he must have been one of the first genuine watchmakers, later historians, even in this present century, also credited him with inventing the mainspring, although we now know this to have been a complete fabrication.

It is a curious thing that all surviving sixteenth-century watches are cased in gilt bronze. There are contemporary inventory references that show that gold and silver were used for this purpose as well, but none have come down to us. It may be that there were restrictions placed upon the use of precious metals for such purposes by the guilds concerned – this happened at a later date, certainly – which made such objects rare even in their own time.

By far the greatest number of extant watches

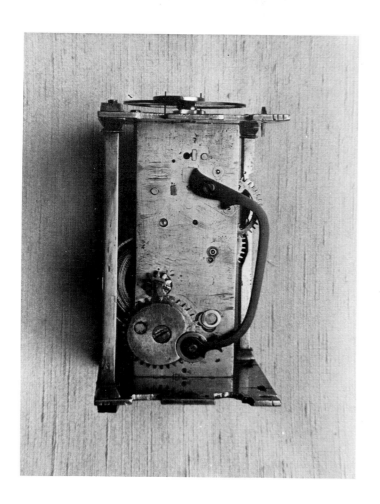

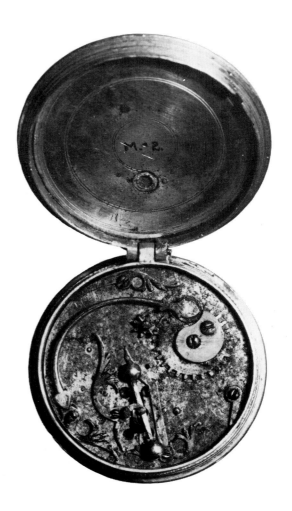

The stackfreed of the clock shown on page 94. The cam is original, but the curved spring and roller are replacements.

Back view of the movement of the watch on the opposite page shows a stackfreed and a foliot with a bristle regulator. Ashmolean Museum, Oxford.

from this period are German, as has been mentioned – and Nuremberg was unquestionably preeminent in this respect from quite early in the sixteenth century. However, research among archives in Italy shows that small clocks – and almost certainly watches too – were being made in that country before 1490, while there was a watchmaking tradition in France from 1525 or a little before. The styles of German and French watches, so far as it is possible to judge – since no French watch survives from before the mid century – were substantially different. There are no French watches in the tambour type of cases; of the mere half dozen or so that predate 1590, nearly all are spherical or oval. Piercing of the case, required to allow the sound of the bell to be heard, is confined to the band and the covers remain solid. The heavy chiselled decoration of German watches is replaced, in the French usage, by fine engraving. Towards the end of the sixteenth century, both France and Germany inclined towards octagonal cases, some of the rather more elegant elongated variety, while from 1590 France produced some of the first watches in oval cases with slightly domed

covers back and front. Although watches were certainly known in other European countries – England, Holland, and Switzerland, in particular – before 1600, the native craft in such countries had barely appeared, so that, in many cases, watches must have been imported into them from one or other of the major producers.

One remaining feature of many – perhaps most – sixteenth-century clocks and watches was the employment of touch-pins. These were placed around the dial, one at each hour, so that after dark, when the generating of any kind of light would have been tiresome and time-consuming, the position of the single hand could be related to its nearest touch-pin; this in turn had to be referred back to the twelve o'clock touch-pin, which was more prominent than the others and clearly distinguishable from them on that account. The same system has prevailed ever since, in watches designed for the benefit of the blind. *Montres à tact*, as the French call them, are but another example of an invention in horology that goes back to the beginnings of the craft, yet has never been bettered.

The Seventeenth Century – The Golden Age of Clocks and Watches

The title of this chapter has no connection with some particular horological application of a precious metal; the phrase is used metaphorically, yet any student in this field will recognise its validity. The hundred-year period between 1600 and 1700 has come to be known as the 'golden age' not only because it offers a far wider spectrum of decorative techniques and materials, and an infinitely higher standard of overall craftsmanship – especially towards the end of the period – than ever before, but also because it saw the birth and ascent to the peak of their prowess of some of the greatest names in the history of the craft. The real uniqueness of this century lies in its production of clocks and watches that were both functional and inherently beautiful, the perfect combination of art and craft. Later periods were to see timepieces become ever more accurate as such, while the quality of their decorative appeal all too noticeably degenerated. Finally, of course, the seventeenth century saw the introduction of possibly the two most significant horological developments of all – the pendulum and the balance spring.

As the century started, the commonest domestic clock was still the iron posted-frame 'Gothic' clock, weight-driven and relatively uncomplicated. Certainly the output of Augsburg, with its preference for spring-driven timepieces, cannot be discounted: too many superb examples remain to please us. But for the average European household – those that could afford it, that is – the iron clock, probably imported from south Germany although perhaps copied locally, gave a better showing than some of the more elaborate timepieces that were available. However, soon after 1600, the English established their own native craft which quickly rose to such prominence as to require proper organisation. One outcome of this was the granting of a Royal Charter in 1631, giving formal approval to the founding of the Worshipful Com-

pany of Clockmakers of the City of London. This was rapid progress for its time – it is difficult indeed to discover native English horologists before the start of the century, the only two names that readily spring to mind being those of Bartholomew Newsam and Randolph Bull, who both made clocks for Queen Elizabeth I and enjoyed the appointment of Royal Clockmaker; yet within thirty years the craft was clamouring for recognition.

The first outcome of this upsurge of activity was the emergence of a purely British style of domestic clock, the lantern clock. Nobody seems to know quite how it got that name – it may well have customarily been hung from a beam in much the way that lanterns were, and it is said that some ships' lanterns were of similar appearance – but it has been conjectured that the word is a corruption of 'latten', or *laiton*, the French word for brass. These clocks are also called 'Cromwellian' clocks, despite the fact that they were in use long before the Protector came to power. The first such clocks were somewhat shorter than the Gothic clocks from which they derived, and there was a large proportion of brass used in their manufacture. The movement continued to be of 'four-poster' construction, with the going train in front and the striking train behind, surmounted by a bell hung from a canopy. The great change was the addition of sheet brass sides, usually easily removable but nevertheless very efficacious in excluding dust.

The lantern clock was made throughout the seventeenth century and into the eighteenth, lasting even longer in provincial usage; and it occurs in the form of 'period reproductions', now either spring-driven or with electric movements, right down to the present day. As seventeenth-century technology progressed, so too did the mechanical design of the lantern clock. Originally these were made with wheel balances and, seemingly, never with a foliot; but soon after the introduction of the pendulum, not only was the wheel balance superseded, but earlier models that incorporated it were converted to the newer form of controller. Early lantern clocks with their original wheel balances are consequently very rarely encountered.

Stylistically, early lantern clocks had a narrow chapter ring, which was confined within the width of the clock frame. As the century progressed, however, the chapter ring became wider, projecting beyond the frame; such clocks are customarily called 'sheep's-head' clocks. Yet another variant, a short-lived fashion lasting about twenty years in the latter half of the seventeenth century, was the 'winged' lantern clock. The pendulum of such clocks was constructed in the shape of an anchor, the flukes acting as the pendulum bob. Extensions – 'wings' – were added to the sides of the case, and sometimes even surmounted with decorative cresting. As the pendulum swung, the flukes appeared momentarily in alternate 'wings', at least demonstrating that the clock was going!

Clockmaking in France, admirable though it was at certain times, enjoyed a rather chequered existence. French craft guilds tended to be organised by localities, and proliferated in numbers between the sixteenth and eighteenth centuries. The first guild of clockmakers was formed in Paris in 1544, but in Blois not until 1597; other centres blossomed at Lyon, Rouen, Dijon and elsewhere. Apart from the mere three royal clockmakers who were allowed in office at any one time – and who were considered outside guild rules and regulations – there were innumerable associated crafts with fringe interests in clockmaking, such as cabinetmakers, gilders, casters, chasers, bellfounders and so forth, all of whose special interests had to be protected. Despite this, and contrary to the practice in other countries, the French clockmakers were able to obtain permission to work in precious metals; this is without doubt the reason why so very few French Renaissance clocks have survived. Once they went out of fashion, they were melted down for the value of their cases, whereas the gilt bronze ones, favoured in Germany and elsewhere, survived in tolerable quantities. Such French examples in base-metal cases as do surface from time to time are mainly of the upright hex-

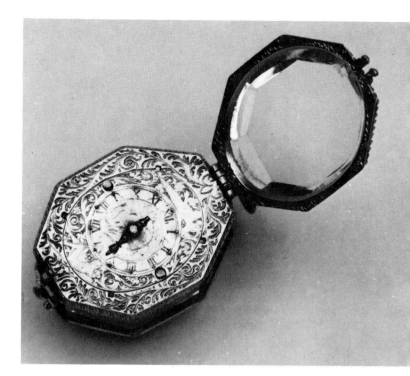

above
Although unsigned, this octagonal crystal-cased watch is probably French and dates from the first decade of the seventeenth century. Museum of the Worshipful Company of Clockmakers, Guildhall, London.

right
Transitional stages between the Gothic and lantern forms of domestic clock are rare, and this example dates from the first quarter of the seventeenth century. The posted frame of forged steel still incorporates Gothic detail. British Museum, London.

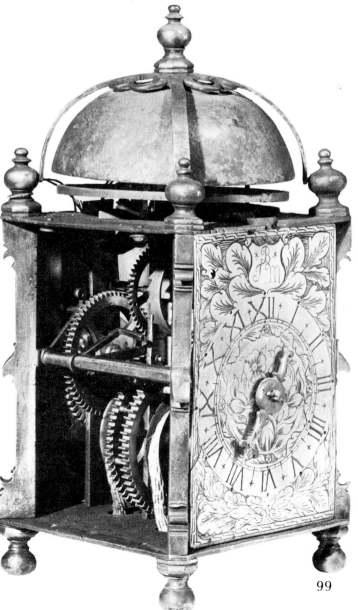

99

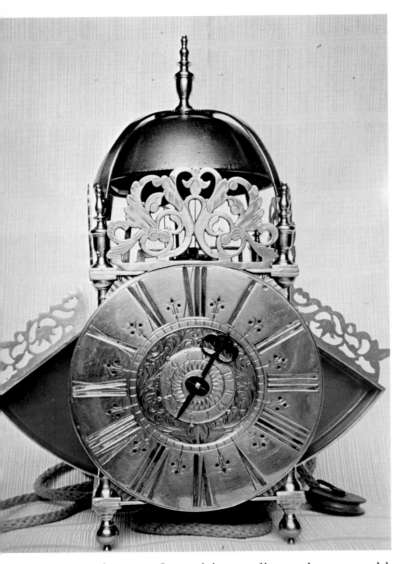

agonal type, of exquisite quality and comparable with anything produced elsewhere. The only traces of their more intrinsically valuable counterparts are the mouth-watering descriptions of them which abound in contemporary documents. Towards the end of the sixteenth century, the French clockmakers tried out various new shapes – at first upright cylinders and squares, and, as always in French artefacts, possessing obvious architectural overtones. However, by the beginning of the seventeenth century the accent was turning squarely towards the production of watches with a consequent decline in the output of clocks, which, to all intents and purposes, died as a French craft industry until after the mid century.

Elsewhere in Europe at this time, too, clockmaking flagged as a craft. The Italian practice tended to be intermittent and fragmented, while Holland was yet to achieve fame and individuality with the rise to prominence of its great physicist, astronomer and mathematician Christiaan Huygens, but again only after mid century.

Why should clockmaking, a relatively new technology, have stumbled so badly at the beginning of the seventeenth century? One explanation that has been advanced, particularly in regard to French clocks, is that carrying a watch for display – and this must have been the principal intention since while they were beautifully made, using the richest materials, they were still appalling timekeepers – became so compulsive among gentlemen of fashion that table clocks, at any rate, became superfluous. There were also extraneous influences. The German industry, for instance, suffered so grievously during the Thirty Years War (1618–48) that it took two hundred years to recover.

There is another 'grey area' in our knowledge of this period, and that concerns exactly how watches were worn. Renaissance watches seem to have been carried on a cord about the neck or, more rarely, at the waist. In England, at any rate, pockets, introduced fifty years earlier, were confined to the breeches until 1675, and watches carried therein would have been subjected to such jarring as to render their already temperamental motions well-nigh inoperative. Yet it is rare indeed to find a watch being visibly worn in a seventeenth-century portrait.

In England, whatever may have been going on elsewhere, the making of clocks – principally lantern clocks – thrived, and alongside it, during the first twenty-five years of the seventeenth century, the making of watches became sufficiently established to see the gradual emergence of a national style which was to last for several decades, as well as to lay the foundations for the supremacy in this field which English watches were to enjoy somewhat later on. At first, they appear to have been based upon French designs – elongated hexagons and ovals of highly engraved gilt brass or silver, sometimes with an added band of contrasting metal. Mechanically very little was to change for seventy-five years, and the surest way of placing a watch from this time in its right category is by its decoration – yet the English national style, for at least three decades from about 1620, was to be devoid of such artifice, at least externally. The 'Puritan' watch, as the style has come to be known, represents a total rejection of everything that had gone before. In round or oval form, and in gilt brass but perhaps more generally in silver, the watch case – and its second, outer case where such is provided – is completely plain, while the dial consists of a simple chapter ring engraved upon an otherwise featureless flat metal surface. The single hand is of steel, with a 'tail' extending back from the centre and balancing the pointer, the whole carrying the barest minimum of turned and chiselled ornament.

The only decoration that was applied to such watches was upon the movement, which largely resembled what had gone before. The balance cocks of such watches were oval, with no sign of a rim to the irregular edge, and they were attached

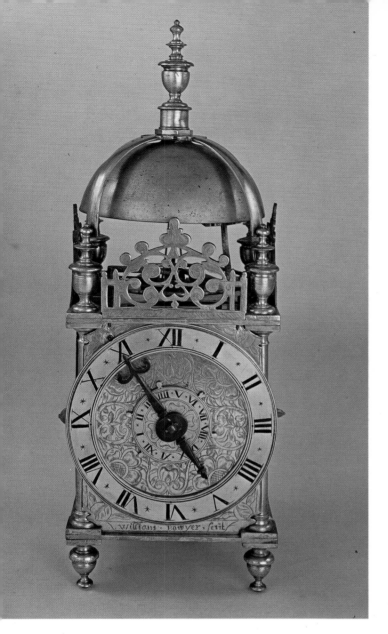

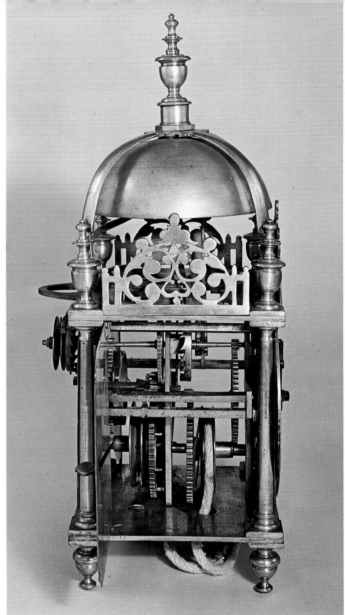

opposite page
This lantern clock, which is unsigned, has wings on either side (sometimes they have cresting on top, as here), in which the anchor-like flukes constituting the pendulum bob appear. This style was short-lived, lasting only about twenty years towards the end of the seventeenth century.

above
This clock, which dates from about 1640, exhibits the narrow chapter ring which is typical of early lantern clocks. It was made by William Bowyer. British Museum, London.

above right
This lateral view of the previous clock, with sides removed to show the movement, reveals the typical fourposter frame, the trains placed one behind the other and alarm mechanism at the rear. The pillars are now brass instead of steel as are the finials and frets. British Museum, London.

to the back plate of the movement by means of a block or tenon, fixed to the plate, which fits into a squared hole cut into the neck of the cock. The tenon and the neck of the cock have been drilled to take a pin which, when in position, makes an adequately firm fixing. Such cocks were decorated with pierced scrollwork and foliage. The mainspring set-up, also located upon the back plate of the watch, was made the site for decorative steelwork, both when this function was performed by the ratchet wheel and click and later, from about 1635, when it was superseded by the worm and wheel arrangement.

The 'Puritan' watch probably reflected the feelings of the times, and it can also be argued that it foreshadowed the English trend towards unadulterated functionalism that was to predominate as the scientific approach to time-measurement took hold. Nevertheless, elsewhere among those nations, mainly European, who were building up a horological heritage, the period from 1625 to 1675 is renowned for producing some of the most fabul-

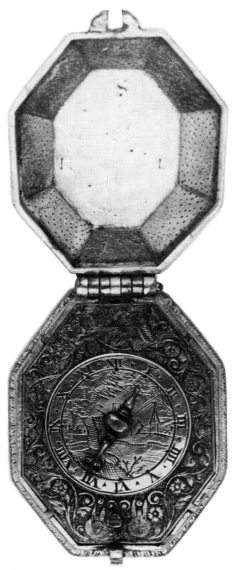

opposite page, above
Signed 'Edm. Bull In Fleetstreet Fecit', this oval watch is engraved in the centre of the dial with Venus and Cupid. It dates from the first quarter of the seventeenth century. Victoria and Albert Museum, London.

opposite page, below
David Ramsay, who was born about 1590 and died about 1654, was the first Master of the Clockmakers' Company in 1632. He was an outstanding watchmaker, and this star watch is one of his finest creations; it was made about 1625. Museum of the Worshipful Company of Clockmakers, Guildhall, London.

left
Another of David Ramsay's watches. The outside of the case is engraved with religious scenes, and the movement is signed 'David Ramsay me fecit'. Victoria and Albert Museum, London.

below
This watch made by Ramsay about 1630 reveals his Scottish background, being signed 'David Ramsay Scotus me fecit'. The octagonal case is in rock crystal mounted in gold. Museum of the Worshipful Company of Clockmakers, Guildhall, London.

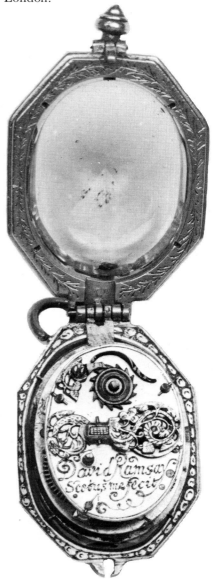

ous watches ever seen. It was the supreme era of the decorative watch, and it may be useful here to review some of the many techniques and materials that were used while this fashion was at its height, although we must not lose sight of the fact that, throughout the whole period, the timekeeping properties of the objects upon which so much expensive craftsmanship was being lavished were, to say the least, minimal. They were, in other words, essentially items of personal jewellery.

There were a number of techniques available for working upon raw metal. One that became popular towards the end of the seventeenth century and throughout much of the eighteenth was repoussé work, in which a design is hammered out from the back, using a variety of different punches. In extreme cases, the relief obtainable can be really three-dimensional. Similar techniques but used upon the front of the metal are known as chasing. Sometimes these two techniques will be found to have been combined on the same watch case, generally upon early rather than later specimens. Classical and allegorical scenes were particularly favoured for depicting by these methods; and where a repoussé watch case is of the very highest quality, it is not unusual to find an additional outer case, consisting simply of two bezels, or rims, hinged together, one of them fitted with a convex glass. In position, the repoussé back of the watch case was covered by the glazed bezel through which it could be examined, yet it was fully protected from accidental damage or from rubbing or scratches in the pocket. Decoration similar to repoussé work can, of course, be cast, although it is difficult to obtain the high quality thereby.

Other methods of decorating metal include piercing, chiselling and engraving. Early German watches combined the first two of these, the depth of the chiselling being sometimes quite unusual; but, except in relatively low relief, chiselling gradually died out, to be superseded by engraving. Cast metal decoration has often to be tidied up by manual means, frequently chiselling, in order to improve the definition of the subject matter.

Enamelling upon metal is a means of decoration of considerable antiquity. In its simplest form, enamel is a special type of colourless glass, known as 'flux', to which colour can be imparted by the addition of metallic oxides. The melting temperature can be varied according to the amounts of the ingredients used, to produce so-called 'hard' or 'soft' enamels possessing different properties, mainly relating to brittleness of surface and retention of colour. Two of the most usual methods of decoration by enamelling are known as cloisonné and champlevé. In the first of these, thin strips or fillets of metal – usually gold – are formed to the outline shape of each colour of the design and fixed in position, often simply being set into a thin layer of enamel covering the whole surface of the article concerned. The compartments thus formed, which will together make up the finished design, are each filled with powdered enamel mixed to give their relevant colours, and the whole object is then fired in a furnace. In champlevé enamelling, the other and commoner form, the compartments are formed by scooping out metal from the object itself, rather than by adding fillets of metal to it; otherwise the process is similar.

A third variant, known as enamel painting, started around 1630. Here there was no attempt to form compartments or cells; a smooth enamel surface was laid down, suitably painted and fired. Because of the expansion of the metal carcase and its possible effect upon the decorated surface, gold was most frequently used; but notwithstanding this, it was usually found desirable to enamel the whole watch case, inside and out, rather than risk cracking. Where this has been done, the reverse protective enamelled surface is called 'contre-émail'. The earliest 'school' of enamel painting was at Blois, closely followed by that at Geneva from about 1650. The most famous watch case

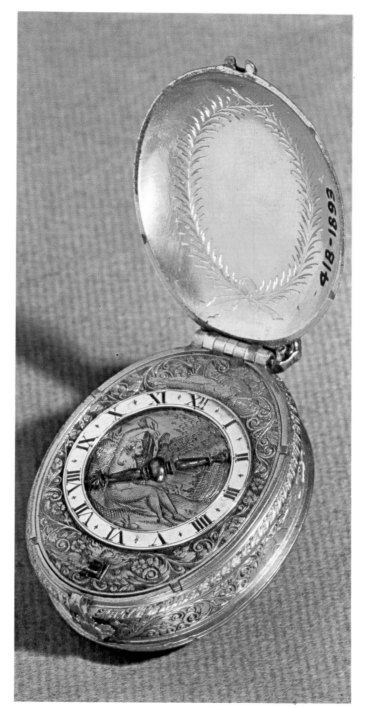

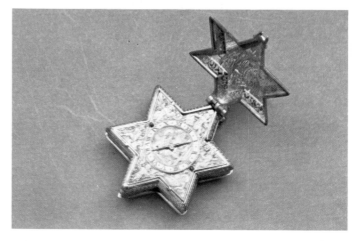

painters in this genre, the Huaud family, originated in the latter city; their watch cases are always signed and have great individuality, although experts consider their work inferior to the very best turned out at Blois.

There were several other processes involving enamelling in use at various times – for example, the painting in enamel pioneered at Limoges, as opposed, that is, to the painting on enamel outlined in the preceding paragraph. Then there were combination procedures like basse-taille. This involves enamelling over an incised pattern, often engine-turned or, as the French expressed it, *guilloché* with geometrical figures; this became very popular in watch cases towards the end of the eighteenth century. Another method used on watch cases is niello, which is effectively a method of filling up the compartments in a champlevé surface, usually of silver or steel, with a black molten filling of various metallic sulphides. The contrast can be very effective.

So far, the carcases of all the watch cases described have been metal, but other materials were used from time to time. One of the richest was

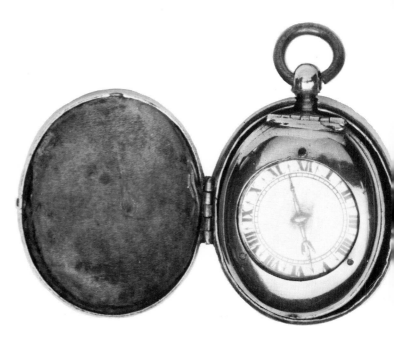

The most commonly encountered oval form of Puritan watch is seen in this example by Edward East which dates from about 1630. Museum of the Worshipful Company of Clockmakers, Guildhall, London.

Edward East, remarkable for the general elegance of his work, did not neglect to make his own signature outstanding, as this example from another of his watches demonstrates.

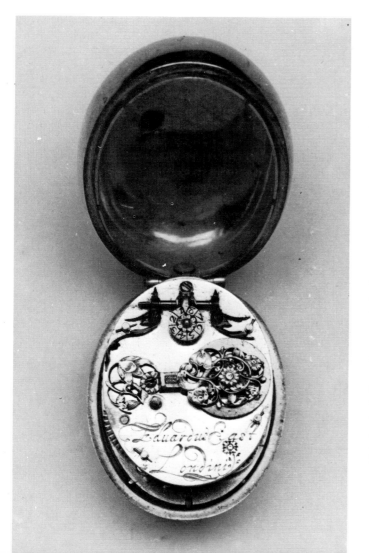

rock crystal, fashioned in a considerable variety of forms, the material itself being generally the clear variety although, occasionally, the rarer smoky type is found. Apart from 'form' watches, to be described in the next paragraph, crystal-cased watches are usually octagonal or round, the two halves of the case set in gilt metal bezels hinged together. Very much more rarely, the bezels are omitted, and the two crystal segments are connected directly by a hinge on one end and a catch on the opposite one. Curiously, crystal is almost never used plain. Round cases are divided into lobes, hexagonal cases are cut with large facets, and so on.

'Form' watches is the term used to describe the multitude of seventeenth-century watches specially cased up to represent something quite different: cross watches, tulip watches, skull watches, book watches and many more. Cases were cast and chiselled in the form of pomegranates, cockleshells, Tudor roses, doves and, in some cases, incorporated rock crystal in combination with silver or gilt metal. Many of these cases were not of the highest quality; but those that were are superb.

Watches like the foregoing were obviously among the most expensive obtainable, but with so much attention being paid to the exotic it would be strange if some change did not rub off on the more everyday product. The English 'Puritan' timepiece remained fairly static until mid century although, with such craftsmen as Edward East putting their names to them, they were as good of their plain and unadulterated kind as it was possible to find. They did aspire to an outer protective case – in order, presumably, to exclude dust since there was nothing decorative to take care of – as did also many of those watches that could be described as works of art. Sometimes, this case was just to deposit them in when not in use – like a jewelbox – but after about 1650, outer cases were made to be worn with the watch, and watches so equipped came to be known as pair-cased watches. These outer cases, in their turn, came to be made in both plain and decorative versions, the latter often employing attractive materials like horn, tortoiseshell and leather moulded to a base-metal carcase, and further decorated with underpainting or inlaying with gold or silver in the fashion known as piqué.

Other details of the watch changed greatly during the seventeenth century. At the beginning, the metal dial plate had a simple hour ring engraved upon it, or the engraving was done on a separate metal ring which was then attached to the plate; occasionally a disc was used in preference to an applied ring. Such rings were narrow, occupying little enough room on the dial plate and the rest of the area was covered in close engraving. Later on, the hour ring became wider, leaving much less room for decoration. Plain white enamel dials started to appear about 1675, but they are nowhere common before 1700 and, in England, not until 1725. Hands are generally of steel and well made, and glasses over the dial came into use at some time during the century, replacing the earlier pierced covers; but since it must always be open to question whether a particular watch glass is original, it is difficult to say when this happened. The recognisably round watch, as opposed to the other shapes that had gone before, became the norm from about mid century.

Up to the middle of the seventeenth century, then, watches according to the English usage were, as a rule, outstanding for their lack of decoration,

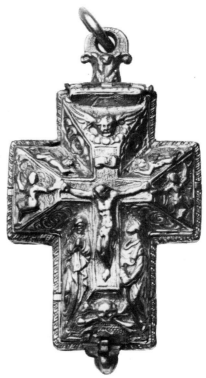

This watch in the shape of a cross, from the second quarter of the seventeenth century, is by Didier Lalemand of Paris and is a typical example of a form watch. British Museum, London.

while the complete reverse applied to those from other manufacturing centres. Clocks came in three principal styles – the lantern clock fitted with its wheel balance, the travelling or coach clock, which was simply a greatly oversize watch, and the table clock with its horizontal dial, largely unchanged from its inception. All such clocks were, of course, survivals from the past, as indeed were the tabernacle clocks with their vertical dials and their three or more trains driving added complications, which were still being made by the Germans and Italians in the style of a century earlier. It was as if the industry was awaiting a sudden flash of inspiration, an invention of genius which would bring the making of clocks and watches to life again after seemingly stultifying for so many decades.

The invention, which was the application of the pendulum to clocks, when at last it came, was in fact the result of applied logic coupled to exceptional scientific acumen, rather than some entirely new concept launched upon an unsuspecting world as a result of an explosion of brilliance never to be repeated. Such inventions are often the best kind. It had been appreciated for a century and more that a pendulum had a capability for keeping time which was much better than any foliot or wheel balance. Galileo, as a young man in 1581, had timed the swinging of a lamp in Pisa cathedral and noted that its period of oscillation – the time it took to complete each swing – was dependent solely on its length and not at all upon whether it was swinging in large or small arcs. This led to the measurement of short periods of time, in such

This mid seventeenth-century watch case combines the techniques of chiselling and engraving upon a carcase that was originally cast. British Museum, London.

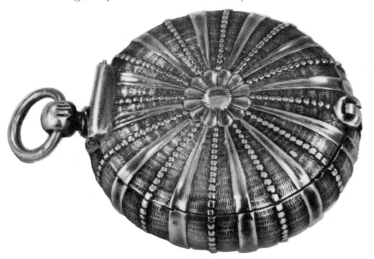

105

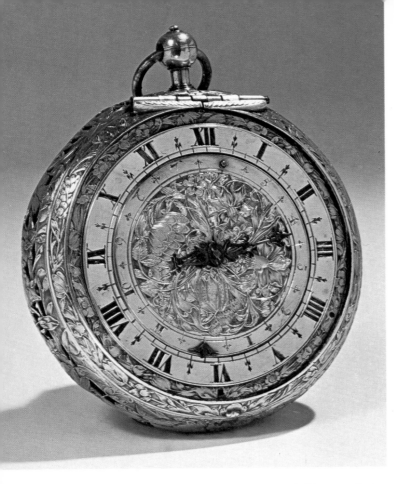

This clock-watch with alarm, a style which East made in various sizes up to and including coach watch, is in a beautifully decorated silver case and an outer case of wood covered with painted leather. Victoria and Albert Museum, London.

As befitted any maker with the Royal Appointment, East made some outstanding watches of which this pear-shaped crystal-cased example is typical. Victoria and Albert Museum, London.

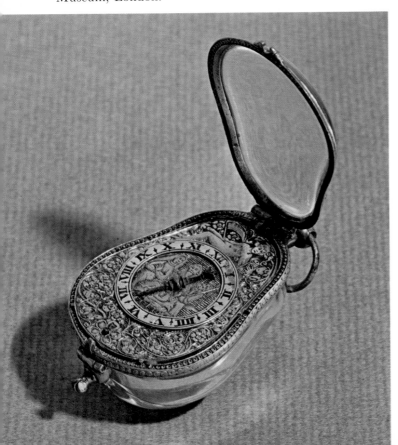

fields as astronomy, being made by counting the number of oscillations of a weight on the end of a cord. Even before this time, the ubiquitous Leonardo da Vinci had sketched pendulums in connection with pumping machinery, while Galileo's son as well as, independently, several experimenters in Italy and Poland were working along the same lines. Finally, the obstacles to harnessing a pendulum to clockwork were overcome, and the problem to all intents and purposes was solved, by Christiaan Huygens, a Dutch physicist.

It is a remarkable quirk of fate that two such brilliant and versatile men as Huygens in Holland and Robert Hooke in England should have shared the same century, let alone almost the same period of it for their life spans. Christiaan Huygens was born at The Hague on 14th April 1629, the son of a poet and statesman of considerable stature. At first he studied law, but then he devoted himself to mathematics and astronomy and quickly built a high reputation. His improvements in telescope lenses led to important gains in observational astronomy, while at the same time he was experimenting to perfect the control mechanism of clocks. He visited England in 1660 and 1663, in the latter year being elected a Fellow of the Royal Society. Subsequently for nearly twenty years he lived under the patronage of Louis XIV of France, and in 1673 published his celebrated work *Horologium Oscillatorium*. In effect, this was the first attempt to apply dynamics to bodies of finite size; later, it was to be of great value to Newton. Other matters to which Huygens applied himself included the wave theory of light – by which he explained reflection and refraction – and polarisation of light, a phenomenon which, despite its discovery by him, he was unable to explain. Huygens died at The Hague, to which he eventually returned, on 8th June 1695, leaving behind him a corpus of work which, when published, occupied twenty-two weighty volumes.

Huygens' great contribution to horology was his investigation of the theory of pendulums – both the ordinary vertical type and the conical, which has a circular instead of a lateral motion – as a result of which he was able to revise Galileo's previous postulation that the only determinant for a pendulum to 'beat' equal periods of time was its length, the size of the arc being of no consequence. This quality, usually called isochronism, is also dependent, so Huygens proved, on the arc described by the pendulum bob being that of a cycloid rather than a pure circle. A cycloid is the curve traced by a point on the circumference of a circle as it rolls along a straight line; in practical terms, a curve of this kind is rather more U-shaped than the curve of a circle.

Huygens translated his ideas into reality by means of pendulum clocks made by a well-known clockmaker at The Hague called Salomon Coster.

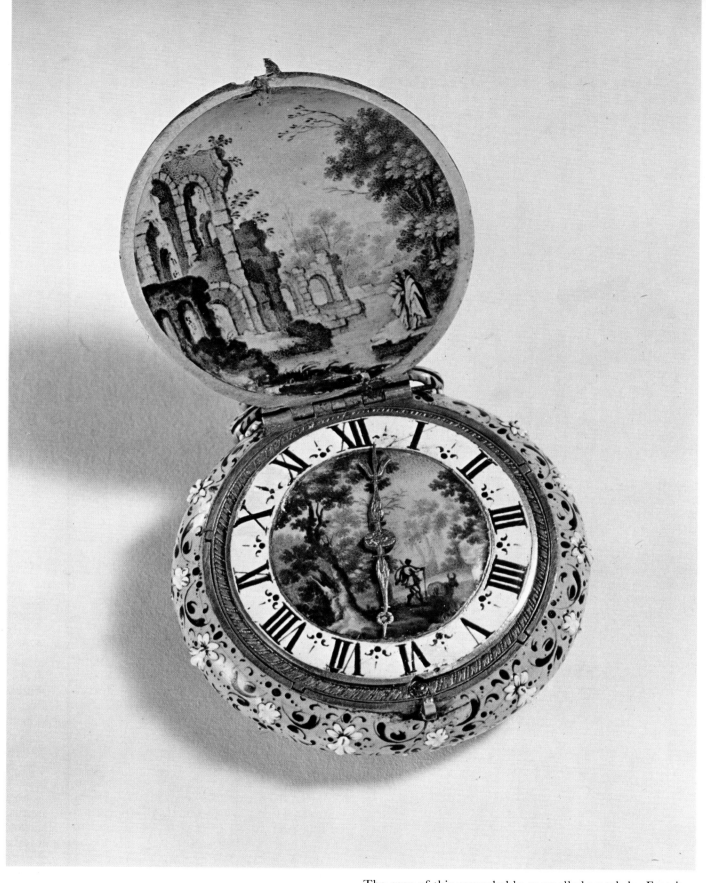

The case of this remarkable enamelled watch by East is
unusually shallow for the period. With a light blue ground
enamelled on gold, the edges of the case are decorated with
small flowers in relief, while the interior pictures are
landscapes with ruined buildings and figures again on a blue
ground. Victoria and Albert Museum, London.

The cycloidal curve of the swinging pendulum bob was achieved by suspending the pendulum on a silk thread hanging between curved 'cheeks' which, in theory, were to cause the arc described by the bob to steepen at each end of its swing. In fact, it was soon discovered that, though theoretically correct, the cycloidal curve caused more problems than it was supposed to solve, and for all normal purposes its effects could be ignored. Finally, Huygens assigned to Coster the right to make pendulum clocks for twenty-one years.

The application of the pendulum of necessity brought about a quite fundamental change in the clock designs obtaining at that time. A vertical pendulum presupposes a movement laid out in a vertical plane, with a vertical dial, as opposed to the horizontal table clocks that had hitherto been so popular. The plates between which the movements of clocks like this were confined would therefore be best described as 'front' and 'back' in place of 'top' and 'bottom'. A whole new generation of clocks was poised upon these mechanical improvements.

More or less coincidentally, John Fromanteel, a member of a famous Dutch clockmaking family based in London, happened to be working for Coster only a matter of days after the Huygens pendulum clock was patented and lost no time in absorbing the requisite technology. Extraordinarily quickly his family in London, headed by Ahasuerus Fromanteel, started advertising the

below left
This form watch by Richard Masterson dates from about 1630, and the silver case is cast in the form of a cockle shell. Museum of the Worshipful Company of Clockmakers, Guildhall, London.

below
The form watch resembling a tulip is found in various sizes, this being quite a small one made by F. Sermand who is probably the same as the maker of the watch on page 110. Its silver case has three crystal windows, and the watch dates from about 1640. Museum of the Worshipful Company of Clockmakers, Guildhall, London.

right
The silver case of this watch by Benjamin Hill is cast in the form of a pomegranate. It dates from the mid seventeenth century. Museum of the Worshipful Company of Clockmakers, Guildhall, London.

far right
Disguised in the form of a dove, the watch is only revealed when the lower part of the body of the bird hinges outwards. Made about 1685, this watch is probably Swiss and is signed 'Soret et Jay'. Museum of the Worshipful Company of Clockmakers, Guildhall, London.

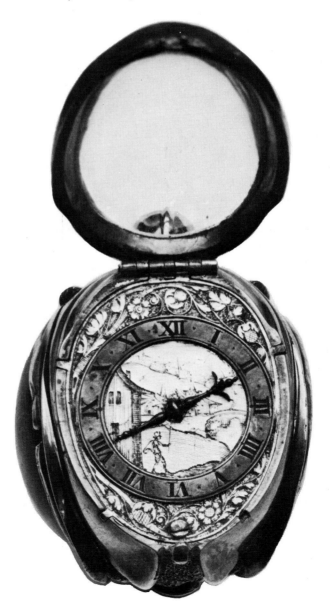

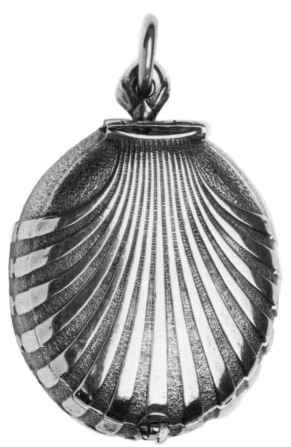

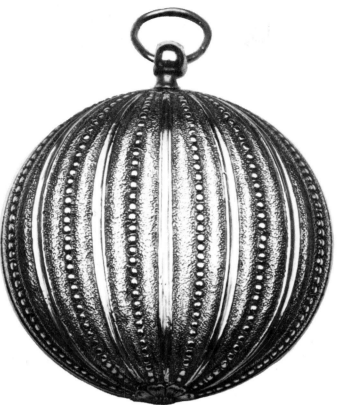

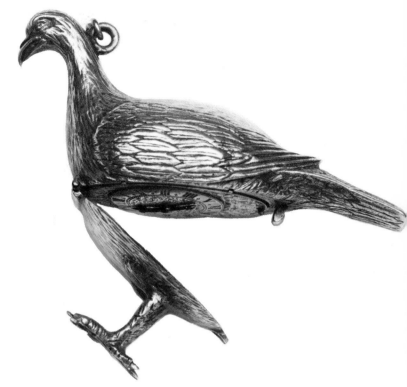

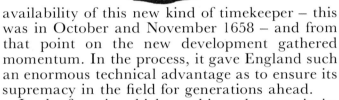

availability of this new kind of timekeeper – this was in October and November 1658 – and from that point on the new development gathered momentum. In the process, it gave England such an enormous technical advantage as to ensure its supremacy in the field for generations ahead.

In the form in which, at this early stage in its history, it was commonly adopted by Fromanteel and many another London clockmaker, the pendulum rod was ten inches long and terminated in a pear-shaped brass bob, which could be screwed up or down the rod to effect regulation. Such pendulums had a period of oscillation of about half a second, and they were applied to two basic types of clocks, one spring-driven and the other powered by weights.

Salomon Coster's first clocks with pendulums were spring-driven, in ebonised black wooden cases with pediment tops, and with two trains placed side by side, for going and striking, both powered by going barrels and both winding through the dial. In England, spring clocks – or bracket clocks as they have come to be known, although many of them never sat on a bracket but on a table or sideboard – and weight-driven hooded wall clocks, both with a strong architectural influence discernible in their design, were the first results of the adoption of the pendulum; they remained in fashion for about fifteen years from 1660 to 1675. The hooded wall clock, by the way, might be described as looking like the top of a grandfather clock, fixed on the wall and with the weights hanging down underneath. These types of clocks did not copy their Dutch progenitors in decorative detail: English clocks never boast velvet-covered dials with applied metal name plaques and chapter rings, but favour gilt metal dial plates, their centres matted or sometimes engraved with the then fashionable tulip type of ornamentation, that flower being adopted instead to reflect the increasing Dutch influence in design. English spring clocks, incidentally, favoured the fusee from the beginning – probably another example of the national emphasis placed upon accurate performance.

Very shortly after these initial styles, the English cherub spandrel appeared to fill the four corners of the dial, outside the chapter ring. In its earliest examples, and especially in those very rare ones where the spandrels have been cast in silver, it is an object of great beauty in its own right. But, like most popular ornamentation, constant copying and insufficient hand-finishing cause deterioration of the effect; this is detectable in English clocks even before the end of the seventeenth century. The other dial feature on English clocks at this time is the maker's signature. Until about 1675 this appears across the bottom of the dial plate, below the chapter ring, and it is frequently in a Latinised form. It might also appear on the otherwise perfectly plain back plate of the movement. Later the name is found in a plaque inside the chapter ring, or on the chapter ring itself – this was eventually the most favoured site for this feature – and after about 1675 back plates became the focus of overall engraved decoration, mainly various arabesque forms and sometimes incorporating a cartouche containing the maker's signature.

Once the architectural styles of clock cases, with their pediment tops and side columns in classic

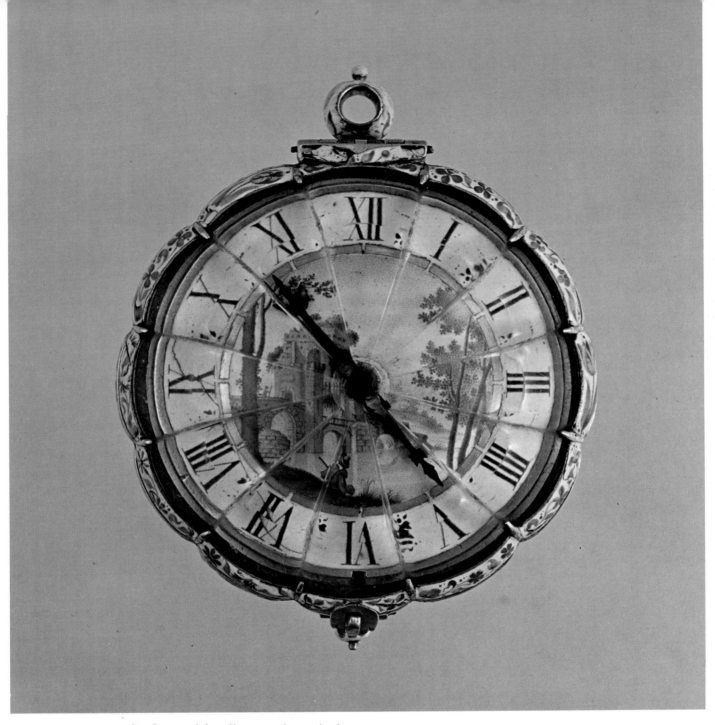

arrangement, and often with gilt metal capitals and bases, the whole upon a suitable plinth, had been superseded – and this was a relatively short-lived style – a more notably English style came into use. It has been said that the period up to about 1680 was the period of experimentation, while makers were struggling to perfect the styling that was appropriate to the new technology; the use of the pendulum clearly bespoke spatial requirements which needed to be reflected in the case design, and it was natural, at first, to seek solutions deriving from a discipline that is wholly concerned with the best use of space, i.e. architecture. However, this was the short answer; the longer one must inevitably have been to discover a recognisable English style, more especially because of the supremacy already gained in the field, which

This watch combines two decorative materials – crystal and enamelling – to great effect. It dates from about 1660 and is by Sermand of Geneva. British Museum, London.

above right
This watch has a square silver-studded leather case and is by Francis Rainsford. Dating from about 1700, it shows the continuing fashion for novelty of shape. Museum of the Worshipful Company of Clockmakers, Guildhall, London.

right
This engraved silver skull contains a watch signed 'Moysant Blois' and has its original shaped protective leather case. Tradition says the watch belonged to Mary Queen of Scots, but the existing mechanism postdates her execution by at least fifteen years. Museum of the Worshipful Company of Clockmakers, Guildhall, London.

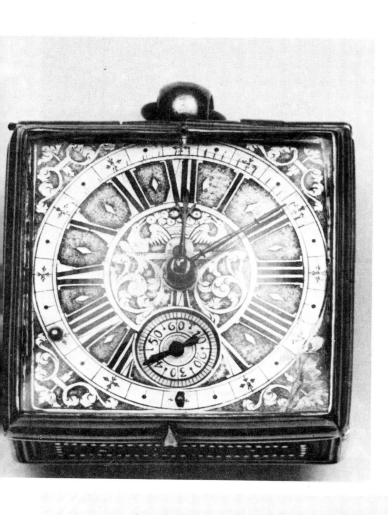

needed to be consolidated. So architectural cases were not made much after 1675, apart from the occasional use of barley-twist pillars and the stepped panel top during the following few years. Instead an essentially upright rectangular case became the norm, with glazed doors front and back, mounted upon a shallow moulded plinth with four simple feet, and surmounted by either a bell or basket top. A handle on the top enabled the clock to be carried most easily from room to room, and especially upstairs to bed at night; for a clock was an expensive item so that only the very rich household would contain more than one. Ebony is by far the commonest wood used for bracket clock cases at this period; of the others occasionally found, walnut is the rarest, while, very infrequently indeed, cases were made entirely of metal, usually gilt.

Case decorations include the fret above the door – to allow the sound of the bell to emerge – which, after about 1685, was made of metal rather than wood, as were also those inserted at the top of the side panels of the case, and sometimes also replaced the glazed rectangles in those panels which had been the original style. Similarly, metal frets with the wood cut away behind them were applied to the front and sides of the shallow domed structure placed lengthwise across the top of the case – the bell top, as it is usually called – which

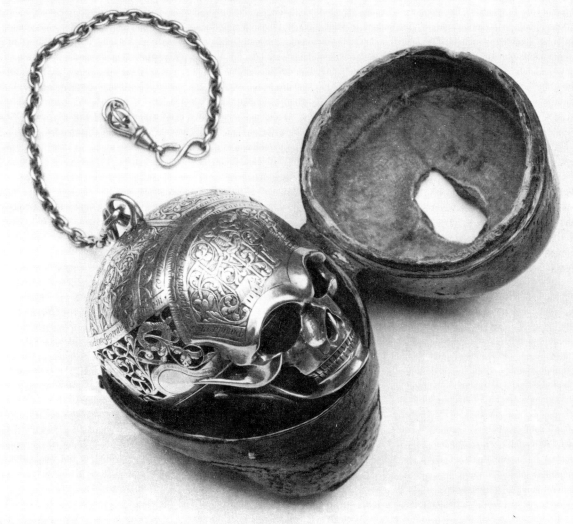

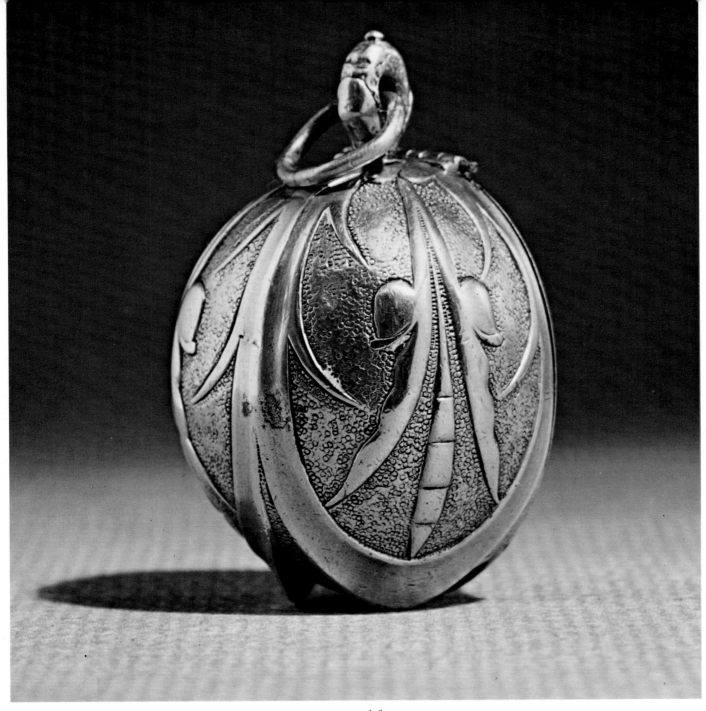

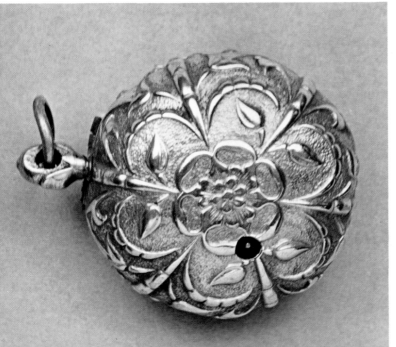

left
The silver gilt case of this watch by William Clay has been cast in the pattern of a Tudor rose which is carried round on to the bezel. The watch dates from about 1640. Museum of the Worshipful Company of Clockmakers, Guildhall, London.

above
Another flower-shaped form watch. The cast silver case shaped like a bud has three outer petals, one of which forms the cover over the dial. The watch itself is by Henry Grendon and dates from the second quarter of the seventeenth century. Victoria and Albert Museum, London.

superseded the architectural top after about 1675; and when occasionally this entire top structure is covered with pierced metal embellishment, it is called a basket top. By the end of the century there were other minor alternatives to this superstructure – a variant of the bell top, known as the inverted bell top, simply added another moulded level to the original, in exactly the same way as did the so-called double basket top – although the great makers, such as Tompion, never allowed ostentation to be confused with elegance. His cases have a restraint which conveys great individuality by comparison with many others of that period, although the foregoing describes in brief the outward appearance of the conventional English bracket clock as it was to remain for a long time to come, albeit with some development of fine detail.

One specialised form of spring clock which has appeared spasmodically from the period under review almost into modern times is the 'night clock'. Most variants of this type substitute a revolving dial with cut-out hour numerals for the conventional hands indicating the time upon a chapter ring. A lamp placed behind the dial at the point where the correct time will always be registered permits of this being read off in the dark, obviating any need to kindle a light. Some of these clocks had a silent escapement, one of the acting surfaces being made of gut. Such clocks, before 1700, are extremely rare.

So much for the English prototype spring clocks. The longcase clock – which is often called in England a grandfather clock, and in America a tall clock – seems to have been a wholly English inspiration, for the earliest known clocks of this kind are all English, and the fashion never seems to have become popular elsewhere, save for its adoption by the Dutch. There are no longcase clocks before 1659, and for the ensuing twelve years or so such clocks all had the short half-seconds pendulum and verge escapement of the bracket clock.

above
The overall enamelling of this watch case is notable for its restraint, the pattern of white flowers and foliage in relief with black markings contrasting with the white enamel dial, the centre of which is decorated similarly to the case. Signed 'Goullons A Paris', the watch dates from the middle of the seventeenth century. Museum of the Worshipful Company of Clockmakers, Guildhall, London.

right
Another watch combining rock crystal with enamelling, this dates from about 1625 and is signed 'John Ramsey fecit'. There is no evidence that this maker was related to the famous David Ramsay, and indeed nothing is known about him except that perhaps he may have worked in Dundee. Museum of the Worshipful Company of Clockmakers, Guildhall, London.

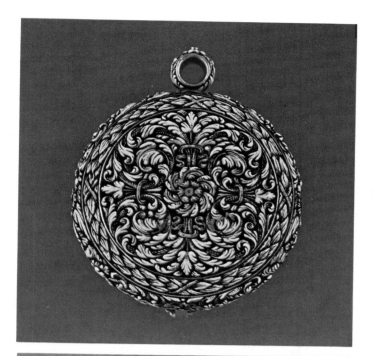

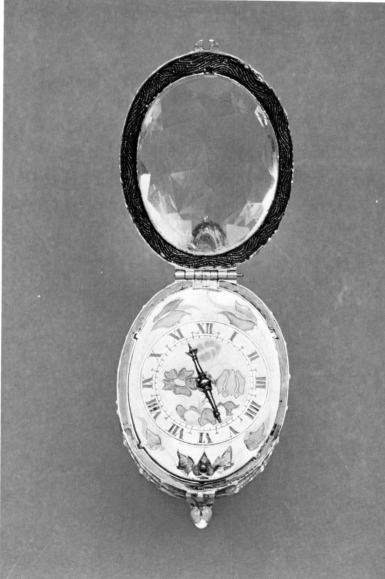

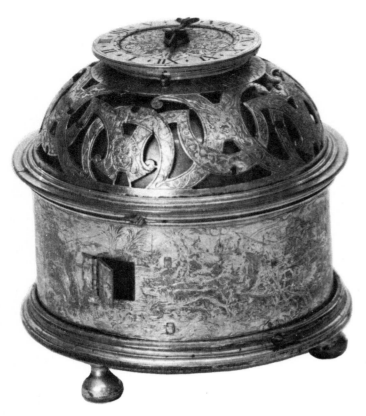
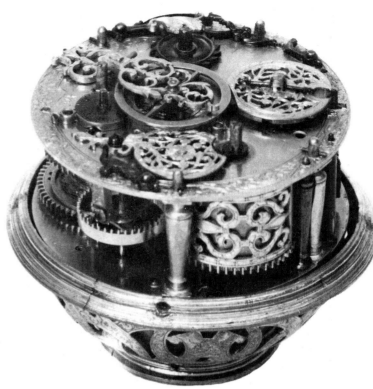

The immediate ancestor of the longcase clock was, of course, the hanging hooded wall clock. Many of these were simple thirty-hour duration mechanisms of the lantern clock type; but once the pendulum had been introduced, eight-day duration became the standard. This required much heavier driving weights than its predecessor, so that the overall mass of the clock may have been too great to suspend from a wall bracket with safety. Certainly hanging clocks of the earlier kind but running eight days continued to be made in the period 1660–75, and all with the then current architectural type of case. At the same time, however, it is likely that a free-standing clock case, which would not only enclose weights, pendulum and mechanism and protect them from dust and interference, but relieve the strain on not always very robust walls, must have been considered highly desirable. Some such considerations are likely to have given rise to the longcase clock.

Until 1675, many of the factors relating to bracket clocks apply also to longcases. Architectural styles prevailed, probably for the reasons of experimentation already postulated. A longcase has three main sections – the plinth, the trunk and the hood – and, in the earliest specimens, it is general to find that the plinth is a plain box-like structure, while the trunk is panelled. At the top of the trunk and around its three exposed sides is a convex moulding, upon which the hood rests – this is an important feature in assigning a period to a clock, for after 1700 these mouldings are almost

invariably concave. The back of the trunk is continued upwards almost to the clock's full height, its outside edges running in grooves in the hood, which has to be slid upwards to obtain access to the mechanism. This was necessary because, at this early period, hoods had no forward-opening door although, subsequently, many were converted, the door becoming usual after about 1700. The lift-up hood was generally lockable by a special device which cannot be released until the trunk door is opened, giving useful additional security.

These early longcase clocks were usually about six feet high, with dials eight to eight and a half inches square. Dial arrangements followed closely those already described for bracket clocks. The half-seconds pendulum almost never occurs with a subsidiary seconds dial; bolt-and-shutter maintaining power is commoner on longcase than on bracket clocks.

Cases in general follow the spring clock fashion in being made of dark wood, usually ebony, more rarely laburnum or lignum vitae. The pure architectural style of the hood, with its triangular portico top and discreet gilt metal embellishment in the tympanum and in the framing of the dial, sometimes extends also to pillars and bases.

There is one other type of longcase clock which deserves brief mention, if only because it may constitute another connecting link with what had gone before. Very much more primitive than those described hitherto, it consists of little more than a posted movement of the lantern clock type, with a duration of thirty hours, which is wound by pulling down a chain or rope inside its longcase. Such clocks were made provincially whenever the long-case was in fashion, and generally with the longer pendulum; but occasionally a famous early maker indulged in such modest work, and there is an example by Thomas Tompion in the collection of the Worshipful Company of Clockmakers in London which is dated at about 1672. It has the short bob pendulum of the time and is housed in a plain black ebonised case of which the hood is topped by uncommon cresting. It also had an alarm train, now missing.

Huygens' application of the pendulum to clock-work was inhibited by the deficiencies of the escapement – the verge – to which it was allied. Thus, however he might strive, by the use of such devices as cycloidal cheeks, to bring it to perfection, the verge escapement itself has inherent mechanical shortcomings the nature of which eluded him; however, it did not elude the English craftsmen who were so assiduously developing his invention. Their contribution was the application of a new clock escapement, to which could be allied the thirty-nine-inch seconds-beating pendulum.

There are two contenders for the claim actually to have invented the anchor escapement, and argument has continued over the years between their respective supporters. The first is a respected craftsman clockmaker, William Clement, who – if indeed he did nothing more – made a clock with this escapement for King's College, Cambridge, which is the oldest specimen of its kind to survive. The clock is signed and dated 1671, and was transferred to the Science Museum in London, where it is shown working, only in the present decade. Clement's claim is substantiated by John Smith, one of the earliest writers in English on horology, who states in his *Horological Disquisitions* of 1694 that Clement was 'the real contriver of the curious kind of long pendulum which is at this day so universally in use among us'. As against this, protagonists of the second claimant point out that Clement never showed any other special merit as an inventor, whereas the anchor escapement was an entirely new and novel departure from what had gone before and thus an invention in every possible sense; and furthermore they draw attention to the fact that Clement seems to have made no attempt to claim the invention as his own during his lifetime, which any craftsman with pride in his work surely would have done.

The second contender for whom credit is claimed in this connection is Robert Hooke. He was mentioned previously as having shared roughly the life-span of Huygens; and in an age in which brilliance almost seems commonplace, he was one of the giant intelligences. Living from 1635 to 1703, he ranged his mind over science and mathematics as those disciplines then existed,

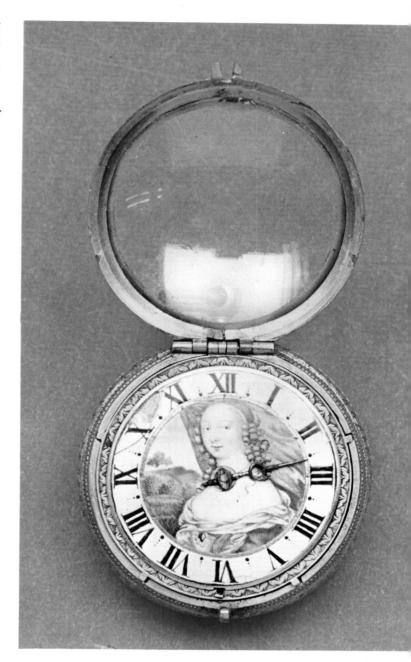

The white enamel chapter ring of this watch surrounds a central enamel portrait said to be that of the Duchesse de Montpensier who was born in 1627. The watch is signed 'Jean Hubert A Rouen' and dates from about 1650. Museum of the Worshipful Company of Clockmakers, Guildhall, London.

opposite page, left
This beautiful small clock dating from the end of the first quarter of the seventeenth century is the work of Henry Archer who was one of the first Wardens of the Clockmakers' Company. The case of the clock was possibly imported from France. Museum of the Worshipful Company of Clockmakers, Guildhall, London.

opposite page, right
The movement of Archer's clock showing the extensive decoration with which it is embellished. Museum of the Worshipful Company of Clockmakers, Guildhall, London.

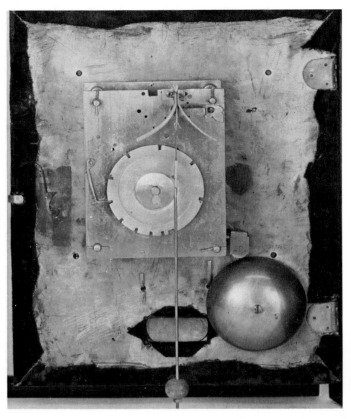

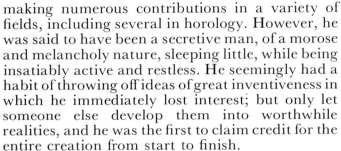

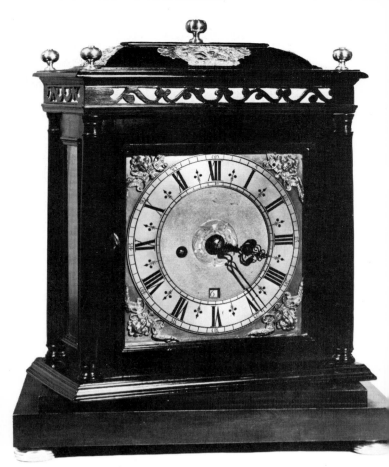

making numerous contributions in a variety of fields, including several in horology. However, he was said to have been a secretive man, of a morose and melancholy nature, sleeping little, while being insatiably active and restless. He seemingly had a habit of throwing off ideas of great inventiveness in which he immediately lost interest; but only let someone else develop them into worthwhile realities, and he was the first to claim credit for the entire creation from start to finish.

Hooke was Curator of Experiments to the Royal Society and sometime Secretary to that august body. He was experimenting with long pendulums as early as 1664, and in 1669 had progressed to one some thirteen feet long and beating once in two seconds, but the escapement was certainly not an anchor. His own diaries do not start before 1672, nor is there mention of the escapement, as such, in any of the Royal Society's Proceedings. Yet it is inconceivable that Hooke played no part whatever in such an important advance in a field in which he was substantially involved. At the present time it might seem most likely that the idea of an anchor escapement started with him and finished, in its fully functional state, with Clement. This is the only theory that meets all the facts as at present understood, but it is to be hoped that more information will eventually come to light on the subject.

Before leaving Robert Hooke, it might be illuminating to review his other contributions to horology. In the field of pendulums, he was the first to postulate the flat steel spring suspension to replace Huygens' silk thread, and he successfully demonstrated this to the Royal Society in 1666. Some years later, in 1672, he produced his wheel-cutting engine, successfully mechanising a procedure which had been hitherto partly manual and consequently liable to some inaccuracy. Finally, he seems to have been the first to suggest using the different coefficients of expansion of brass and steel as the basis for compensating against temperature changes in horological mechanisms, although it was to be another half century before this device underwent further development.

The incorporation of the one-second pendulum and anchor escapement in longcase clocks caused their dimensions to increase in almost all directions. Thus after 1675 the eight-inch square dial grew to ten inches, where it remained for almost the remainder of the century, although before 1700 eleven- and even twelve-inch dials began to appear. Heights of cases grew to seven feet, aided by the fashion for higher ceilings; this extra height in the clock case was achieved by adding to it a shallow domed top equivalent to the bell top of a bracket clock. This feature, accompanied often by finials at the two forward corners and with sometimes a third on top, is nevertheless not as pleasing as the flat top, embellished on occasion with cresting, the latter being just an alternative method of accomplishing the same objective.

Details of the hood and dial settled down by 1690. The use of columns at either side of the dial followed the same progress as in the bracket clock, alighting eventually upon the slim round column that was to last throughout the ensuing century.

116

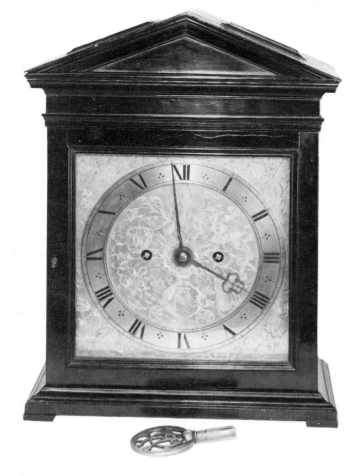

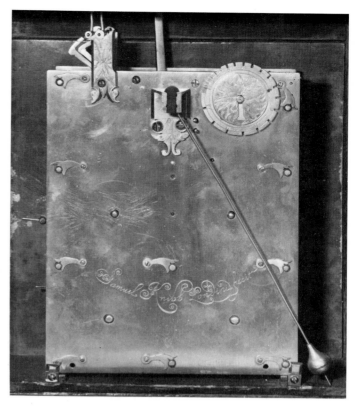

above

This table clock with its fine architectural case, was made by Samuel Knibb; the narrow chapter ring, all-over engraved dial and fine simple hands suggest the period round 1665. Museum of the Worshipful Company of Clockmakers, Guildhall, London.

right

The back plate of the movement of Knibb's clock bears no decoration but the maker's signature in a beautiful flowing style, together with some engraving on the count wheel. Museum of the Worshipful Company of Clockmakers, Guildhall, London.

far left

This clock signed 'Pieter Visbach Fecit Hagae met priuilege' gives a good impression of the first clocks made for Huygens – to whom the 'privilege' refers – by Salomon Coster. The silk suspension to the pendulum and the cycloidal cheeks are typical of such early Dutch pendulum movements. Museum of the Worshipful Company of Clockmakers, Guildhall, London.

left

Even relatively little-known makers turned out fine clocks in the last quarter of the seventeenth century, as this specimen by Edward Bird shows.

From about the same date, too, the maker's signature appeared upon the chapter ring rather than upon the dial plate. The lift-up hood lasted until about 1700, even with the taller generation of clocks. Seconds dials became customary, of course, almost as soon as the seconds pendulum was introduced. The larger dials required a rather bulkier corner ornament than the hitherto ubiquitous cherub spandrel, so that designs embracing two cherubs supporting a crown, or sometimes a woman's head within an arabesque arrangement, are commonly encountered.

Unlike the bracket clock, ebony and ebonised finishes for the longcase clock faded out of popularity in the final quarter of the seventeenth century. Olivewood and walnut succeeded them, together with special effects like the 'oyster' pattern, which is veneer cut across the grain of the wood, in this case often laburnum. Panels of inlaid decoration and, after 1690, all-over inlay were much favoured. The earliest variety of this kind of decoration, known as parquetry, is very rare in clocks; it involves building up patterns with straight edges – such as diamonds, squares and similar shapes – and arranging them as a design. It was followed by marquetry, the usual type of such embellishment on clock cases, in which complicated designs of birds, flowers and other motifs were built up from veneers of different coloured woods, the colours often being obtained by staining, and sometimes with the additional use of ivory and bone.

The trunk of the longcase was of necessity closely related to the pendulum, its proportions

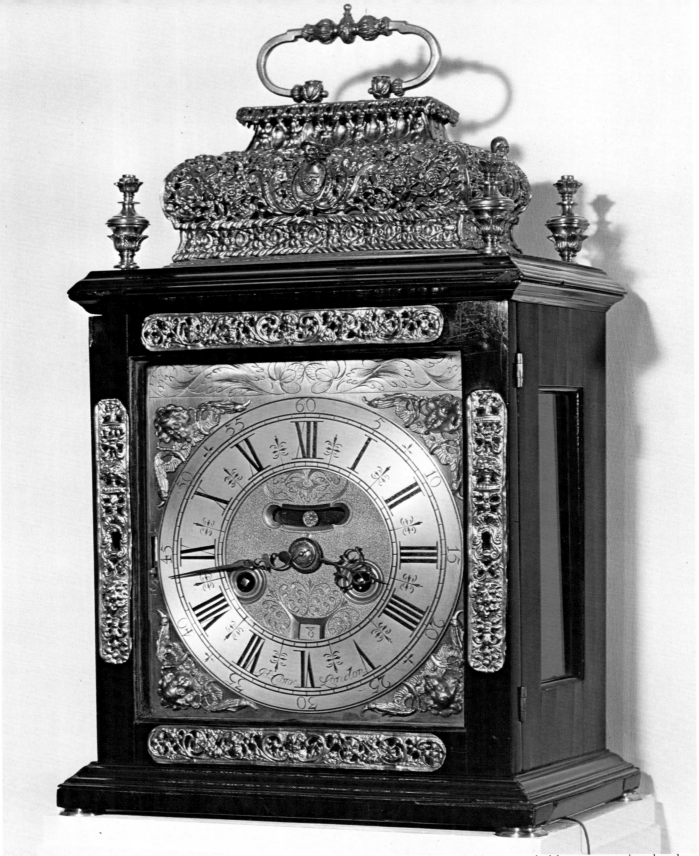

This magnificent basket-top spring clock possesses a strangely asymmetrical dial, with the apertures for the winding squares apparently displaced to the left. There is also a substantial engraved band above the dial which might seem to serve no obvious purpose. However, there exists a second clock by the same maker, John Clowes of London, which is virtually identical to this one, and which has these same curious features. The overall displacement seems to have resulted from certain unusual mechanical elements in the movement, and this was probably not appreciated at the design stage.

right
The architectural design of this hooded wall clock, with its pointed pediment, specially turned columns and rising hood, is typical of the period about 1680. Made by William Clement, it has a striking movement that runs for eight days. British Museum, London.

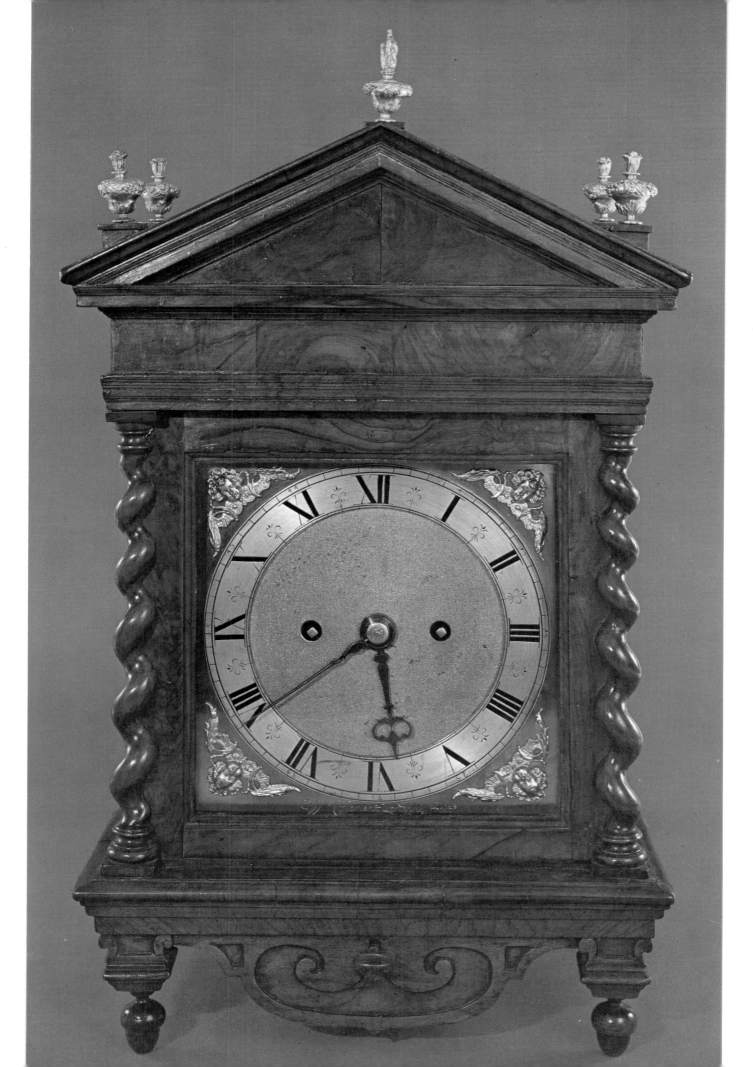

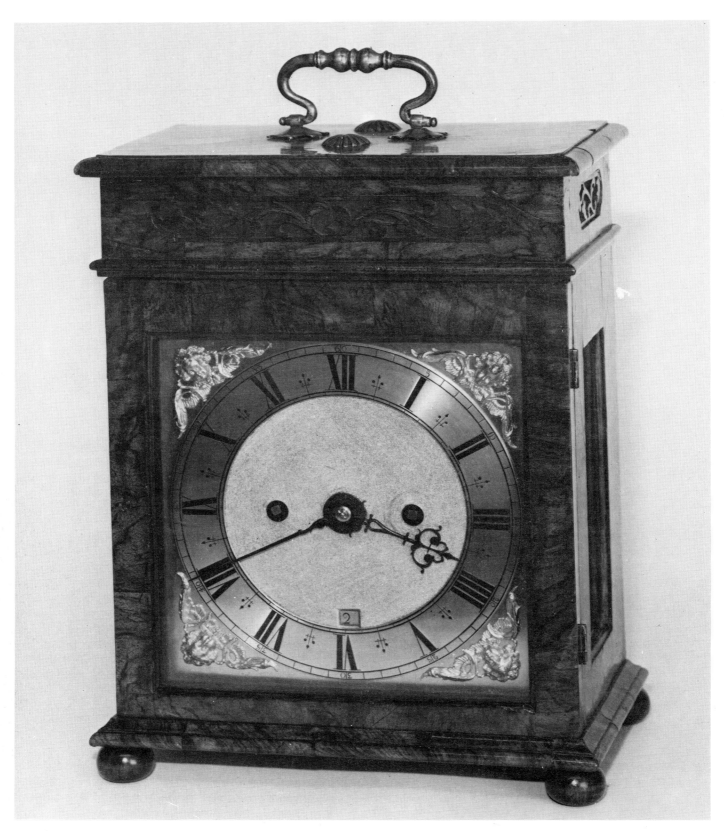

reflecting the length and arc of swing. Square-topped trunk doors further extended the lines of the square dials – for the arch had not yet invaded the clockcase – and, as if to encourage inspection, it is common to find a bull's-eye glass, called a lenticle, set into the trunk door at the level of the pendulum bob, and through which it can be seen swinging.

Rare among clocks in this final quarter of the seventeenth century were some interesting experimental examples by William Clement and several other makers, still striving to improve the performance of the pendulum. In these, a pendulum having a length of sixty-one inches and

left
This clock by 'Henry Jones in ye Temple' is in a most unusual walnut case. The period is about 1675. Museum of the Worshipful Company of Clockmakers, Guildhall, London.

right
Another unusual case houses this eight-day spring clock with striking train which is signed 'Edwardus East Londini', and dates from about 1670. British Museum, London.

beating 1¼ seconds was employed. Inevitably, the pendulum bob of such clocks was swinging within the plinth; some such clocks, therefore, have another door at that level, to give access to the bob for adjustment and regulation, done by raising or lowering it on the rod by means of a rating nut. At the very least a lenticle is set into the plinth, for purposes of observation. An obvious feature of such clocks, too, is the seconds dial, divided into forty-eight instead of sixty. No further clocks of this type were made after about 1700.

The seventeenth century saw the first appearance in England of the kind of superb native craftsmanship that was needed to breathe life into the inventions of contemporary scientists such as Huygens and Hooke. Strangely, most of the great workmen from this period spanned the end of the century, many only reaching the peak of their attainment in the succeeding one. One, however, lived out his life wholly within these five score years. He was Edward East.

East was born in 1602 and lived to the ripe old age of ninety-five. He came originally from Southill in Bedfordshire which, by a curious coincidence, is only a few miles from Northill, birthplace of Thomas Tompion. He was apprenticed to a goldsmith, being admitted to the Freedom in 1627; but switched shortly after, to become the junior member of the first Court of Assistants of the Clockmakers' Company, newly formed in 1631. He was Master of the Company in 1645 and 1652. His work is characterised by its extreme elegance and simplicity, enhanced by his ability to work in precious metals gained from his training as a goldsmith. He became Royal Clockmaker, first to Charles I and later to Charles II. The latter regularly presented watches by East as prizes for tennis played in the Mall, London. East seems to have spent the last few years of his life at Hampton in Middlesex.

By contrast, a second Royal Clockmaker of the Caroline era remains something of a mystery.

Robert Seignior was born in 1645, the son of a tailor. Entering into an apprenticeship in 1660, under John Nicasius – a well-known craftsman of the day – he was duly admitted to the Freedom in 1667. He never subsequently served any office in the Company, and his output must have been minimal; a bare handful of clocks and watches bearing his signature seem to have survived. Yet all are of the highest quality. Furthermore, he was a friend of Hooke and Tompion, figuring in the diary of the former. In 1674 he was granted a Royal Warrant 'without ffee, until the Death, Surrender or other Determinacion of Edward East. And then to enjoy the same place with ffee . . .' However, he never did enjoy the 'profitts, allowances and priviledges thereto belonginge', for he died in 1686, and East survived him by more than a decade.

One of the unusual features of clockmaking in the seventeenth century was the way the craft seemed to attract whole families to its practice. The Fromanteels were one example. Edward East lived so long that for years it was believed that there must be at least two of him. But perhaps the best-known craft family of that period were the Knibbs. Samuel Knibb, born in 1626, started as a clockmaker at Newport Pagnell, becoming accredited to the Clockmakers' Company in 1663, soon

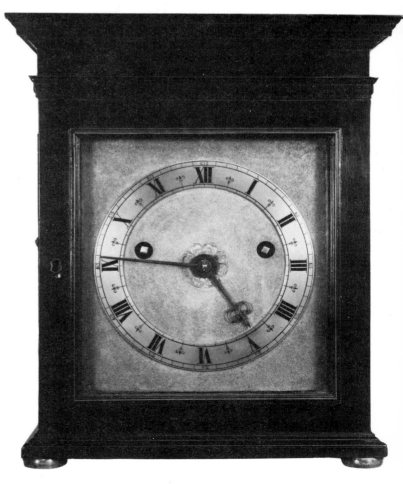

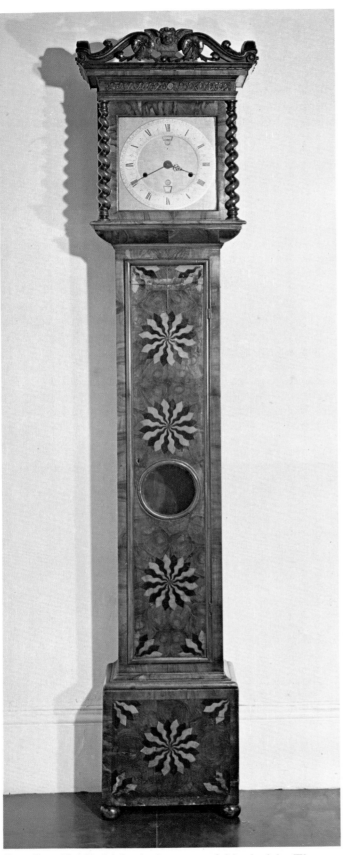

Standing 6ft 10in high, the longcase of this clock by Thomas Tompion, which dates from about 1680, is a superb example of the use of olivewood inlaid with star medallions in ebony and satinwood. The movement is of one month duration. British Museum, London.

after he moved to London. The very few clocks identified as made by him are of the finest quality. His cousin Joseph (1640–1711), having been apprenticed to him from 1655 to 1662, set up in business at Oxford, where his first clocks reflected the influence of Fromanteel's work which he had certainly acquired from his time with Samuel. However, he soon revealed evidence of his own original thought. Meantime, in 1664, he took as apprentice his own younger brother John (1650–1722), and in 1668 another cousin Peter. The work of Joseph Knibb remains outstanding, even among the general excellence of the work of the other members of his family; he seems to have prospered certainly up to 1697, when he retired to Hanslop, continuing to make a few clocks until he died in 1711.

The greatest craftsman of his day – indeed, his admirers would say, the greatest of all time – was Thomas Tompion, who has often been called the 'father of English clockmaking'. As has been said already, he was born at Northill in Bedfordshire close to Edward East's birthplace, although not until 1639. Little is known about his activities until his admission in 1671 to the Clockmakers' Company, of which he became Master in 1703. Tompion's reputation rests entirely upon his supreme abilities as a craftsman and designer of complex clocks; his standards were emulated by many another fine London maker, albeit not always with complete success, but there is no doubt that the supremacy enjoyed by English horologists of his time owes more to his example than to anyone else's. By contrast, his name is not connected with any specific invention directed to improving timekeeping, and in this regard his friend and partner George Graham exerted a more lasting influence. Tompion became known to Robert Hooke soon after arriving in London and was subsequently commissioned to make clocks and watches of special design for him. Curiously, he never seems to have enjoyed the Royal Warrant although, for example, he made a fine equation clock for William III. Tompion worked with two partners during the latter years of his life. Edward Banger, a relative by marriage, joined him in 1701, the partnership lasting about seven years; a number of works bear their joint signatures. George Graham, another relative by marriage, had worked for Tompion since 1696 and was subsequently taken into partnership. They too maintained all the standards in their work which Tompion had initiated. Finally, Tompion died in 1713, being buried in Westminster abbey and, nearly forty years later, his grave was reopened to receive the body of his last partner, George Graham.

In fact, Graham survived until 1751, thus playing a large part in maintaining the craft practices and standards pioneered by East and Tompion. Many other fine seventeenth-century makers lived

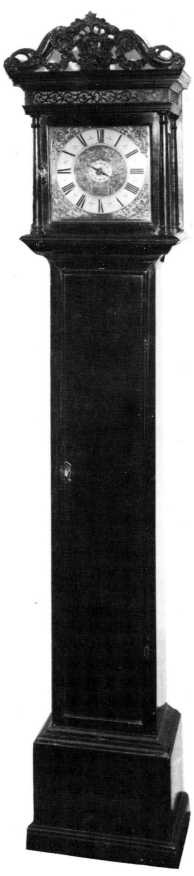

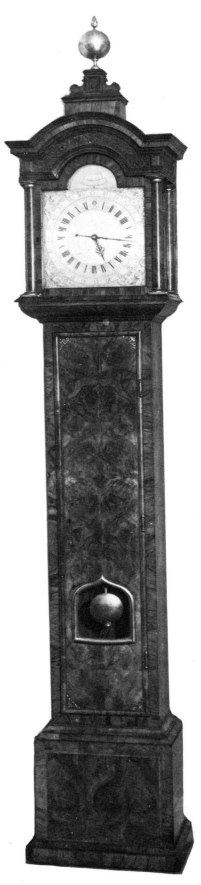

The ebonised pinewood longcase surmounted by cresting encloses a posted movement signed 'Tho. Tompion, Londini fecit'. It is an early example of this master craftsman's work which appears to date from about 1672. Museum of the Worshipful Company of Clockmakers, Guildhall, London.

Made about 1695 for William III, this year clock by Thomas Tompion incorporates the first examples both of equation work and of a break-arch dial. Royal Collection.

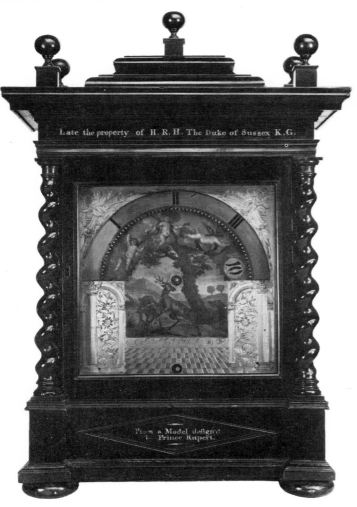

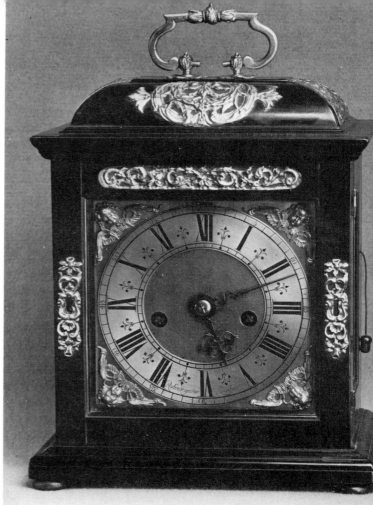

on well into the eighteenth century – Daniel Quare until 1724, Joseph Williamson until 1725, the Windmills family even longer – and it may be more convenient to consider these in the succeeding chapter. They provided a continuity within the craft at a time when nothing could have been more important.

Although it will be dealt with more fully in a later chapter, an important milestone in the history of chronometry took place during the last quarter of the seventeenth century and will be mentioned now in order to preserve events in their correct sequence. In 1675, in order to initiate studies in astronomy directed to aiding navigation, Charles II established an observatory in Greenwich Park, installing as his first Astronomer Royal – a title which prevails to the present time – a certain John Flamsteed. An outstanding feature of this new observatory was the pair of year-duration weight-driven clocks commissioned from Tompion. The need for accurate timekeeping in observatory circumstances such as these being so great, the famous craftsman went to enormous lengths, within the limitations of horological knowledge then current, to achieve precision. Thus their long duration was intended to avoid errors due to frequent winding, while their fourteen-foot pendulums, beating two seconds, reduced considerably the small cumulative error deriving from pendulums with a shorter period. These two clocks

must certainly be numbered among the world's great timekeepers since, as scientific instruments, they played their part in advancing human knowledge in the fields of astronomy and navigation.

The application of the pendulum to clocks was exactly matched, in the latter half of the seventeenth century, by the invention and application of the balance spring to watches. In their different ways both offered the same facility, a means of regulating the timekeeping without altering the main driving force of the timepiece. This latter method, at the best of times, can provide only a coarse adjustment.

There is no doubt that the perceived advantages of the one improvement led directly to the other, and indeed, the dramatis personae are the same. Huygens published, in 1675, his claim to the invention of the balance spring, only to be met with a counter-claim from Hooke, stating that he had originated the same device in 1658. The craftsmen of the day sat on the sidelines watching the course of events, except for Tompion, personally involved by Hooke, who claimed he had commissioned him to make a watch with such a spring. The two designs, even so, were not identical. Huygens' spring had a pinion built in to enable the balance to make much larger vibrations – an arrangement which is usually called a 'pirouette' – whereas Hooke's much simpler arrangement is virtually the same as the one in use to this day. The dispute

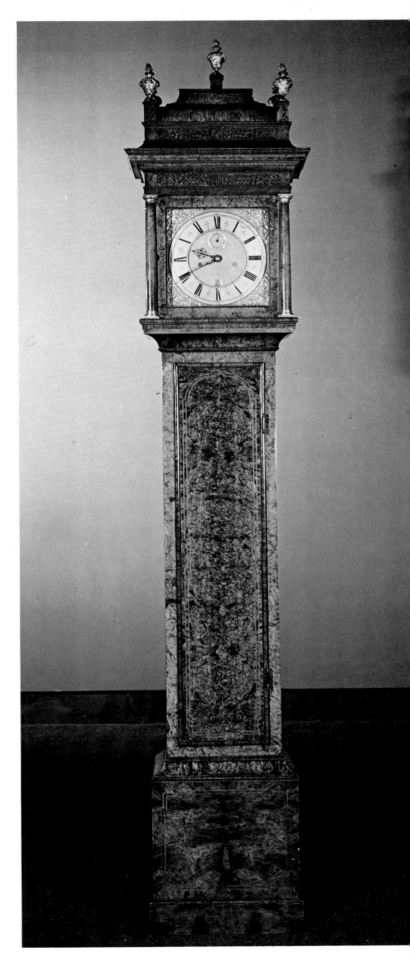

has never been finally settled; but whereas Hooke's
design was implemented at once, Huygens' device
is very rarely encountered and not in examples
made directly under his aegis. It is a fact that
Tompion was making watches with balance
springs soon after 1675, and that George Graham
subsequently quoted Tompion as authority for
crediting the invention to Hooke.

In the next fifteen years a number of events had
their effect upon watchmaking. The waistcoat
came into fashion, so that watches ceased to be
hung round the neck or from the waist and were
stowed comfortably away, where they would be
likely to come to far less harm in wear than formerly. This was a happy conjunction of events
because, while previously the timekeeping was
haphazard and size was of no importance, so that
many watches were quite small, the new balance
spring watches tended at first to be uniformly large
and would have been a nuisance if permitted to
swing loose.

Another significant event had political and
religious origins. Watchmaking in continental
Europe had had spasmodic beginnings – in
France, and in Germany until her problems with
the Thirty Years War, in Switzerland after 1550 or
thereabouts, and in Britain rather later. The two
latter centres at least offered a haven to Protestants
as well as a prosperous market for fine timepieces,
and had already benefited from the great craft
skills of the Huguenots, who, in their efforts to
escape persecution, had settled in both countries
and were peacefully plying their trades. This
movement was suddenly given unexpected and
enormous impetus by the revocation in 1685 of the
Edict of Nantes by Louis XIV of France, which
had protected Protestants there. As a result,
Huguenots already settled in England and Switzerland were augmented by the sudden arrival as
refugees of thousands of their French contemporaries.

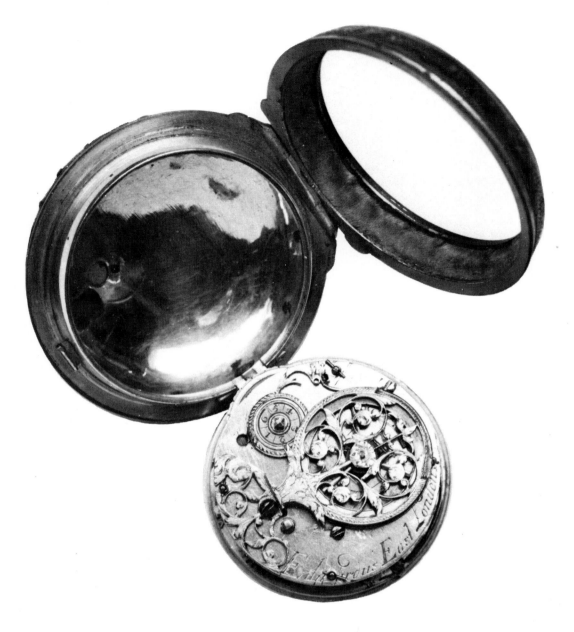

With a balance spring of only two turns and a cock with irregularly shaped foot, this watch movement of Edward East's was made about 1680 and reflects the earliest stage in the application of the balance spring. Museum of the Worshipful Company of Clockmakers, Guildhall, London.

Both pendulum and balance spring do much more for their respective timekeepers than simply supply, as mentioned earlier, a convenient vehicle for effective regulation to obtain accurate performance. The pendulum is continually moving from one extreme to another – from the outermost points of its swing, whence it has been impelled by the escapement, to its zero vertical position, under the influence of gravity – and this overall action is a rhythmic one. Similarly, the effect upon a watch escapement of incorporating a balance spring is to make the action rhythmic and consistent: just like a pendulum under the influence of gravity, the balance spring is continually trying to return the balance wheel to zero – in this case, its natural position of rest. Previously, the action, already

inherently erratic, could be violently affected by sudden movement or positional changes. Henceforth the watch could be made to perform rhythmically – and accurately – when positioned in any plane, and whether static or mobile.

As the benefits of the balance spring became obvious, very many earlier watches were 'converted', a procedure which the modern purist collector often deplores, but which must have made an enormous difference to watch-users at that time. But the increased accuracy obtainable now made it worthwhile to indicate minutes as well as hours, and this of itself occasioned some most interesting developments.

The employment of two hands on a watch dial to tell us the time is such a familiar arrangement, which it is entirely second nature for us to read,

Daniel Quare made a few magnificent year equation clocks similar to this example in a walnut case standing 9ft 10in high, which is reputed to have been made for Hampton Court Palace about 1695. British Museum, London.

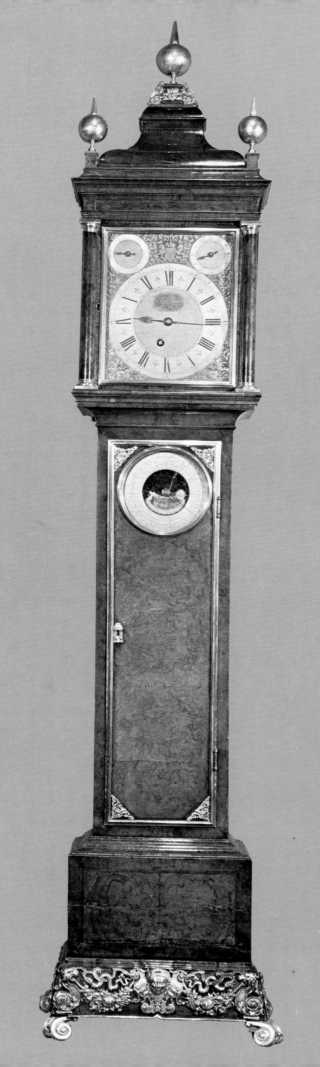

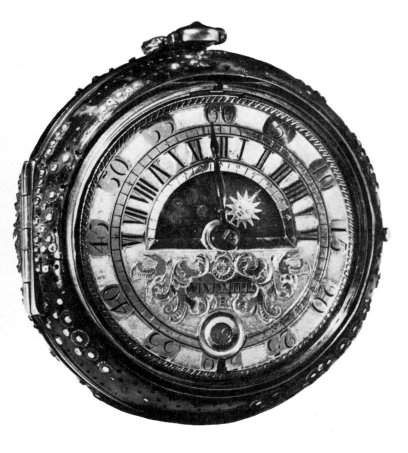

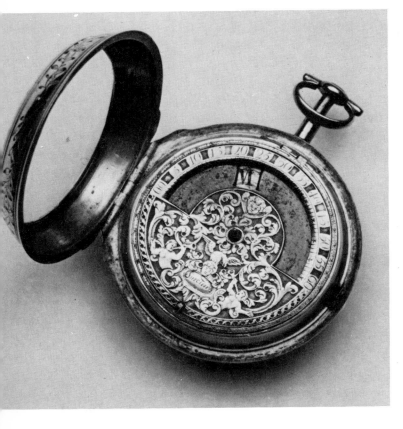

that it is difficult to appreciate the extent of the problem for people who had never been brought up to enjoy this amenity. Children learn to tell the time with both hours and minutes, as part of a normal upbringing, but the need to educate whole nations in such a technique must have been comparable to the recent British experience of adopting decimal coinage and 'going metric'. The conventional system of concentric hour and minute hands soon caught on – even though the mechanical arrangements under the dial to accommodate them are sufficiently ingenious as to suggest that they cannot have been invented overnight – but this was seen by watchmakers at the time as merely one of a number of dial arrangements with which they were experimenting to find the most practical, convenient and easily assimilable. Of the others, some are very rare, while one system at least is fairly common and might therefore be considered the 'runner up' to the two-handed method.

This is the variation known as the 'sun and moon' dial. The upper half of the dial contains a semicircular aperture, around the curved edge of which are engraved the hours starting from VI at one side, arriving at XII – in the place where it would be on a conventional dial – and extending on to VI again at the far side. Behind this aperture is a revolving disc, upon which, diametrically opposite each other, are engraved representations of the sun and the moon, and this disc revolves once in twenty-four hours. Thus, at sunrise – say at six a.m. – the sun appears at the extreme left-hand edge of the aperture, indicating the hours through the day to six p.m. As it disappears from view on the far side, the moon rises at the VI on the near side, performing the same function through the night hours until the whole procedure starts again at six a.m. the following morning. The minutes are indicated separately upon a minute band running around the extreme outer edge of the dial, upon which the five-minute figures are usually engraved upon polished plaques, the long minute hand revolving from the centre in the normal way. This kind of watch may be said to be unusual in showing day and night hours separately, even if such information is self-evident.

Another type of dial utilising a cut-out aperture is called the 'wandering hour' watch. This time, around the edge of the semicircular opening are shown the minutes from 0 to 60, the five-minute divisions again being shown on polished plaques. Revolving behind this aperture is once again a disc, with two circular 'windows' cut into it directly opposite one another. Behind this disc and pivoted to it are two small discs, one engraved with the even hours, the other with the odd, in such a way that as the parent disc rotates, whichever window happens to be in view upon the dial shows the correct hour against the minute band. Supposing this to be an 'odd' hour, the next – even – hour

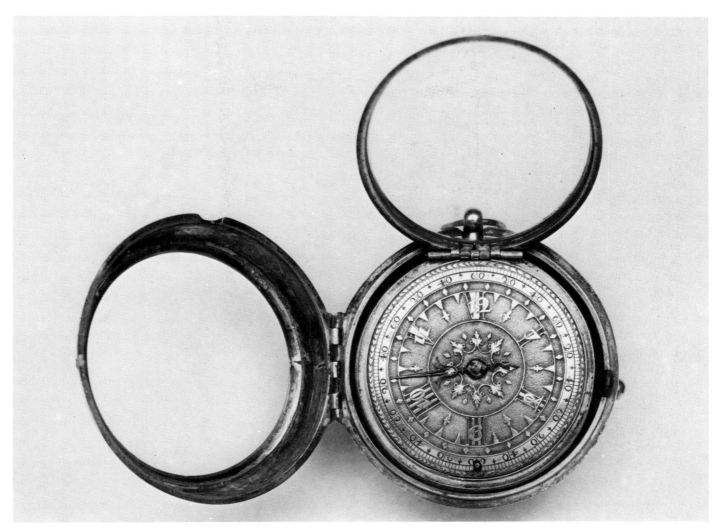

A dial divided into six hours instead of twelve provided much more space for the accurate reading of an outer ring calibrated in minutes, all with the use of a single hand. This example from about 1680 is signed 'Will Bertram London'. Museum of the Worshipful Company of Clockmakers, Guildhall, London.

opposite page, above
The commonest of the experimental dials associated with early efforts to indicate minutes, this sun and moon dial watch is by Joseph Windmills and was made about 1700.

opposite page, below
Another experimental dial from the same period was the 'wandering hour', and this specimen signed 'Sinclare Dublin 146' dates from about 1690. Museum of the Worshipful Company of Clockmakers, Guildhall, London.

will have been set up meantime beneath the opposite circular window but, of course, will remain out of view until the current hour has passed the '60' mark on the minute band. This type of watch was probably inspired by the night clock of this period.

A third variation used experimentally to show minutes had the main dial divided into only six hours instead of the conventional twelve. Therefore, on the 'six-hour dial' watch, the single hand revolved twice in each twelve-hour period; but, since each hour division was necessarily twice as large as on the normal dial, it was correspondingly much easier to divide them to show minutes, calibrated in twenty minute divisions upon a polished outer band. In order to cope with the hours 7–12 on watches of this kind, it is usual for 1–6 to be shown in large Roman numerals, with 7–12 in smaller Arabic numerals superimposed upon them.

These and other similarly eccentric forms of dial devoted solely to ascertaining the best way to indicate minutes are found not only upon English watches but also upon watches from other parts of Europe. Most may be dated between 1680 and 1700, although outside Britain some of the versions died a long death. It is not unknown, for instance,

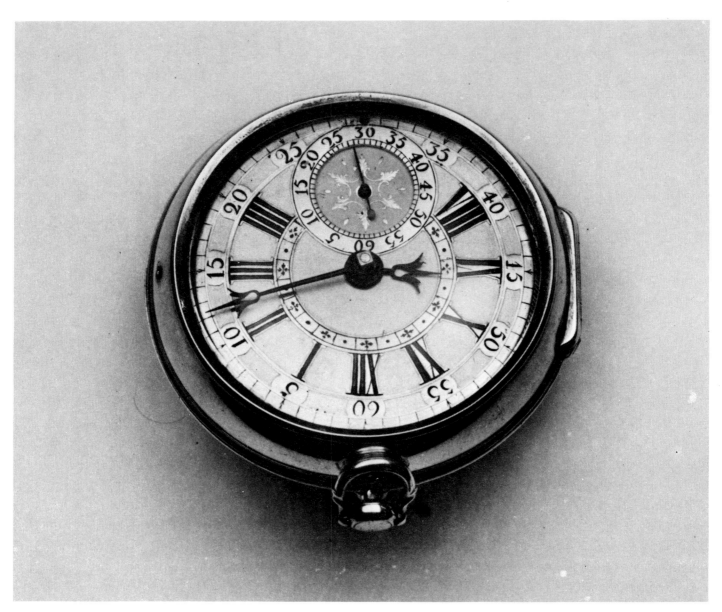

A large and beautifully made watch by Benjamin Bell of London. Its outstanding feature is the outsize subsidiary seconds dial and steel tulip hands. Its date is about 1690. Museum of the Worshipful Company of Clockmakers, Guildhall, London.

to find a six-hour dial watch with an enamel, as opposed to an all-metal, dial. Like many another manifestation in horology, too, it is probably true to say that the 'novelty' watch, as a concept, was newfangled several centuries back, and that nothing wholly new or original has been seen since.

Before leaving watches with such strange dials as some of these, brief mention must be made of the 'pendulum watch' – almost a contradiction in terms – which occurred for a short time around 1700. This variety of watch is always supposed to have been inspired by the universal belief among non-scientific people in the quasi-magical properties of the pendulum. The movement of such

watches was so arranged as to reveal the balance vibrating, either through an aperture cut into the balance cock or, a much to be deplored practice, by moving the escapement to just beneath the dial, through which an opening was cut to reveal the balance wheel. In both cases a spurious 'bob' was added to one arm of the balance wheel, and this, seen swinging backwards and forwards through the opening, whether in front of or behind the movement, was intended to give the impression that a pendulum was at work. Nowadays such an example of misplaced ingenuity would simply be dismissed as a gimmick, and probably it was originally intended mainly to boost sales. Even so, Dutch makers as well as some French ones exten-

This fine spring clock was made by Thomas Tompion about 1700. The subsidiary dials in the upper corners are for regulation and strike/silent. Museum of the Worshipful Company of Clockmakers, Guildhall, London.

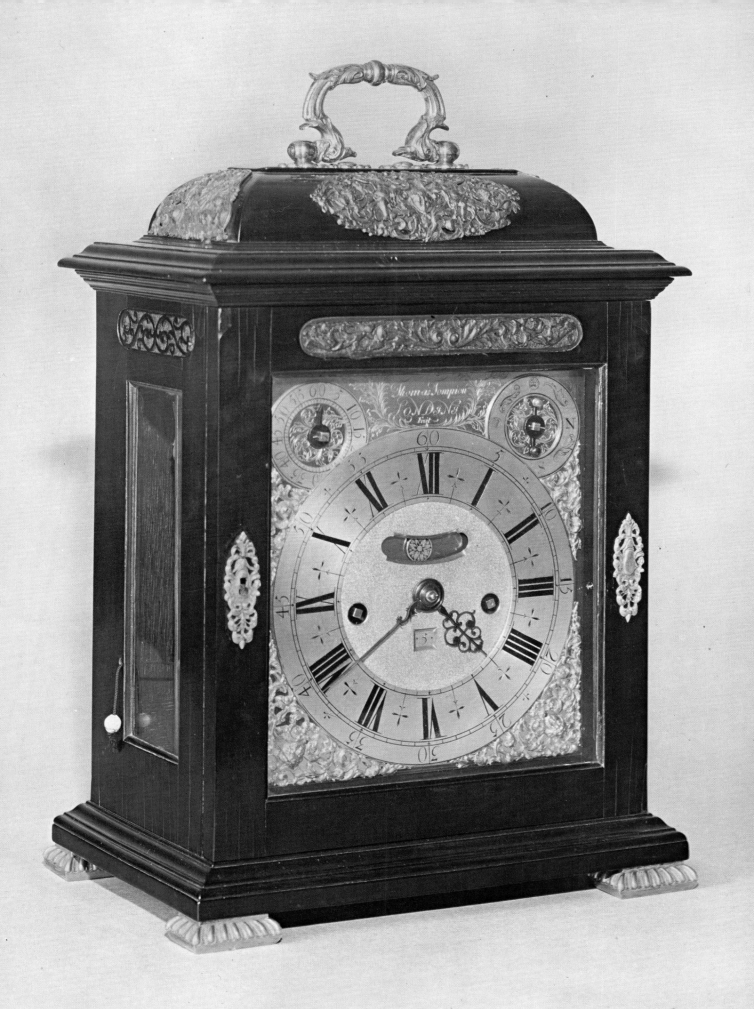

sively adopted the practice of the cut-out balance cock to show a 'bob' swinging on the back of the watch movement during the eighteenth century.

As the title of this third chapter indicates, the most decorative watches predate 1700. The last quarter of the century saw the beginnings of the popularity of repoussé work for outer cases, at this early stage often no more than flutes radiating from a central boss. Tortoiseshell was another favoured material, being decorated with silver or gold piqué work. Silver and gold filigree is also known but very rare. Stone or crystal is only found – and then exceptionally rarely – framed in otherwise gold cases; cornelians particularly were employed in this style.

So far as other European styles were concerned – and the foregoing has tended to concentrate upon English styles in view of their importance in the history of the craft at this time – certain features are prominent and should be noted. Dutch watches came to favour the so-called 'arcaded' minute band – that is to say, instead of being a complete circle it was broken by twelve equally spaced arches. This feature is even reflected in watches made by English makers for export to that country and is immediately detectable. French dials were quite different from usage elsewhere in that the hour numerals were displayed upon separate enamel plaques, which were in turn mounted upon a decorated metal dial plate. This rather heavy arrangement nevertheless suited the style of French watch known as the 'oignon', a near spherical single-cased watch with overall engraving, generally made in gilt metal, which can suffer badly from wear. Enamel cases are now rare except in France and Switzerland.

The movements of English, French and Dutch watches cannot be easily confused once their styles have been noted. French watches for a long time before and after 1700 employed a winding system actuated by a square projecting through the dial centre. The balance wheel is protected not by a cock, but by a balance bridge, the latter being fixed to the back plate of the movement by two screws, one each side, rather than the single fixing through the cock foot favoured in England. This bridge is generally very large and is the focus for all the decoration applied to the back of the movement; the only other feature visible on such movements is the small regulation dial, simply retained in position by a small bar or arm rather than forming part of a slide plate. On Dutch watches either a cock or a bridge may be found, but, in the latter case, the design is quite different from that of the French. The Dutch bridge will often have two projecting arms through which it is screwed down into position; it is much smaller in size than the French, and the dial for regulating more prominent, eventually being incorporated into a slide plate in the English style.

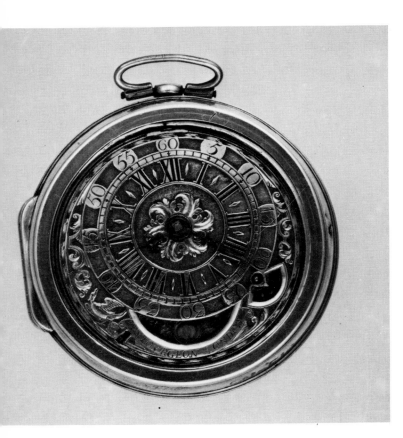

About 1700 a short-lived fashion arose presumably directed at the more gullible and purporting to show watches controlled by a pendulum. This was nothing more than a metal disc fixed to the crossbar of the balance which, as in this case, was sometimes sited to show through an aperture cut in the dial. This watch was made by David Lesturgeon of London. British Museum, London.

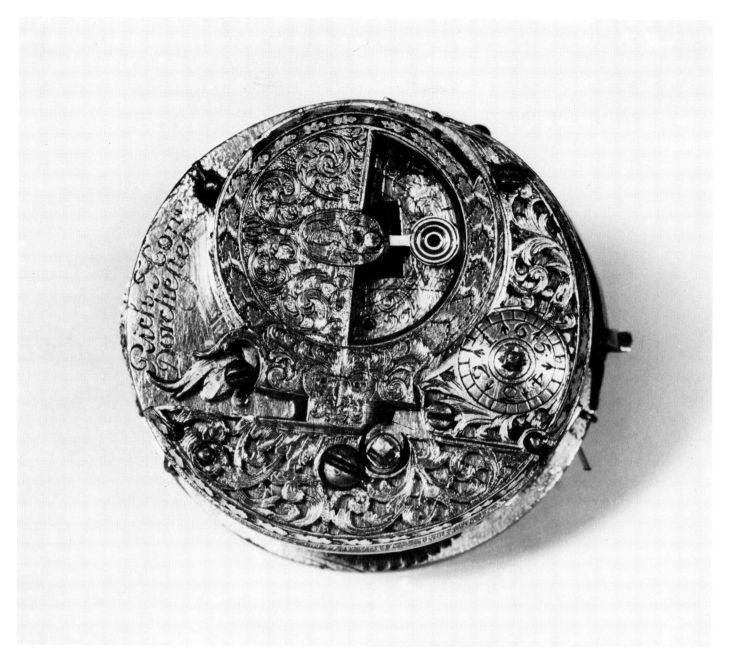

The other version of the pendulum watch involved cutting an aperture in the cock table to allow the disc on the crossbar of the balance to show through. This version is by Richard Howe, Dorchester, who died in 1713.

Another aspect of clock- and watchmaking to which little attention is paid, but which is of signal importance in any general study, is methods of production. Thomas Tompion, most of whose working life was spent in the seventeenth century, is credited with producing altogether around six thousand watches and six hundred clocks – at least, this is the number that may be supposed to have borne his signature, even if they have not all survived. A presentday craftsman, handmaking a single watch – even with all the benefits of modern machine tools and precision equipment – takes upwards of two thousand hours upon the task.

Therefore clearly Tompion employed a workshop of skilled men who must have specialised in their tasks. In other words, even by the later seventeenth century, there must have been considerable division of labour. Furthermore, from long before this time there are clear indications that certain parts of watches, especially dials, were imported from one country to another – it is not uncommon to find an English and a French watch from the earlier part of the seventeenth century with dials as identical as hand-produced parts can ever be; clearly they came from the same workshop. Research has not, as yet, thrown much light upon exactly when a single craftsman ceased to make every part of the watch or clock carrying his name, but in the event it may well turn out to be very much earlier than most students would consider likely.

Progress Towards Precision - The Eighteenth Century

By the year 1700, most of the fundamental inventions necessary to the construction of a timekeeper with modest pretensions to accuracy had been perfected. The pendulum had been applied to clocks for sufficiently long a period as to have run itself in; the corresponding device for watches, the balance spring, although of more recent origin, was also now in general use everywhere. For clocks, the anchor escapement had revolutionised timekeeping, and a static clock with a pendulum beating seconds coupled to this escapement was, of its kind, every bit as good a timekeeper as would normally be required for ordinary household purposes at the present day, three hundred years later. Many period clocks with this mechanism are still cherished domestic possessions, performing both a decorative and a functional role effectively, and their owners would certainly not swap them for something more up to date.

The only substantial gap in the technology was a better escapement for watches. The verge escapement, the earliest known for both clocks and watches, had been superseded in the former; but there was still no alternative for use in the latter. The verge is in many ways an admirable escapement – and, even at the present time and despite enormous research, much misunderstood by a lot of antiquarians. It is robust and relatively fault-free, going for long periods without maintenance or any kind of attention. It is constrained simply by its design – during its cycle of operation, it is not at any point wholly detached from its balance mechanism, so that the latter is never able to swing free of its influence. In theory, the more 'detached' from contact with the escapement, apart from the moment of impulse, that a balance – or, for that matter, a pendulum – is, the better the timekeeping. So it is not surprising that the eighteenth century should turn out to be the century of escapements, among much else – for the changing

life of the ordinary individual, as well as the demands of certain branches of science, was going to require rather more precise time-measurement than had been necessary before.

The second half of the seventeenth century had given England a technological lead that was to last substantially throughout the eighteenth century as well. As has been indicated, other European countries had had their problems. What was the situation in the principal centres of clock- and watch-making outside Britain?

In France, from the beginning, a clock was always seen to be – and deliberately designed as – part of the furniture first, and as a timekeeper only second. French clockmaking underwent a traumatic decline in the middle of the seventeenth century, and when it as dramatically revived following the successful introduction of the pendulum, the first native style to appear was the 'pendule religieuse'. This style was at first clearly modelled upon Salomon Coster's first clocks, and mirrors the strongly architectural approach, although it was not long before they achieved an individuality as well as a splendour which is all their own. Made either to stand on feet or to hang on the wall, these clocks became the standard domestic French design until well into the eighteenth century, although some canister clocks were still being made almost until 1700. These clocks were the forerunners of the famous round French clock movements that became increasingly popular in the eighteenth century, and which achieved virtually a monopoly of production in the nineteenth. The French equivalents of the finest English practitioners, all of them working in Paris, were the families of Thuret and Martinot, Louis Baronneau, Nicolas Gribelin and Pierre Gaudron. Of the cabinetmakers of the day – who were much involved in the casing-up of clocks – mention must be made of André Charles Boulle, famous for the

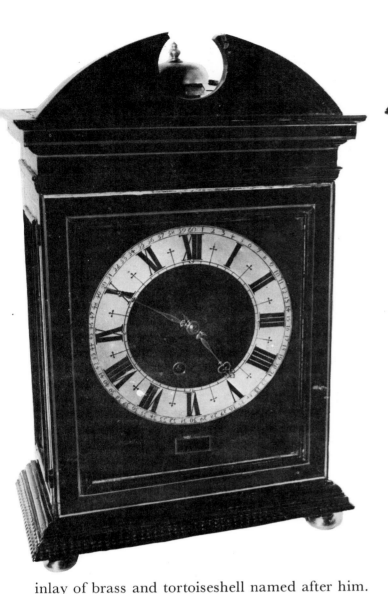

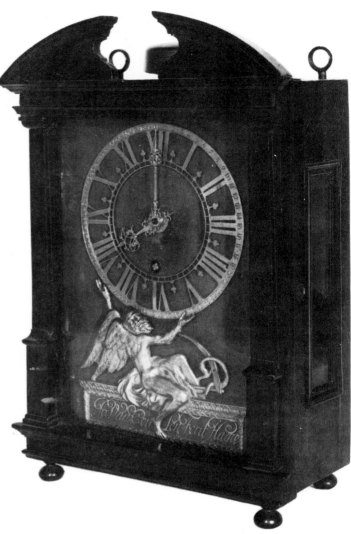

inlay of brass and tortoiseshell named after him.

The 'religieuse' – supposed, incidentally, to have been so named because in shape it resembled a French nun in her habit – underwent substantial development in the latter part of the seventeenth century, the architectural style gradually disappearing in favour of more free-ranging decoration, which included basket and inverted bell tops, with highly embellished side columns, the whole often surmounted by a gilt figure as opposed to the earlier vases or finials. Such clocks gradually merged into what has come to be known as the 'Grand Style', in which the rectangular basic shape has given way entirely to an arched form; and this quite rapid evolution laid the foundation for the galaxy of styles, exuberant often, yet always elegant according to the French taste, which was to burst upon the world in the eighteenth century. Invariably, however, the French clock was first a piece of furniture. Thus, the French equivalent of a longcase clock required that it should look like a mantel clock standing upon a pedestal – which, of course, was actually the lower part of the case and housed the pendulum. Even when, later on, long-

left
left
The similarity between this French clock and the previously illustrated Dutch one will be obvious. This earliest type of pendule religieuse by De l'Héritier of Paris dates from about 1675; it has a verge escapement and quarter repeating on three bells. Netherlands Clock Museum, Utrecht.

above
A typical early Haagse klokje by Jan van Ceulen of The Hague. This example was made in the late seventeenth century. Science Museum, London.

case clocks were made in one piece, they looked nothing like those to be found in England. Straight lines disappeared finally in the Régence period (1715–23) to be replaced by curves, which gradually developed into the true Rococo style of Louis XV. The mantel clock and such hitherto unknown types as the 'cartel' clock, a wall clock in a frame of highly gilt carved wood or cast bronze, kept pace with the ever increasing tendency to elaborate decoration, utilising groups of figures and animals – Philippe Caffieri is a particularly celebrated artist in this regard – allied to a wide range of decorative techniques. Boulle has already been

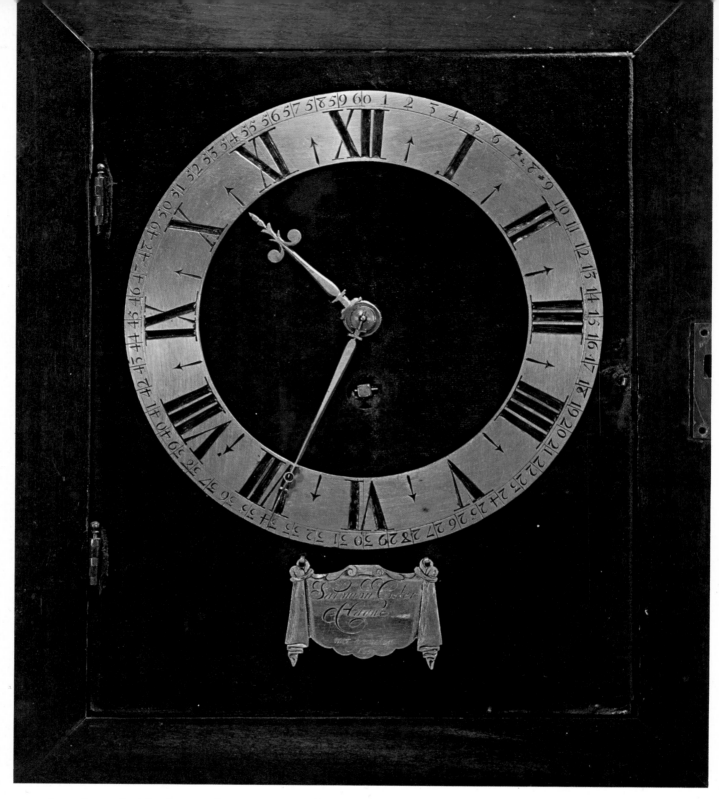

mentioned, and this form of marquetry of tortoiseshell and brass enjoyed huge popularity. Gilding was contrasted with bronze in the castings for cases, which come in infinite variety. Another form of decoration to become very popular towards the middle of the century was 'Vernis Martin', a form of lacquerwork which added the ingredients of colour range, hitherto lacking, to the armoury of the Rococo designers.

Eventually, however, the passion for Rococo passed, and the second half of the eighteenth century saw a return to symmetry and the straight

The earliest type of Dutch pendulum clock, a Haagse klokje, made by Salomon Coster in 1657 to Huygens' direction. The chapter ring and cartouche containing the name are set upon a ground of blue velvet. Every minute is numbered. Netherlands Clock Museum, Utrecht.

right
The cartel clock epitomises the exuberance of French clockmaking in the mid eighteenth century. This example has a case made by C. Cressent and a movement inscribed 'Guiot, Paris'. Wallace Collection, London.

136

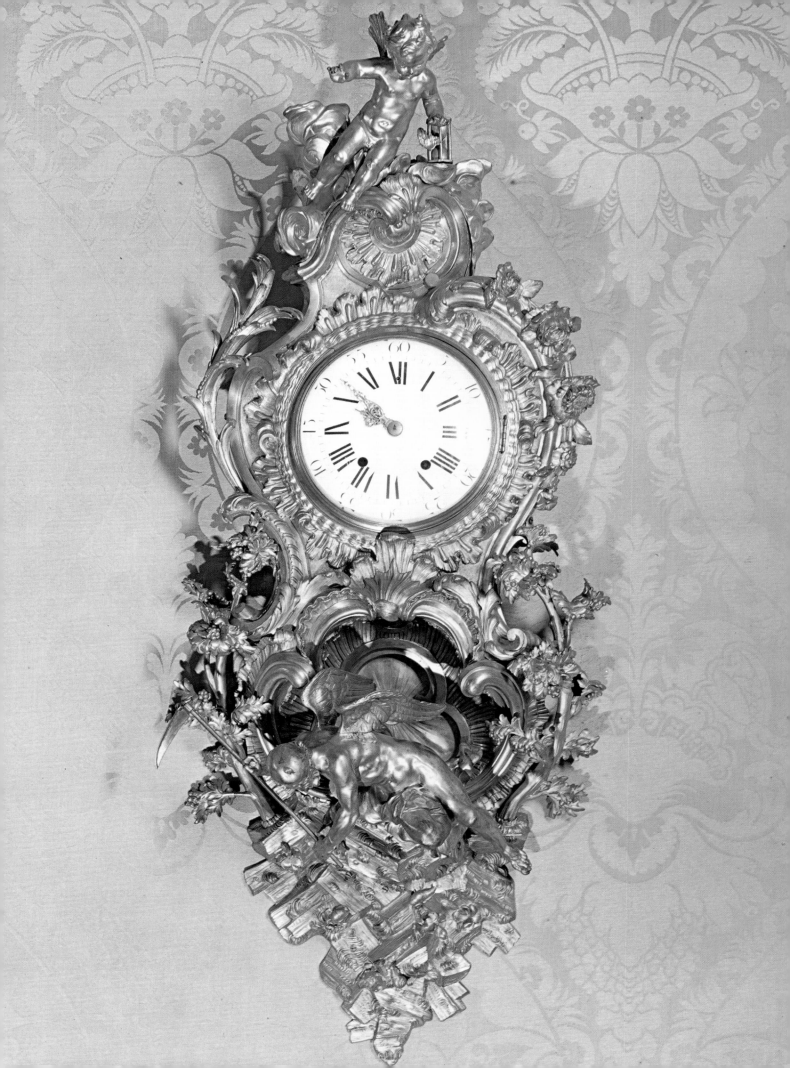

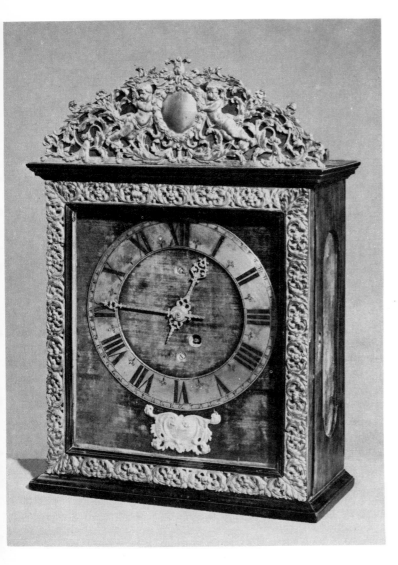

A pendule religieuse by the famous Paris maker Isaac Thuret, about 1675. Science Museum, London.

line, fine workmanship and a great reduction in elaborate decoration. Bracket clocks were largely superseded by mantel clocks, and white marble, with gilt bronze applied decoration, became fashionable. Dials generally were made smaller and of one-piece white enamel, instead of the style previously favoured, in which the hour and five-minute numerals appear as raised enamel plaques on a gilt metal plate, the centre also being of enamel. Several new types of clock appeared – for example, the 'column' clock, in which the central element, the clock itself, is slung beneath a portico top supported upon side columns. Another particularly graceful version is usually called the 'lyre' clock.

Contrary to popular belief, Switzerland has always concentrated upon watches rather than clocks, but even though she was making these in Geneva as early as the sixteenth century, her influence has always been indirect, and she was very late in formulating anything that could be described as a national style. In the earlier periods she is best known for the work of her émigré craftsmen, like the Vulliamys and Emery, who went to England, and Lepine, Berthoud and Breguet, who worked in France. Throughout the eighteenth century most of her production was for export, and was not of the highest quality.

Holland failed to take advantage of the tremendous potential lead given to them by Huygens' genius. However, there must have been much cross-fertilisation of ideas between the Dutch and the English; for example, the longcase clock, generally thought to have originated in London, was very quickly copied and adapted for use in Holland. Seventeenth-century Dutch longcase clocks are much like their English equivalents, except that they follow Coster's style in cladding the dial in velvet; but by the eighteenth century they have veered away, great emphasis being placed upon complications of every kind, with music, phases of the moon and tidal dials becoming quite commonplace and often allied to simple automata which either moved continuously in phase with the escapement or only when the music or striking trains were in action. Typical of such visual additions to the clock's normal function was the ship rocking on the waves, the windmill with rotating sails and the fisherman catching a fish. At the same time, Dutch longcases became much more elaborate – and, many people would say, much less elegant – than their English counterparts. The bases became bulbous, with elaborate paw feet and hoods surmounted by all kinds of exotic figures: Atlas holding the world, with trumpeting angels on either flank, is a typical example.

Perhaps more essentially Dutch than the longcase clock could ever be are a range of hanging weight-driven wall clocks whose detailed design as well as outward appearance differ according to the localities from which they originate and the periods when they were made. First and nowadays most prized is the Zaandam clock, from the industrialised district of Zaan, north of Amsterdam. Zaandam clocks are noted for their highly finished wooden cases with glazed sides, dials backed with velvet showing off with distinction the silver chapter rings, and hollow wall cases which accommodate the pendulum. This type of clock was made from about 1670 until the middle of the following century.

A simpler version of the Zaandam clock originating from Friesland is known as the 'stoelklok'. Appearing first about 1700, it is supported upon a wall bracket with a roof above to exclude dust; sometimes a linen runner is added to this latter feature, hanging down on either side. Both dial and bracket of such clocks would be brightly

This clock is known as the Avignon clock because that city presented it to the Marquis de Rochechouart in 1771. Here the clock is enveloped in statuary rather than separated from it. Wallace Collection, London.

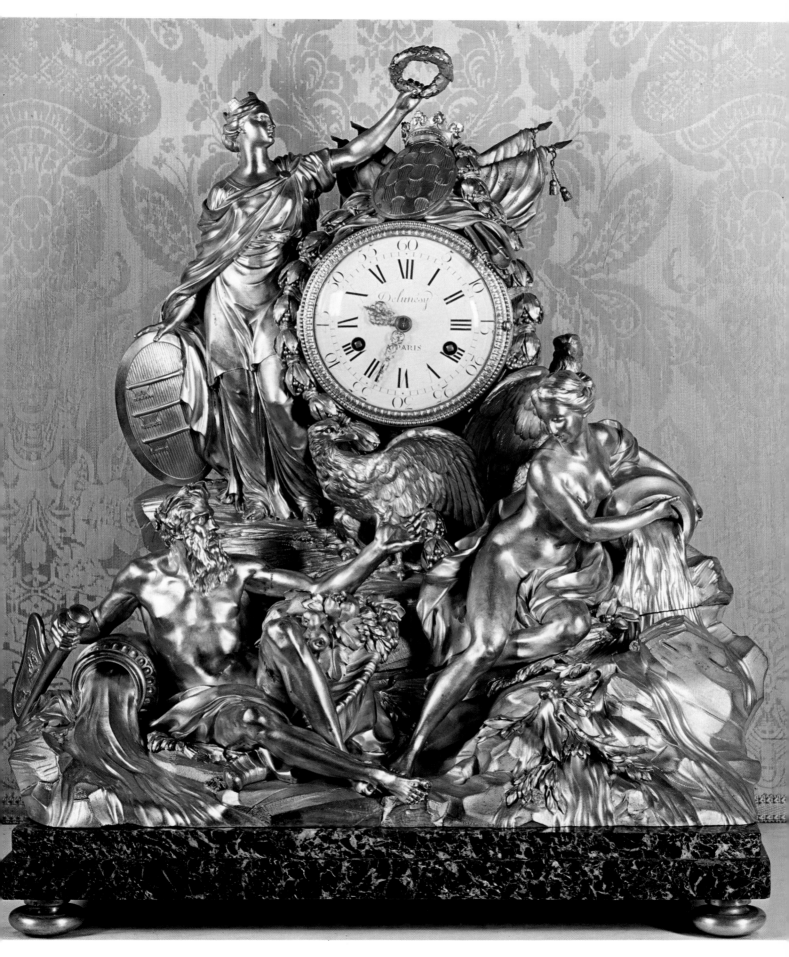

139

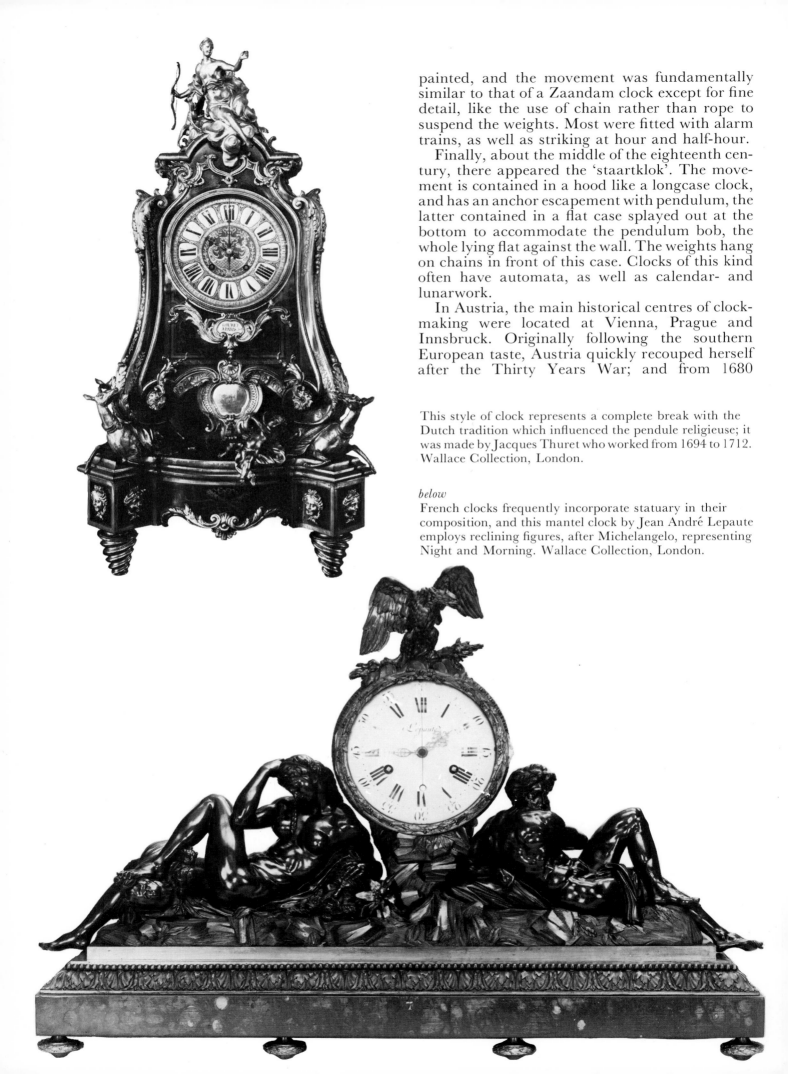

painted, and the movement was fundamentally similar to that of a Zaandam clock except for fine detail, like the use of chain rather than rope to suspend the weights. Most were fitted with alarm trains, as well as striking at hour and half-hour.

Finally, about the middle of the eighteenth century, there appeared the 'staartklok'. The movement is contained in a hood like a longcase clock, and has an anchor escapement with pendulum, the latter contained in a flat case splayed out at the bottom to accommodate the pendulum bob, the whole lying flat against the wall. The weights hang on chains in front of this case. Clocks of this kind often have automata, as well as calendar- and lunarwork.

In Austria, the main historical centres of clockmaking were located at Vienna, Prague and Innsbruck. Originally following the southern European taste, Austria quickly recouped herself after the Thirty Years War; and from 1680

This style of clock represents a complete break with the Dutch tradition which influenced the pendule religieuse; it was made by Jacques Thuret who worked from 1694 to 1712. Wallace Collection, London.

below
French clocks frequently incorporate statuary in their composition, and this mantel clock by Jean André Lepaute employs reclining figures, after Michelangelo, representing Night and Morning. Wallace Collection, London.

onwards, for at least a century, the English influence is clearly marked. Starting with posted movements, sometimes allied to complicated astronomical trains as well as conventional time-measuring machinery, the Austrian spring clock, by the early part of the eighteenth century, followed English patterns but coupled them with Austrian Baroque ornamentation. The Austrian longcase clock, however, favoured the bulbous style of French provincial work. It was not until about 1780 that a truly native style emerged. This was the 'Stutzuhr', and consisted essentially of a substantial base from which sprang the clock upon a slender support, with flanking ormolu ornamentation and often surmounted by a gilt figure, or sometimes an imperial eagle. Beneath the clock, in the space above the plinth, swings the pendulum bob, and behind it is generally a mirror. The effect can be most attractive.

Finally, mention must be made of clockmaking in the Black Forest. The great feature of clocks from this area is the use of wood for every part of the mechanism, except in those rare places where it simply cannot be made to work. The reason was economic – the peasants in that locality, taking to clockmaking in the middle of the seventeenth century, had of necessity to use readily available local materials, among which brass and steel did not figure. Their first clocks, then, had a foliot balance and a single hand; and, apart from the verge itself, the escape wheel teeth – which were simply metal pegs – and the pins forming the leaves of the lantern pinions, everything was wooden. Power was provided by a stone driving weight. These clocks had painted wooden dials, and only later were their movements boxed in. Striking mechanism was not added until about 1730, nor was the pendulum substituted for the primitive foliot until roughly the same period. Indeed, specimens still incorporating the latter form of controller are found as late as 1760. The popular feature peculiar to Black Forest clocks is the cuckoo bird call to sound the hours, which, contrary to popular belief, is not of Swiss origin. Although cuckoo clocks were undoubtedly made in the eighteenth century, few have survived that can be dated prior to about 1840, and they more properly belong, therefore, in a later chapter.

So inevitably it is necessary to return to England to find the mechanical ingenuity that was so necessary to propel horology in the direction in which developments in other branches of science and technology were to demand that it should go. For, while the French experimented with extremes of decoration on clocks and furniture alike, the Dutch regionalised their styles and the Austrians adapted other national styles to their own usage, it was the English who continued to experiment with mechanical improvements to make time-measurement ever more accurate and reliable, as

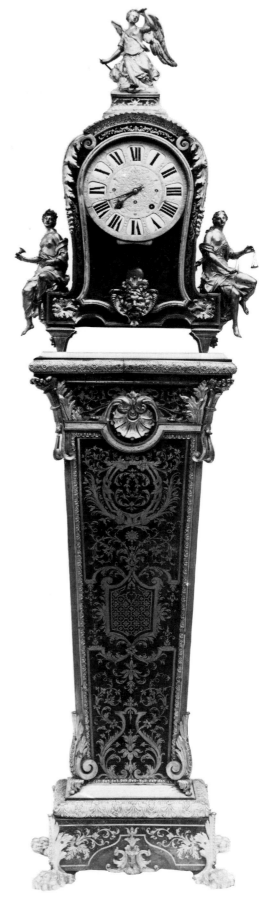

Another French clock style, the pedestal clock, is shown in this example by Vidal à Paris about 1750. Wallace Collection, London.

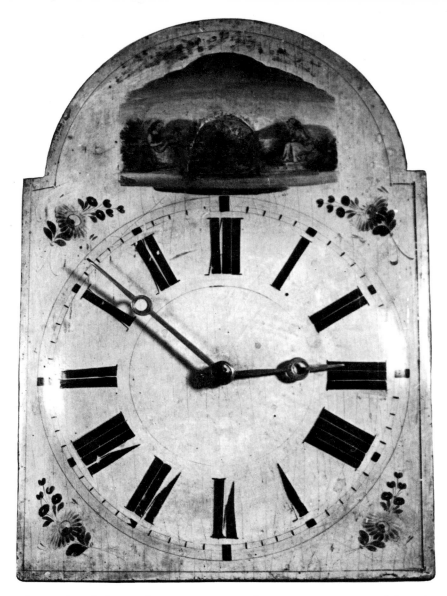

well as to retain throughout the eighteenth century the supremacy which their skills had earned them in the previous one.

An instance of this is the provision of special mechanism to indicate the equation of time. This, it will be remembered, is the name given to the difference – which varies from day to day – between solar time, as read from a sundial, and mean time; and the facility depends upon a specially designed cam, called the 'kidney piece' because of its shape, connected to the main mechanism.

The first equation clocks all bear famous English craftsmen's names – Tompion, Quare and Williamson – and the last-named claimed to have invented the principle involved. Tompion, however, can claim to have been first in the field with a clock for William III made about 1695; and the likelihood is that both he and Williamson, who claimed also to have made such clocks for Quare, obtained the idea of the kidney piece from Huygens. The great Dutch physicist wrote a letter to his brother Constantan, then working for William III, in which he explained the principle he had evolved, and it is conceivable that this was the starting point for both Tompion and Williamson.

Astronomy was catching the popular fancy then much as it does today; but it was also serving a much more serious purpose. The equation clock was an example of the scientific solution to a commonly encountered problem, for people had noticed, since the advent of the anchor escapement and the much more accurate performance of their clocks stemming from it, what a substantial effect the equation represented: the sun could be as much as a quarter of an hour fast or slow, by comparison with their clocks. More serious purposes were served by astronomical clocks such as those built, forty years or so apart, by Samuel Watson and Henry Bridges.

Samuel Watson was Mathematician in Ordinary to Charles II. Relatively little is known about him, his claim to fame resting upon at least three astronomical spring clocks, all different in design, one of them made for the King, and one or both of the other two reputed to have belonged to Sir Isaac Newton. These were the first such clocks to have been made for a very long time; and apart from the creation of Richard of Wallingford, known to us only by literary reference. Watson's were the first such masterpieces by an English craftsman.

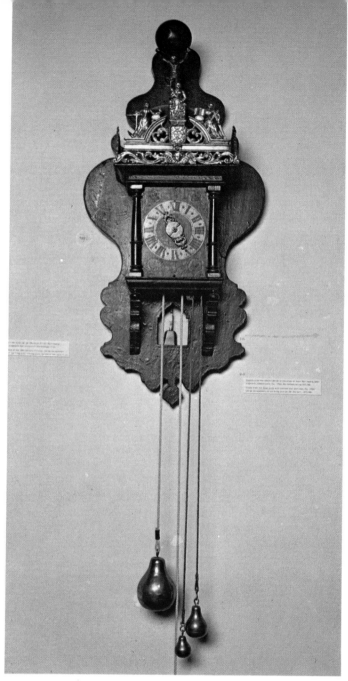

Zaanse clocks originated in a district north of Amsterdam, near the River Zaan, and were made for something over fifty years from about 1670. This example by Groot dates from the latter end of that period. Netherlands Clock Museum, Utrecht.

opposite page
The simplest European clocks – they were constructed almost wholly of wood – originated from the Black Forest and were virtually a cottage industry. This nineteenth-century 30-hour example has a shield dial.

right
This typical late seventeenth-century Dutch longcase clock, an eight-day example, incorporates Dutch striking and alarm and is signed 'Jac. Hasius, Amsterdam'. British Museum, London.

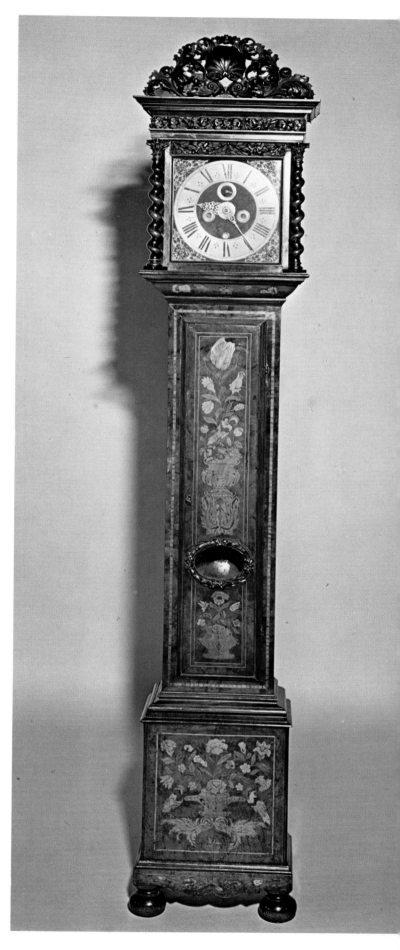

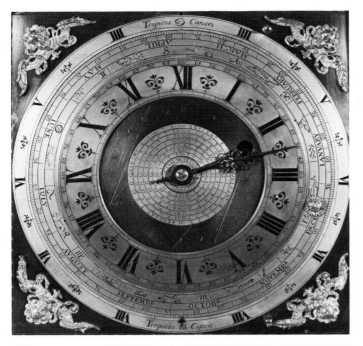

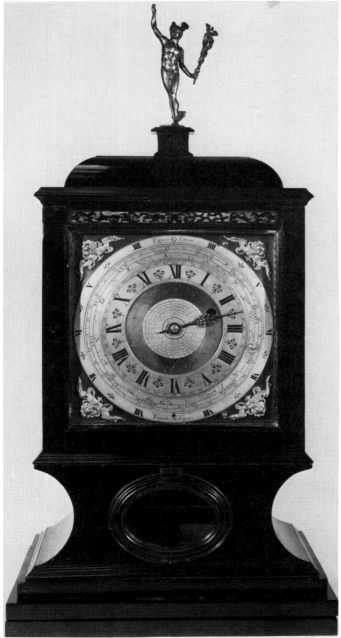

below

Three astronomical table clocks by Samuel Watson and dating from the late seventeenth century are recorded. This one belongs to the Clockmakers' Company. Museum of the Worshipful Company of Clockmakers, Guildhall, London.

left

The dial of the Watson astronomical clock demonstrates the complexities which he was able to incorporate into his creations. This clock is reputed to have belonged to Sir Isaac Newton. Museum of the Worshipful Company of Clockmakers, Guildhall, London.

Watson's royal clock was ordered by Charles II in 1683 and was probably completed about 1690. However, his original client having died before completion – and his successor abdicated – Watson was left with this highly complex machine on his hands. He apparently even went so far as to offer it as the first prize in a raffle, but seemingly this never took place for it had passed into the hands of the Queen by 1694. It is in the Library of Windsor Castle.

The main dial of this clock is twenty inches square, divided into four quarters, in each of which is a sub-dial. Taking them in order, that at top left is for the sun and planets revolving around the central earth according to Ptolemaic theory. At top right, the lunar dial has the earth at its centre, with the moon so arranged that, in its motions, its white side always faces the earth. The sun, revolving around the earth, is represented now only by the pin which used to carry its effigy. The left-hand lower dial indicates the year of the solar cycle and the Dominical Letter – by the shorter of the two pointers – as well as the day of the month, and the month of the year. On its right, the fourth sub-dial shows the Metonic Cycle or Golden Number, as well as the Epact. As for the time, that is shown only to the nearest quarter-hour by the small central dial.

Watson's two other astronomical clocks appear to date from the last ten years of the seventeenth century, and their provenance has been dealt with in detail by the late H. Alan Lloyd in an article in the *Horological Journal* for December 1948, pp. 750–59. It seems likely that both may have belonged to Sir Isaac Newton although they cannot be identified with certainty from existing inventories of his belongings. Even so, they establish without any doubt Watson's claim to have been the first maker of complicated astronomical clocks in England; previously, the limit in such designs had been the provision of a lunar dial and calendarwork.

The fashion that he started continued during the eighteenth century with a group of clocks by different makers, which varied in their essential purpose from the academically serious to the popularly scientific. Some of them fall into the category

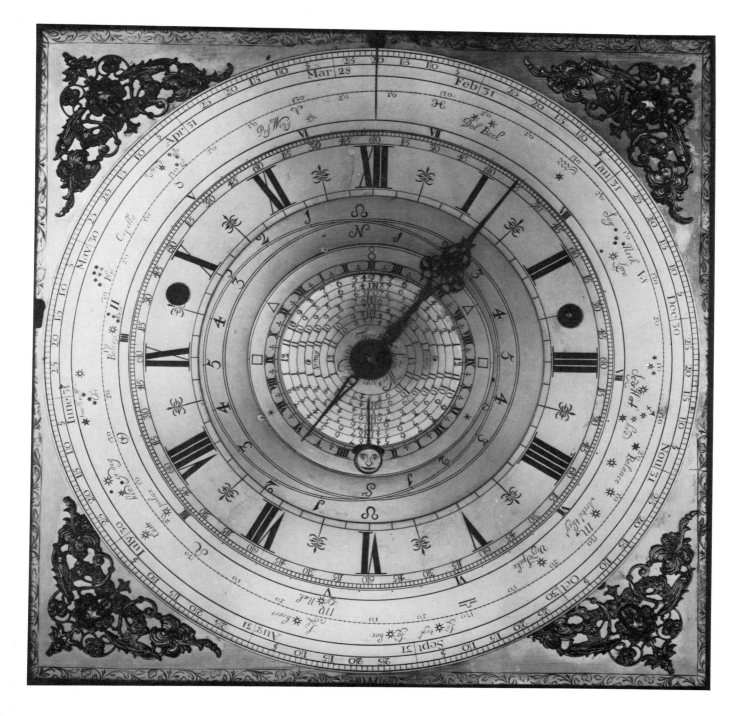

Careful inspection of this second of Watson's complicated clocks will reveal differences from that previously illustrated. None of the three clocks is identical one with another. Science Museum, London.

which we should nowadays describe as exhibition pieces, but their purpose went rather further than pure novelty. In England at this time, among educated and even less educated people, curiosity was at last being aroused concerning the world – and even the universe – around them. Natural philosophy, a broad term covering the sciences of natural phenomena, was becoming the focus of attention not only of the well-informed professional but also of the amateur and the dilettante. Many of those who fit into the latter two categories were nonetheless highly intelligent and enthusiastic students, and, certainly in horology and astronomy, there are plenty of examples of important contributions to knowledge and understanding being made by just such people.

Outstanding among the group of clocks just mentioned is one known as the 'Microcosm'. It was of monumental size – ten feet high and standing upon a base six feet wide – and it was made by Henry Bridges of Waltham Abbey about 1734. His tombstone gives his age at his death in 1754 as fifty-seven, and apparently he was an architect; thus he is a good example of the brilliant amateur contributing to the scientific stream. Otherwise virtually nothing has come to light about him. The clock itself could not have been attempted unless

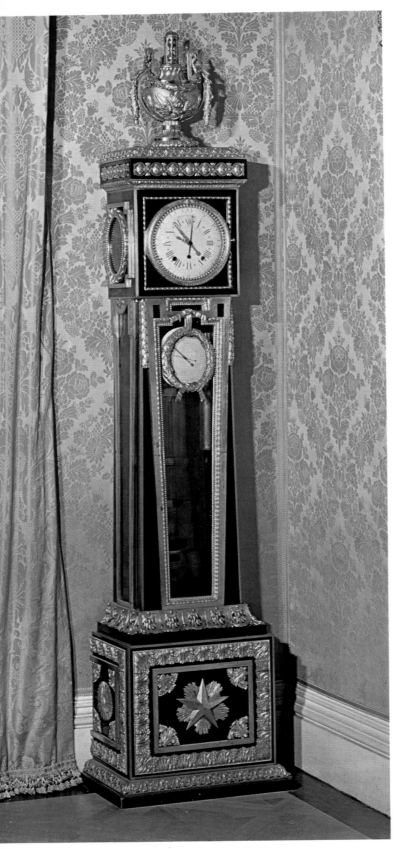

French clock of about 1770 by Ferdinand Berthoud, veneered in oak and ebony with a wheel barometer beneath the dial. Wallace Collection, London.

the maker had become an exceptionally competent workman in horological and allied skills; and its purpose seems to have been mainly to provide a source of income, by its exhibition. Thus, it is known that it was on view at the Mitre, near Charing Cross in London, towards the end of 1741, while in 1756 it had been taken to colonial America, where it was seen in Philadelphia as well as in New York.

The astronomical 'heart' of the Bridges 'Microcosm' consists of the two large dials, set one above the other; the top dial is based on the Ptolemaic system of celestial motions, and the bottom one on the Copernican. This is believed to be the only clock to embrace both systems, and it is perhaps strange – although in keeping with the new-found popular approach to science of the time – that allied to such academic profundities were the most elaborate automata, the whole being accompanied by music from an organ that either performed automatically or could be played from a keyboard. It is said that the mechanism embodied some twelve hundred wheels and pinions.

When the clock was exhibited, a descriptive leaflet entitled *A succinct Description of that Elaborate Pile of Art, called the Microcosm* was offered for sale; this of itself seems to have run to at least seven editions. The cost of viewing the clock varied from location to location, sometimes being as low as sixpence, yet on occasion as high as four shillings and sixpence. Immediately after Bridges' death the clock seems to have passed into the possession of one Edward Davies, for whom at least one edition of the descriptive leaflet was published. After returning from America – its final appearance there seems to have been in Boston – it was shown at Chester and Glasgow, and then seems to have disappeared completely. Eventually the astronomical movement was found in Paris in 1938 by the late Courtenay Ilbert, covered with a tarpaulin on the landing of a staircase in a furniture warehouse, and brought back to London by him, where it can now be seen in the British Museum. No trace has ever been found of the elaborate case or the automata.

An example of the more wholly 'exhibition' type of clock was that made by Jacob Lovelace of Exeter. Said to have taken over thirty years to build – Lovelace's dates in the eighteenth century are uncertain, although it is known that he was sixty when he died – this also was a monumental clock, measuring ten feet by five feet and weighing half a ton. It embraced all sorts of automata, including a moving panorama, an organ, a bird organ – whatever that may have been – and a belfry with six ringers, 'who ring a merry peal ad libitum'. The more serious content of the clock included a 'Perpetual Almanack' which was said to need regulation only every 130 years, the equation of time, and a leap year index revolving once every four years.

146

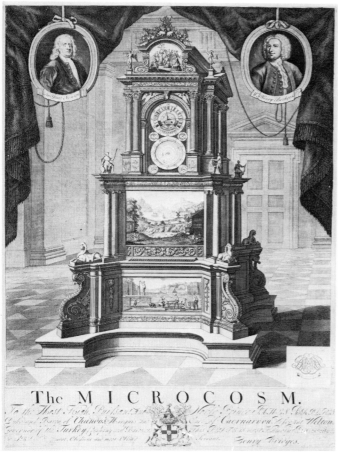

The MICROCOSM.

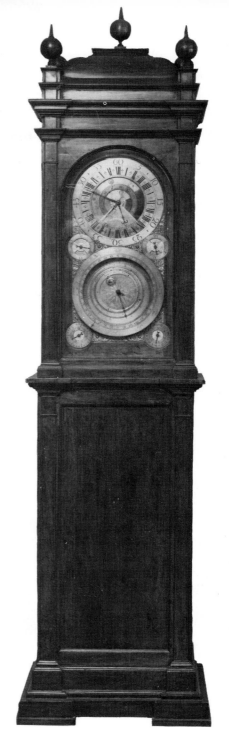

Another rather ingenious indication is located within the main twenty-four-hour clock dial, and shows the sun 'seen in his course, with the time of rising and setting by an Horizon receding or advancing as the days lengthen or shorten'. Within the same area was also located the age and phases of the moon.

The Lovelace clock is said to have turned up in a garret some while after his death, and thence to have passed into the possession of various persons in Exeter and thereabouts. It was frequently exhibited in the nineteenth century, notably at the Great Exhibition of 1851, and in 1888 it was proposed to purchase it for the City of London, but this was not carried through. By the time of the Second World War, it had found its way to the William Brown Street Museum in Liverpool,

above
This broadsheet was issued to advertise the 'Microcosm'. Even given artist's licence, there can be no doubt that originally this clock must have been most impressive. Museum of the Worshipful Company of Clockmakers, Guildhall, London.

above right
This is all that now remains of Henry Bridges' 'Microcosm' which was discovered by the late Courtenay Ilbert in Paris. British Museum, London.

where it was believed to have been totally destroyed by a bomb. However, of recent years, parts of it have come to light again, namely the complicated dial, some of the chiming train, and an odd ornament from the case. Curiously, it would seem that the clock was never officially photographed during its 'lifetime' as a complete entity, and the only representation of it that is left is the rare lithograph by Hackett which was published in 1833. It would seem, from comparison with those parts that have so far been recovered that this rendering must have been fairly accurate.

Another clock with pretensions to being a scientific instrument, albeit not in the astronomical sphere, is James Cox's 'perpetual motion' clock. Cox was an exceptionally able maker of compli-

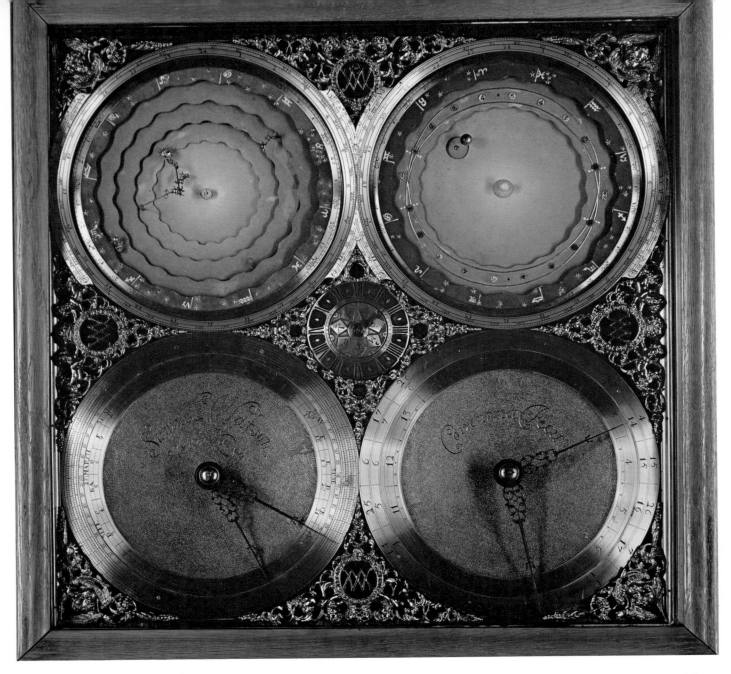

The remaining Watson clock has a dial layout totally different from the other two and is dealt with on page 144. Royal Collection.

cated musical automata clocks, invariably housed in the most lavishly ornamented cases, and frequently destined for China, where such extravagances were much to the taste of the rulers of that country. Cox had his workshop for many years in Shoe Lane, in the City of London, and, among other enterprises, he pioneered the Spring Gardens Museum at Charing Cross, which closed after a life of some six years, towards the end of 1774. The objects on show in this museum were of his own creation, and at the end there were some fifty-six of them; the fee for viewing was half a guinea. Cox obtained a private Act of Parliament enabling him to dispose of his museum exhibits, after its closure, by public lottery, and much of the information about them derives from the catalogues published in this connection. Cox himself died in 1788.

His 'perpetual motion' clock, exhibit no. 47 according to one catalogue, sets out to solve the insoluble, at a time when the concept of perpetual motion had caught the public imagination, and when indeed other clockmakers had tried – on paper, at least – to provide their own answers to a problem that almost seems to have overtones of the alchemist about it. Most of the other solutions were deliberately fraudulent, such as the one which wound a clock by the action of opening and shutting a door. Cox seems to have been serious about his, certainly to the extent of producing a most interesting as well as workable piece of machinery, which illustrated a principle – the use of small changes in barometric pressure to wind a clock – not finally adopted, despite its obvious utility, until the advent of the 'Atmos' clock nearly two centuries later.

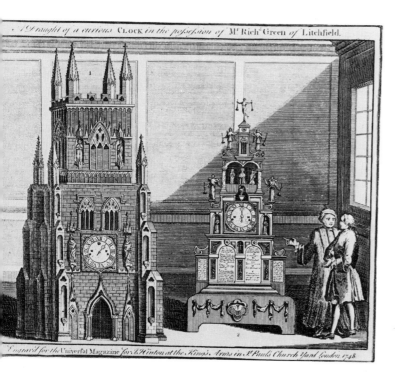

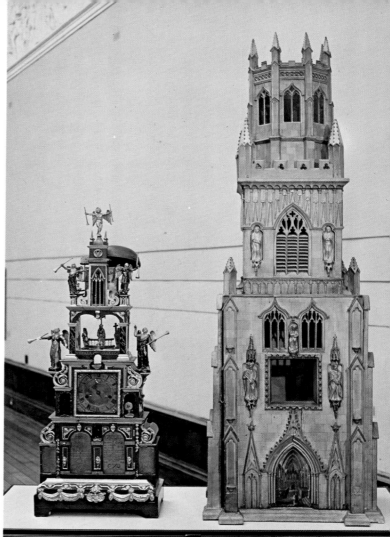

Artist's licence has clearly been used in this print of Richard Greene's Lichfield clock which appears to tower over its observers.

The mechanism of Greene's Lichfield clock has been slightly modified over the years, and it has been fitted with a pedestal and superstructure. Described in contemporary accounts as an altar clock, it carries no indication of who made it. Victoria Museum and Art Gallery, City of Bath.

The date of Cox's clock is about 1760. Without going into the greatest detail, the winding arrangement depends upon two huge reservoirs of mercury – the weight of the liquid metal involved is about 150lb, of which the cost at the present time would be prohibitive – and these are in a state of unstable equilibrium, a kind of 'see-saw' action being involved. Even a small change in barometric pressure upsets the balance, which is enlarged by a lever system as well as given a uni-directional momentum, and applied to raising the weight which actually drives the tiny clock mechanism. The latter is, in fact, of the scale and substance of a watch. It appears that the mechanism worked well, and that the driving weight was almost always fully wound. Whether or not James Cox really believed that he had found an answer to the quest for perpetual motion must remain in doubt; the charge of half a guinea to inspect his museum was designed to prevent 'undue masses of the curious' from causing damage by congestion, and, presumably, reduced numbers enabled him to control their proximity to the clock to a nicety. Furthermore, despite his protestations that everything was clearly visible and that there were no hidden mysteries, the particular device which converts the upward or downward movement of the lever sys-

tem into a one-directional winding facility had been very carefully boxed in and hidden away. This might have been to stop professional competitors from cashing in on his invention, of course; we shall never know for certain.

One more unusual English clock in this general category – although completely outclassed by those already described – does deserve brief mention. It is usually referred to as 'Greene's Lichfield clock', although Greene was not the maker but the owner.

Richard Greene (1716–1793) was trained as an apothecary and surgeon, but seems to have abandoned any professional ambitions in such directions quite early in life, to devote himself to the amassing of curiosities and objects of unusual interest in every conceivable sphere of human knowledge or activity. He spent his entire life in Lichfield, of which he became Sheriff in 1758 and eventually one of that city's Aldermen. He was the first to set up a printing press there, but his fame undoubtedly rests upon his museum, to which visitors came from far and wide; even the great Dr Johnson, accompanied as ever by the voluble Boswell, inspected it on at least two occasions.

Among the vast mass of miscellanea set out in cases, closets, hanging from ceilings and so forth,

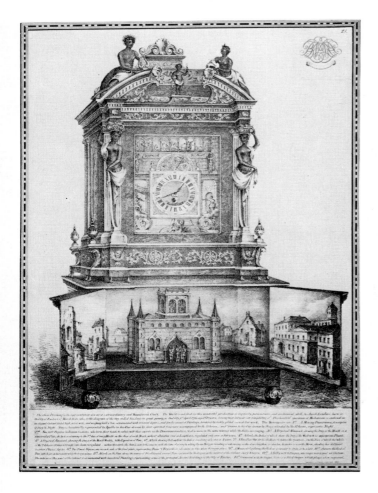

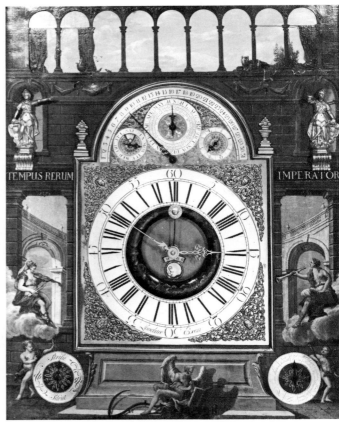

was a timepiece described as a musical altar clock. There is no indication, either upon the clock itself or from documentary references, as to who made it, although additions and improvements both to the structure and to the musical mechanism have been recorded. The clock is first described in the *Universal Magazine* of 1748, and is of good provincial workmanship; but it lacks that extra finish which always denotes the London practice.

The altar clock itself is about four feet high; but in 1768 it was provided with a pedestal and an outer superstructure which, when both are in position, give a total height in excess of nine feet. The prevailing religious flavour of the work is reflected in the various tablets, mainly of silvered brass, upon which appear the Ten Commandments, the Lord's Prayer and the Creed; this is further supported by statues of St John the Evangelist and St Peter, placed in niches either side of the clock dial, and there are a number of other statues positioned elsewhere on the clock. Above this again, a pavilion adorned with angels and cherubim contains an effigy of Pontius Pilate washing his hands, and around him process continuously three figures representing Christ going to his Crucifixion, the Virgin Mary and Simon the Cyrenian bearing the Cross, the trio making one complete revolution each minute. The clock is spring-driven; it incor-

above left
This 1833 lithograph of the exhibition clock constructed by Jacob Lovelace of Exeter is probably the only complete pictorial representation of this machine. Museum of the Worshipful Company of Clockmakers, Guildhall, London.

above
Of recent years parts of the Lovelace clock – thought to have been entirely destroyed – have been recovered and make an interesting comparison with the print of this same subject. Merseyside County Museum, Liverpool.

porates simple calendar- and lunarwork. Besides striking the hours on a large bell positioned at the back and just below the topmost figure on the pinnacle – which is said to represent 'Fame, with wings expanded, holding a sword in each hand' – the clock has a musical action playing every three hours or at will. It is interesting that the pin-barrel operating the musical action has been repricked, presumably as part of the 1768 refurbishing, so that, where there were once eight tunes, now there are only five. The history of the clock once Greene died and his museum was dispersed – much of it was sold off between 1799 and 1821 – is not well established; but eventually it was bequeathed to the Victoria Art Gallery, in Bath, when that was opened in 1900.

This astronomical organ clock is the only one of Henry Jenkins's monumental masterpieces at present known to exist (see page 154). While the curious observer sits at the hinged bureau flap thoughtfully provided to support his notebook, the organ beguiles him with a selection of twelve tunes – six on each of the two interchangeable pin-barrels. In the opening exposed by the flap can be seen the two weights driving the main going and striking trains of the clock, while behind and to their right is the massive weight that powers the organ action. The reserve pin-barrel is stored on a shelf at top left of the opening.

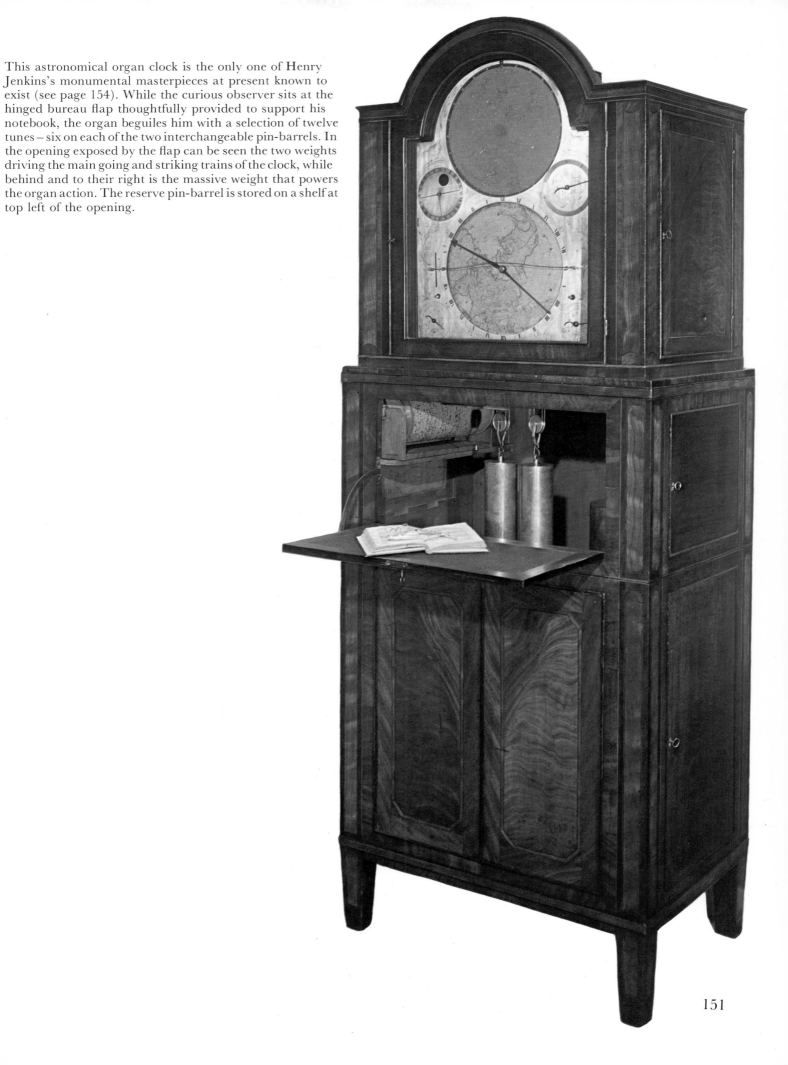

Such are a representative sample of the variety of interesting and important large clocks being made for public approbation in England during the eighteenth century – for the only one of those described which could reasonably fit into any ordinary household would have been James Cox's clock. There were other clocks of this kind which have either disappeared altogether or of which little is known. Christopher Pinchbeck (1670–1732) made astronomical and musical clocks, as well as inventing the zinc-copper alloy which was used as a cheap substitute for gold, and which is usually called 'pinchbeck'. In his advertising, in 1731, he refers to his shop 'at the Musical Clock in Fleet Street', and there is an illustration of a typically large ornate machine complete with automata on at least three levels, which, it is reasonable to suppose, was one of his own productions. It seems unlikely that this clock can still exist, despite the remarkable survival rate that such mechanisms seem to enjoy, even if they are, in some cases, only partial entities. Indeed his son, also Christopher, made a superb astronomical clock for George III about 1768 which is still in the royal collection.

Another mystery surrounds the work of Henry Jenkins, who is said by Britten, in the sixth edition of *Old Clocks and Watches and their Makers*, to have flourished from 1760 to 1780 in various locations in London. This same craftsman published a book in 1778, entitled *A Description of several Astronomical and Geographical Clocks with an account of their motions and uses*, from which it is clear that he had made several extra-complicated astronomical clocks, with musical and other parts incorporated, and was in all respects a considerable craftsman. Yet until quite recently, he was known for one or two domestic clocks with astronomical complications, and his monumental clocks were thought to have perished.

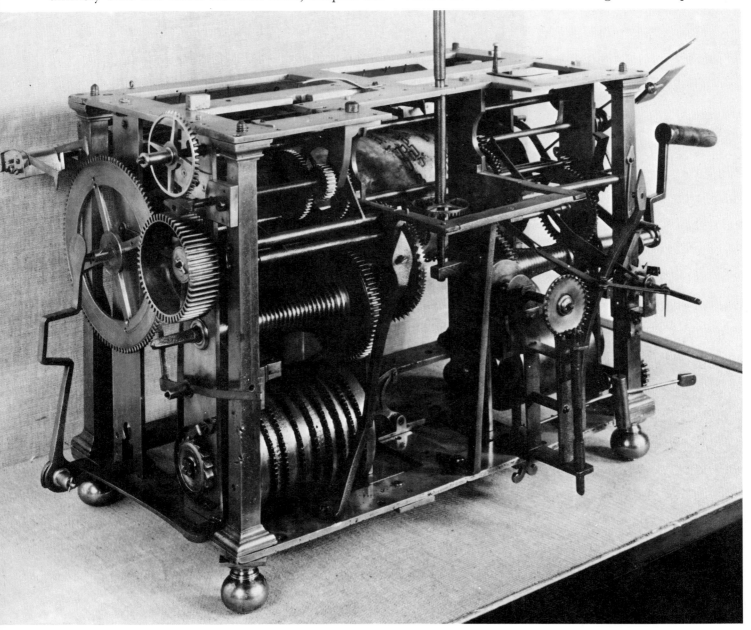

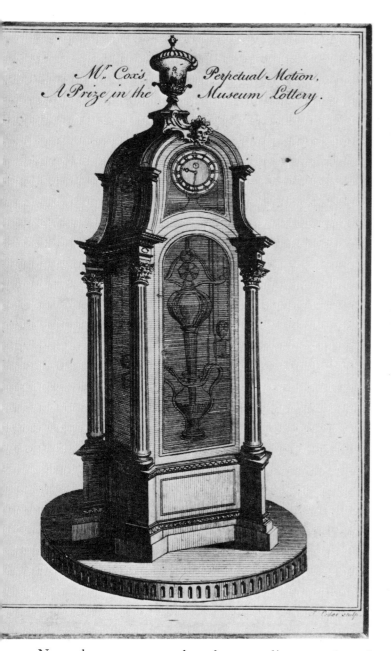

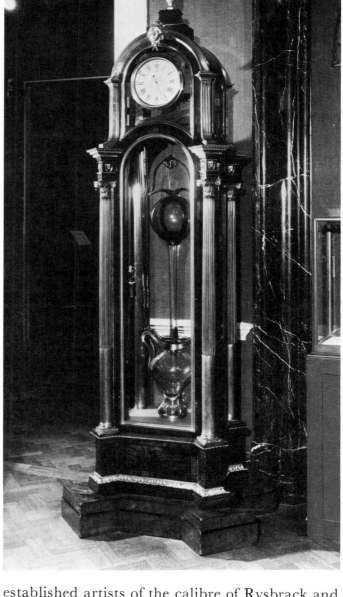

Now, however, one has been rediscovered and restored to much of its original splendour and performance (see illustrations on pages 151, 154).

There remain two makers whose work should be mentioned, on account of their ingenuity and fine craftsmanship; in each case representative specimens still exist by which they can be judged. Charles Clay died in 1740. The date of his birth, somewhere in the West Riding of Yorkshire – for the family turns up in the registers of several villages within a few miles of Huddersfield – remains unknown. His claim to fame rests upon the design and production of a small handful of musical – usually organ – clocks, of which the finest, described by its maker as 'The Temple of the Four Grand Monarchies of the World', remains to this day in the collection of the Queen, at Kensington Palace in London. It says much for Clay's importance in his own time that he was able to invite

established artists of the calibre of Rysbrack and Roubiliac, leading Baroque sculptors in the England of that period, as well as musicians like

above left
James Cox's celebrated experimental clock, whether or not he really believed in perpetual motion, received much attention in his lifetime as witness this contemporary print.

above
James Cox's clock, to judge by contemporary illustrations of it, is one of the best preserved of all experimental English clocks surviving from this period. Victoria and Albert Museum, London.

opposite page
The musical movement of the Lovelace clock after restoration.

153

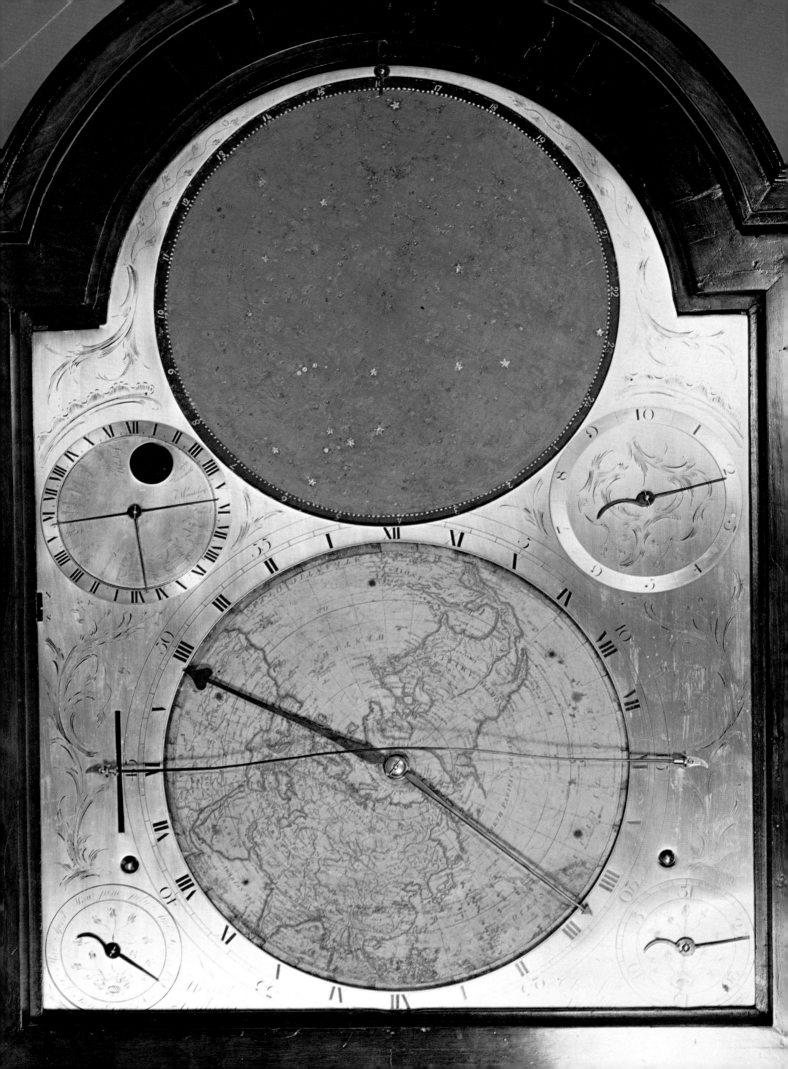

Handel and Geminiani, to help him with the appropriate elements of his clock. Equally sad is the fact that, though the outer structure exists intact, so that one can appreciate what it must once have been, it is only a shell, for the whole of the interior has been gutted – probably by the Victorian clockmaker Vulliamy, who made a habit of such things – and the pedestal which contained the musical action has been replaced by an open-work stand on legs, wholly out of keeping with the object it supports. Even the small integral clock has been replaced. Of his other work, there is a fine clock in the royal palace in Naples, which is reasonably well preserved – including its tiny pipe-organ – although not working. Historically, the Duke of Sussex, a great horolophile, who had many clocks among his possessions when these came to be auctioned by Christie's on 4th July 1843, had a Clay organ clock; and in the description accompanying this lot, no. 127, Clay is described as having lived 'in the latter part of the reign of George I and the beginning of the reign of George II, and was a very celebrated maker of machine-organs'. Perhaps the only entirely complete and working example of his work to be seen in recent times was sold by auction in London in 1972. This particular clock seems to have been taken, soon after it was finished, to Amsterdam, where it became part of a notable collection; after that, it went to Portugal where it has remained ever since. It was clear that this clock must also have been one of Clay's important productions, for both the musical and artistic elements show unmistakable signs of collaboration with at least some of the celebrities already mentioned.

The second maker of whom mention must be made is Alexander Cumming. Born in Edinburgh about 1732, he died in 1814. He was an uncle of John Grant who was one of his apprentices, and went on to become one of the great precision clock- and watchmakers of the time. Cumming made a number of fine clocks and watches during his lifetime, being elected a Fellow of the Royal Society, as well as publishing a treatise entitled *The Elements of Clock and Watch Work* in 1766. He is probably best known, however, for his interest in coupling the phenomenon of barometric pressure with clockwork – not, like James Cox, to produce perpetual motion, but for more academically scientific ends, to produce the first successful self-

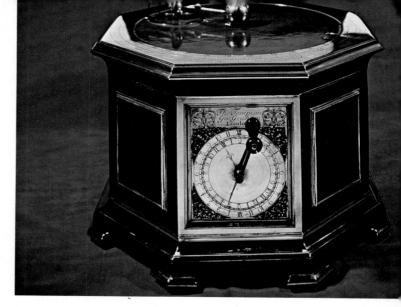

Apart from the clocks and watches they made in partnership, Tompion and Graham occasionally set their names to something rather more unusual like this orrery which shows visually the motions of the earth and moon around the sun. Museum of the History of Science, Oxford.

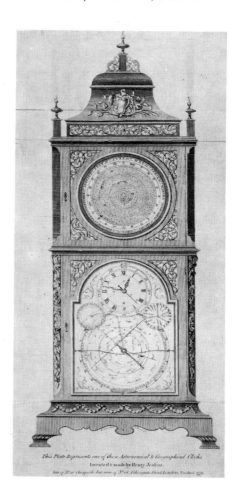

The dial of Henry Jenkins's clock reveals this maker's modest signature – Henry Jenkins, Cheapside, London – which is just discernible at the bottom of the dial-plate, left and right of centre. The dial itself transmits a variety of information, from the age of the moon and high tide at a range of different coastal towns, to the varying lengths of day and night throughout the year. Jenkins published his own description of his highly complicated clocks in 1760, with a second edition in 1778.

The frontispiece from Henry Jenkins's book *A Description of several Astronomical and Geographical Clocks . . .* , as it appeared in the second edition of 1778, gives a clear indication of this maker's individual style. It bears marked similarities to the clock previously illustrated, although clearly it is not the same instrument.

155

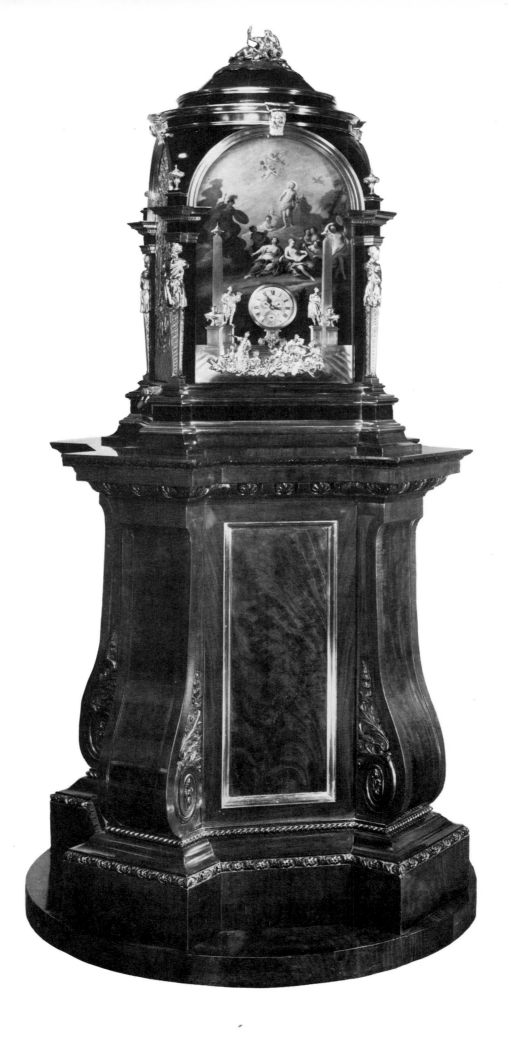

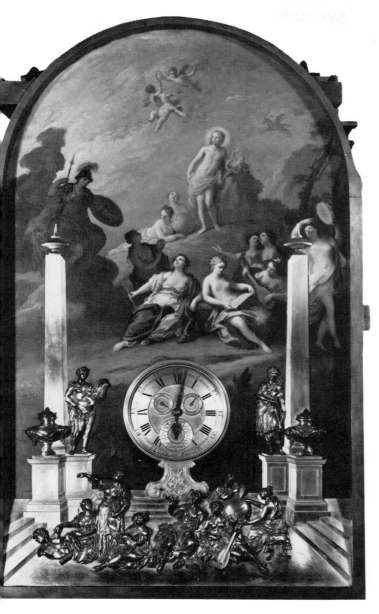

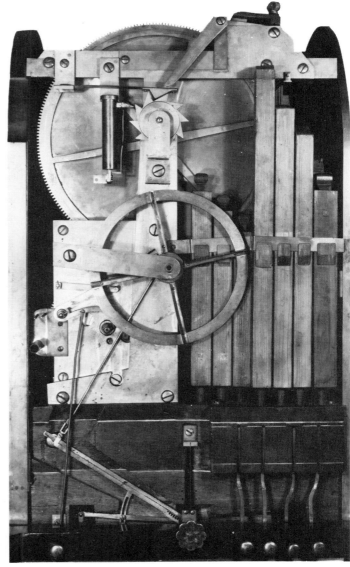

above
This detail of the dial of Clay's organ clock reveals painting by Jacopo Amigoni.

above right
The organ incorporated into Clay's clock plays ten tunes on a range of 96 wood pipes, the whole being controlled by a 13½in diameter pin-barrel.

left
Charles Clay was celebrated for his complicated musical clocks, in the execution of which he invariably invited other artists and craftsmen of stature to collaborate. This one, dating from about 1740, is perhaps the only complete example of his work remaining.

recording barograph. In 1765 he sold his first model to George III – it remains in the royal collection to this day – for which he was paid no less than £1,178, as well as an annual retainer of £150 for maintaining it. The following year he made a second instrument for his own use. These clocks display many fine original features, including a gravity escapement of Cumming's own design, which is fully explained in his published treatise.

Such is a brief outline of the more extrovert manifestations of horological ingenuity and excellence that took place in Britain throughout the eighteenth century. While these may seem to have occurred in a veritable explosion – and, for a small country, they represent a vigorous activity on quite a grand scale – it would be wrong to imply that nothing corresponding to this output was going on elsewhere. Vienna, for instance, was the centre for a small coterie of craftsmen building superb complicated clocks with an individuality all of their own. In the Bavarian National Museum can be found perhaps the finest example of this school, a

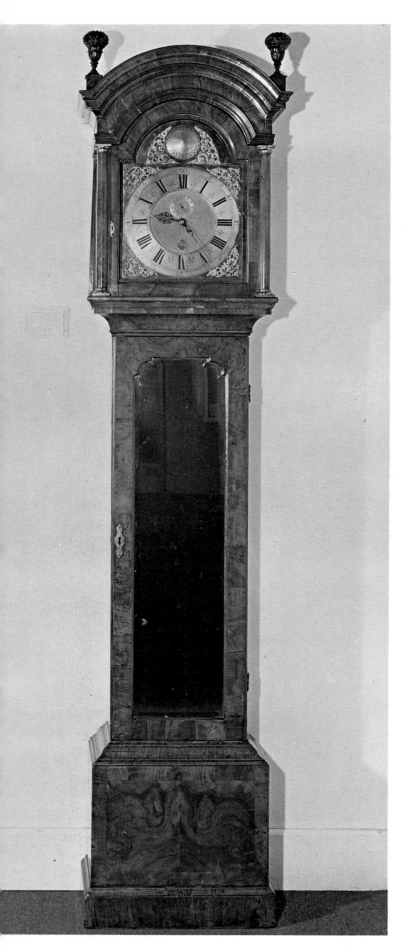

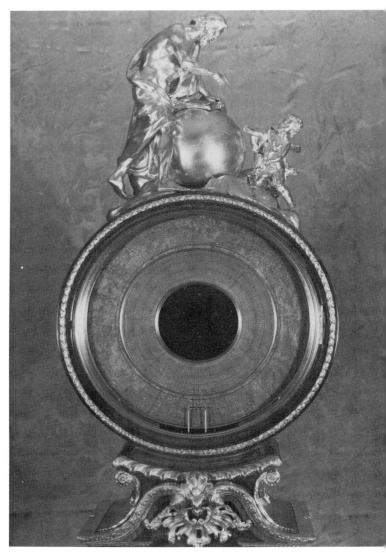

Alexander Cumming applied the idea of connecting clockwork and barometric pressure. This shows the dial of the self-recording barograph which he made for King George III in 1765. Royal Collection.

left
This year-duration clock was made by William Webster about 1720 and incorporates a slightly arched Vauxhall glass mirror into the trunk door. British Museum, London.

opposite page, top
The clock made by Aurelius in Vienna between 1760 and 1770 is depicted in this general view. Some authorities maintain that the clock case is the finest of its kind ever made. The clock is now in the Bavarian National Museum.

opposite page, below
The quality of the workmanship on the dial of the Aurelius clock is higher than even this photograph might indicate, while the complexity is self-evident.

monumental clock by an Augustinian friar, usually known as Aureliano, who taught mathematics and philosophy and, during the period 1760 to 1770, built this clock with his own hands. In essence it is an exceptionally complex astronomical clock, housed in a case, by an unknown maker, of a quality unequalled in any other known example.

Another Viennese clockmaker of eminence was David Caetano, a pupil of Aureliano, who built a month-duration astronomical clock of even greater complexity than that of his master. Completed in 1769, this clock is now in the Vienna Clock Museum. Work of the finest quality, though on a smaller scale than that of the two massive clocks just mentioned, was also coming from such other well-known makers operating in Vienna as Mathias Ratzenhofer, whose working life spanned the turn of the eighteenth and nineteenth centuries, followed early in the nineteenth by craftsmen of the merit of Brandl and Joseph Ettel.

Whatever else may be said, by way of wonder and amazement, about some of the clocks just touched upon, they contributed very little, in practical terms, to the timekeeping needs of the man in the street, being more often than not designed for some loftier scientific purpose which fell right outside his ken, or else simply as an exhibition novelty. Nevertheless, at a different level, a great deal was going on – mainly, but not wholly, in England – to refine the design and improve the performance of ordinary domestic timekeepers. This still resulted partly from the initiative of rich patrons – who had always hitherto been the springboard from which technological improvements had leapt upon the community, since a bottomless purse can be a great incentive to a comparatively impoverished craftsman – and partly from a gradually changing pattern of life, with the Industrial Revolution just around the corner. But the main impulse, as might be expected, was generated by scientific and humanitarian needs, such as that of accurate navigation, and the astronomical and horological implications associated therewith.

However, improvements occurred only at a very leisurely pace. In domestic clocks, for example, relatively little happened during the first twenty-five years of the eighteenth century. Longcase clocks gradually got larger – the six-foot case of the previous period grew to a norm of between seven and eight and a half feet, while dials expanded from ten inches square to eleven or twelve. Hoods were removed by being pulled forward on runners, and all had front-opening doors; the lift-up hood had disappeared altogether by 1700. On the top, flattened domes with three ball finials become usual and, where mouldings appear, these are now generally concave instead of convex. Marquetry inlay was popular, especially in the all-over seaweed pattern, but the finest clocks were mostly

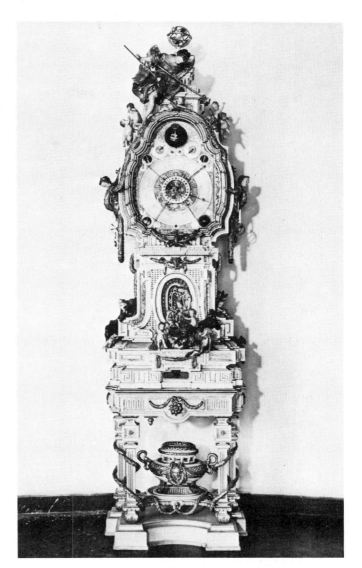

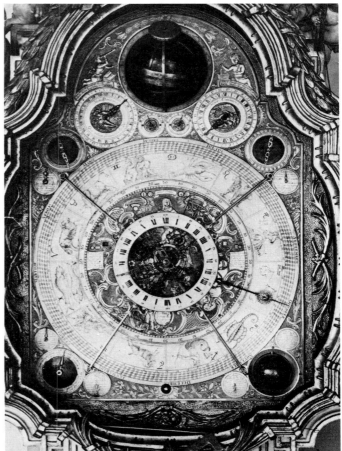

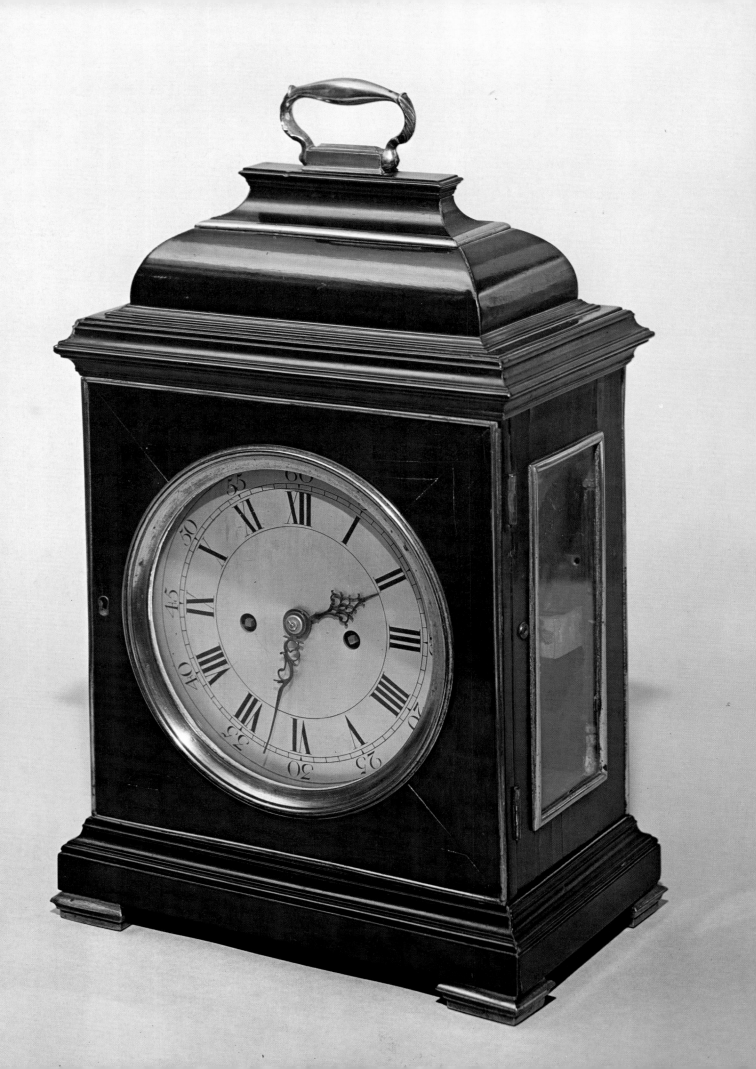

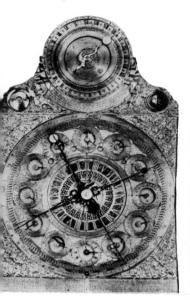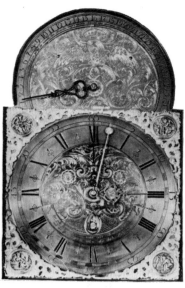

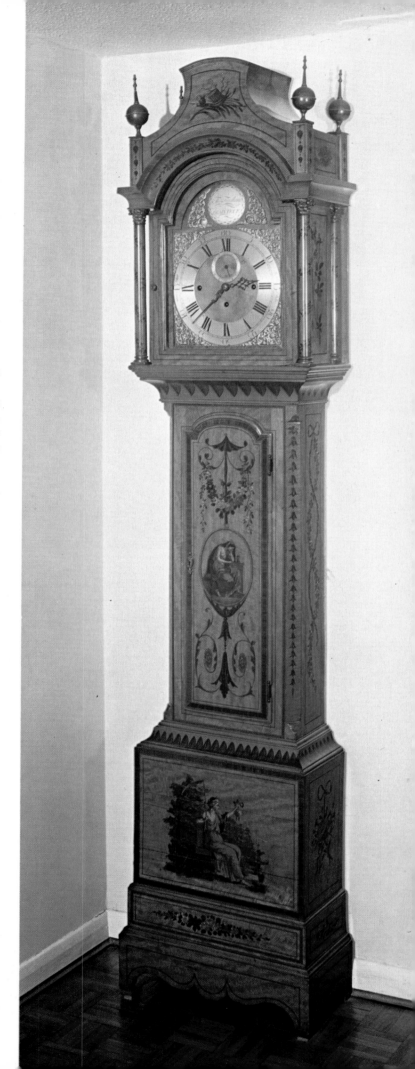

housed in walnut. Lacquer is another finish in vogue at this time.

This period saw the rise to eminence of George Graham, who achieved a degree of elegance in his clocks that would be difficult to surpass. He also perfected the only mechanical innovation of note that occurred, the dead-beat escapement. Technical complexities apart, this escapement can always be distinguished from its near relation, the anchor escapement, by its lack of recoil in action. Observation of the seconds hand on any ordinary longcase clock reveals that, as it advances from division to division on the dial, each forward movement is immediately preceded by a momentary retreat, which is the recoil. With a dead-beat escapement, however, each forward motion of the hand is divided from the next following only by a pause: the hand is described as beating 'dead' seconds. Graham perfected his escapement in 1715, and his mercury pendulum in 1726: he utilised the consequential change in the volume of a body of mercury as a means of compensating for alterations to the length of a pendulum caused by changes in the ambient temperature, one of the principal causes

above
David Caetano was a pupil of Aurelius. He constructed a month weight-driven clock whose complexities needed dials at both front (left) and back (right). Clock Museum, Vienna.

left
Another innovation attributed to Ellicott about 1750 radically changed the appearance of the bracket clock by substituting a round dial for a rectangular one and by doing away with the necessity for spandrels. Museum of the Worshipful Company of Clockmakers, Guildhall, London.

right
Essentially of the period round 1790, this unusual painted satinwood eight-day longcase clock is by John Fordham of Braintree. During the nineteenth century the movement was modified by the addition of an eight-bell chime, necessitating a new dial centre and chapter ring.

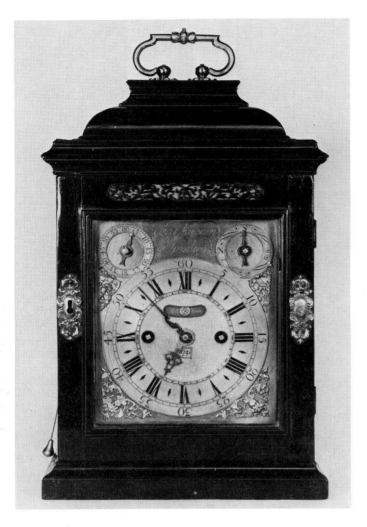

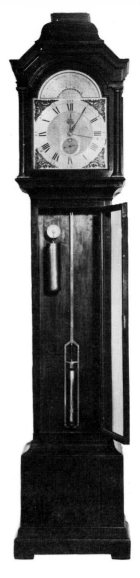

This small bracket clock by George Graham was made some years after Tompion's death but still bears the unmistakeable hallmarks of the quality and individuality which they conferred upon their clocks. It stands only 13in high. British Museum, London.

Made about 1740 and standing 7ft 8in high, this fine mahogany longcase equation regulator clock by George Graham has his 'dead-beat' escapement and mercury compensated pendulum. It is of one month duration. See also page 31. British Museum, London.

of inaccurate timekeeping in ordinary clocks. These two innovations combined in the same clock formed the basis of the famous Graham 'regulator', which was in all essentials the finest clock of its type – that is, as an accurate timekeeper for observatory and other scientific purposes – until the last few years of the nineteenth century. Regulator clocks were simply timekeepers: any complication, even such as striking, which might possibly have upset the performance of the going train, was rigidly excluded. Despite these considerable advances, Graham made relatively few clocks and must have concentrated his attention mainly upon the roughly six thousand watches which carried his signature.

Spring clocks in England underwent relatively little change during the first half of the eighteenth century. Black was still the favourite colour for the wood of the case, which as a consequence was either ebony or ebonised pearwood, although for the more high-grade pieces walnut remained the

preference. Lacquer became increasingly popular, and dimensions overall started to increase. The most noticeable change in the style of bracket clocks throughout this time was the gradual appearance, starting about 1710, of the break-arch dial and case. This had been first introduced by Tompion fifteen years before in one special clock, his longcase year-duration clock with equation of time, made for William III; and when first introduced into bracket clocks, it was mainly employed to accommodate a strike-silent control or calendarwork. The other outward change of style that started during this time, but was not at all common before 1750, was the substitution of a round, instead of a square, window in the front door, which effectively eliminated spandrels and produced a somewhat severe effect. However, a new style had become highly desirable, the previous one having done duty with so little change for so long.

Longcase clocks, to judge from survivng examples, seem to have gone into a temporary decline in the two decades immediately prior to the mid century. The break-arch dial and hood, when seen in the longcase, predispose towards some change in the shape of the trunk door, the top of which was now generally arched, while the corners of the case are usually chamfered. Walnut, lacquer and japanning were customary for London clocks, while oak remained popular in the country; mahogany is almost unknown at this period. The top of the hood passed through a number of styles almost simultaneously; the break-arch top has been mentioned, but the inverted bell top was also fashionable, while country makers even tried to revert to an earlier fashion with an architectural flavour imparted by the broken pediment. This, however, gradually degenerated into a more Baroque form. Mechanically, mention has been made of Graham's important contributions to escapements and temperature compensation. Harrison, whose genius will be more fully described in the next chapter, made similarly substantial contributions in the same areas, his form of compensation being based upon the 'gridiron' concept. John Ellicott, not only a renowned clockmaker but also a Fellow of the Royal Society, devised yet another version of a compensated pendulum, using the same principle of the differential expansion of metals, although it seems to have found little favour with other makers.

The second half of the eighteenth century saw England's ascendancy in the specialised form of time-measurement known as chronometry, and much of the native talent of its best craftsmen was devoted to solving the complex problems associated with that discipline. Consequently, developments in the ordinary domestic clock were slow to occur and do not amount to substantial change until late in the century. While the popularity of the longcase declined in the south, it suddenly blossomed forth in the northern counties, from about 1760. Mahogany, a wood almost unknown in clock cases before that date, quickly gained popularity and monopolised the field. Virtually all other woods and finishes – except the countryman's oak for simple clocks – died out. Northern styles at first followed those last in vogue in London, and only later deviated into the broad proportions which have been generally considered a debased form, albeit sometimes very well constructed. Bracket clocks continued much in their previous form, and still with the verge escapement; the anchor, as modified for this type of clock, was not generally adopted until after 1800.

Growing alongside these traditional styles there gradually evolved a whole new series of shapes and sizes of clocks, a burgeoning comparable with what was happening in France; but these were only starting to take the fancy of the ordinary customer in the last two decades or so, and did not

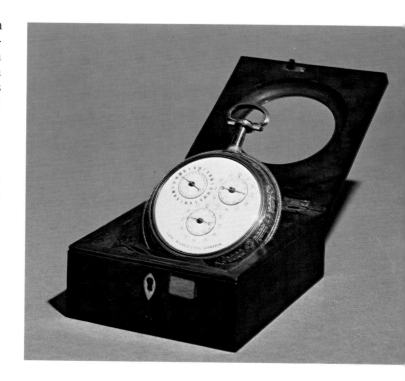

This large travelling clock – its diameter is 3¾ in – was made by George Margetts about 1790. The three dials read hours, minutes and seconds respectively, the last two showing both mean and sidereal time. The polished wood protective outer box for this clock is a recent discovery. While possible not contemporary, it is unlikely to date from long after the beginning of the nineteenth century. Museum of the Worshipful Company of Clockmakers, Guildhall, London.

become really established until the following one. Thus, for longcases, a Chippendale design in which the clock itself sits atop a tapering case, something like an inverted obelisk, while exceedingly rare, is by no means unknown. This style is quite reminiscent of what was happening to such clocks in France. In more conventional styles, it was the dial that changed, either to a simple silvered and engraved plate, or to one painted white with numerals picked out in black. These fashions date from about 1775. Regulator clocks, in the style set by Graham, were not greatly different from other longcase clocks; but during the latter part of the eighteenth century these became much more severe and totally undecorated. Square silvered dial plates have the display of hours, minutes and seconds separated by splitting into sub-dials, and such an arrangement is usually called a regulator dial, even when it is used on a watch. The purpose is to avoid the additional friction resulting from having motionwork under the dial to support the usual arrangement of concentric hour and minute hands.

As for bracket clocks, we have already noted the style, pioneered by John Ellicott about 1750, in which the square front door has a round dial window and no spandrels. About 1770 the conventional bell top started to give way to a break-arch

163

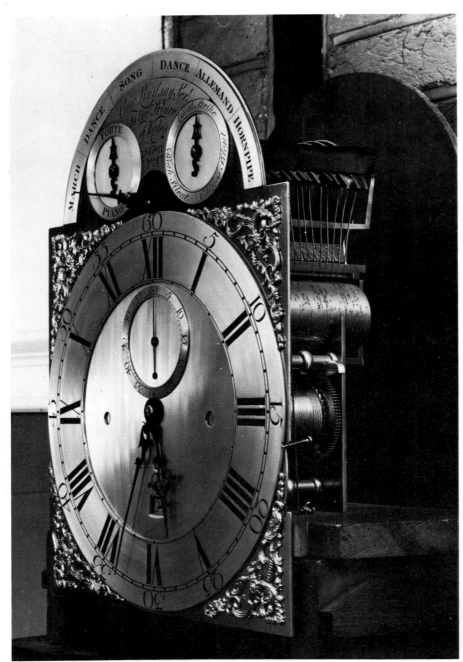

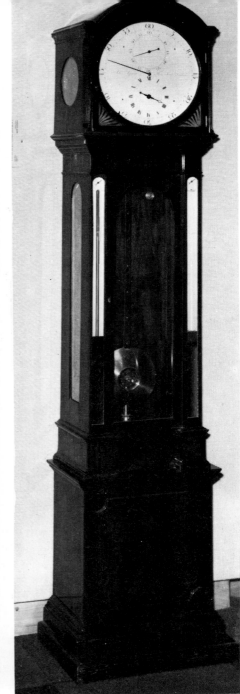

top, a style which developed and extended well into the nineteenth century. Repeating facilities in bracket clocks had all but disappeared by 1750, but musical and organ clocks became popular. Such clocks can have as many as four trains, for going, striking, chiming and music. An entirely different form of clock – more, perhaps, for a mantel than a bracket – was the balloon clock. This first appeared as early as 1760 but took a long time to come into prominence; then it stayed in fashion until about 1810. These clocks are generally plain, with at most a panel of inlay below the dial and a pronounced waist.

Two other forms of clock remain to be mentioned. Coach clocks, the outsize watches made for the traveller to hang up *en route*, which were pioneered by such makers as Edward East in the

seventeenth century, continued to be made throughout the eighteenth. Almost invariably, they now have a pull-repeat facility.

The other type of clock is that popularly called the 'Act of Parliament' clock, after William Pitt's levy of 1797 on all clocks and watches. This so diminished the market for these commodities that innkeepers provided their customers with the right time, as an additional service, using a particular style of clock which, though quite attractive, could be cheaply made. A very large number of such clocks survive, and they can often be dated to several decades before the single year that Pitt's levy was enforced. Their popular name is clearly incorrect, therefore, and they were simply inn clocks of the second half of the eighteenth century. Mostly of mediocre quality, they include the occa-

164

far left

George Lindsay, who held the Royal Warrant from George III, was arguably the finest maker of musical clocks of his time. On pages 52 and 53 will be found an illustration of one of his organ clocks, spring-driven. This large weight-driven longcase clock has a third (musical) train which plays a selection of six tunes on twelve bells, but using thirteen hammers. The extra hammer permits a fast staccato effect on one of the bells.

left

Spring-driven regulator clocks are rare, and this one by John Grant, a famous London maker at the turn of the eighteenth and nineteenth centuries, is said to have been for his own use. It is of one month duration and has an unusual gravity escapement. Museum of the Worshipful Company of Clockmakers, Guildhall, London.

right

Grant chose to employ Ellicott's design of compensated pendulum for his regulator clock, and this close-up shows the pendulum bob which encloses the arrangement of a brass and iron component acting upon hinged levers. Museum of the Worshipful Company of Clockmakers, Guildhall, London.

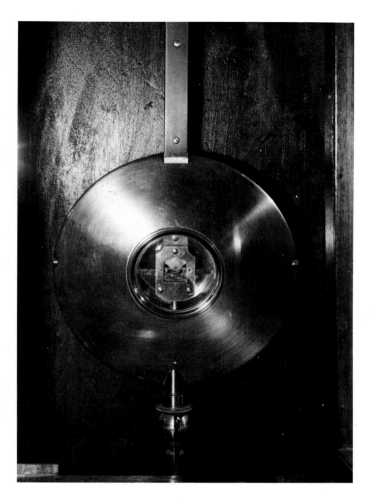

sional specimen that is exceptionally fine, both in design and in execution.

When the progress of watchmaking in the eighteenth century is examined, it is clear that two attitudes of mind are at work. The English, preoccupied with precision timekeeping as part of their efforts in the field of chronometry, are poised to make many important mechanical discoveries applicable to watchwork. The French, on the other hand, are more concerned with the ultimate appearance of the watch and will direct their energies to improving this, so that eventually they can claim to have influenced its final metamorphosis into the modern watch.

Very little of any consequence happened, either mechanically or in any other respect, to the watch during the first half of the eighteenth century. The escapement, the heart of the 'movement', was probably still the verge although Graham had long since perfected his cylinder escapement, and used nothing else in his watches after 1727. Pair-cases, plain and unadulterated, with enamel or – now rather more infrequently – metal dials, were the norm. As the century progressed, watches became a little smaller and the dials lighter in concept, with minute figures gradually disappearing altogether. Seconds hands were often pivoted from the centre, which added sophistication to the appearance of the watch; but in no form were seconds hands yet common. Multiple dials were employed whenever complex astronomical, calendar or stopwatch information was to be displayed; in the last-named category, the stop action brought the entire watch to a halt, an arrangement which persisted throughout the whole century.

The thick pair-case watch was universally used in England certainly until 1775, and was still being made for another seventy-five years. Even when the best London practice was to dispense with it, the substitute did nothing to make the watch thinner; the first 'consular' cases were almost indistinguishable from pair-cases, and the movement was still hinged to swing out, but there was just one case instead of two. The French, however, moved rapidly towards the thinner watch in the last quarter of the century, and these were often wound through the dial to obviate the need of a double-backed case. Watch cases were now often completely plain, gold or silver, and such enamel work as is found has greatly degenerated from what had gone before. Similarly, repoussé decoration, at its best by mid century, persisted in increasingly debased forms until 1775. Guilloche, or engine-turning, started to come into its own from about 1770 and, in combination with over-enamelling, often edged with half pearls or paste, can produce a superb effect.

Mechanically, the second half of the eighteenth century saw the cylinder escapement further refined, in both England and France, by making part or the whole of the cylinder out of ruby. As made originally in steel, the cylinder is very susceptible to wear; with its bearing surfaces made of ruby in the English usage pioneered by Ellicott

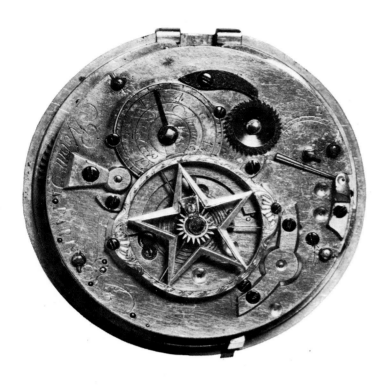

At the end of the eighteenth century, a small handful of English and French watchmakers recommenced experiments with the lever escapement. Robert Robin working in Paris made a number of such watches about 1790.

and Arnold, or completely out of that same precious hardstone, as subsequently developed by Breguet, it seems almost impossible to wear the escapement out. However, the brittle nature of the stone makes accidental damage likely to have more serious consequences than with the earlier version.

Having some relationship to the cylinder escapement – they are all three so arranged that their escape wheels operate in a horizontal plane – are, first, the virgule and, secondly, the duplex. The virgule is only found in French watches and, as developed about 1780 by Jean Antoine Lepine, enjoyed a short vogue of only about twenty years. Today it is a collector's item indeed and only rarely encountered. Theoretical advantages of the virgule were largely offset by its inherent fragility, the difficulty of making it and its inability to hold oil. As a result, it wears quickly, so that its performance rapidly deteriorates. An even rarer version of the virgule known as the double virgule has survived in very few examples indeed, and these are almost exclusively in museums.

The third of the horizontally designed escapements is the duplex. To a greater or lesser degree it possessed all the faults inherent in the virgule: it too was fragile and difficult to make and to keep lubricated. But it was capable of providing great precision in performance, when built by the most skilled hands. Certain London makers specialised

in it almost to the exclusion of other escapements, most notably James McCabe, who was himself turning out fine examples towards the end of the eighteenth century while his successors continued the fashion even towards the middle of the nineteenth. The duplex seems to have acquired such a reputation during its heyday that it became the preferred escapement for the highest quality watches, despite the advent of the detent and the lever. And this reputation would not be contradicted by present-day experience, for there still remain plenty of fine watches with duplex escapements which, carefully maintained, give as good a performance now as when new, perhaps a century and a half ago.

The detent escapement was, of course, developed directly from the inventive 'stream' that was tackling the longitude problem and the navigational need for a high-performance timekeeper. While it can be perfectly well adapted to a pocket watch, the timing of its development was such that it could hardly have been available in any quantity for ordinary domestic use before 1800: all supplies were diverted to become deck watches for marine use.

The remaining escapement was the detached lever, invented during the eighteenth century and destined eventually to become the most important of them all, though unrecognised at its true value by its inventor and discarded. Thomas Mudge, a famous and inventive horologist with a particular interest in the field of chronometry, completed his prototype lever watch in 1759; George III, for whom it was made, gave it to Queen Charlotte, and it has remained in the royal collection to this day. It has often been called 'the most famous watch in the world'.

Mudge had the advantage of knowing about a prior invention, called the 'rack lever', which originated in France; and he must have recognised that the great disadvantage of the escapement in that form was the rack and pinion which continually connected the escapement to the train. It was his flash of inspiration to redesign that particular part of the mechanism, eliminating this feature altogether. He believed in his escapement to the extent of writing that in watches it could answer its purpose better than any other watch escapement then available. But he also conceded that it was very difficult to make, and few craftsmen would attempt it, let alone succeed.

This remarkable specimen can only be described as a skeleton clock, although it is quite unlike a normal one. Dated 1776, it is signed 'Jas. Merlin, Inventor' and therefore has associations with James Cox, for whom Merlin was principal mechanic. Unusual technical features of the clock include a dead-beat verge escapement with a crown wheel of sixty teeth, while the connection between the verge arbor and the centre wheel is by means of a worm pinion.

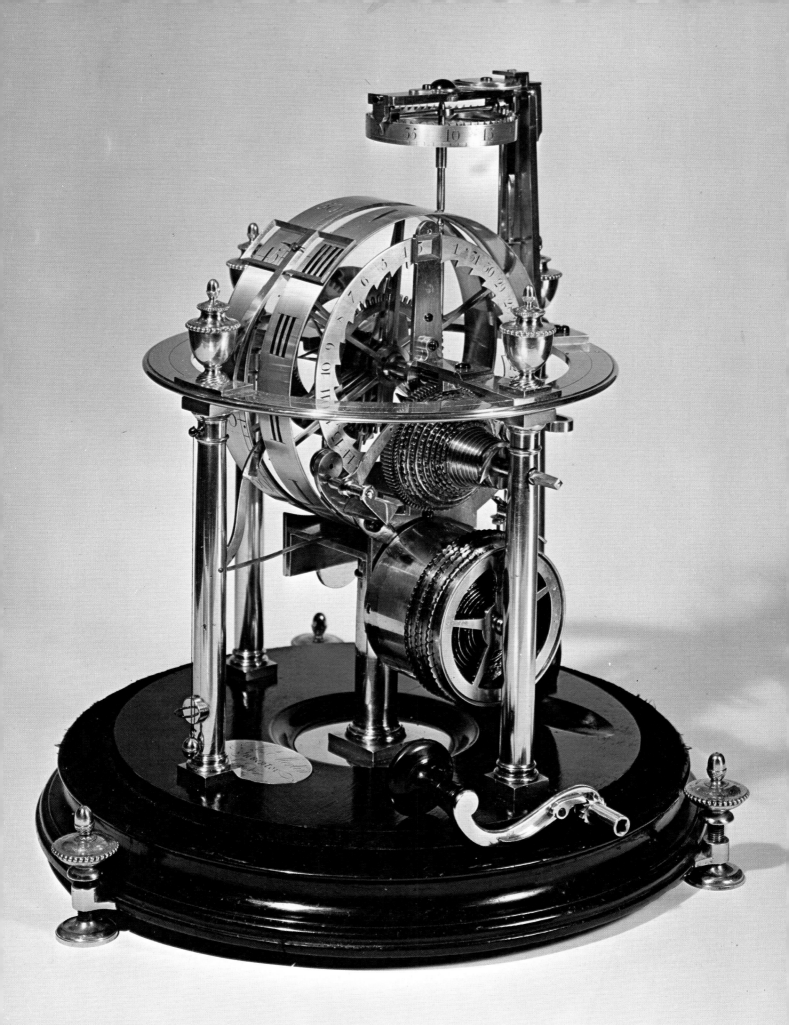

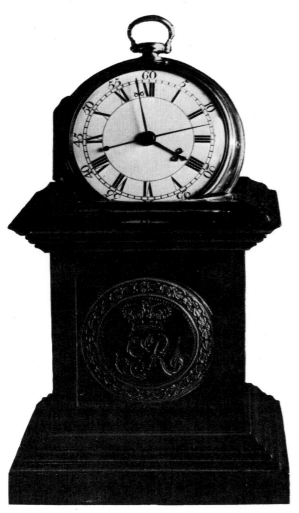

In fact, apart from Mudge's original watch, the lever escapement was the subject of further experiment in a very few watches made by a small handful of the best watchmakers towards the end of the century. Josiah Emery holds pride of place in this regard, although Leroux and Grant, as well as one or two others, produced their own versions of this mechanism, and similar experimentation was going on independently in France, by such makers as Robert Robin. It would be true to say, however, that the generality of watchmakers ignored the lever escapement until well into the nineteenth century, and the fully developed version, as handed down to our own times – which is known as the table-roller lever – did not become commonplace until at least 1830.

Technical features such as the balance spring were undergoing modification and improvement throughout this period, but they had at least been introduced. On the other hand, the other innovation of great importance in watchmaking was the equivalent to the temperature-compensated pendulum in clocks, the compensated balance. This refinement can hardly have been necessary until well into the nineteenth century for ordinary pocket watches which, in other respects, were not sufficiently accurate to justify such sophistication. But the chronometermakers did need it, and where they went the watchmakers were not slow to follow.

The first pocket watch with a lever escapement was made by Thomas Mudge for George III in 1759, but it was not for another sixty years or more that the escapement was to become commonplace. Royal Collection.

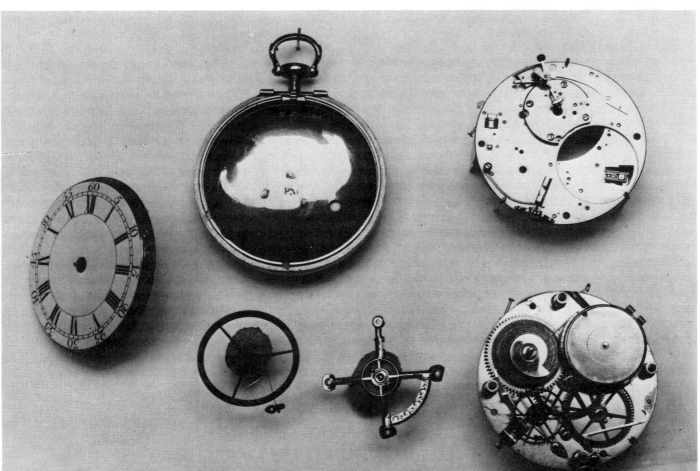

Marine Chronometry - 1675 to 1820

There is nothing mysterious about a chronometer: it is simply a special kind of timekeeper for use on board ship, where it is an important navigational aid.

In the usage of most English-speaking countries, the definition of a chronometer requires that it must have a particular type of detached escapement, which is known as the detent – or, sometimes, just as the chronometer – escapement. In Switzerland, however, a chronometer tends to be any timekeeper that has successfully passed stringent observatory tests. Marine chronometers are generally housed in brass drum-shaped cases, which in turn are slung in gimbals – so that, whatever the motion of the ship, the chronometer remains level – and these are fitted in a mahogany box with a glass-topped lid, as well as an outer solid lid. The time can be read, therefore, with the minimum of disturbance. The same specially accurate detent escapement was also fitted into watches, and in the early days these tended to be a little on the large side, when they were known as 'deck watches'; they too were often contained in specially fitted mahogany boxes with sliding lids, although not in gimbals. The original purpose of the deck watch was to enable the ship's 'box chronometer' – an alternative and self-explanatory term – to be set to time accurately, when the ship was in port, without having actually to move it from its normal position; the going of any timekeeper is affected to a greater or lesser degree by extraneous motion, and in the case of the ship's navigating timekeeper this was avoided at all costs. So the deck watch instead was taken to the nearest observatory where it was set to time by the regulator clock – which itself would be checked regularly by the observatory's transit instrument – and then brought back to the ship, where its time would be compared with the marine chronometer, and the latter adjusted as required.

But why was such an irksome procedure necessary? To appreciate this, it is important to understand one of the greatest hazards facing the mariners of those days, not a new hazard by any means but one that, in the more prosperous trading times of the seventeenth and eighteenth centuries was costing not only lives, then considered reasonably expendable, but also valuable cargoes, which were not. This hazard was simply the inability of a ship's captain, once out of sight of land, to be able to plot with any degree of certainty exactly where his ship was positioned. Some of the great voyages of discovery which took place before and during this time must, for their success, have depended upon a large slice of luck, however brilliant may have been the navigators conducting them. The alternatives to making a desired landfall were the likelihood of shipwreck or, perhaps even worse, slow death from diseases of dietary deficiency like scurvy.

Plotting a position at sea follows much the same pattern as on dry land; and anyone who has ever done any mapreading knows that, for the latter, one needs two coordinates. These are imaginary lines, one running north to south, the other east to west, and any position can be expressed in terms of the point at which two such lines cross. At sea, any navigator must know his latitude – that is, the distance north or south of that imaginary circle we call the Equator – as well as his longitude, which is his distance east or west of an imaginary meridian passing through the two Poles, before he can plot his position on a chart. Latitude is relatively easy to determine, by observation of the altitude above the horizon of certain of the heavenly bodies. Longitude is much more difficult, and any reliable calculation needs the services of an accurate timekeeper recording mean time on an internationally recognised meridian, such as Greenwich – which is Longitude 0° – for comparison with the

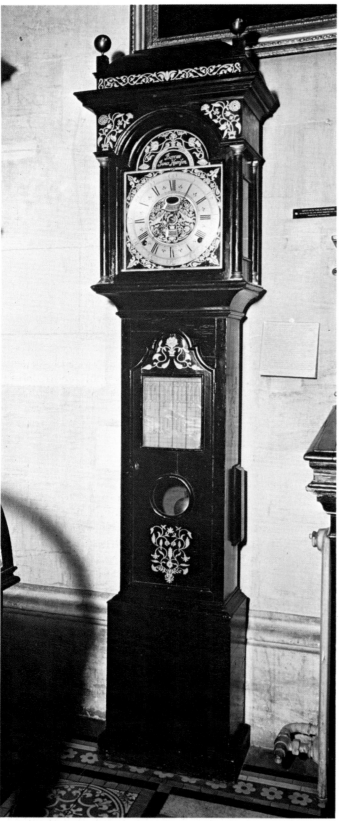

This high-performance longcase clock, signed by John Harrison's younger brother James and dated 1728, incorporates two of the innovations for which Harrison is celebrated – his grasshopper escapement and gridiron compensated pendulum. The movement is constructed almost wholly of wood. Museum of the Worshipful Company of Clockmakers, Guildhall, London.

local time of a ship, as again found by observation. When it was first decided to tackle this problem, neither the prime meridian nor an accurate marine timekeeper existed.

The first serious attempts to study and rectify this situation began in 1675, when Charles II established by Royal Warrant an observatory in his royal park at Greenwich, 'in order to the finding out of the longitude of places, and for perfecting navigation and astronomy'. Several first-class brains were involved in this matter from the start; the architect of the observatory was none other than Sir Christopher Wren, while the first 'observator' – forerunner of the office of Astronomer Royal – was a young man called John Flamsteed.

Flamsteed was a clergyman from Derbyshire; but he had already made quite a reputation for himself as an astronomer and mathematician before he started 'to measure distances in ye heavens' towards the end of 1676. The job cannot have been a sinecure for, although the Royal Warrant took care of Flamsteed's salary and even extended to that of an assistant, there was no provision whatever for purchasing equipment, so that, for the rest of his working life – and he died in 1719 – Flamsteed had to beg, borrow or buy out of his own pocket everything that he needed. At one time he was even taking in his students, giving them food, lodging and tuition, in order to make ends meet. Yet nothing deterred him. He seemed somehow to be able always to acquire what was necessary for his work, and over the years he amassed a formidable body of some 40,000 observations. These formed the basis of his star catalogue, a monumental work which was not published until after his death but which effectively established him as the founder of modern positional astronomy.

Notwithstanding all this activity – which was valuable in other directions – little was accomplished towards the principal objective of improving navigation. So in 1714 the Government offered a reward, by Act of Parliament, for 'such person or persons as shall discover the Longitude'. The prize was graduated according to the accuracy achieved, ranging from an upper limit of £20,000 if within half a degree, to £10,000 within a degree, upon a trial voyage from Britain to the West Indies. Translated into terms of precision timekeeping, a chronometer, to win the top prize on the six-week voyage involved, would need to keep time within three seconds a day; although this type of accuracy was within the capacity of the best static pendulum-controlled clocks at that time, such machines would have been quite useless at sea where the motion of the ship would have fundamentally disturbed their timekeeping. It required something special in the way of a timepiece to withstand such elemental forces and

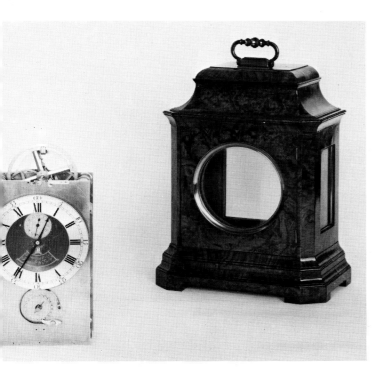

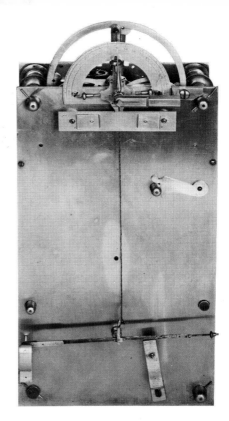

Henry Sully, an Englishman who spent nearly all his working life in France and who died in 1728, designed this marine clock about 1724, and it was subsequently sent to George Graham for inspection. Museum of the Worshipful Company of Clockmakers, Guildhall, London.

This view of the movement of Sully's marine clock shows the big balance which in its oscillations acts upon a horizontal pendulum to which it is attached by a silk cord. Museum of the Worshipful Company of Clockmakers, Guildhall, London.

still keep good time; and such an instrument was not, in the event, to be proven in use for nearly half a century after the prize was first offered.

Despite what might now seem the obvious disadvantages of the pendulum in marine use, the earliest attempts to make a timekeeper for use at sea depended upon one, albeit specially designed. Huygens, already the pioneer of the pendulum and the balance spring, tried his hand at this as early as 1660, but the performance of his timekeeper was so erratic as to be worthless. Others, including Henry Sully, a very able innovator, worked along similar lines; but any attempt to associate any kind of pendulum with a ship was bound to fail, and the answer was eventually to be found in a balance controlled by a spring.

The great English pioneer – among a number of pioneers of stature, for England was to make an international reputation for herself in this field of 'the Longitude' – was John Harrison. Born into the trade of carpenter in the village of Barrow in Lincolnshire in 1693, Harrison and his younger brother James early in life started building simple clocks almost entirely out of wood. By 1726, what is more, they had constructed two regulator clocks of the most ingenious design, again employing wood as almost their sole raw material. Being carpenters, however, as well as inventors, they would

know how to make the most of the natural properties of their chosen medium; thus, for example, they used lignum vitae as an anti-friction agent, for this wood is considered self-lubricating. Their pendulums were of the temperature-compensating design usually described, on account of its appearance, as 'Harrison's gridiron'; the principle was so to arrange a grid of alternating rods of brass and steel that their changes in length with variations in temperature to all intents and purposes cancelled each other out, leaving the effective length of the pendulum unaltered. Their escapements, of the kind descriptively known as a 'grasshopper', were nearly silent in action and the most accurate – even though also the most complex and fragile – then available. These clocks – both of them still in existence, and still capable of giving an excellent account of themselves – had other highly sophisticated and quite new features that were also attributable entirely to the genius of the Harrisons, and without doubt, at the time, they must have been the most accurate clocks in the world. John Harrison himself noted that they kept time 'without the variation of more than a single second in a month'. What is more, in order to test the accuracy of their regulators, the Harrisons were not content with their own equation of time calculations – perhaps they distrusted the inherent accuracy of a

Harrison finally encapsulated his ideas on marine timekeeping within the two large watches known as H.4 and H.5, the first being completed in 1759 and the second in 1770. H.4 (left): National Maritime Museum, Greenwich. H.5 (right): Museum of the Worshipful Company of Clockmakers, Guildhall, London. H.5 was only completed when Harrison had reached the age of seventy-seven, and in appearance it is very severe by comparison with the decoration applied to H.4 (left, below).

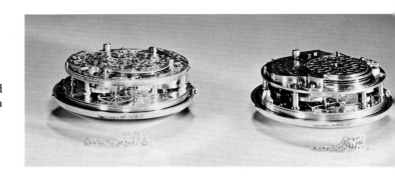

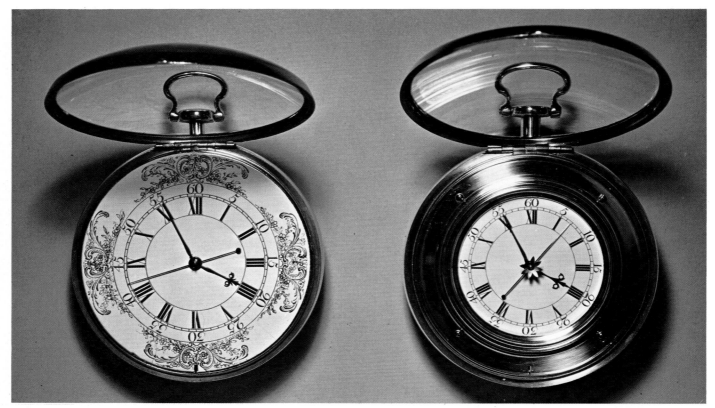

sundial, with which such calculations had to be used – and instead made their own 'transit' observations of a suitable star.

Perhaps their experience with these two high-precision clocks led the Harrisons to decide to enter into the search for a longitude timekeeper. In any event, they early realised that they could no longer work in wood, and that they would need capital to underwrite the expensive purchases of brass and steel from which they would have to construct their machines. Luckily for them, the Board of Longitude – the body appointed to oversee the working of the Act of Parliament relating to the quest for the longitude, to make trials of timekeepers and to recommend the award of prizes – could advance money against the completion of designs thought to be particularly promising, in order thereby to alleviate just such circumstances as were facing the Harrisons.

Accordingly, John Harrison came to London for an interview with Dr Halley, who was not only Astronomer Royal – there is a well-known comet named after him – but also a member of the Board of Longitude with particular responsibility for dealing with the inventors in the field. Halley sent Harrison on to see George Graham who, as both a Fellow of the Royal Society and a celebrated practising clockmaker, could give an expert opinion on the technical aspects of Harrison's work. Despite Harrison's thoroughly distrustful and truculent attitude of mind – like many another genius, he always thought others were trying to steal his plans – and even though he was always so inarticulate, to judge from surviving manuscripts, as to be quite unable to explain intelligibly to others what he was striving to accomplish, Graham was greatly impressed. It is said that they talked for ten hours non-stop, as a result of which Graham encouraged Harrison to build his marine timekeeper, to this end lending him money from his own pocket interest-free, and undertaking that, if the result turned out well, he and Dr Halley would support his approach to the Board of Longitude for development money to continue the good work.

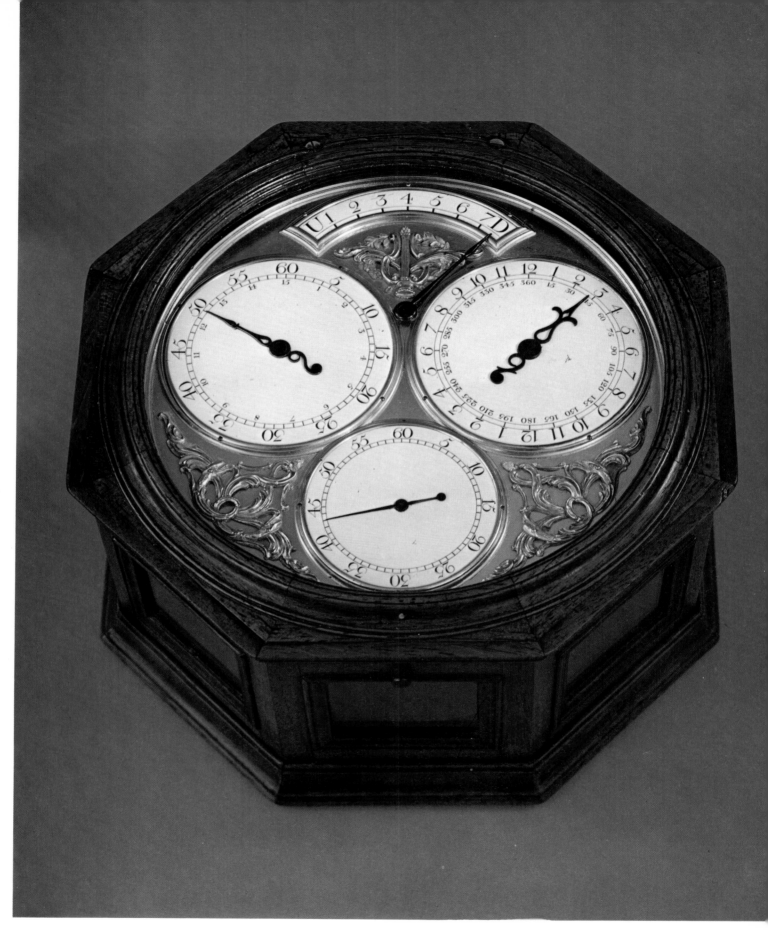

Following Harrison's pioneering work, another innovator was Thomas Mudge who made three marine timekeepers of highly sophisticated design and obtained an award of £3,000 for his work. British Museum, London.

It took Harrison five years to build this first sea-going clock, and Graham's money was not of itself sufficient to finance the operation. However, other money seems to have been forthcoming, both from private individuals and from the East India Company, mindful, as always, of any way of reducing its losses at sea. Known as 'H.1', this first marine chronometer was a monumental machine by any standards, weighing about 72lb and occupying space equivalent to a cube of almost two feet.

H.1 had been completed probably about 1735, and was then tested on board a barge in local waters in order to fine-tune it. Accompanied by John Harrison, the great clock was next sent on a voyage from Portsmouth to Lisbon and back, in 1736, when the longitude calculated by reference to the timekeeper gave a position sixty miles nearer the correct one than the captain's own reckoning.

Despite its cumbersome bulk, H.1 set an entirely new standard in maritime time-measurement, and it has been calculated that, had the clock been assessed according to the standards which were eventually formulated as being the most accurate and informative concerning the performance of such a timepiece, it would at least have qualified for third prize from the Board of Longitude. Even so, that body was by no means unimpressed, and when Harrison asked for £500 as a grant-in-aid to build a second, improved timekeeper, the Board at once agreed. Being always canny about spending public money, however, it insisted that both H.1 and H.2, when completed, should be handed over to the nation.

Except for the escape wheel, all the wheels of H.1 were made of wood, and one of its exceptional characteristics is that it requires no lubrication whatsoever. H.2, which was essentially a refined version of H.1, was made with brass throughout but, in the event, was even more massive than H.1, weighing 103lb. Both brothers worked on H.2, which was finished in 1739, but it was never tried at sea since John Harrison seems to have determined to do even better before exposing his work to public scrutiny again.

At about this time too – and it may have had some bearing on John Harrison's attitude to the testing of H.2 – it seems that the brothers ceased their fruitful collaboration, and James Harrison gave up his interest in marine clocks altogether. John meantime had virtually abandoned H.2 and was already at work upon H.3; in 1741 he told the Board of Longitude that it would be ready for a trial voyage to the West Indies in two years and was given a further £500 on the strength of this assertion.

However, it actually took Harrison seventeen years to finish H.3, which was ready by 1757. Even then he was not satisfied, and asked that the trial be delayed while he finished yet a fourth – and

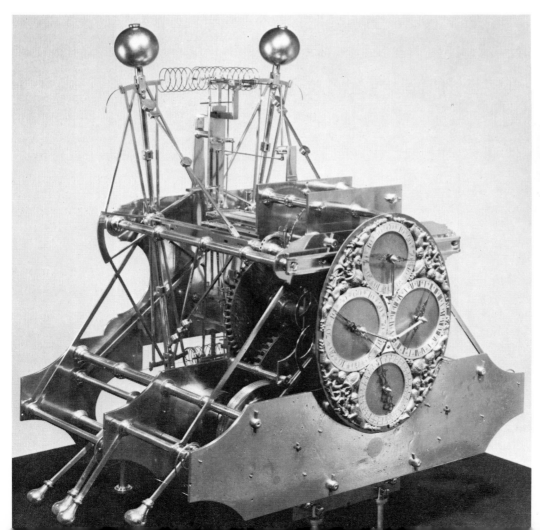

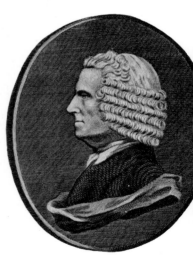

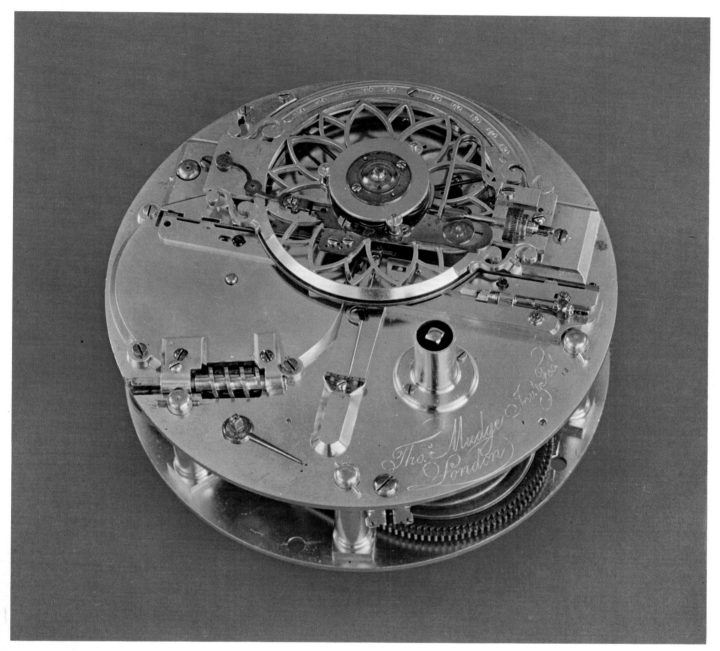

The chronometers Mudge made himself performed well although they were too complicated for large-scale production, and the copies commissioned by his son after Mudge's death did not stand comparison with the originals. This shows the back view of Mudge's marine timekeeper. British Museum, London.

left
Several representations of John Harrison exist including a cameo portrait by Tassie, and a mezzotint. This engraving from the *European Magazine* was published in 1788 and is perhaps less well known than some of the others.

far left
This first of Harrison's massive marine timekeepers was tested in 1736 on a voyage to Lisbon and was found to have an almost negligible error. National Maritime Museum, Greenwich.

much smaller – timekeeper. This was originally to have been an ancillary to the larger clock; but when it was completed, Harrison maintained that it would be a serviceable marine timepiece in its own right and that its performance was every bit as good as that of H.3.

H.4 was, in fact, much closer to the tradition of the travelling coach clock than anything Harrison had produced previously. It was, in effect, a large silver pair-cased watch, some 5·2 inches in over-all diameter, and it must have made a strange stable-mate for the three huge machines that had preceded it. Anyhow, when the time came to equip the trial ship, Harrison determined that H.4 should go on its own, and he himself, being then sixty-seven years old and perhaps no longer really fit for the privations of a long sea-voyage, stood down in favour of his son William.

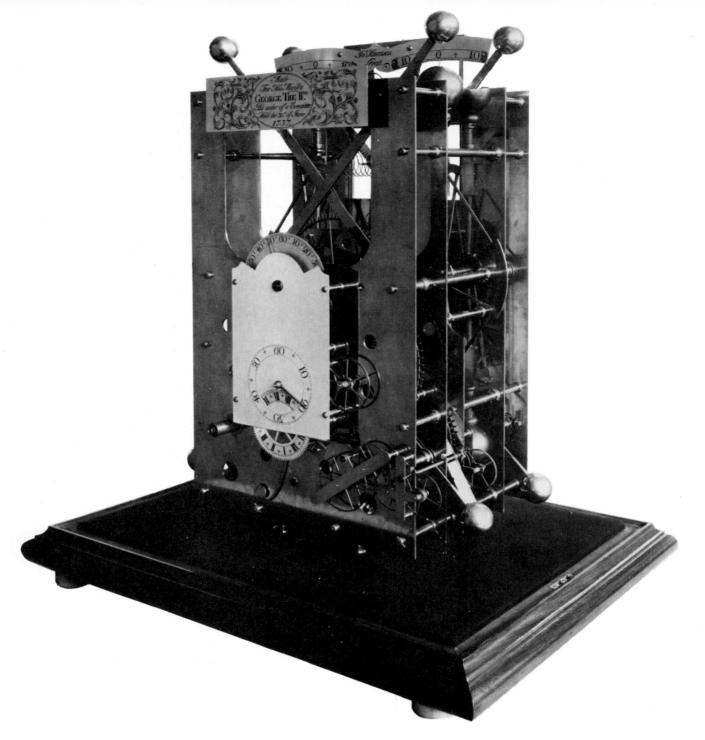

This machine constituted Harrison's second design of marine timekeeper and was finished in 1739. National Maritime Museum, Greenwich.

So, on 18th November 1761, this most famous of Harrison's timekeepers was taken on board H.M.S. *Deptford*, which set sail from Portsmouth in bad weather, with the timekeeper resting on a cushion in the captain's cabin. Ten days out, amid conflicting opinions from the ship's navigator and other officers on board, William Harrison predicted the time at which they would sight a particular island in the area of Madeira. When this turned out to be correct, the ship's company were nothing if not impressed. Upon arrival in Jamaica it was found that the watch had performed well within the most stringent limits required; and even when brought back again, in fearsome weather, to Britain, it still proved more accurate than anything else in the field.

However, the Board of Longitude, hitherto helpful and sympathetic to Harrison – he had had a number of small sums of money as grants from them to sustain his work – now seem to have turned against him. There followed years of wrangling and argument, much of it petty, with Harrison issuing pamphlets and getting up petitions in an effort to get himself a fair hearing, while the Board remained implacable in its antagonism to his demands. One of the chief protagonists was the Rev. Nevil Maskelyne, a member of the Board and eventually Astronomer Royal, who advocated an alternative method of finding the longitude based on lunar distances, and it was clear that for much of the time he carried the Board with him. It was not until 21st June 1773 that Parliament agreed to pay Harrison further money, bringing his total prize to £18,750; he had also had some £4,000 in grants over the years. He remained bitter and resentful to the end, which was not far away. He died at the age of eighty-three in 1776.

Looking back over the lifetime of this man, the major part of which he had willingly devoted to solving the longitude problem, one must marvel at his single-minded genius – especially in the light of his unpromising start in life – and clearly he must also have possessed the greatest determination, to enable him to carry on in the face of such adversity. Being deprived of the prize for so long meant that, for years, he was constantly short of money and living with his family in poverty since he could not work on his timekeepers as well as earn enough by some other means to support them. The demands made upon him by the Board of Longitude must strike anybody as going far beyond anything the Act required, let alone authorised them to do; they continuously demanded that Harrison hand over to them all his timekeepers, provide detailed drawings of them, make further copies to ensure they were capable of quantity production, and so on. Many of these demands came when Harrison was an old man – indeed, he made a fifth timekeeper, H.5, which he did not finish until he was seventy-nine – and even though he had the support of George III, who tested H.5 in his own private observatory in Richmond Park, it seemed he simply could not prevail. He may well have been a difficult and cantankerous man with whom to deal, but he deserved better treatment at the hands of his own country, whose reputation was to be enhanced by his inventions, than he ever received.

The single most powerful reason why his timekeepers were not fully appreciated in his own time – and this applies particularly to H.1, as its performance was appraised in 1736 – was the lack of understanding of corrections for rate. It was universally supposed at that time that a precision timekeeper must keep exact time day after day, whereas in practice, it is much better for a 'rate' to be laid down – that is to say, for it to be established with certainty that a timekeeper will gain or lose a certain number of seconds each day without fail – and for this correction to be applied consistently when making calculations from the timekeeper. If H.1 had been corrected by this means, its performance would have been seen to have been running within about three seconds a day, or within the lower limit for the prize money.

Harrison's five marine timekeepers were lost sight of for many years in the cellars of the Admiralty in London, but were rediscovered between the wars by Lt-Cdr R. T. Gould, who painstakingly

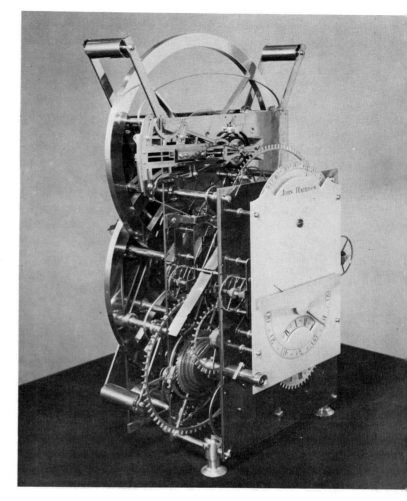

The third and last of Harrison's great machines won for him the Gold Medal of the Royal Society in 1749, but he was still not satisfied with its capabilities. National Maritime Museum, Greenwich.

restored them all to working order, an enterprise which occupied him for seventeen years. H.1, H.2, H.3 and H.4 are in the custody of the National Maritime Museum at Greenwich, where they can be seen working with all their original vigour. H.5 belongs to the Worshipful Company of Clockmakers and is on display with the rest of their collection at Guildhall, in the City of London.

While Harrison was undoubtedly the great inventive genius in the pioneering days of marine chronometry, he was surrounded – and was succeeded – by others of far more than average ability, both as designers and craftsmen. One of the more productive aspects of the Longitude Act, although it provoked a great deal of jealous animosity and petty bickering between all the leading makers of the time – for the prize was so big that few wanted to be left out of the running – was that it inspired such an atmosphere of competitiveness as to spark off every vestige of inventive ingenuity contained within the craft. The English, from very early times, were far more interested in accurate timekeeping than in any of the more flamboyant

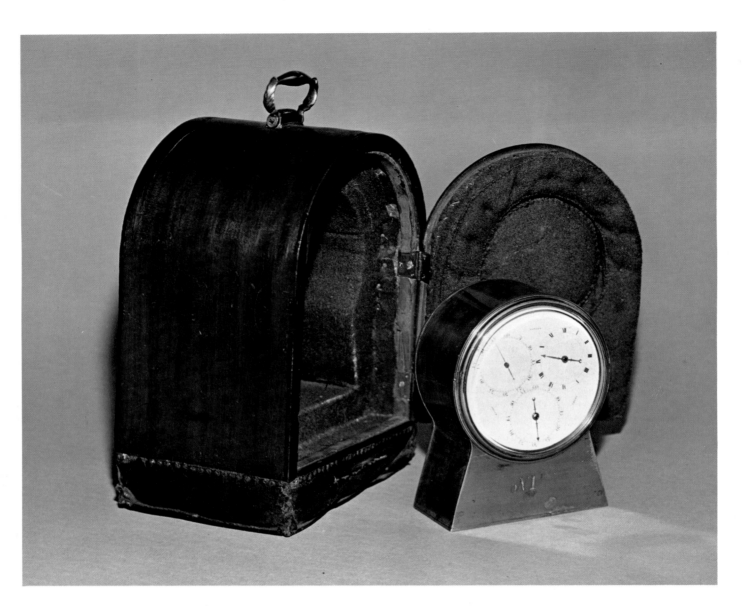

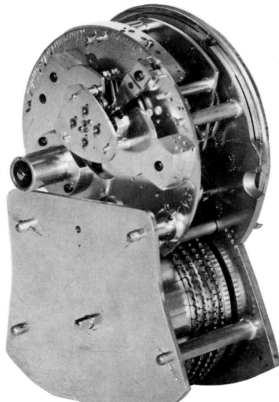

Josiah Emery, an ex-patriate Swiss working in London, made four experimental chronometers, of which this is one, which he submitted for trial at Greenwich in 1792. Museum of the Worshipful Company of Clockmakers, Guildhall, London.

left
Emery's chronometer had a constant-force escapement and such advanced features as friction rollers for the balance arbor instead of the normal pivot holes. Museum of the Worshipful Company of Clockmakers, Guildhall, London.

opposite page, above
This fine deck watch by John Arnold dates from about 1776 and has his earliest form of detent escapement, the pivoted detent. Museum of the Worshipful Company of Clockmakers, Guildhall, London.

opposite page, below
This outstanding pocket chronometer by Larcum Kendall was made in 1786. It has a pivoted detent escapement, and noticeable on the back plate is the spiral bimetallic compensation curb. Museum of the Worshipful Company of Clockmakers, Guildhall, London.

approaches to horology – which, for instance, tended to put almost equal emphasis upon decoration – so that, in this sort of climate, they positively flourished.

One of these contemporaries was Thomas Mudge, whose major contribution to horology must be the original concept of the lever escapement, even though, as we have seen, he discounted its value. Born in 1715 he lived to a ripe old age, dying in 1794. He was a member of the technical committee which examined Harrison's timekeeper H.4 on behalf of the Board of Longitude. Harrison had had to dismantle his machine in front of the committee and explain the finer points of its working, so that they could determine its 'general utility', which probably meant how easy it would be to produce it in quantity. But Mudge had his own quite different ideas about the design of a marine timekeeper. He accordingly appears to have largely abandoned what must have been a most profitable business making high-grade clocks and watches, to concentrate upon his chronometers, of which he made only three. The first was completed in 1774. His chronometers were marvels of sophisticated mechanical complexity, which was one of their greatest drawbacks, since, while Mudge himself was a craftsman of supreme ability, head and shoulders above even the best of his contemporaries, any practical chronometer design had to be capable of replication by men of more modest talents. His three chronometers – two of them Mudge called 'Green' and 'Blue' after the colours of their cases – performed well while Mudge himself was available to supervise them, although even so they did not surpass Harrison's timekeeper. As Mudge himself became too old to continue the practical side of the work, his son organised a consortium of the best available craftsmen to copy his father's design of timekeeper, and between twenty and thirty of these marvellous machines seem to have been made. Mudge senior just lived long enough to see the first of them completed and running; his part in the project had been intended to be that of technical adviser, instructing the craftsmen involved on his own methods for making chronometers. As it was, none of the copies ever even approximated in performance to the originals, and the scheme eventually failed. The Mudges were not wholly ignored by an ungrateful nation for their contributions to finding the longitude: they received £2,500 from Parliament, although little enough encouragement from the Board of Longitude itself.

One other craftsman might be mentioned, from these same very formative years, if only to underline how great a fount of talent was available in England then. Larcum Kendall, another member of the technical committee that examined H.4, was subsequently paid £450 by the Board of Longitude to make a copy of it. The workmanship of this copy

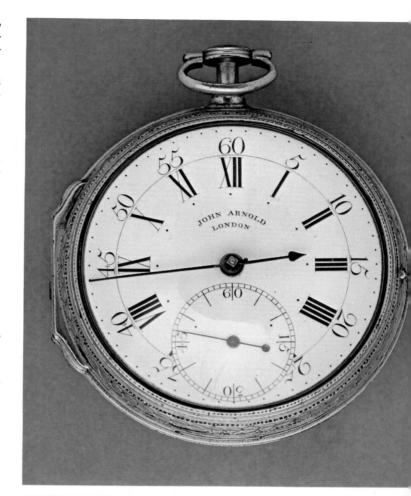

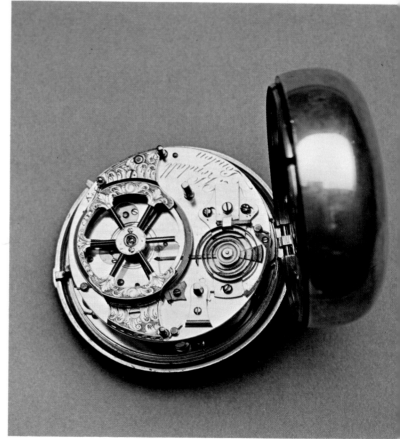

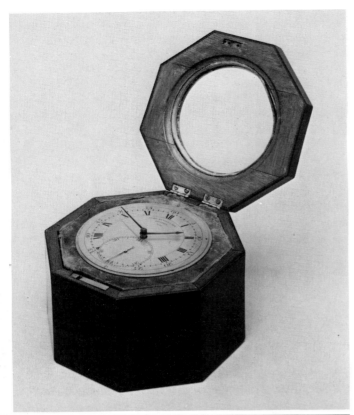

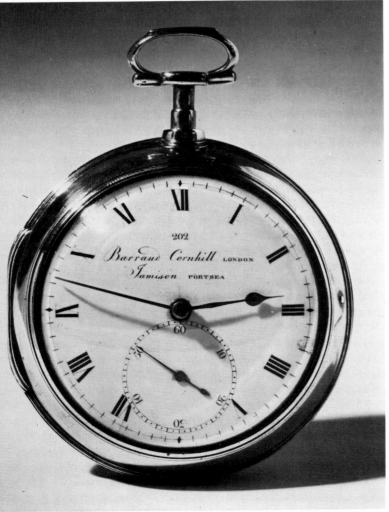

was superior to that of the original – even Harrison, who did not customarily bestow compliments, acknowledged this – and the instrument performed superbly over a three-year voyage in the hands of Captain Cook.

Both Harrison and Mudge, in their different ways, had clearly demonstrated that the longitude problem was capable of solution, and the final conversion of their pioneering efforts into a form that was eminently practical, in that it could be produced in fair quantity and at a fair price, yet met all the technical requirements, was carried out at the inventive hands of two great English chronometermakers. Their work overlaps to some extent; and by this time a number of important and highly skilled makers in London were hard on their heels, so that, where they led, others were quick to follow.

John Arnold was born in 1736 and made his first chronometer in 1770. However, it was not until some years later that his experimentation enabled him to turn out a design for a chronometer that was wholly successful. His special contributions in this area include his design of spring detent escapement – that particular feature which, it will be remembered, distinguishes a chronometer from any other variety of timekeeper – as well as a succession of designs for bi-metallic compensated balances. He was also the first to fit his instruments with helical balance springs, which were often made of gold. His great inventiveness came to a head in the early 1780s with several important patents; and the quality of his work may be gauged by the performance of one of his pocket chronometers, worn over a period of thirteen months at around this time. Its total error was only 2 minutes 33 seconds, and its daily rate never varied more than 2 seconds.

Arnold died in 1799, but his work was ably carried on by his son John Roger Arnold. The Arnold chronometer factory at Chigwell, in Essex, turned out a steady stream of high quality timepieces. For ten years from 1830, Arnold junior had as his partner Edward Dent, a most able craftsman; and when he eventually died, in 1843, the firm was bought up by Charles Frodsham, so that the continuity of its reputation for high-grade work was assured. In its own day – and despite the acrimonious, even malicious, criticisms of Earnshaw – there is no doubt that the Arnold establishment, whether under the supervision of father or son, was generally considered to be the chronometermakers of choice.

The second of the two great English chronometermakers of this period, as has just been hinted, was Thomas Earnshaw. He was a very different person indeed from John Arnold: jealous, very deprived as a young man and often forced, because of his comparative poverty, to work for other people, whom he always suspected were out

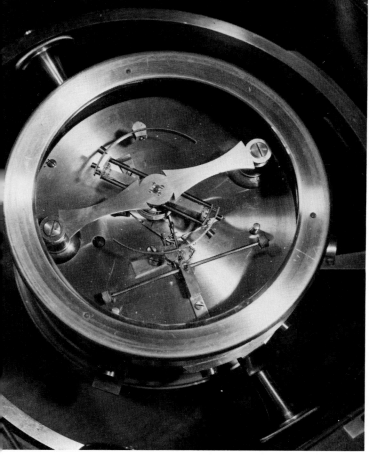

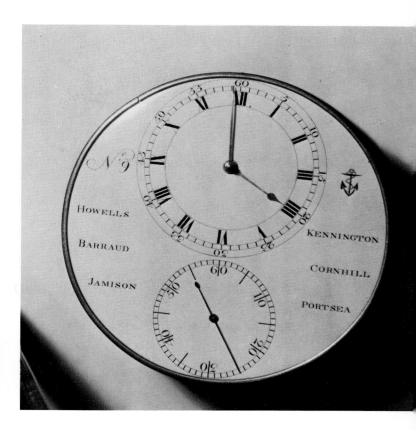

to steal his inventions. He was born in 1749, and
his influence stretches well into the nineteenth century, as he did not die until 1829. He, like his
competitor Arnold – and there was always much
rivalry between them – invented a form of spring
detent escapement but, being unable to afford to
patent it, arranged with a craftsman in rather
better circumstances than himself, one Thomas
Wright of the Poultry, in the City of London, to do
it for him. However, Wright left it rather late, by
which time Arnold had already produced his
arrangement, which was very similar indeed to
Earnshaw's. Much acrimony followed. Earnshaw
accused another maker called John Brockbank, for
whom he had once worked and to whom he had
shown his invention, of having betrayed him to
Arnold. It is clear that the two inventions must
have been arrived at almost simultaneously, but
whether this was coincidental or there was some
element of treachery or collusion will probably
never be known.

The technical differences between Arnold's and
Earnshaw's escapements are perhaps best
summed up by saying that Arnold's has the
theoretical edge, but Earnshaw's works out best in
practice. Both makers solved the problem of quantity production, at a reasonable price, of a technically more than adequate marine timekeeper; and
where Arnold contributed in the design of balances
and balance springs, Earnshaw solved the difficult
technical problem of making bi-metallic elements
by fusion – previously the brass and steel strips
were just riveted together. Thus honours must be
about equal.

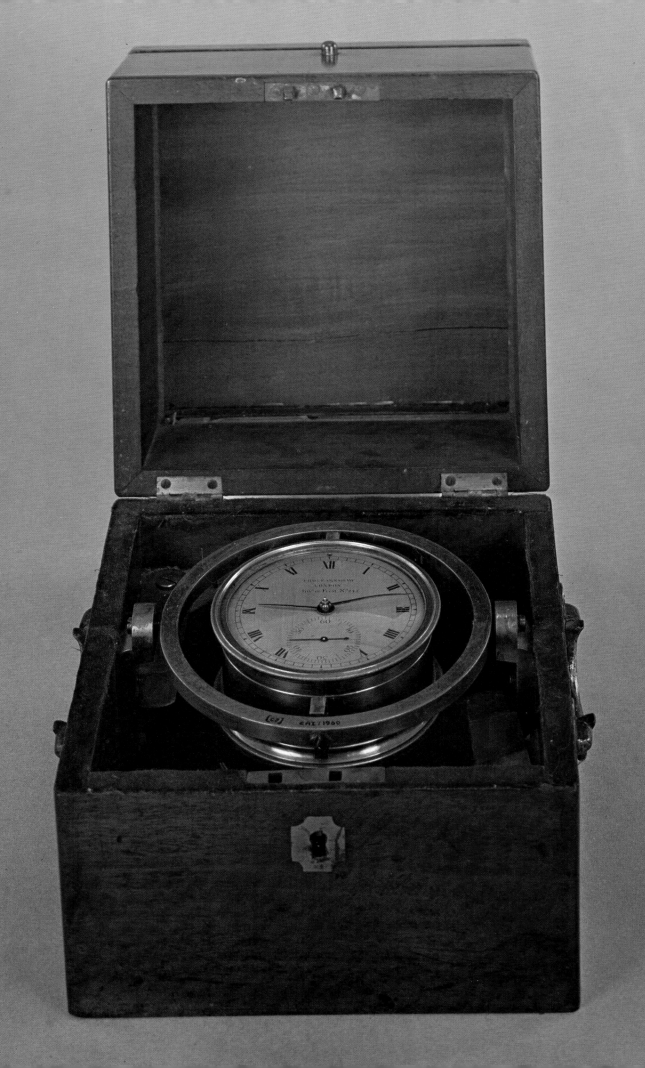

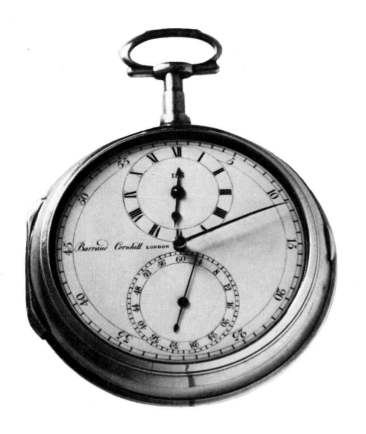

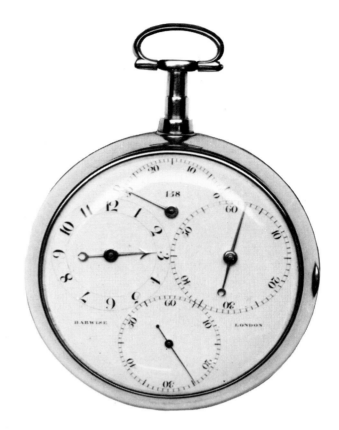

above
Chronometermakers at the end of the eighteenth century seem to have made a practice of modernising their past manufactures if and when the opportunity arose. Among other things, Barraud always took any chance to remove his former partner Jamison's name from both dial and movement. This example was made by them in 1797 and is interesting because its regulator dial numbers seconds in fours instead of the conventional fives.

above right
The dial of this pocket chronometer by John Barwise, made in 1800, shows a different version of the regulator dial incorporating three subsidiaries for hours, minutes and seconds respectively. The sector at the top is an up-and-down indicator. Museum of the Worshipful Company of Clockmakers, Guildhall, London.

left
This early example of a marine chronometer by Thomas Earnshaw dates from about 1795. It is numbered 245 although Earnshaw's numbering has not so far been properly rationalised. British Museum, London.

England was not, of course, the only country to try to solve the longitude problem. France, in particular, had its pioneers, notably Pierre Le Roy. Son of a famous horologist father, and born in 1717, he started to experiment with timekeeping at sea in the 1740s; by 1766 he was demonstrating to Louis XV his fully developed timekeeper. It was a superb machine with a number of original features: temperature compensation, for instance, was achieved by using on the balance a thermome-ter filled partly with mercury and partly with alcohol. As the surrounding temperature dropped, the mercury moved towards the rim of the balance, slowing it down, and vice versa. Le Roy's timekeeper, in sea trials, just about equalled H.4 in performance.

Le Roy died in 1785, but another French pioneer, Ferdinand Berthoud, survived him by twenty years. Berthoud arrived at the design of a spring detent escapement at much the same time as Arnold and Earnshaw in England, but his principal claim to fame rests upon his experimental machines. He hardly ever seems to have made two alike; and his accompanying technical writing is of value.

In England, by the death of Earnshaw, chronometers had become commonplace; and, what is more, they eventually settled into a pattern, which has remained largely unaltered to the present day, based upon his design. Arnold and Earnshaw had among their contemporaries craftsmen of high calibre: men like Barraud and Brockbank, Jamison, Margetts, Pennington, and, of course, Emery, together with a few others. These were succeeded in the nineteenth century by even more skilled people, for the Victorian era was nothing if not the peak period for mechanical excellence. It is sad indeed that very little of this special expertise still exists today, where radio time signals and beacons as well as electronic gadgetry has largely superseded the handmade precision timekeeper that first solved the longitude problem.

The Industrial Revolution – The Nineteenth Century and Beyond

As a social and technological phenomenon, the Industrial Revolution had no very clear beginning or ending. Some people regard it wholly as a spin-off from the development of steam power, in which case it is entirely technological; others see it solely in terms of the progression from an agricultural base to an industrial one, and the enormous re-education programme that that must have involved. However it is seen, in human terms it represents one of the greatest upheavals mankind has experienced – on the small scale if one considers only Britain, but gradually spreading to affect much of the world.

Most will agree, however, that this evolutionary process – or whatever one may choose to call it – started in the eighteenth century and extended well towards the middle of the nineteenth. Some even argue that it is still going on. It wrought change throughout the whole of society, for nobody was entirely immune or insulated from its effects.

In the horological field, as the eighteenth century drew to a close, there had not yet arisen the nationwide demand for cheap timekeepers that

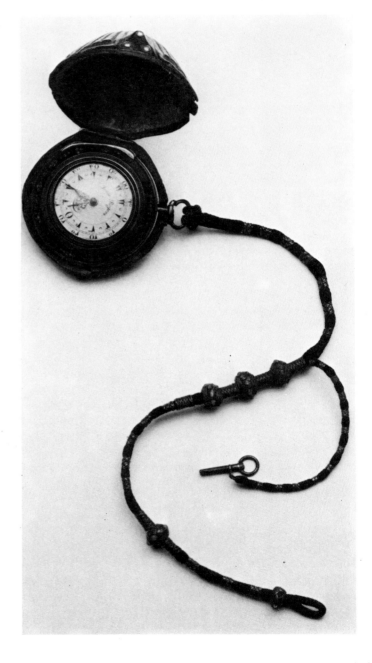

right
Turkey was one of the principal export markets for English watches at the turn of the eighteenth and nineteenth centuries. The example shown is by Isaac Rogers and has no fewer than four cases. The two innermost are of plain silver, hallmarked 1780. Next comes a case covered in tortoiseshell, and finally a protective wooden outer case shaped like a cone. The watch is complete with its original carrying cord, ornamented with silver wire.

opposite page
A good example of the clocks that were made in small batches for such markets as China and India, this musical table clock was made for Barraud of London, whose name it bears, by the firm of Thwaites & Reed about 1767. There are Chinese characters on the back plate and those presumably of a repairer under the dial. Museum of the Worshipful Company of Clockmakers, Guildhall, London.

184

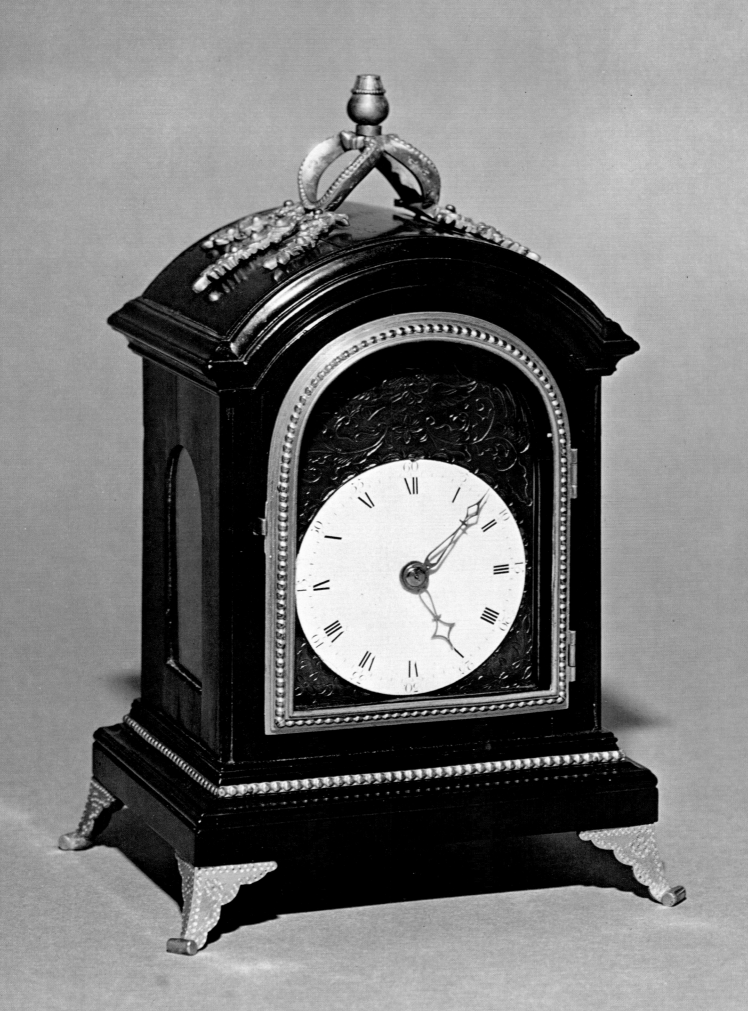

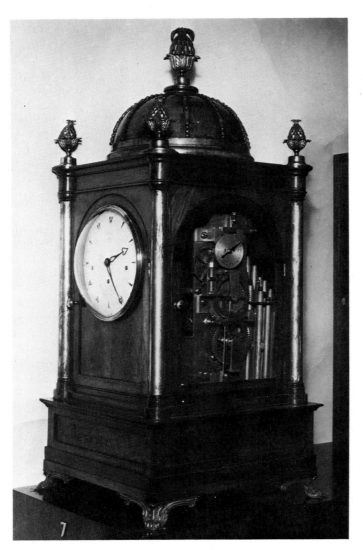

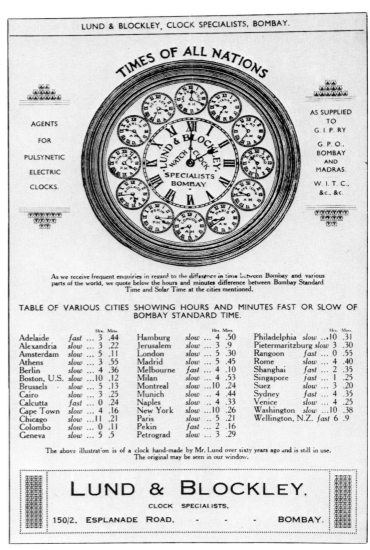

was rapidly to follow in the wake of the railways. The clockmakers, however, were quite content – those that were not engaged in the chronometry competition, that is – to cater for the needs, such as they were, that existed nationally while busily developing their extensive and highly lucrative export market.

It is difficult to say how and when Britain's huge turnover in hand-finished clocks and watches for foreign markets started. It undoubtedly sprang from the enormous reputation for workmanship of the highest quality that followed the technological gains achieved in the seventeenth and early eighteenth centuries. By 1800 the principal markets seem to have been the continent of Europe – where, for decades, English and especially London-made products had been the subject of massive local forgery, so revered were the genuine articles – the Near East, especially Turkey, and, in the Far East, India and China. In those days the exporting craftsman went to enormous lengths to ascertain exactly what his customers required, and then to meet it in every minute detail, a factor allegedly ignored by many modern British exporters. The result has been an extensive heritage of English-

made export watches and clocks which embrace features imposed upon them by their foreign buyers.

It is often said that the products the English exported were only those that were not good enough for the home market. It seems more likely that, being realists, they adjusted the quality of such goods according to the price they could obtain and the variety demanded; for it is certainly not true to say that no pieces of the best kind were exported – far from it. Looking first at the Far Eastern markets, the Chinese seem to have had an insatiable appetite for clocks of the most elaborately decorated kind, which had also to possess novelty or entertainment value. Thus, automata – often not in any human image, but using revolving jewelled spirals, glass water-simulating spouts and falls, rotating finials and cupolas that are made in segments and splay out as they fly round – were all-important, as was the provision of music to accompany them. The casework also had to be embellished in what, to the English taste at that time, must have seemed a most vulgar manner; it is quite customary to find the nominal maker of such clocks has built into his structure imported Swiss

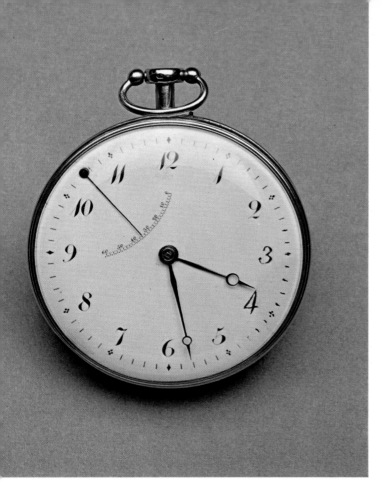

This is probably the oldest surviving *perpetuelle* or self-winding watch since it came from the workshop of A.-L. Breguet, the supreme craftsman, in 1783. On the back of the gold case is the initial 'N' surmounted by a crown, and although its earliest history is by no means certain, it is said to have belonged originally to Czar Nicholas I of Russia. Museum of the Worshipful Company of Clockmakers, Guildhall, London.

right
The back of the movement of the Breguet *perpetuelle* reveals noticeably the heartshaped counterpoised weight which operates the self-winding mechanism and also the tuned steel gongs on which the quarter-repeating action sounds. Museum of the Worshipful Company of Clockmakers, Guildhall, London.

opposite page, left
Inscribed 'Vulliamy London Clock and Watchmaker to the King of the British Empire', this large mahogany organ clock was made about 1820, and from the Turkish numerals on the dial its intended market is self-evident. Vulliamy was, of course, watchmaker to George III. British Museum, London.

opposite page, right
An ephemeral fragment from the early twentieth century, this leaflet advertises the Bombay office of a well-known firm of London clockmakers, Messrs Lund & Blockley.

enamels, usually from Geneva, as well as sundry other components not generally used in products for the home market. At the end of the eighteenth century, these highly decorated – or perhaps grossly over-decorated – but beautifully constructed pieces, whose functional qualities left nothing to be desired, were not only purchased direct by the Chinese; it was taken for granted that any British ambassador to the Chinese court who wished to make his mark with the Emperor would present such a clock as a gift. The Honourable East India Company did likewise in order, no doubt, to sweeten relations. Yet is is clear that the Chinese valued such devices wholly as sophisticated toys of the time, not as timekeepers; and indeed, many far more ordinary kinds of timepiece were delivered to the Chinese market for much of the eighteenth century, from both Britain and other European countries. There is a detailed account of the intricacies of the Chinese market for timekeepers in Professor Cipolla's *Clocks and Culture: 1300–1700*.

India was, of course, particularly susceptible to the absorption of large quantities of English-made timekeepers as simply another manifestation of its Empire status. The East India Company handled clocks and watches until it was finally wound up just after the mid nineteenth century. By that time, most English manufacturers of any repute had either opened their own offices in the subcontinent or had appointed local agents. Even though clock- and watchmaking in England was still a craft-based manufacture – as will be seen, it did not finally abandon this method in favour of mass-production until the twentieth century – there were firms operating in the Clerkenwell area of London who made clock movements in quantity for the trade, probably from late in the eighteenth.

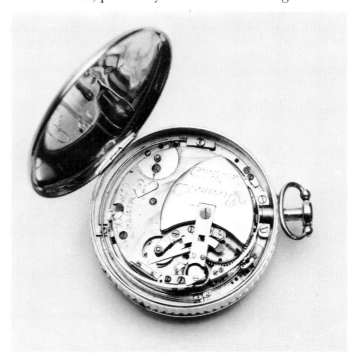

right
Dating from about 1800, this typical Breguet *souscription* movement is a few years earlier than the other (opposite). Museum of the Worshipful Company of Clockmakers, Guildhall, London.

opposite page, left
Another early example of Breguet's work, this watch was once thought to be a forgery, but it is now recognised as a genuine Breguet watch dating from about 1784. Museum of the Worshipful Company of Clockmakers, Guildhall, London.

opposite page, right
Although typical in other respects, this Breguet *souscription* watch of about 1805, has more than the ordinary number of divisions between the hours and there is no secret signature on the dial. Museum of the Worshipful Company of Clockmakers, Guildhall, London.

From the fragmentary records of such firms that have survived, it is not uncommon to find orders received for dozens or half-dozens of movements 'to suit the India market' or 'according to the Chinese taste'.

Coming nearer home, it is curious to note that, whether or not the Islamic peoples were instrumental in transmitting any original knowledge of clockwork to Western cultures, by the eighteenth century English craftsmen were supplying a large number of fine timepieces to the Near East, and particularly to Turkey. It is not at all uncommon, therefore, to find good London-made clocks and watches with dials inscribed with numerals in Turkish characters, and sometimes the maker even went to the trouble of having his signature translated into the vernacular as well. Watches made for the Turkish market left this country with at least three cases, instead of the customary pair, and were often fitted with yet a fourth on arrival at their final destination. This extraordinary protection may have been simply to exclude dust and dirt in a country where such inconveniences were part of the way of life to a larger extent than in Europe. The generality of Turkish watches are cased in silver, the two inner ones being plain, the third usually covered with tortoiseshell having a row of decorative pins bordering the edge. When, outside all this, the Turks added another case, it was completely in their own tradition, so that it is as unlike the rest of the watch as can be imagined.

Finally, a word about British exports to Europe. The popularity of English clocks and watches stemmed from their reliability, which in turn derived from the traditional English interest in performance rather than appearance; so they were extensively copied, but they were also bought in quantity and much sought after. One of the most thriving European markets was Holland; timepieces intended for that country will always be found to have the arcaded minute band which was so much favoured there. The forgeries of English work, incidentally – and they are likely to be encountered from time to time – are almost invariably very easy to detect. It never seemed to occur to those that produced them that they might study what they were attempting to emulate in order at least to attempt a facsimile. Mis-spellings of makers' names, styles wholly out of keeping with English practice, forged hallmarks on cases that will withstand only a cursory glance before they are detected – such is the common trend among these articles. For the very reason that they are usually so unlike what they purport to be, although

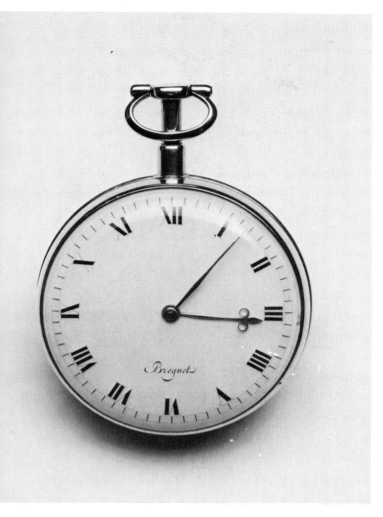

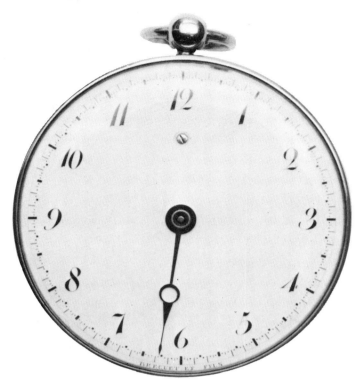

often of good quality in their own right, they make an interesting subject for specialised study.

This was the commercial export situation in the English clock and watch industry, then, as the nineteenth century commenced. It was not to remain for very much longer in such an obviously healthy state.

Technologically, as has been seen, the development of precise time-measurement as a navigational aid spanned the second half of the eighteenth century and much of the first half of the nineteenth, and in the midst of this period there flourished a remarkable French craftsman-designer, whom many consider to have been the greatest genius in this field ever to have lived. Abraham-Louis Breguet was born at Neuchâtel in Switzerland in 1747 and died in 1823, and during his working life produced some of the most elegant, as well as the most superbly designed and constructed, timepieces the world has ever known. He made a substantial contribution, by way of original invention, to the progress of accurate time-measurement, but more particularly, perhaps, he seemed to have at his disposal a never-ending supply of creative designs for his work, so that virtually every object that left his atelier was unique. This is not strictly true, of course: his 'Souscription'

watches, for which clients subscribed in advance just as one might do for a luxury edition of some special book, were made in series. But otherwise his capacity to please his richer patrons with special productions seems to have been inexhaustible. Today, as might be expected, his watches and clocks are highly sought after by collectors, and fetch very large sums of money. The majority of them doubtless perform every bit as well as when they were first made and, as his epitaph, can thus stand comparison with that accorded to any other great man.

The nineteenth century saw the emergence and development of mass-production methods for the manufacture of clocks and watches, which in turn generated the greatest tensions in the trade in Britain that had ever been known. Rightly or wrongly, the craftsmen who had been nurtured all their lives in a tradition of quality and pride in workmanship, coupled with a small batch-production system and hand-finishing, could not bring themselves to change the habits of a lifetime which, in the process, would inevitably have meant surrendering something of the individuality which they could impart to their product. The trade maintained outwardly that mass-produced timepieces could never compete with the quality article either in

189

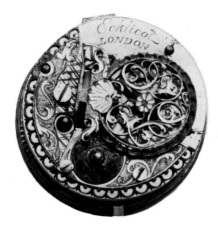

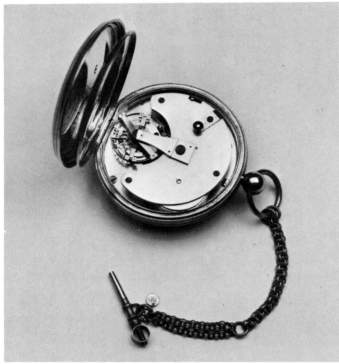

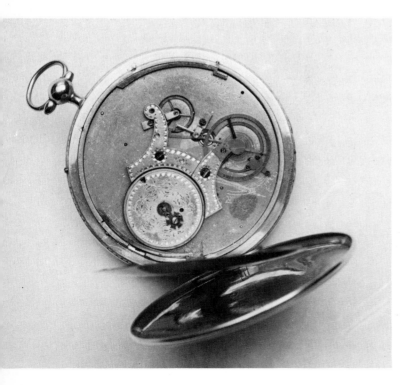

performance, reliability, finish or in any other important characteristic and steadfastly refused to move from that entrenched position. In so doing, they were deliberately swimming against the stream that was being followed by most of the other manufacturing nations, or the ones, at any rate, who were significant in the world horological scene. Principal among these were to be the Americans, the French, the Germans, especially the Black Forest cottage industry, and eventually the Swiss. The result of this inflexibility was that, by 1842, England had become the world's largest market for cheap imported clocks, and eight years later the annual figure for such imports had reached a record peak of 228,000. The home trade, needless to say, was in complete chaos, and unemployment rife.

So it is a sad fact that the typical household clock in Britain in the last century was foreign. From the 1840s onwards, cheap American-manufactured brass clocks, derived from a design that had originated in Germany, were selling at ridiculously low prices, while the Black Forest product – of rudimentary construction, with wood used for as many components as possible in place of the much more expensive brass – also rapidly gained acceptance. The most popular version of this last type, known as the postman's alarm, had a mainly wooden movement behind a circular painted dial, which was encircled by a hinged and polished hardwood bezel holding the protective convex glass. Centrally positioned on this dial was a small

top
The work of London watchmakers was extensively forged on the continent throughout the eighteenth century, but it is not difficult to detect. Purporting to be a watch by John Ellicott, this movement is signed 'Ecklicot, London' and is of late eighteenth-century vintage. Museum of the Worshipful Company of Clockmakers, Guildhall, London.

centre
This Breguet watch incorporates his device, the tourbillon, which is intended to counteract position errors. The escapement is a lever, and the tourbillon rotates in one minute. Museum of the Worshipful Company of Clockmakers, Guildhall, London.

left
Probably Swiss and of the early nineteenth century, this watch is falsely signed 'Breguet', but it is a fine watch in its own right, incorporating a pin-wheel lever escapement. Museum of the Worshipful Company of Clockmakers, Guildhall, London.

right
Very much more elegant than the average English skeleton clock, this mid nineteenth-century specimen is unsigned, of eight-day duration and notable for the two large spring barrels on the same arbor which drive the two-train movement. Museum of the Worshipful Company of Clockmakers, Guildhall, London.

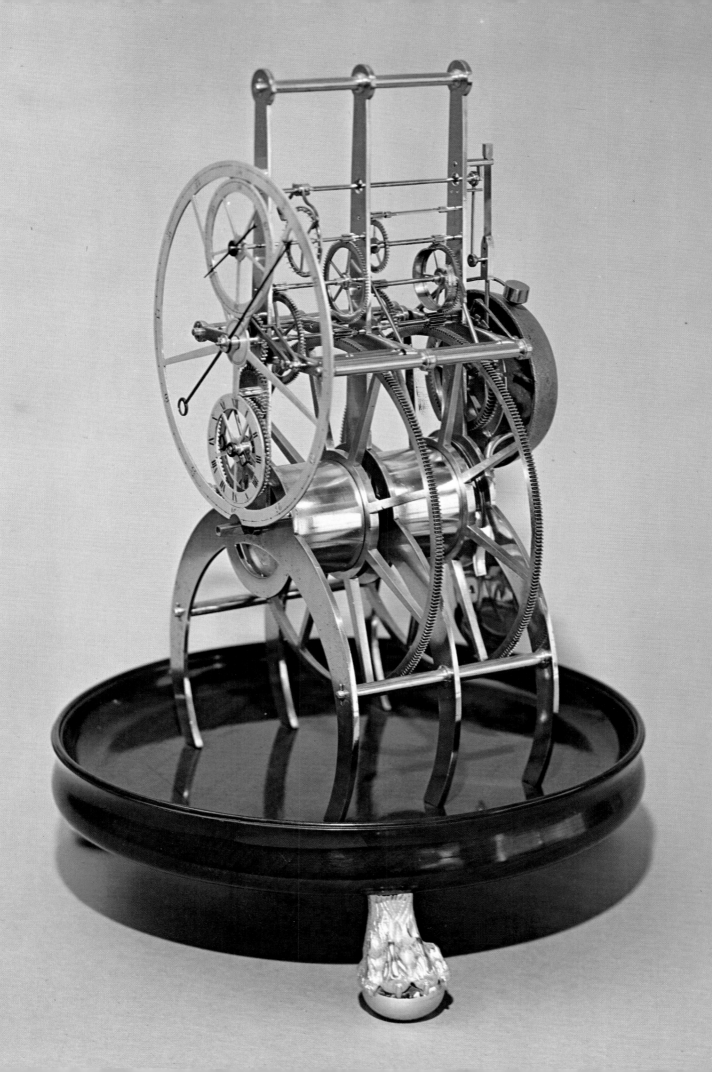

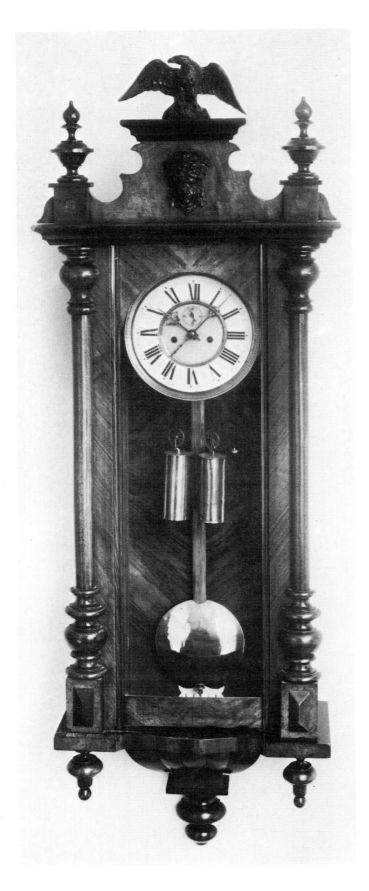

Dating from about 1890, this Vienna regulator clock has the name of the maker, 'Lenzkirch', stamped across the back of the wings of the eagle which surmounts it.

alarm dial, and the whole mechanism was weight-driven, elementary and trouble-free. Other versions of the Black Forest clocks included the ubiquitous cuckoo clock, often – incorrectly – attributed to the Swiss.

Another foreign import was the French clock. Their standard factory-made product, a clock mechanism contained within small circular plates, had been so perfected that, even with such seemingly outdated features as locking-plate striking, it must have been the most accurate mass-produced clock made anywhere in the world. The other popular clock for which the French must take credit – even though it, too, was made elsewhere – the carriage clock, or *pendule de voyage*, became very popular in a range of qualities from the cheapest to the best, and was often sold through agents whose very English names contrast quaintly with a place of origin such as 'Paris'. The very few – mainly London – craftsmen who made a wholly English carriage clock, reserved the style for their best quality and most sophisticated mechanisms, so that such a clock emanating from the firm of, say, McCabe, Frodsham, Dent or Vulliamy will be a timekeeper of excellence. Towards the end of the century, Victor Kullberg (1824–1890), a Swedish craftsman who settled in London, produced some eight-day chronometer carriage clocks of unrivalled elegance and performance.

Finally, by the last quarter of the century, there had come into circulation a clock known always as a 'Vienna regulator', although at various times it was copied outside Austria by, among others, the Germans and Americans. These clocks contained certain anachronisms: for example, because of the shortened pendulums in some models, their seconds hands rotate once in forty-five instead of sixty seconds, and are therefore solely for decoration. Yet, despite such idiosyncrasies, there is usually built-in maintaining power, to keep the clock going while the weights are being wound up, and both pendulum crutch and escapement pallets can generally be adjusted. Vienna regulators are capable of a most impressive performance, given good conditions, and the best of them embrace far higher standards of quality than their detractors will ever give them credit for. Indeed, one well-known firm in this field, Lenzkirch, are said to have finally closed down when they felt that, for various reasons, they could not maintain the superior performance of which their clocks had been capable. Nevertheless, the term 'regulator' applied to such clocks was, strictly speaking, a misnomer.

So, apart from the specially produced London-made carriage clocks just mentioned, what was the native English clock style during the nineteenth century? Indeed, was there one at all?

For a start, the traditional longcase clock of London quality seems to have met a sudden end in popularity and virtually to have become extinct about 1820, although there are provincial examples from later than this. It was not resurrected again until about 1900. The craft did, however, continue to turn out sufficient hand-finished movements to keep things ticking over. It was correctly thought that there would always be a demand for such work, from the wealthier members of the community and from institutions of various sorts, and many such movements went into three-quarter-length clocks which hung from, or rested upon, a bracket fixed to the wall. These often looked like a longcase clock without its base, and the cases tended to be ornately carved and pretentious, claiming to follow such revived styles as Egyptian, Gothic, Jacobean, Louis Quatorze or Quinze, and others. It can honestly be said of such clocks that they were made superbly well: like so much other nineteenth-century craftsmanship, an enormous fount of skill and knowledge was applied to products that, artistically, were unworthy of it. Thus many, if not most, survive to the present time and function supremely well: it is virtually impossible to wear them out.

The same strictures apply equally to the mantel, bracket or table equivalents of the three-quarter wall clock; they were usually designed in 'improved' versions of earlier styles, with more elaborate decoration incorporating caryatid figures, frets, mounts and finials of every sort and

The most commonly encountered Black Forest clock in England is the so-called postman's alarm of which this is a typical example. It was imported into Britain by the firm of Camerer Cuss & Co. who are still in existence.

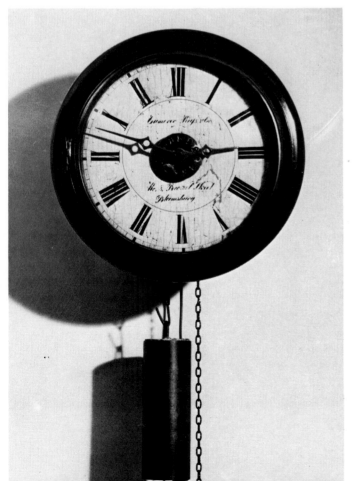

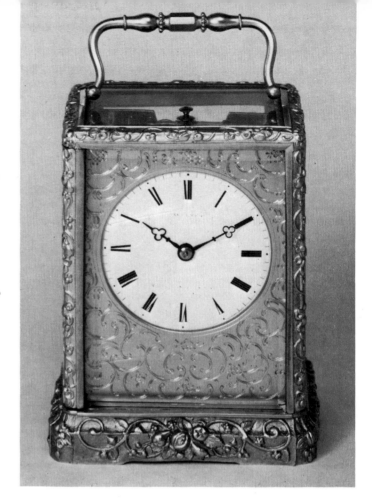

An attractive carriage clock made about 1840 and signed 'J. B. Beguin à Paris 5', it strikes the hours and half-hours and also repeats on a bell. The club-tooth lever escapement has jewelled pallets. Museum of the Worshipful Company of Clockmakers, Guildhall, London.

kind, the whole on a robust and indestructible scale. The largest of these were an inescapable feature of the library, hall or dining-room of any large house, or the directors' quarters of an institution; the more imposing the environment, the larger and more ornate the clock. Alongside such ostentatious English styles, there was also a resurgence of interest in materials like buhl and papier-mâché, and these found favour in revived versions of usually French designs from the previous century.

If there was a typically nineteenth-century native clock design then it was that known as the English dial clock. This is the spring-driven clock, so familiar on railway stations and other public places, but also seen in smaller versions in kitchens and offices but not generally in living-rooms, of which the outstanding feature is simply a painted iron dial, normally not bigger than fourteen inches in diameter, protected by a convex glass set into a hinged brass bezel and all within a turned mahogany surround. These clocks had substantial movements with heavy pendulums, and perform universally well. Sometimes they are fitted with longer pendulums, necessitating an extended

193

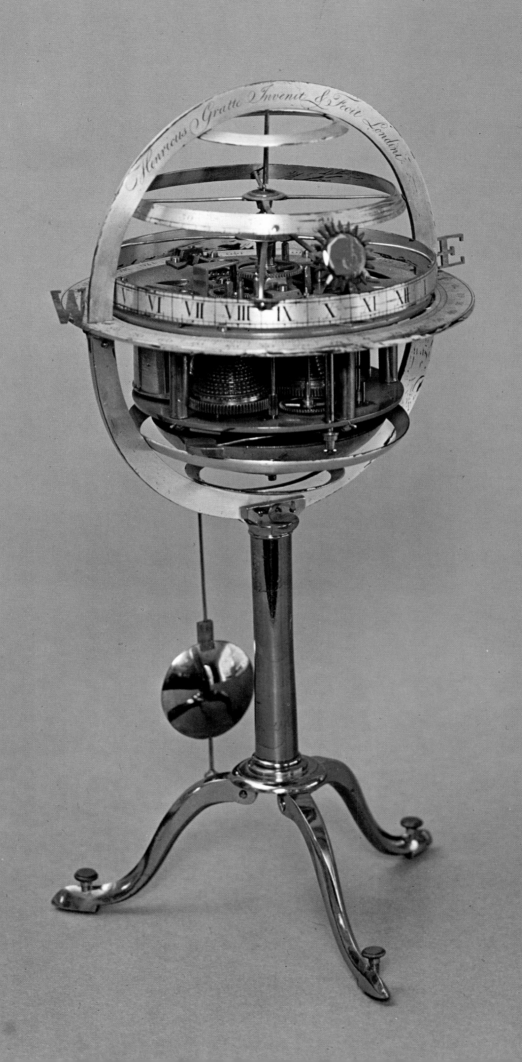

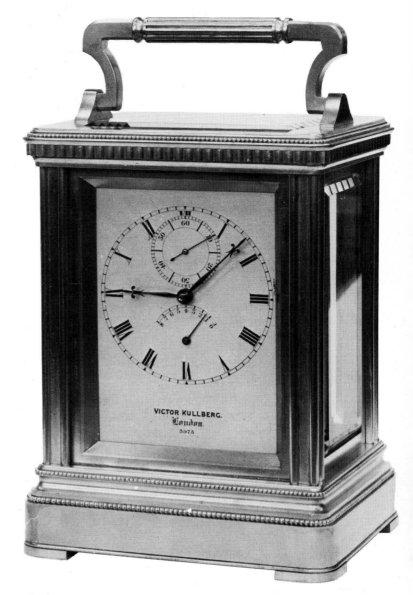

trunk below the otherwise round profile of the clock, and this variety is known as a 'drop dial'. The English dial has quite a long history, certainly back into the eighteenth century when the dials were silvered on brass, rather than painted iron, and the escapement was a verge, often planted with the rest of the movement between triangular-shaped plates.

Another variety of nineteenth-century English clock is that form known as a skeleton clock, so called because the whole movement is positioned between skeletonised plates and everything is clearly visible through its protecting glass dome. The early history of this form is not clear: it may have derived simply from 'skeletonising' some other kind of clock in order, for the sake of novelty, to display the movement. But it is certain that skeleton clocks are not the masterpieces of apprentices to the craft, as was once thought. The lace-like plates are sometimes just patterns in symmetry, but often deliberately made to represent a building, usually a cathedral. There is a French style called a skeleton clock, much less solid and plebian and obviously a different design altogether, so that the English version, in fashion from about 1860, can be considered a distinctive type.

Although the domestic longcase clock went into eclipse at this time, the scientific equivalent, the regulator clock, continued to be produced by the best firms, in small quantities but to the highest standards. Such clocks went either to observatories and similar scientific institutions, or were installed by clock- and watchmakers to regulate their stock as well as, perhaps, to time those clocks and watches temporarily in their care while undergoing overhaul. The cases of regulator clocks have always been strictly utilitarian and devoid of any kind of decoration whatsoever; so, even if they had been widely available, they would not have appealed to the average Victorian household.

Mention of that remarkable Queen brings to mind that the most famous tower clock in the world, Big Ben, which looks down upon the Houses of Parliament at Westminster, was constructed and erected during her reign. The designer of the clock, Edmund Beckett Denison, was born in 1816, succeeded to his father's baronetcy as Sir Edmund Beckett in 1874, was given a peerage under the title of Baron Grimthorpe in 1886, and died in 1905. His was perhaps one of the last minds that could range, with equal success, over several completely unrelated fields and reach the top in every one; nowadays, progress has made it difficult enough for any man to aspire to succeed in one field, let alone several. Beckett was a very successful lawyer – a Queen's Counsel, no less – as well as an architect of no mean pretensions, an astronomer and a horologist of great ability and inventive capacity. The Westminster clock was built by Frederick Dent to Beckett's designs in 1854, bench-tested for five years, and finally installed at the top of its tower in 1859; and there is much excellent literature available about it, including Beckett's own work on the subject, in which is included his detailed description of the double three-legged gravity escapement he developed especially for the clock. The title 'Big Ben', although it is generally applied nowadays to

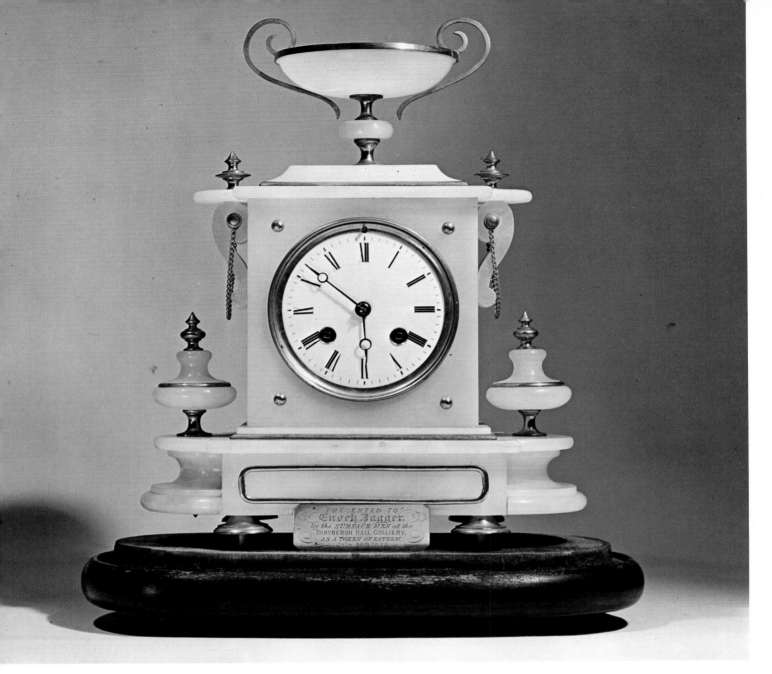

the clock as such, is strictly the name of the great
hour-bell, weighing nearly thirteen and a half tons,
and so called after Sir Benjamin Hall, the Com-
missioner of Works who placed the order for its
casting.

Big Ben has been subjected to most of the minor
irritants that plague large public clocks from time
to time – invasions of birds and accumulations of
snow, among others. Over the 117 years that it has
occupied the tower at Westminster, there have
been about thirty stoppages from such causes,
none of long duration. However, in the early hours
of 5th August 1976 Big Ben suffered a major
breakdown, far and away its most serious to date.
The rates of chiming and striking of the great clock
are controlled by giant fly-governors, whose vanes
rotate against the resistance of the air. On this
occasion the fly-shaft on the quarter-chiming train
fractured. Effectively this released the train to run
out of control under the power provided by a

This French clock in its alabaster and gilt case was presented
to the author's grandfather in 1875 by the surface men of the
colliery of which he was manager. It is typical of the
factory-made but good quality clock of the period.

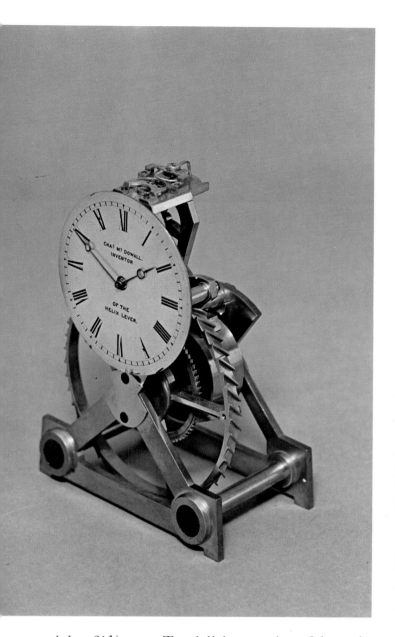

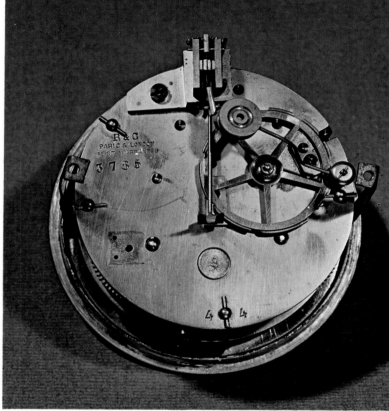

Charles MacDowall, who was born in Wakefield and died aged 82 in London in 1872, was a clever horologist with a taste for the novel approach. He made skeleton clocks with oblique-toothed gearing and invented the 'helix lever'. Museum of the Worshipful Company of Clockmakers, Guildhall, London.

weight of 1¼ tons. Total disintegration of the train followed, as the weight plunged to the bottom of the tower, and the remainder of the clock did not escape unharmed. The main frame was fractured in several places and had to be bolted together with steel plates and supported by lifting jacks. The damage to the clock room itself caused by large fragments of flying metal resembled the effects of a bomb explosion – indeed, this was the first thought of those who entered therein immediately after the accident. It has been possible, thanks to the great skill and ingenuity of those responsible for the clock, to restart Big Ben and to restore the hour-striking action, which was also damaged quite severely, but it is likely to be many months before its famous quarter chimes will be heard again. If, as seems likely, the causative factor was metal fatigue, then conceivably the whole future of the original mechanism may be at a stake. Certainly radiographic and magnetic flaw investigations

The movement of the French presentation clock represents the stage of development reached by the factory-made round French clock movement towards the end of the nineteenth century. Notable features are locking plate striking, long considered obsolete in other countries, and the particular type of pendulum adjustment attributed to Brocot.

197

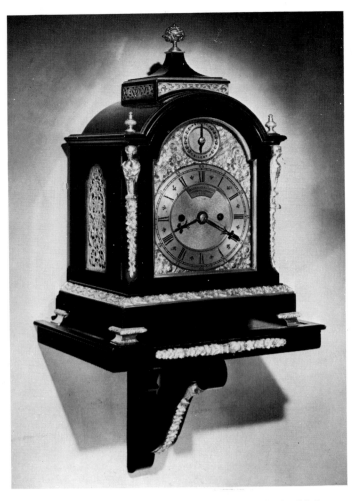

Large and elaborate bracket clocks of this kind which was made by Barraud & Lund about 1885, were considered essential in boardrooms, libraries and similar institutions.

tics possessed by tower clocks from earlier periods, nevertheless they are exceptionally reliable timekeepers and possess much of merit in their various parts.

Big Ben was, of course, a unique clock – and despite its all-pervading aroma of impending standardisation and mass-production, the nineteenth century did see some other outstanding custom-built clocks produced, both in England and elsewhere. Mention has been made earlier of the third Strasbourg cathedral clock, built by Schwilgué and opened in 1842. The great French clockmakers like Breguet, already recognised as outstanding by 1800, and others such as Berthoud and Janvier, were exerting an international influence in Europe, so that countries like Austria produced one or two superb craftsmen making clocks of astonishing individuality. Mathias Ratzenhofer, for instance, made a series of three remarkable productions in the form of a vase of flowers, a wheelbarrow full of flowers and a sunflower clock. They were all exquisite in concept as well as in execution. In Britain, pride of place for horological novelty in the nineteenth century probably belongs to William Congreve, an artillery officer at Woolwich whose principal claim to fame is perhaps his invention of a military rocket. Congreve almost certainly never knew of previous attempts in Europe to use a rolling ball as a time standard; if he did, he clearly thought it worthwhile to try the system again. Thus, in 1808, he completed and patented his rolling ball clock, of the tipping platform type, which has been studiously copied by various firms subsequently, though on a very small scale. He seems only to have made one clock of this kind himself, and it appears to be the only one that is weight-driven. There is little doubt that, even if the basic principle was not original, the finished product was a great improvement on anything of the same kind that had gone before, although it needed the most delicate adjustment to make it give of its best.

What was happening in clockmaking elsewhere in Europe? The Black Forest is perhaps a good starting point. A cottage industry adopted by peasants in the middle of the seventeenth century, it progressed very slowly throughout the eighteenth, the thrifty craftsmen continuing to use wood as far as possible for every component, at least until the second half of that century, when at last brass wheels started to become usual. These were mounted upon wooden arbors, however; brass arbors and plates were not to appear until well after 1800. The cuckoo clock first appeared probably between 1730 and 1740, at about the time that the foliot balance was replaced by the pendulum; but very few such clocks that date prior to 1840 have survived, and the familiar 'chalet' style did not appear before 1850. The craft product that had started in such a modest and rudimentary

have revealed serious invisible faults in at least two of the remaining wheels. How fascinating it would be if Beckett himself were still alive to apply his inventive mind to the many problems involved.

Although Beckett devoted a great deal of time to horology, being an accomplished theorist and an author of technical and literary stature, he cannot really rank as a professional horologist, since he can only have derived a very small part of his income, if indeed any, from such activities. His work on clocks is usually held up as a prime example of the great contribution that the gifted amateur has to offer in this field. He was elected President of the British Horological Institute in 1868 – an honorary post, of course – and, with his architect's aspect now to the fore, designed their headquarters building in Northampton Square, Clerkenwell, which the Institute continued to occupy until very recently. Although they were not attributable solely to Beckett's influence in the trade, it is interesting to note that Victoria's reign saw the construction of some fine large public clocks, mainly in churches; and although these may not always exhibit the individual characteris-

way, however, gathered momentum fast as the market for inexpensive timekeepers opened up, so that Black Forest clocks were sold in large quantities in England, even against competition from cheap mid-nineteenth-century American imports.

In France, the nineteenth century saw the start of a process of simplification – certainly so far as the casework was concerned – which was consistent with a gradual turn-over to factory production. Statuary, always a focal point in the more elaborate French productions, now became a subsidiary factor, being placed apart from the clock movement rather than having the latter built into it. The clock would be covered, too, with a glass shade to exclude dust, although this feature disappeared towards the end of the century, by which time cases of polished marble or slate were much in vogue. The great advantage of the round French clock movement was that it was adaptable to so many different kinds of cases to meet all needs; and, from its beginnings in the eighteenth century, it was to become perhaps the finest commercially produced timekeeper ever made. By the end of the century, the Americans were copying the styles of the most popular French clocks but fitting them with modified movements of their own, in the end reaching an all-time low-quality version little better than a common alarm clock.

By about 1900, the French and Germans were in possession of most of the European market for clocks. The Germans, apart from their Black Forest output, had tried out so-called 'four hundred day' clocks with large balances suspended on a fine steel wire and rotating in a horizontal plane – torsion balances, as they are known. They also made their own versions of the Vienna regulator, both weight-driven and spring-driven, although the genuine Austrian article was itself common enough.

Any account of the nineteenth-century mechanical clock must necessarily be incomplete without brief mention of the nightwatchman's clock. Presumably brought into being as a direct result of the

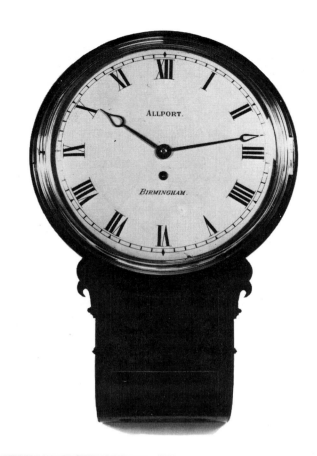

above
The earliest English dial clocks were fitted with a verge escapement and short bob pendulum; but when the longer pendulum associated with the anchor escapement came into fashion, it proved necessary to add an extension to the clock case to accommodate the extra length. This version is known as a drop dial, and Samuel Allport, maker of the example shown here, flourished in Birmingham from 1828 to 1860.

right
Regarded as a novelty clock, this unsigned French timepiece of about 1835 nevertheless demonstrates a scientific principle, that of the conical pendulum. A horizontal arm rotated by the clock train maintains continuous contact with a projection on the bottom of the pendulum weight, which is suspended above it by a thread, giving a continuous circular motion. Museum of the Worshipful Company of Clockmakers, Guildhall, London.

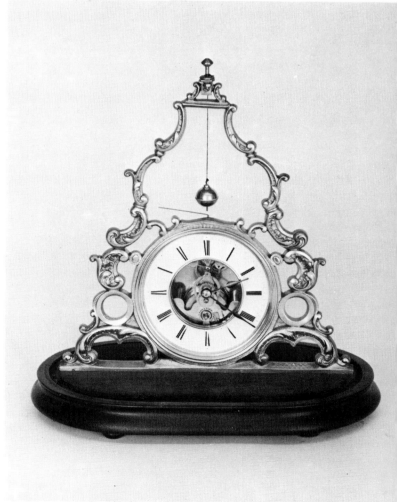

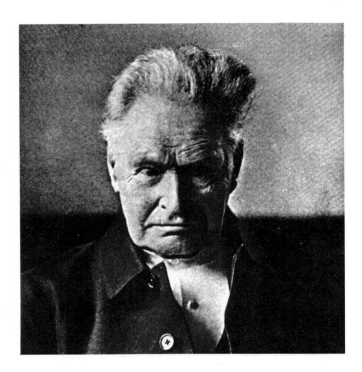

The slightly eccentric genius who designed the Westminster clock 'Big Ben', Lord Grimthorpe is seen here in old age. He died in 1905.

Industrial Revolution, these clocks had their beginnings in the eighteenth century with the designs of John Whitehurst of Derby, but were still to be found throughout much of the succeeding one. They took several forms, one of which is generally found in a long plain wainscot oak case, similar to but rather shorter than the average long-case clock. The mechanism works by employing a single fixed hand, which registers the time against a rotating dial, calibrated in hours and quarters. Around the edge of the dial, at half-hourly intervals, are set metal pins, one of which the watchman had to depress when he went his rounds. Only one pin at a time could be operated, and then only when it was in exactly the right position in relation to the actual time. To re-set the pins necessitated unlocking the clock. Thus the watchman had to be by the clock at precisely the right moment or the clock would note his absence by leaving a pin projecting; this accounts for the other name by which such devices were known, the 'tell-tale' clock. Another common form of watchman's clock, apparently known as Hahn's Time Detector – and, in modernised form, used to the present day – is essentially a locked clock, built into a drum-shaped case. The clock, in fact, houses a printed paper disc divided into hours, which it causes to rotate – in other words, it is a rotating dial which, once used, constitutes a permanent record and can be replaced with a fresh unused one for the next period. The watchman carries the clock with him on his rounds, and, at each station that he has to visit, there will be chained to the wall a key which he must insert into a keyhole on the band of his clock and turn once. Since each key differs from all

the others at the various stations, this makes an appropriate impression on the rotating paper disc, revealing the time recorded as well as the actual station being visited. It is not even possible to open the clock at the end of a shift, to replace the dial disc with a new one, without this fact, too, being automatically recorded.

There was one other noteworthy instance, incidentally, in which locked timekeepers have played a part in daily routine operations. In England up to 1846, the public mail – the Royal Mail, as it is known – was carried by horse-drawn coach in the custody of a guard who had to carry with him a large watch, set to time by an official before he started out, and then locked in a specially made box, so that it could not be tampered with. The journey timings were recorded by local postmasters on a time-bill, as the mail coach passed through their areas, the locked watch having to be produced for this purpose each time. A glazed aperture in the box lid permitted of the dial being read without any need to unlock the container itself. Most of these special watches with their boxes were made for the General Post Office by George Littlewort, who had premises in Cannon Street and had been granted a patent for his particular design, in which the wood box was heavily reinforced with brass. These watches usually were of long duration, going for at least three days before winding was necessary.

Before turning to the evolution of the watch in the period under review, there is one other unique development which should be examined, and that is the first appearance of the electric clock. Alexander Bain, with his original patent no. 9754 granted in 1843, is generally considered to be the pioneer in this field, and his device used an electric current solely for driving a pendulum, the transmission to the hands remaining mechanical. He was anticipated by Steinheil in Germany, with his patent of 1839, but this was only concerned with the transmission of time signals to secondary clocks. It was not long before the application of electricity in this field was greatly expanded, however, with slave clocks being automatically brought to time by impulses transmitted by a master clock, and time signals from observatories being received by land-line at points very far distant. In London, in the second half of the nineteenth century, first the firm of Barraud & Lund and then, from 1876, the Standard Time Company, under the direction of John Lund, a specialist in electrical horology, had installed a network of land-lines over the roof-tops from its headquarters to outlying jewellers and watch- and clockmakers, as well as to other business firms to whom a knowledge of the right time was of special importance. Standard Time itself received an hourly time-signal by line direct from Greenwich Observatory, which it simultaneously retransmit-

right

A watchman's 'telltale' clock originally located in one of the big banks in the City of London. The dial bears the signature 'Barrauds, Cornhill, London', and it is possible to place its date at 1816. The dial revolves against a fixed pointer which can be seen above 12 o'clock, and the pins to be depressed by the watchman are clearly visible around its edge.

below

The cuckoo attachment to Black Forest clocks at first was incorporated into the painted shield-shaped dials of their wall clocks, and the chalet type of cuckoo clock does not appear before about 1850.

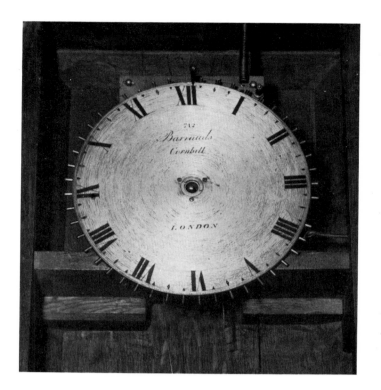

ted. This basic system, even using much of the original control equipment, was in use until destroyed by bombing during the Second World War; even then, it was partially rebuilt and continued to give a similar service, albeit on a more restricted scale, until economic considerations finally forced it to close down only as recently as 1964.

It will be obvious that, from considerations of scale alone, the watch presents a multitude of different – and generally more difficult – problems in its manufacture than the clock. Manual dexterity, when hand-working watch parts as opposed to those for a clock has to be much more sensitive and highly developed to avoid a disaster that can, in extreme cases, negate several days' work. By the nineteenth century, however, the evolution of the watch was being adequately paced by development of the quite sophisticated technology needed to manufacture it. Mass-production aside – and this was an essentially American phenomenon which will be dealt with in the next chapter – skilled craftsmen in Victorian England had brought the mechanical arts to a zenith, and were able to use hand tools, often of their own making, as well as a variety of hand- or foot-powered machine tools, to fashion complex multi-component assemblies to a degree of precision and to smaller tolerances than at any previous time in history. In a sense, this remarkable progress towards precision workmanship was just a logical further step in what was already a long heritage. Seventeenth-century invention produced a timekeeper that kept going, even though haphazardly; in the eighteenth, the target was reliability coupled with ever more precision in performance, and this spilled over into the nineteenth and even the twentieth centuries. Once the main principles of precision mechanical timekeeping had been established, however, there was at last time to devote to the convenience of the user, in such matters as winding mechanisms – the ubiquitous key-winding system was so unwieldy by comparison with the nowadays commonplace button-wind or, in watchmakers' parlance, 'keyless' system – as well as in the method of activating ancillary motions such as chronographs and

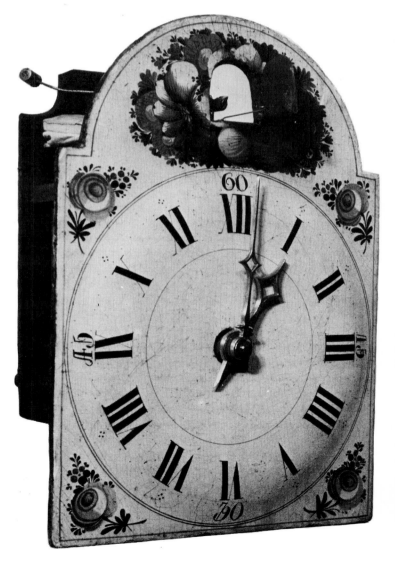

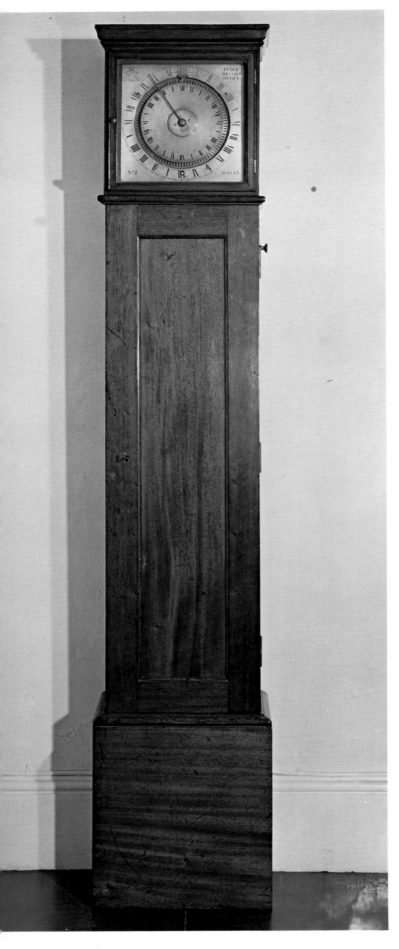

repeatingwork. Such were the preoccupations of makers towards the end of the nineteenth century.

At the beginning, however – by 1800 – the verge was probably still the most common design of watch escapement, followed closely by the cylinder. The duplex was just coming into favour, for those who wanted a quality watch but could not, perhaps, afford a pocket chronometer. The lever, which was eventually to assert itself as the finest escapement for watches, was still something of an anachronism; invented, abandoned, reinvented in the 1780s and 1790s, and abandoned again apart from its close cousin, the rack lever, it was ripe for yet a further appearance. The rack lever had many attributes comparable with the eventual form that the escapement was to assume; yet, because of its rack and pinion, it was not in the technical sense a 'detached' escapement, being always in contact with the train throughout its cycle of operation. In the second decade of the century two intermediate forms of detached lever, known respectively as Massey's crank-roller and Savage's two-pin lever, appeared and continued to be made for some time, although very shortly thereafter the first true version of the English lever, called the table-roller lever, made its appearance. This would have been about 1825, and it very quickly established itself, undergoing only one other modification, in the latter half of the century, to incorporate a double roller, which did not affect the action of the escapement. By mid century or shortly thereafter, then, the lever watch had superseded the duplex and the detent – the pocket chronometer was always a fragile machine to carry on the person – while the cylinder was obsolescent except in its cheap imported version. The only other escapement still being made was the verge, and this continued until about 1900, although principally in the provinces. It seems curiously appropriate that the oldest mechanical escapement known to mankind should have had such an incredibly long life, yet, for those who did not need the most precise timekeeping, it was a robust device, reliable in service and easy of maintenance.

The first attempts to devise an easier system of winding up the watch and to dispense with the inconvenient watch key, were made in 1820 by Thomas Prest, foreman at Arnolds, the chronometermakers at Chigwell in Essex, although the celebrated John Arnold senior, the founder, was long since dead by this time. Although it employed a button on the pendant similar to the modern system, Prest's design possessed certain technical disadvantages and was never popular during his lifetime. Other approaches to the problem involved what is usu-

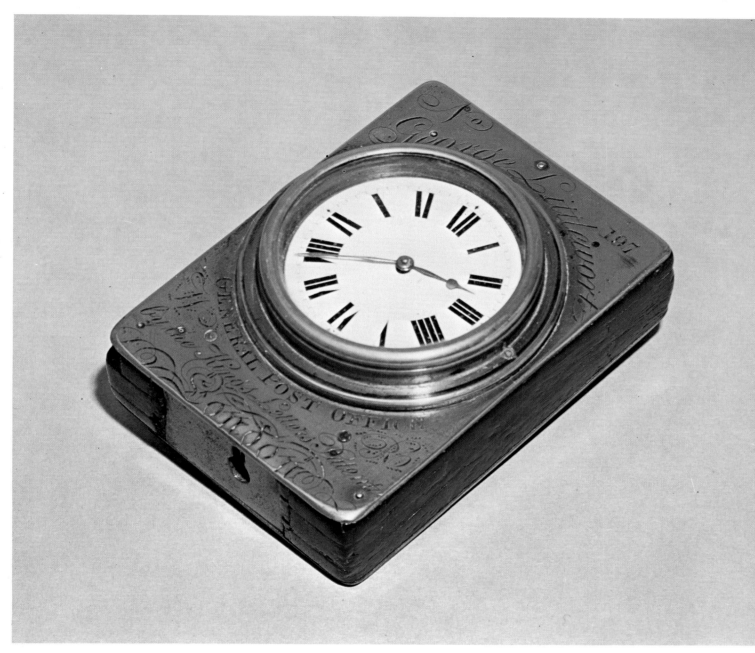

George Littlewort patented a special type of lockable three-day duration watch for use by the guards on mail coaches. Museum of the Worshipful Company of Clockmakers, Guildhall, London.

ally called 'pump-winding', that is, a push-pull action applied to the pendant knob. A certain A. Burdess, a Coventry maker, devised a system by which a lever, pivoted to the back plate, engages with a ratchet arrangement acting upon the fusee arbor. The lever projects through the watch case, and can be pumped up and down, the ratchet engaging – and therefore turning the fusee – on the downward stroke, and then free-wheeling on the upward. His watches also possessed an unusual system for hand-setting, having a wheel with a milled edge projecting outside the rim of the movement, yet being in constant engagement with the minute wheel. The additional friction caused to the motionwork thereby must surely have made the arrangement most unserviceable. A number of other winding systems were tried out, especially towards the end of the nineteenth century; many of

these employed a button, but often it had to be wound while pressure was applied simultaneously to a push-piece located beside the pendant on the band of the case. Failure to do this meant that the winding train was not engaged, and the button just turned freely between the fingers. A variation of this system utilised two push-pieces, one each side of the pendant. Pressure on one together with operation of the winding button, wound the watch; pressure upon the other gave the facility to set the hands, just as in the system which was eventually universally adopted. The height of absurdity in attempts by the watch trade to dispense with the

203

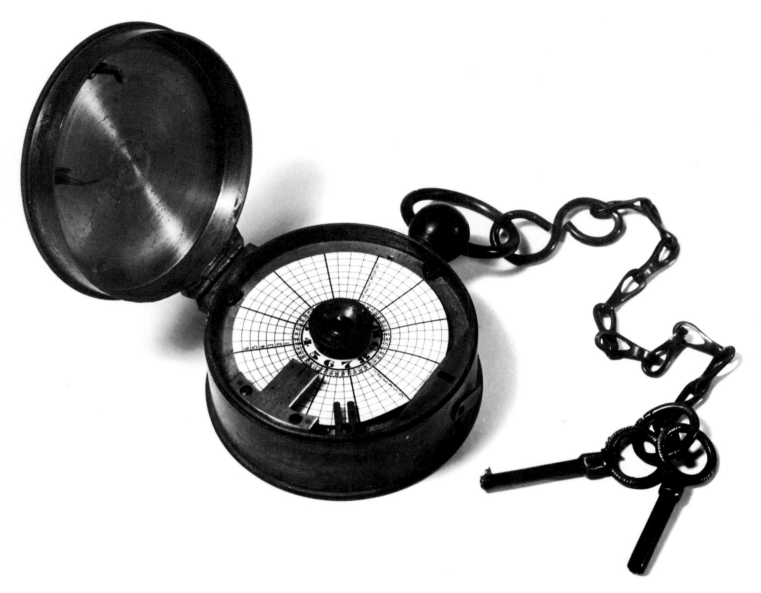

Another version of the watchman's clock was carried by the watchman himself. This one is called 'Hahn's Patent Time Detector'. The working of this clock is described in the text on page 200.

key-wind system was probably reached as late as 1870, when the firm of Barraud & Lund marketed watches whose pendants were topped by buttons looking exactly like those fitted to keyless watches. However, when the button was pulled, it came free of the pendant, only to reveal that attached underneath it – and concealed within the pendant when not in use – was a key!

It may sound, from the foregoing, as if the English watch trade had been somewhat obstinate as well as stupid in their development of keyless winding. They had their problems, though, not the least of which was their long-established belief – almost a creed, one might say – that one prerequisite for accuracy in watches was a fusee. Although many fusee keyless watches were made, and suc-

cessfully – these are held in high esteem by collectors today – it is in general much more difficult to adapt the fusee watch for keyless winding than the going barrel watch. Eventually, this consideration was to seal the fate of the fusee, which was abandoned towards the end of the century. Foreign manufacturers had by then been using the going barrel successfully for a long time, and it must have been hard for the English trade to have to yield on such a basic principle; yet force of circumstances gave them little choice.

There were other technical advances going on alongside those mentioned, so that it was almost a case of consolidating the fundamental inventions in watchmaking to produce the article that was perfect in all respects – appearance, reliability, performance and convenience of use. Thus, although the table-roller lever watch, once established, became the standard good-quality watch, there were still those makers – James Ferguson Cole, for example – who sought to improve the escapement even further. Yet another ingenious maker, Thomas Cummins – until recently, relatively unappreciated – was not only one of the first to use the lever escapement in quantity after its revival, but also employed it in special watches of the very highest quality, starting about 1822. Yet inventiveness did not always produce the results expected. For example, Breguet, although not first in the field, had adapted the principle of the pedometer to produce an automatic watch – he called them '*montres perpetuelles*' – but this fashion, even by such a master, had only a relatively short life. Next, Harwood suited the same principle to the wristwatch in 1923. Even then, the fashion was short-lived, and automatic watches have not become really popular until recent times.

In the latter half of the nineteenth century, apart from standardising, in the end, a functional keyless winding system, a rather better arrangement was devised for operating additional motions on watches – chronographwork, for example, or repetition actions. This took the form of slides, as they are called, built into the band of the case and operated by a thumbnail. Such action was more positive, as well as more suitable for the thinner plainer designs of late nineteenth-century watches, than anything that had been tried before, especially now that the elongated pendant, reminiscent of the old pair-case watch, had disappeared. As to additional complexities, the minute repeater became fairly commonplace – musical watches had had a short vogue earlier in the century, but again the fashion did not last – as well as various types of stopwatch and chronograph mechanisms. Much complicated repeating, musical, chronograph and similar work was made in Switzerland and imported into Britain where it was fitted quite happily to English-made watches.

But how did the appearance of the watch change in the period under review? The pair-cased watch was still the norm in 1800 and was to continue for some decades still in the provinces, even if London usage was changing. The first real hunter and half-hunter watch cases – even these often have a pair-case *en suite* – have the thick profile of the styles that preceded them and, for some reason, were mostly made in Birmingham around 1802–04. The first single-cased watches – these are often called 'consular' cases – looked like pair-cases; the glazed bezel opened and the hinged movement swung outwards, as if one were opening the inner of pair-cases. Behind the movement but integral with the rest, the case is double-backed, the outer one hinged and opening to permit winding through the inner, which is, of course, fixed. This type of single case gradually evolved into that which prevailed throughout most of Victoria's reign; in this the pendant had shrunk to become a mere knob on the case, with the bow pivoted in it. The band of such cases, and sometimes a border

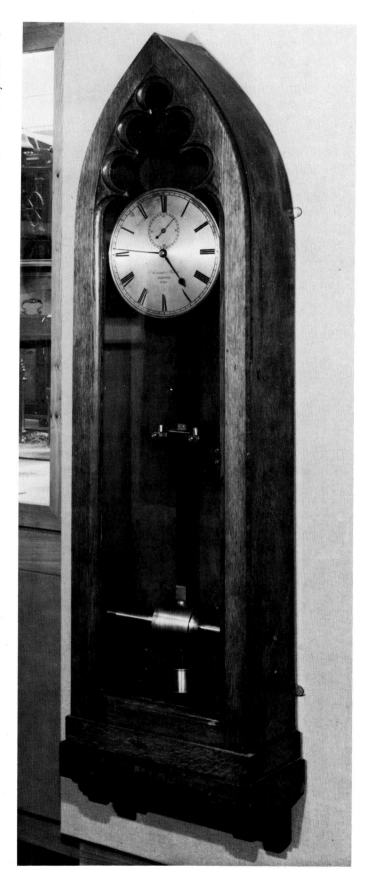

The Scotsman Alexander Bain was the first to apply electricity to drive the pendulum of a clock, an invention which he patented in 1840. Museum of the Worshipful Company of Clockmakers, Guildhall, London.

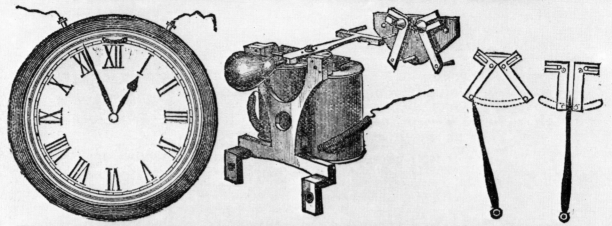
round the back as well, were knurled, and later engine-turned designs became customary. For a while around the mid century, cases with cast decoration, usually with a floral motif, became common, and these coincided with a sudden return for a time to metal dials instead of the enamel ones which had been in use since the previous century. Where gold was the metal involved, it was not unusual to find applied decoration in different coloured alloys, the whole usually being described as in 'four-colour gold'. Metal dials were soon discarded in favour of enamel ones, however, and, as the century continued, the heavy gold open-faced ('O.F.') watch, as well as the hunter and half-hunter, became popular. Of the latter styles, of course, the hunter has a solid cover over the dial which has to be opened before the time can be read, while in the half-hunter a hole is cut in the centre of the cover, of sufficient size to allow the directions of the hands to be ascertained, these being read against a ring of hour numerals engraved around the edge of this aperture. Initially there was some tendency to overdecorate these handsome watches: either the cases were cast to provide relief all over, or sometimes just an elaborated monogram or at least an ugly cartouche waiting to contain one, were provided. But by the

last two decades of the century such watches had evolved into the plain, functional and generally high-grade timekeepers which our grandparents and their parents were accustomed to wear.

The other radical change which took place in the pocket watch during the last century was the gradual disappearance of any decoration on the movement. The original purpose of decorating movements, presumably, was to make them a focus for the admiration of both their owners and those who were allowed to examine them, while at the same time, perhaps, drawing attention away from their indifferent capabilities as timekeepers: it will be remembered that such decoration was applied from a very early stage in the evolution of the watch, long before it could realistically be considered as anything more than an ingenious toy for the rich. By 1800, such decoration had already become degenerate by comparison with what had gone before, but there was still plenty of it: the watch cock, for instance, was still likely to be the site of all-over engraving of a kind, even though piercing, as an added attraction, had been discarded. The shape of the cock, too, remained as it had been – a round 'table' above the balance, joined to a splayed 'foot', which was screwed to the movement. However, two influences seemed to be

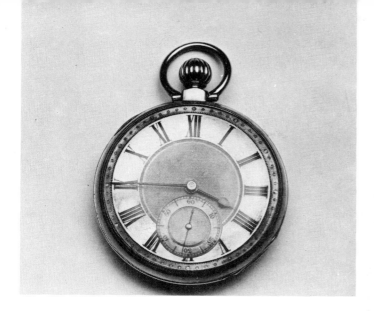

left

The firm of Barraud & Lund were among the first to use electricity to synchronise 'slave' clocks with a regulator, and this advertisement for their process appeared in the *Horological Journal* in January 1878. This method was in use on the railways by 1892.

right

This small watch, presumably intended for a lady, originated from a famous London watchmaking firm, James McCabe. It incorporates a duplex escapement and dates from 1835, that is, during the last decade in which this form of controller continued to be made.

The common English watch in 1800 was still the ubiquitous verge. This example by Barraud, which has a subsidiary calendar dial, is typical of the best quality practice at that time, this particular one having been made in 1797.

This watch by John Roger Arnold, son of the famous chronometermaker, is fitted with the early system of keyless winding developed in 1820 by Thomas Prest, Arnold's foreman. Museum of the Worshipful Company of Clockmakers, Guildhall, London.

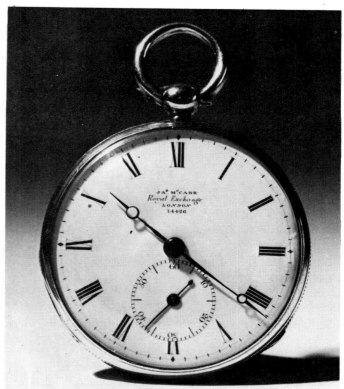

at work during the first three decades of the century. The high-precision watch movement – the pocket chronometer, that is – was quickly to become completely plain, as well as needing modification to the shape of its watch cock to suit the helical balance spring.

It was almost as if the makers mutually decided that precision and decoration did not mix: in fact, they do not, in the sense that the last thing a proud craftsman in this field wants is for some nosey busybody to be constantly prying into his precision machine, and doubtless affecting its performance by letting in dust and moisture. Thomas Earnshaw, in fact, was so adamant on this point that many of his pocket chronometer movements are screwed into their cases and need special tools to extract them. Breguet took a like view.

Another influence, which in a sense seemed to be going in the opposing direction, was experimentation in the shape of the watch cock probably as part of the general trend towards a much thinner watch. The traditional English hand-finished watch was robust, heavy and thick, all characteristics which supported its good and reliable performance. However, the demand was for a change, sparked off, no doubt, by the French, who were making watches of a thinness and elegance which

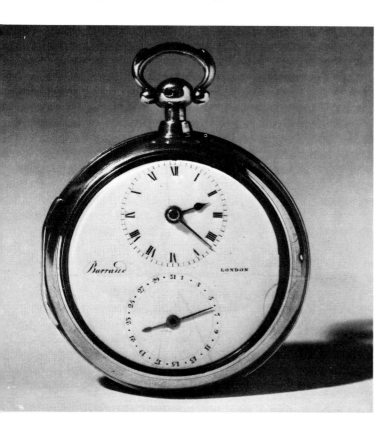

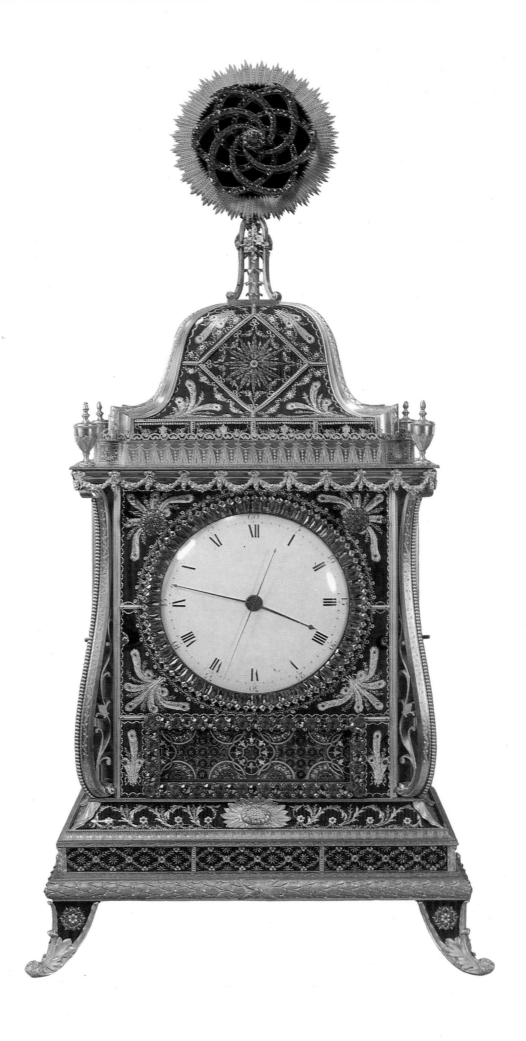

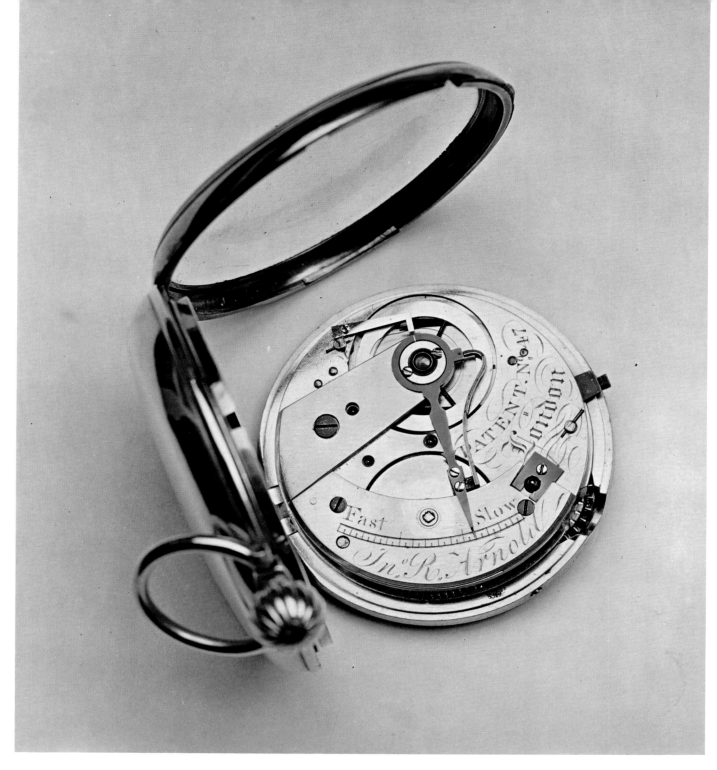

The movement of the Arnold watch also reveals the particular type of 'sugar-tongs' compensation curb, favoured by the younger Arnold. The escapement is a ruby cylinder. Museum of the Worshipful Company of Clockmakers, Guildhall, London.

left
Made by Henry Borell of London, this elaborate enamelled and gem-set automaton clock was a present from George III to the Emperor Ch'ien-lung of China in about 1790. At the hour a small door opens below the dial, and ships move about on simulated waves. Jürg Stuker Gallery, Berne.

must have been much envied by their cousins across the Channel. The full-plate watch – in which the train is planted between two solid plates with the balance mounted outside them, pivoting in its cock which is screwed to the back of the movement – had, perforce, to give way to something thinner and therefore more sophisticated, but without detracting from any of its finer advantages, such as performance. The eventual solution, of course, was to cut away part of the back plate and drop the balance into the cavity so formed. It still required its own cock, but this time screwed to the underside of the front plate. Experiments in this direction were going forward among London

209

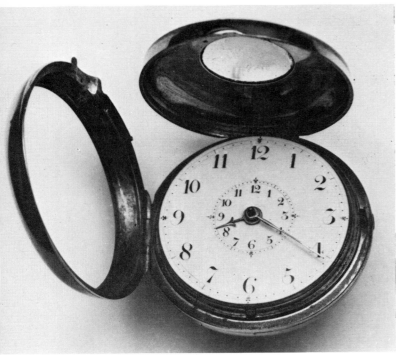

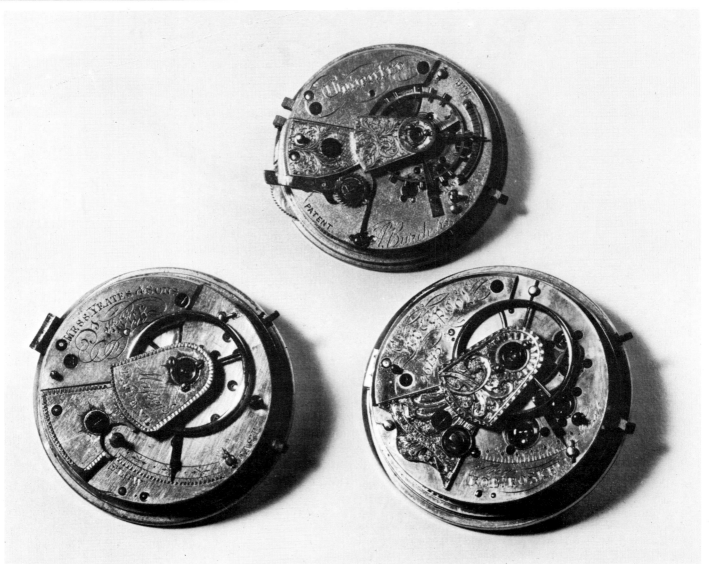

makers as early as the 1820s, so that three-quarter plate movements became commonplace and the so-called half-plate rather less so, although the full-plate movement continued in country practice for the rest of the century and even beyond. As to decoration, this continued throughout the short period of trial to find a new watch cock shape, and for some time after the rounded-wedge-shaped cock table had been adopted. Finally, decoration became completely perfunctory and haphazard – there was even one short period in which a circular raised area on the back plate immediately above the spring barrel became the site of engraved decoration – before eventually disappearing altogether.

The only other European watchmaking countries of any consequence in the last century were France and Switzerland. The French, led by such style-setters as Breguet, Motel and others, set their sights on high-quality thin watches of the greatest elegance and, certainly at the beginning of the century, placed themselves alongside the English in their insistence upon the best standards. The Swiss, curiously enough, had made little impression on the world horological scene before 1800, having managed to 'export' only some of their finest craftsmen to other countries so that it almost seems that, for the first quarter of the century, they still marked time while waiting for the advent of mass-production. In the end, the French and the Swiss took the same road, while the English clung obstinately to their illusions about the hand-finished watch, even though in this sphere too they had been largely overtaken by the French. The Swiss meanwhile made something of a speciality of novelty during the early decades of the century: musical and repeating watches, with automata ranging from simple *jaquemarts* simulating the striking of bells beside a cut-away dial to other very much more complicated actions. Soon, however, the pace was to be set by pioneers like Frédéric Japy, whose engineering skill provided so many of the first machine tools in Switzerland, and Favre-Jacot who opened the first watch factory. One of the side effects of this fundamental change in methods of production was the gradual replacement of the former common Swiss full-plate verge movement with the much more readily quantity-produced Lepine calibre – in which there is really only one plate, all the train wheels and other components being pivoted in cocks screwed to it – together with the cylinder escapement. The Swiss maintained this style for the remainder of the century, and the French also adopted it.

When the Great Exhibition opened in London in 1851, the Swiss made a great impression with their display; sadly, there was only one English firm, Rotherhams of Coventry, who had employed steam-powered machinery in making their exhibits. This followed a lone attempt, a few years previously, by a Swiss called P. F. Ingold to make

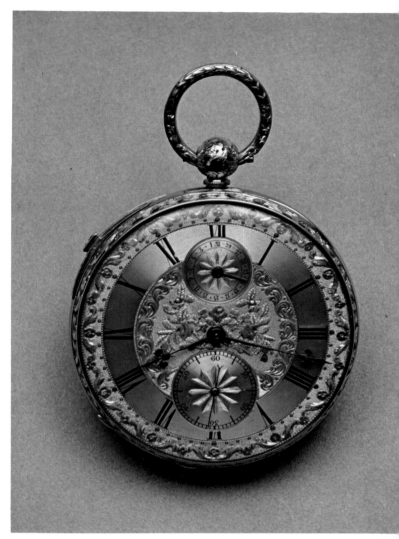

watches in England using machine tools. It was instantly and vociferously opposed by the trade in Clerkenwell and Coventry, who successfully crushed it. In fact, Ingold had had contacts with America, the fount of mass-production methods, and nobody will ever be able to assess accurately how much damage must have been done by the English craft to its own future livelihood by this inward-looking unprogressive attitude. The extraordinary thing is that, rather than admit the error of its ways, the craft continued to hold to its hidebound attitude which it did not finally abandon until the late 1920s, when the economic depression made life on the former system impossible. Fine watches, at such times, are made to be broken up for the intrinsic value of their precious-metal cases, not bought new over the counter!

In terms of horological achievement, how can one sum up the nineteenth and twentieth centuries? Certain it is that nothing very new was discovered, for there was little of fundamental significance still awaiting invention in the respective arts, if one ignores the ordinary mains electric clock working synchronously with the alternating current, which after all is only an electric motor with gearing. All-embracing fashions in art – such as Art Nouveau and Art Deco – were reflected, certainly, in clocks; but although other objects in these styles have made their mark, the horological applications seem mostly to have failed to survive. However it may be presented or disguised, there has already been a precedent for almost every complexity or additional action; thus automatic watches were an eighteenth-century development, calendar watches even earlier, alarm watches earlier still. Stopwatches, chronographs, timers, call them what you will, there is nothing even comparatively recent about them: they have been around for centuries! The only peculiarly twentieth-century feature, or fashion if you prefer it, has been the wristwatch, attributed to the First World War period when it was much more convenient than a pocket watch; since some early examples seem to have been made up by fitting ladies' fob watches with lugs either side to take a silk or leather strap it may even have preceded that great human débâcle by a few years. But it hardly rates as an epoch-making discovery such as, for example, the first successful application of the pendulum.

There were important fringe inventions, nevertheless – not of a mechanical nature them-

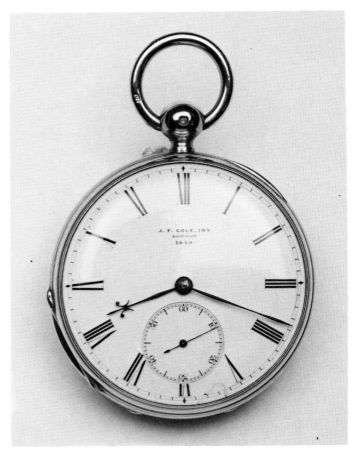

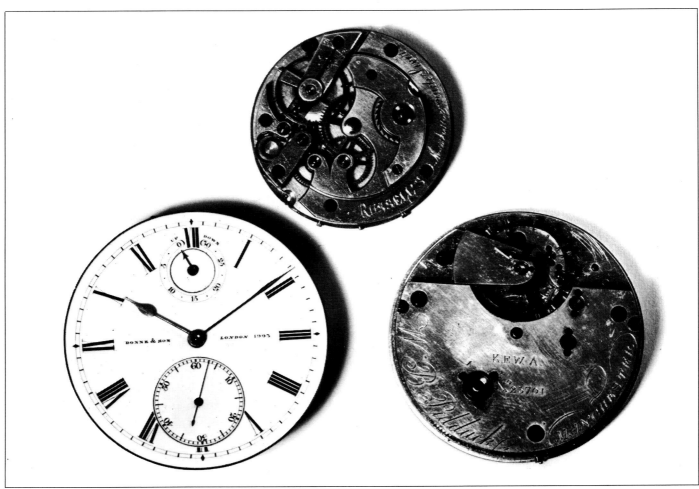

left
James Ferguson Cole experimented towards the middle of the nineteenth century in an effort to improve the already well-established lever escapement. This watch was made in 1848. Museum of the Worshipful Company of Clockmakers, Guildhall, London.

below left
These three lever movements dating from late in the nineteenth century, include an example by W. D. Pidduck of Manchester, which obtained an 'A' rating at Kew Observatory, another by Donne & Son which has an up-and-down indicator, and a 'machine-made lever' from the well-known Liverpool firm of Thomas Russell.

selves, but of the greatest use in mechanical devices. In 1920, for instance, the Nobel Prize was awarded to Charles-Edouard Guillaume (1861–1938), who was at that time Director of the International Bureau of Weights and Measures in Paris, for discovering certain nickel-steel alloys that were virtually impervious to changes in temperature. Called by their inventor 'Invar' and 'Elinvar', they replaced almost overnight all previous systems for temperature compensation. The two other major developments in the last seventy years have been the free-pendulum clock perfected by W. H. Shortt in 1921 – an electro-mechanical device of astonishing accuracy, and only overtaken by the electronics-based quartz crystal clock, invented in America in 1929.

Even though the English craft of the fine watch might appear to have presided over its own funeral, there is one consolation to be derived from such seeming obstinacy. Those directly involved sadly reaped no benefit, for it is only now just starting to pay off. Because the tradition of the hand-finished watch lasted so much longer in England than elsewhere – for it was still possible to have one made to suit one's taste less than fifty years ago – many such fine watches must still be in circulation, and certainly some are eminently fit for collection. Such quality pieces help to offset the dearth of any other interesting twentieth-century developments. Wristwatches, *per se*, are not very attractive objects, but doubtless they also will become collector's items in the end; and it is amusing to speculate how long it is going to take, in view of the speed with which at the present time fashions in collecting are catching up with history!

below left
This early leather wristwatch strap, believed to date from about 1908, is designed to contain a small pocket watch, thus converting it for wearing on the wrist. Museum of the Worshipful Company of Clockmakers, Guildhall, London.

below
The first application of the self-winding principle to wristwatches, this specimen by John Harwood, who made his prototype six years before, dates from about 1928. The Depression forced the firm into liquidation shortly afterwards. Museum of the Worshipful Company of Clockmakers, Guildhall, London.

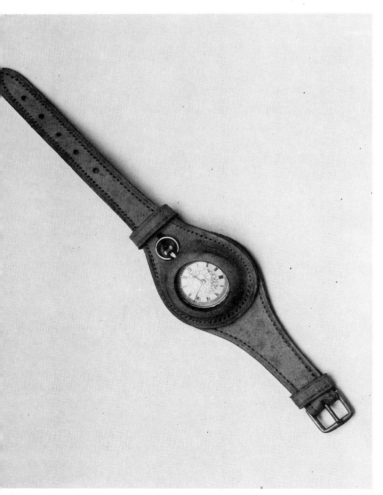

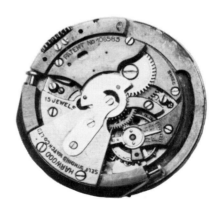

East Meets West

Anybody taking up the study of horology seriously reads certain standard works of reference, visits museum collections, joins appropriate organisations and perhaps, if his means will allow, starts to collect items which particularly appeal to him. There is a very dangerous tendency, once this stage has been reached – and it may take five months or fifteen years, depending upon individual circumstances – to lapse into a state of euphoria based on the wholly erroneous belief that all the basic knowledge necessary to enjoy and appreciate every aspect of the art, craft and science of the subject has now been carefully explored and assimilated. In fact, the student has become an expert, or so he thinks.

The only real expert in horology is the one who recognises that there is no such animal, since it is not possible to become one within the capacity of one mind and one human life-span. The infinite ingenuity of man in things mechanical has made it absolutely certain that no one person will ever be able to locate, let alone examine, every permutation of mechanical components in the form of a timepiece that has ever been constructed, to say nothing of the limitless combinations of complications that are frequently associated with such objects. Without doing that, nobody has any right to claim comprehensive knowledge of the subject. Even to the present time, the world's big auction houses, and even the most prominent specialist dealers in the field, continue to turn up from time to time horological objects the exact like of which have not been seen before by the majority, if not indeed by any, of those claiming expertise in such things. Naturally the degree of novelty varies from one item to another: it is rare for anything to come to light so exceptionally unique as materially to affect the recorded course of horological history, yet it does happen. Perhaps this is one of the characteristics that makes horology such an exciting subject for study.

The most convincing way to demonstrate the precept set out above is probably to consider in some detail two totally different horological cultures, at the same time recognising that, in dealing with such a universally experienced phenomenon as the passage and measurement of time, these are but two among many that possess marked differences one from another. Like time itself, there is a quality of the infinite about the range of instrumentation associated with it, not to mention such arbitrary characteristics as the periods into which time is divided.

Japan

For all its modern commercial and technical achievement, in the matter of time-measurement Japan presents an extraordinary paradox. It is only a little over a century – the exact year was 1873 – since she abandoned a method of time-measurement and a complicated calendar that had been long since outmoded, and changed to the European system. But the paradox extends even further. Once the change had been made, most of the obsolete timepieces were exported as novelties, so that they have now become extremely rare in their country of origin, although common enough in advanced Western countries. Finally, and as if this was not enough, Japanese clockmakers of the pre-1873 era were innately conservative, so that accurate dating of many of their wares within a span of two and a half centuries is an impossible task, even if one encounters them.

This Japanese 'lantern' striking clock on its lacquered stand has a steel movement with a single foliot. The hand revolves against the fixed lacquered dial, and the engraved panels enclosing the case are of silvered brass. British Museum, London.

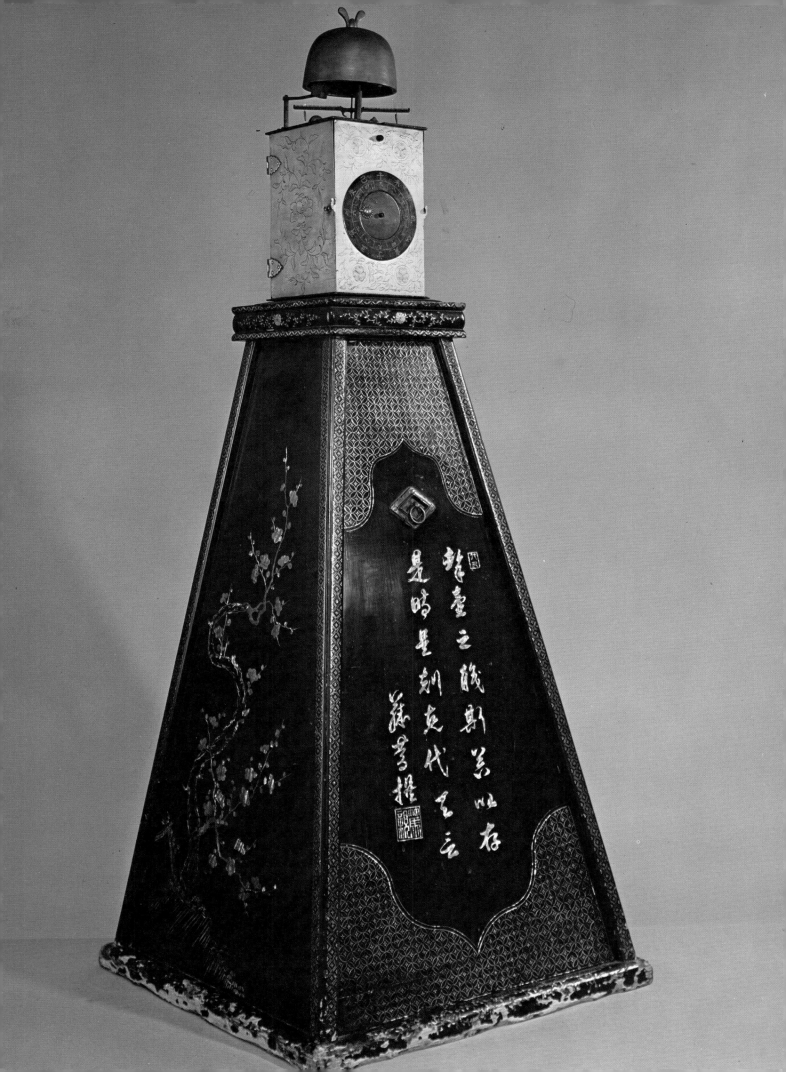

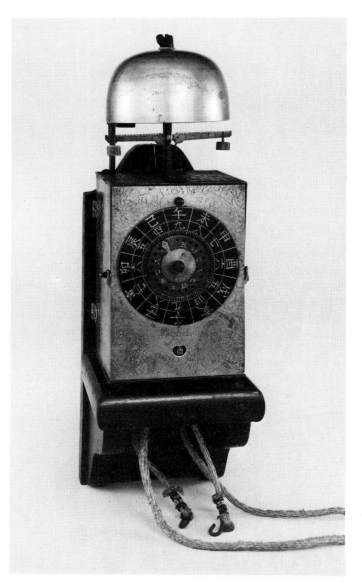

There are a number of other problems connected with any proper study of old Japanese horology which it is as well to recognise from the beginning. It will be obvious that the flimsy construction – by Western standards – of Japanese houses, built without solid walls and with rooms divided by movable partitions, precludes the accommodation of heavy weight-driven wall timepieces or brackets of any kind. Furthermore, the Japanese, unlike other cultures, do not favour heavy items of furniture such as chests of drawers, cabinets or even mantelpieces. Indeed, normally their rooms – certainly those in which they entertain guests – are absolutely empty save for some special object, which will have been brought in temporarily for the occasion, to suit some particu-

Another version of the lantern clock encloses it within a wall-bracket and glazed hood. This example has a revolving dial with adjustable numerals. British Museum, London.

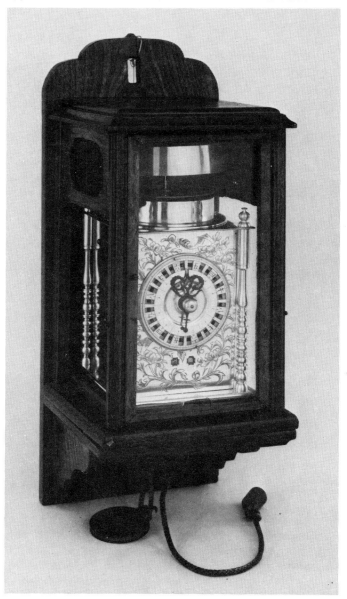

Another Japanese lantern clock, this one has more elaborate decoration than the previous example, indicating a somewhat later date. British Museum, London.

The aspiring student horologist from any Western culture who wants to learn about Japanese practice faces an enormous obstacle from the beginning. There is no work in his own language to guide his studies and provide the groundwork. Actually this is not entirely true, as will be seen from the Further Reading list on page 254; but, taking the English language as an example, the most authoritative work on Japanese horology forms part only of a general dissertation on clockwork that was published nearly fifty years ago, has long since gone out of print and is now, in fact, both scarce and expensive on the secondhand market. But, more important, it has never been updated in the light of recent research, if indeed any substantial corpus of such has so far been undertaken. It could be a prolific field for the right person to explore.

lar mood and which may be enhanced by other temporary features specially arranged in its vicinity. Finally, of course, clocks in long cases, so that their dials were six feet or more from the floor, would serve little purpose in surroundings in which people customarily sat on the ground.

It is clear from the foregoing that any clock which must, of its very nature, form a permanent part of the domestic scene, would be anathema to the Japanese who had no taste for permanence in their surroundings; and it will not be surprising, therefore, to discover that clocks were mainly confined to the temples and to the homes of nobles and the very rich, where it was customary to keep a clockmaker occupied with their continual adjustments, as the calendar demanded. It is certainly true that even educated Japanese have been largely ignorant of these relics of a bygone age, and a British diplomat writing early in the present century of his experiences in Japan in the third quarter of the previous one, mentioned that neither clocks nor punctuality were common, and it was always very difficult to be certain about the time of day.

So, strangely, the best evidence as to the antecedents of Japanese clocks must perforce come from the instruments themselves, and from the occasional references in the literature of that land. Of the latter, one volume of a three-volume treatise on mechanical toys and clocks which was published towards the end of the eighteenth century is relevant; a more recent account devoted wholly to Japanese horology was published in 1924. Both will be found in the Further Reading list.

It is rather beyond the scope of this book to deal at any length with the history of Japan from the time when it first accepted mechanical timekeeping devices, even if this were known with any accuracy. Did clocks arrive with the Portuguese, when they first reached Japan about 1542? Or did they emanate from the Spanish, or possibly the Dutch, who, of all the European merchant countries, seem to have devised the most effective, albeit short-lived, trading arrangements with Japan? Even Britain's East India Company traded with Japan for ten years early in the seventeenth century but, being uncompetitive, finally abandoned the market. However this may be, there is evidence that Japanese craftsmen, who were very skilled indeed in the working of metals, slavishly copied the crude sixteenth-century domestic clock that was current in Europe and almost certainly did so under the supervision of European masters.

This, however, at once focussed attention on a key problem. The Japanese divided the day according to a method which had its origins in China, not into twice twelve hours, each of equal length, as customary in the West. The Chinese system reckoned time according to the 'natural' day, starting at dusk. Each period from dusk to

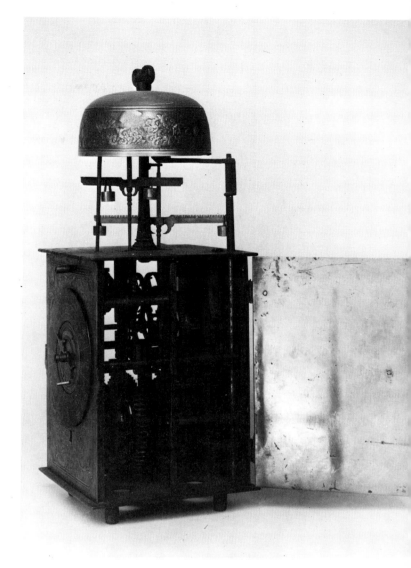

Features of this lantern clock include double foliot, striking and alarm. The hand revolves against a lacquered chapter ring. British Museum, London.

dawn and from dawn to dusk was divided into six equal divisions; but, owing to the seasonal variation in the length of the periods, the length of such divisions varied according to the time of year. These divisions – which we may, for ease of expression, loosely call 'hours' henceforth, although it will be understood that they are of constantly varying length – were sounded in temples by strokes upon a bell, ranging in descending order from nine to four. To complicate the matter even further, each hour not only equated with a specific number of bell strokes but also with a sign of the Chinese zodiac. The hour was, in fact, designated by its zodiacal name, and since some of these signs were considered lucky and others not, it needed only a glance at the clock to see if the time was propitious for any special course of action. Although generally the divisions on clock dials incorporated both number and sign, there are examples which exhibit only the one or the other, while yet a third

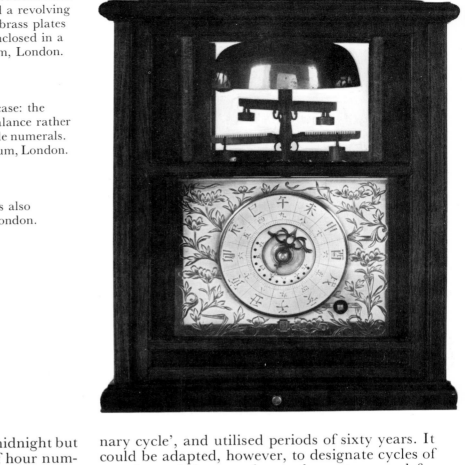

variety retains the signs for noon and midnight but numerals for the rest. As to this use of hour numbers, it is not out of keeping with Oriental tradition, which so often seems to organise things in a reverse order to that used in the West, that the Japanese should count their hours backwards. It is more difficult to say why the numbers 9 through to 4 should have been chosen. Several theories have been advanced, based on numerological considerations, but there is no evidence to support one against another. It does seem certain that the numbers 1, 2 and 3 were reserved for temple use in a different, probably liturgical context, while 9 possessed supposed magic properties and was therefore reserved to indicate the two invariable moments of each day, midday and midnight.

It has already been mentioned that clocks had to be continually adjusted as the calendar of the seasons influenced the precise lengths of the two periods of each day. But the Japanese calendar itself – the system for determining chronological dates – was excessively complicated; indeed, there were three different methods, all in use together. One consisted of counting by the years of the reigns of Emperors, in much the same manner as British Acts of Parliament are still dated. The second depended upon reckoning by a period of indeterminate length and dating from some important event after which the period was named. The third and final system is generally termed the 'sexage-

nary cycle', and utilised periods of sixty years. It could be adapted, however, to designate cycles of months and days, and was the system used for calendar indications by clockwork.

Clocks made by native craftsmen in Japan fell into three broad classes, two of which, although not strictly comparable with any Western counterpart, are frequently categorised by the same stylistic terms.

The first style, which is usually called a 'lantern' clock, covers any weight-driven clock supported on a stand on the floor or on a bracket, or suspended by a loop. Its sides are encased by plates, not unlike the European clock which is known by the same name, and it is surmounted by a bell. This is the oldest style of Japanese clock; it was made continuously from the early seventeenth century until the whole mode of timekeeping was changed in 1873, the only development of significance being from about 1830 when changes to the structure occurred as a result of the desire to increase the area available for decoration. The stands for such clocks varied from a truncated cone to a more table-like version with cabriole legs, in every case the weights hanging inside it and clearly visible.

Portable spring-driven clocks enclosed within a glazed wooden case, and resting either upon a bracket or a suitable piece of furniture, are sometimes designated 'bracket clocks'. Drummond

218

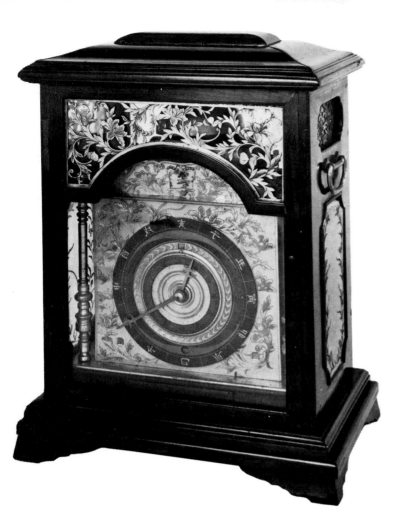
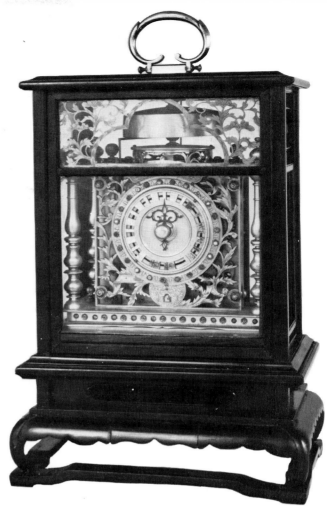

Robertson did not consider that any of those he had encountered had been made prior to about 1830. Much embellishment was lavished upon the visible plates of the movements of these clocks, and most of them have a wheel balance and a balance spring. The striking system is also peculiar, in that it is a compromise between locking-plate and rack striking, using elements of both.

Finally, there is the weight-driven 'pillar clock', to which no European clock even approximates, so called because it was long, narrow, very lightly constructed and could be attached to the main upright of a building in a wholly unobtrusive way which the Japanese, with their delight in unoccupied space, would not find offensive. This was the cheapest quality clock of the three styles, and also seems to have been introduced about 1830. It varies in length from one to four feet, with the movement contained in a glazed box at the top, and the pillar or column below the movement is hollow. The weight moves up and down inside this structure, and a pointer attached to it, which projects through a slit running the length of the front of the column, indicates the time against movable division marks, permitting adjustment as necessary for the variable periods of night and day. The remarkable feature of such clocks is that, at first sight, their construction could not conceivably permit of any striking mechanism. This deficiency was overcome by the ingenious expedient of using

the striking train as the weight to drive the going train. It was then only necessary to fit each division mark with an internal pin which unlocks the train as the weight reaches it. There were, nevertheless, certain drawbacks to the system, the solutions to which are regrettably much clumsier than the original concept.

The necessity for frequent alteration of the calibrations of the clock in Japan produced some interesting devices which will not be found on any Western timekeepers. Several of these depended upon the special characteristics of the foliot balance, which was retained for at least two centuries after it had been abandoned elsewhere in the world. Thus one early form of clock had no provision for maintaining Japanese time other than by the unsubtle and inconvenient method of moving the weights on the foliot arms every sunrise and sunset.

The obvious system for coping with a situation like this was by movable hour divisions, and further to facilitate additional complications like striking, these were usually located upon a rotating hour circle which indicated the time against a fixed pointer. The hour markers themselves were planted friction-tight in a groove running around the circle so that their relative positions could be adjusted at will. Each had a pin projecting from its back, so that as the divisions were moved, the pins inevitably moved with them. Then, when the hour

219

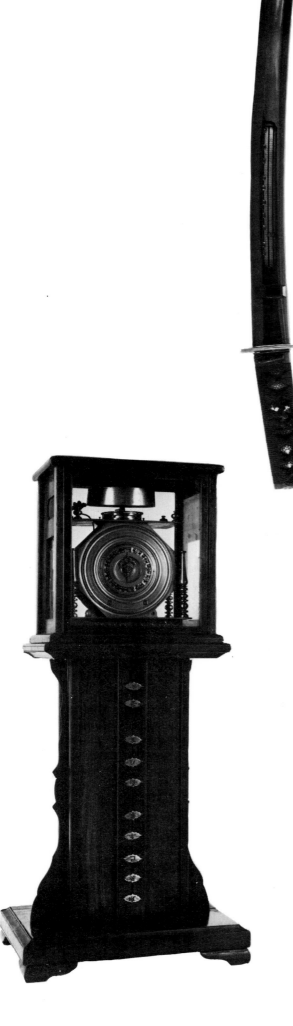

circle rotated, the pins as they passed the fixed pointer would release the striking train, and the hour would sound.

Towards the end of the seventeenth century probably the most ingenious approach to this problem was evolved. This required two entirely separate verges and foliots, one for the day and one for the night; each verge was linked to its own escape wheel, but these were mounted back to back upon a common arbor, and effectively each escapement was capable of being engaged with or disengaged from the going train by means of a flexible mounting for the lower pivots of the verges. The change-over was performed automatically twice a day by the clock itself, simply by means of a cam actuated by the locking-plate. All that was necessary then was to set up the weights on each foliot to reproduce the rate required for the day and night hours of the current half-month – that was the period during which they remained constant. The clock did the rest.

Although it sounds cumbersome, so was the time-measuring system employed by the Japanese – and despite the clear advantages, if only in terms of convenience of operation, of the double foliot arrangement, single foliot clocks were still being made in Japan well into the nineteenth century. The Japanese, as a result, probably developed the foliot controller to as great a degree of proficiency as it was inherently capable of attaining; the arms, for example, generally have between thirty and thirty-five notches, often with engraved gradations for ease of adjustment. Such clocks, even so, usually required winding twice a day.

The striking trains of Japanese clocks indicated the six primary divisions of day and night – counting backwards from nine to four – and occasionally there will be found provision for striking a half-division. The locking-plate system adapted quite easily to this, remembering that it could only be unlocked when the movable hour divisions on their rotating dial reached their correct position oppo-

left
Described by Drummond Robertson as a 'fancy' clock, this Japanese timepiece is a combination of the lantern and pillar clock, and reading the time by either method is possible. British Museum, London.

above
Another so-called 'fancy' clock, this example might better be described as a sword clock. The principle is much the same as a pillar clock. British Museum, London.

right
This clock has a double foliot, a steel striking movement and a brass case engraved with flower sprays. The wooden stand is decorated with lacquer. British Museum, London.

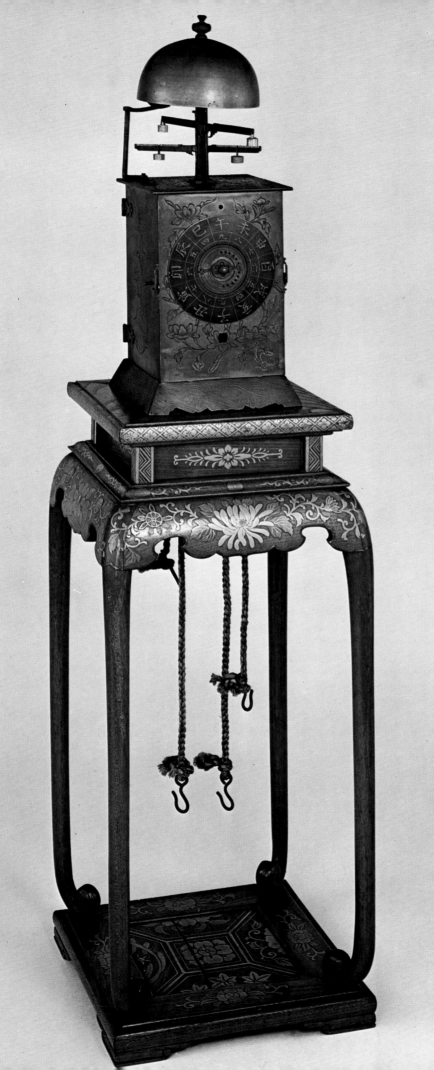

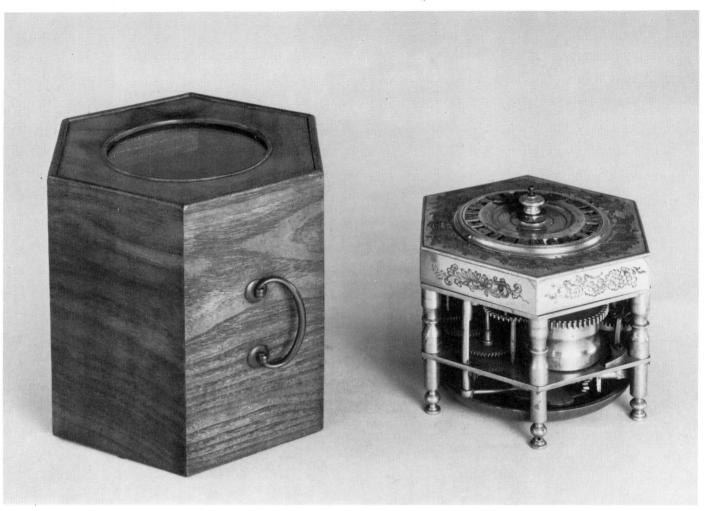

A hexagonal travelling clock with wood outer case, this timepiece is only 3in wide. British Museum, London.

below
Described as a 'doctor's clock', this timekeeper is one of the nearest Japanese equivalents to a watch. The extreme outer measurements including the protective Shitân-wood case, are about 5½in x 1in. The movement is spring-driven with a balance. British Museum, London.

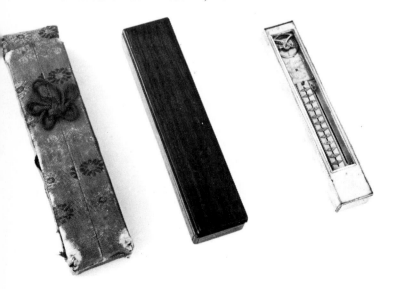

site the fixed pointer. Alarm trains and calendar-work were sometimes added, but not until after about 1700. The former utilised that primitive but nonetheless effective means by which a peg is inserted in the appropriate hour division at which the alarm is required to go off, and when the correct moment is reached the peg trips the alarm train.

Japanese timepieces are hardly ever signed or dated; and the use of specific materials in the construction is of little help as a guide to dating. The national garment, the kimono, provided no receptacle capable of housing anything like a pocket watch as it is known in the Western world, although small portable clocks disguised to resemble the inro, or medicine box, and attached to the girdle are known. There are other versions of tiny clocks, spring-driven naturally, which may have been carried similarly; and indeed, although attention has been principally focussed upon the three common categories of Japanese domestic clock, other styles – which Drummond Robertson refers to as 'fancy clocks' – will occasionally be found. Similarly, the Japanese seemingly made some large astronomical and other complicated and specialised clocks, but they must be so rare that it is unlikely one will ever be encountered.

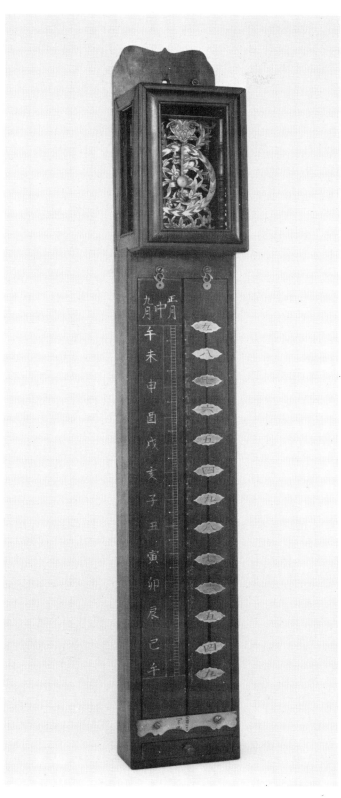

An elaborate example of the pillar clock with two time scales, one fixed and one moveable. At the top, the skeletonised movement is enclosed in a glazed Shitân-wood hood. British Museum, London.

right
In another development of the Japanese lantern clock, the weights are enclosed within a pedestal case such as this one in red lacquer. British Museum, London.

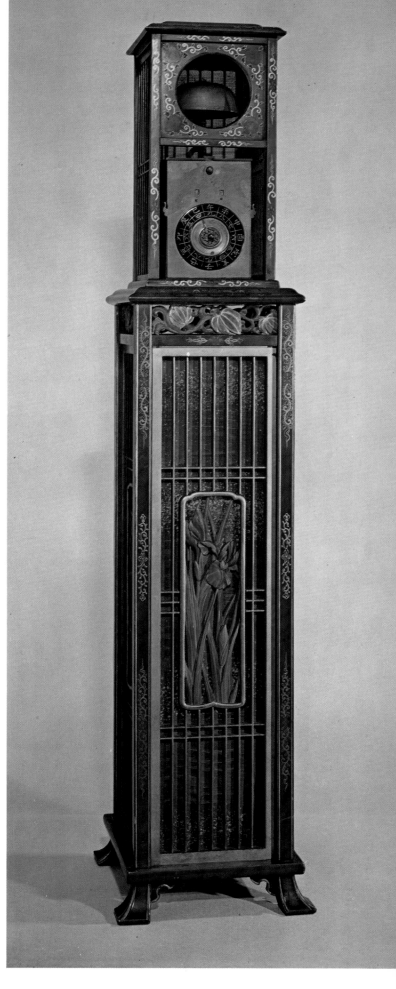

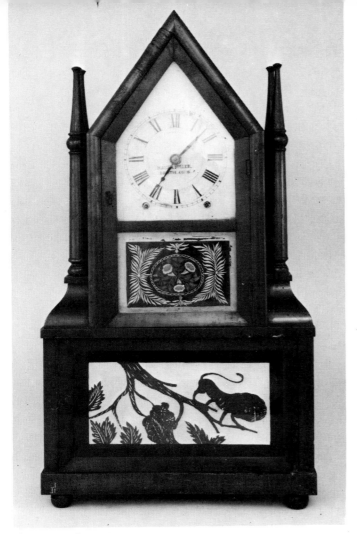

America

The most important single feature of the American horological heritage must be its single-handed pioneering development of mass-production methods, which were subsequently and so successfully adopted by the Swiss. Nevertheless, there was a craft tradition in America long before quantity and standardisation became important criteria in the field of horological manufacture.

The dividing line, very roughly, is the year 1800. Before that time, isolated craftsmen working very much in the English tradition, made some remarkably fine clocks, mainly longcases, and generally employing wood for both case and movement since brass was a scarce and expensive commodity. Among the earliest clockmakers working in America may be mentioned Abel Cottey, who set up in Philadelphia in 1682 and developed a considerable business making clocks that, with their flat-topped hoods, were indistinguishable from their English predecessors. In fact, Philadelphia and surrounding areas became well-known for clocks throughout the eighteenth century, as production gradually expanded. The second quarter of that century saw the introduction of break-arch dials and shallow domed tops, the cases themselves remaining largely undecorated. Then, from about 1760, the English provincial style of hood surmounted by curling 'horns' became popular

and remained in vogue throughout the rest of the century. Towards the end of that time, however, a kind of cresting of irregular outline was introduced, known colloquially as 'whale's-tails'. As brass became more readily available, the custom arose for thirty-hour duration movements still to be made of wood, but eight-day and longer-running mechanisms were fashioned in the more expensive material.

While the War of Independence (1775–83) was being fought, clockmaking in America came to a sudden halt, the craftsmen presumably being better occupied in other ways. However, when life returned to normal again, the longcase clock was now thought something of an extravagance – it was certainly expensive by the standards of those times – and a number of makers occupied themselves with the problem of producing a smaller and less costly timekeeper for ordinary domestic use. Hitherto American clockmaking had very much followed the English pattern, but now for the first time the Americans were on the point of creating a wholly native style, which in various manifestations was to remain popular for a long time to come.

There are four major types of American clocks, and at this point it will be useful to list them. The tower clock takes precedence, as being the earliest type of clock of which there are records, apart from a few domestic clocks that had been imported. There are any number of seventeenth- and eighteenth-century references to tower clocks, and as the years rolled by various famous names in American clockmaking history added such clocks to the repertoire of their manufactures. These included such giants as Simon Willard, Eli and Samuel Terry, and Seth Thomas.

Next come tall clocks, the American terminology for the English longcase. As has been mentioned Pennsylvania predominated in this particular manufacture, although such clocks were made all over the eastern seaboard. The earliest had metal dials about ten and a half inches square; lack of decoration throughout can probably be attributed to Quaker influence. Later, the dials became even larger. A derivation of the tall clock, often called the dwarf tall clock despite the apparent contradiction in terms, attained a height of not more than four feet. Very few seem to have been made, mainly in the early nineteenth century.

The third type of American clock is the wall clock. This came in a number of different shapes and styles, the earliest being the so-called 'wagon-wall'; such clocks are, to all intents and purposes, tall clock movements without any casing. Then came the 'banjo' clock, a style which, at its best, is both graceful and functional; many connoisseurs hold this to be the greatest artistic achievement by the Americans in the field of horology. The 'lyre' clock is much like the style just

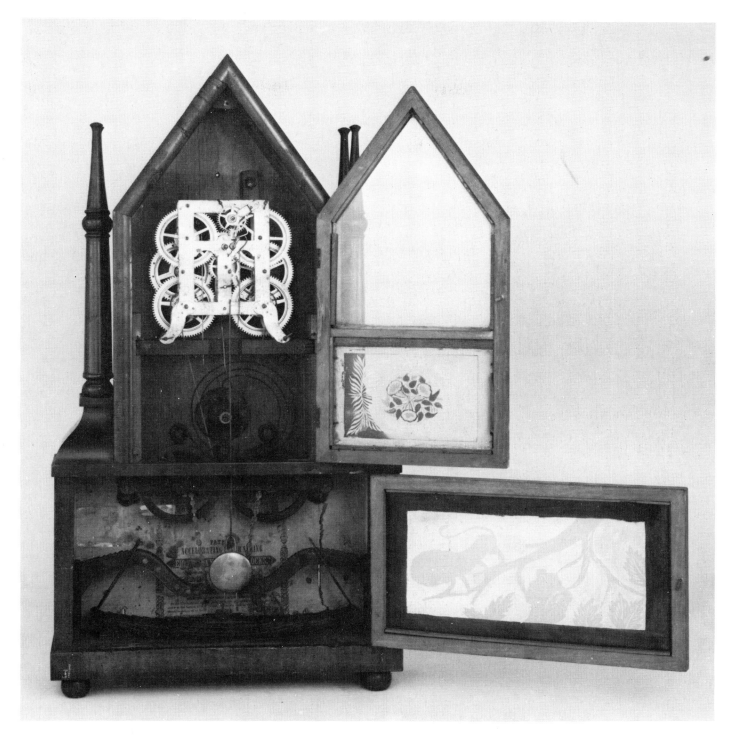

mentioned except that its trunk is shaped like a lyre, while the 'girandole' has a circular base where the 'banjo' has a rectangular one.

Lastly, the American shelf clock derived directly from the early American producers' desire to find a more convenient and less expensive substitute for the tall clock. The earliest were made by the Willards and others after the War of Independence, while perhaps the finest development of this style was that introduced by Eli Terry in 1817 and known as the 'pillar and scroll' clock. Another clock style which, at its best, has an unsophisticated, even naive, attractiveness that is completely

opposite page
Made by Birge & Fuller of Bristol, Connecticut, about 1835, this style is known as the 'steeple on steeple'. The eight-day movement is driven by a wagon spring. British Museum, London.

above
This view of the movement of the steeple clock shows the wagon spring, which is flexed when the clock is wound up. British Museum, London.

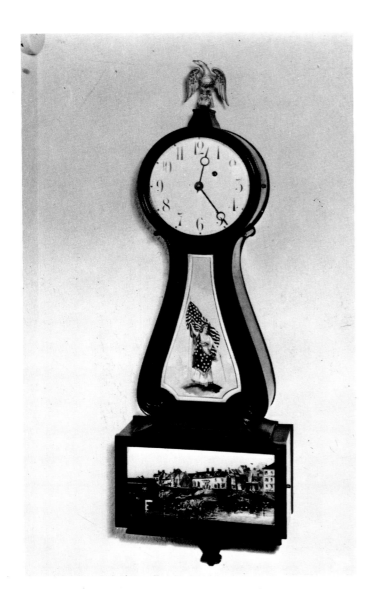

Lyre clock, a variant of the banjo clock, made in the first quarter of the nineteenth century.

unique, the 'pillar and scroll' was as subject to the transience of fashion as any other artefact, and from a peak of popularity in 1825 it went into a decline, being replaced in the 1830s by the so-called 'bronze looking-glass clock' for the invention of which Chauncey Jerome claimed credit. At about this time, too, there appeared the OG clock, the name deriving from the wavelike moulding ('ogee') of its rectangular case; this continued to be made until 1914. It was the largest-selling product of the Connecticut branch of the industry.

It is a curious reflection on the state of the industry in America during the last century that even shelf clocks had to be weight-driven until 1845, when springs became available as a power source at reasonable cost. From that moment on, individual makers marketed a stream of different styles dictated by their own whims and, doubtless, by local demand. There are far too many of these for anything like a comprehensive list to be given in the space available, but among the more popular may be mentioned the steeple clock, the beehive, and the acorn. Finally, there came the age of novelty – 'gimmickry' might be the best description to use – during the last two decades of the century. Negro automata figures with blinking eyes, and rejoicing in such titles as 'Topsey' and 'Sambo', clocks with conical pendulums, clocks in which the escapement causes a piece of weighted thread to wind and rewind itself continuously round a post, clocks in 'Marblized' cases somewhat resembling the Victorian attachment to polished slate – these and a host of others heralded the aesthetic decline of the American clock business, although doubtless it continued to be profitable.

Before turning to American watches, mention must be made of the phenomenon of mass-production and the key American figures in the clock industry concerned with it. Eli Terry (1772–1852), already referred to in connection with the 'pillar and scroll' clock, was the first man to produce cheap clocks in quantity, at first with wood but later with brass movements. In 1806, he took upon himself the production of a single order for four thousand clocks and devised not only the factory to make them in, but also the sales techniques for distributing and retailing them. In fact, he changed the whole system of clock purveying of those days in which, first, the clock was ordered and only then was it made by hand and sold to the client. Henceforth, clocks were to be made first, then ordered and sold subsequently. This was an important milestone in the commercial development of America.

The secret was that machines making identical parts could produce a hundred in the time it would take a craftsman to make one. At the peak of Terry's production of his 1806 order, clocks were being made at the rate of about sixty a day. Not only did Terry continue to develop his own quantity production and aggressive selling methods, but other inventive craftsmen were not slow to follow in his wake. Hydraulic power was used extensively to drive machinery, and by the 1820s clockmaking was at the peak of its boom, so much so that clocks were used in place of money as a form of currency. Even houses could be bought for sufficient clock movements. But inevitably the tide turned; by 1837, depression conditions brought clockmaking to a complete standstill and terminated for ever the demand for the wooden clock movement.

Boom conditions returned again the following year, however, after the introduction of yet another low-priced model, and by 1845 Connecticut clocks

A product of the Forestville Manufacturing Company is this 'acorn' clock of about 1850. British Museum, London.

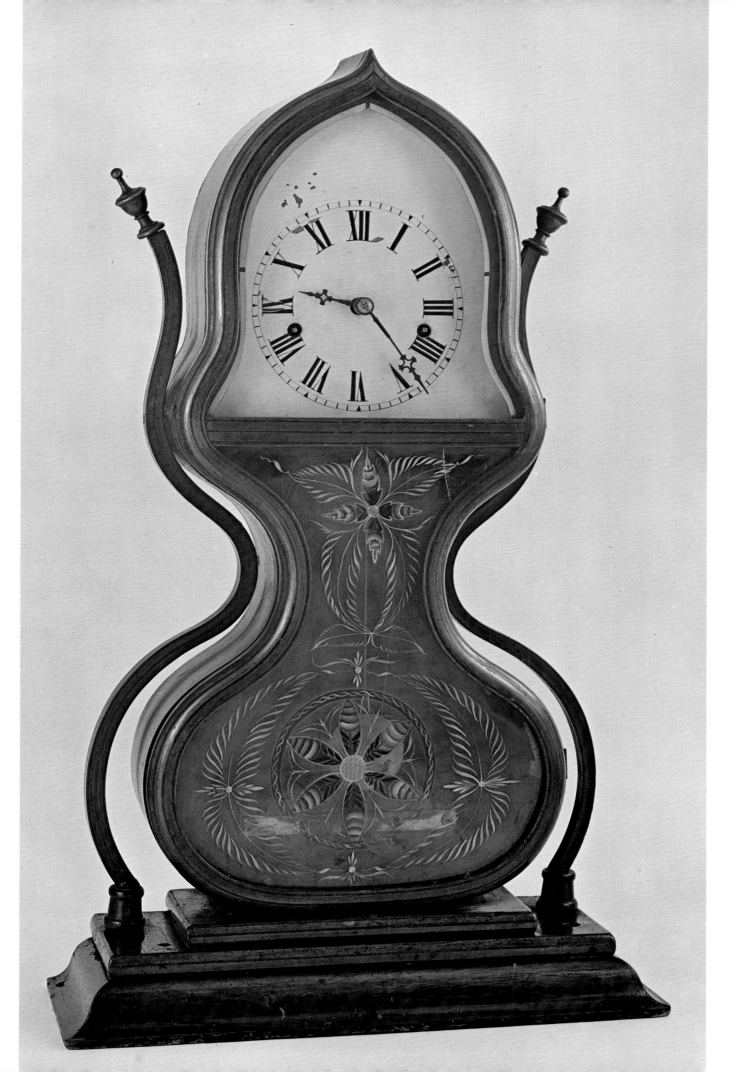

had cornered the market with an output of nearly one million clocks a year. This period saw the introduction into England of cheap brass weight-driven shelf clocks from the factories of one Chauncey Jerome, a leading Connecticut maker. This very prosperous period continued until 1857 when financial panic brought about another well-known manifestation of American commercial and industrial enterprise, consolidation. Clockmaking started to become concentrated within fewer and larger units, a trend that has continued to the present time. There are many illustrious names in

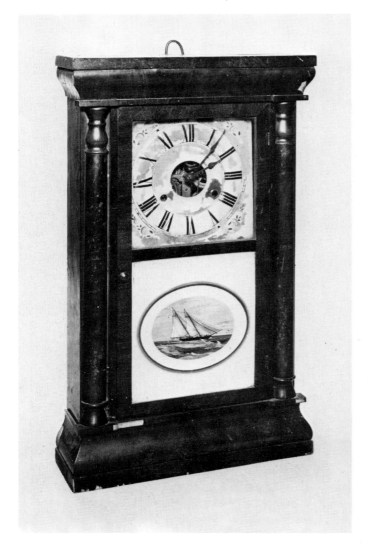

Shelf clock made by Seth Thomas about 1840 in Thomaston, Conn.

right
A fine banjo clock of about 1840 by A. Willard jr. American Museum in Britain, Claverton Manor, Bath.

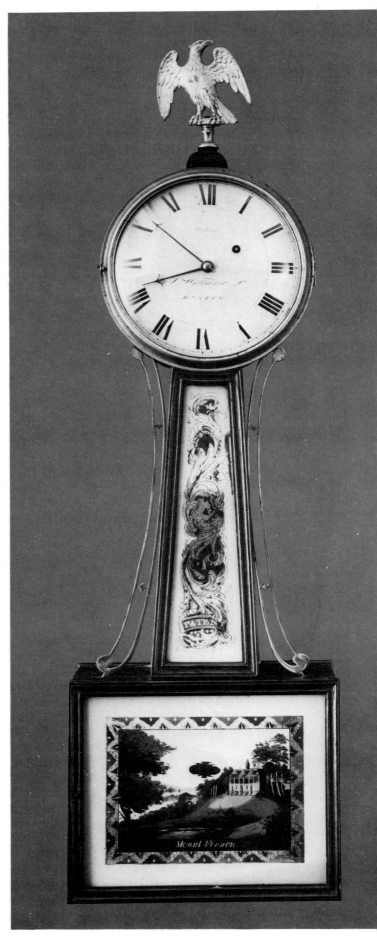

228

American clockmaking from both before and after the introduction of quantity production on factory lines. The Willards, Simon and Aaron, made many fine clocks of various styles, of which their 'banjo' is perhaps the most revered. Simon is said to have produced some four thousand of this model between 1802 and 1840. Gideon Roberts made another kind of wall clock, the 'wag-on-wall', in quantity and owned an assembly plant in Richmond, Virginia, after 1800; but it is not yet determined whether he used mass-production principles for his manufactures. Seth Thomas brought even greater commercialism to bear in the industry by buying the rights to certain patented designs of clocks from such as Eli Terry and producing them in quantity. He founded the Seth Thomas Clock Company in Plymouth, Connecticut, in 1853 employing some nine hundred operatives; the firm exists to this day.

The story of watchmaking in America is shorter – if no less dynamic – than that of clock manufacture. Although precise evidence is somewhat lacking, it would appear that, prior to about 1850, there was little native production in America, and those watches that survive are nearly always European imports even if they may have American names on the dials and movements. It is possible, too, that parts were brought into the country, and the assembly and finishing carried out locally. There is a record of a factory in Norwich, Connecticut, belonging to Thomas Harland, that is said to have produced two hundred watches and forty clocks annually, around 1800, but none of them is now known to exist. Luther Goddard is the first big name in American watchmaking. He began making watches in Shrewsbury, Massachusetts, in 1809 to counteract a shortage produced by tariff restrictions on the imported product and continued until a couple of years after the embargo was lifted in 1815, when he found himself no longer able to compete with the excessively low prices, whereupon he returned to gospel preaching. Even so, it has never been discovered whether his business – in which he certainly employed other watchmakers – was mainly that of assembling foreign-made parts, or whether the whole manufacture took place on American soil. A second attempt to quantity-produce watches – they only made between eight hundred and one thousand altogether – was started by the brothers Henry and J. F. Pitkin between 1837 and 1841. They started in East Hartford and finished in New York City. Jacob Custer of Norristown, Pennsylvania, is also reputed to have made a number of watches in 1843.

But the real start of the American mass-production watch came in 1850 with the founding of the Waltham Watch Company by Edward Howard and Aaron Dennison. They designed special machinery for volume production and laid the

The 'OG' clock is so named because of the ogee configuration of the wooden moulding in which it is framed. This eight-day example was made by E. N. Welch Manufacturing Company of Forestville, Connecticut. It was clearly made with export to Britain in mind, since it attempts to portray the royal arms in its lower panel.

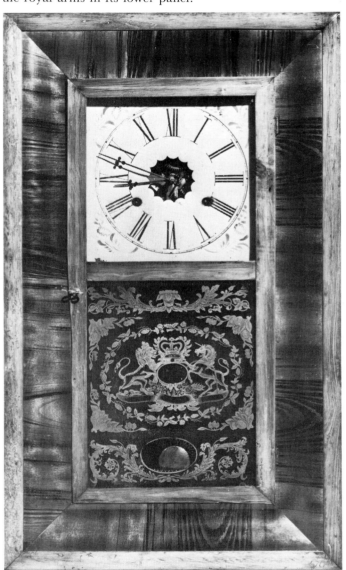

basis of a business which survived successfully for exactly one hundred years, closing down in 1950. Another famous watch 'name', Elgin, started life in 1864 as the National Watch Company (of Elgin, Illinois), but pressure from the consuming public is said to have caused the incorporation of the location into the firm's name in 1874. It continued to make fine watches until the early 1960s.

Such watches as these were by no means cheap, however, and American brilliance next applied itself to the design and mass-production of the really inexpensive commodity. The Auburndale

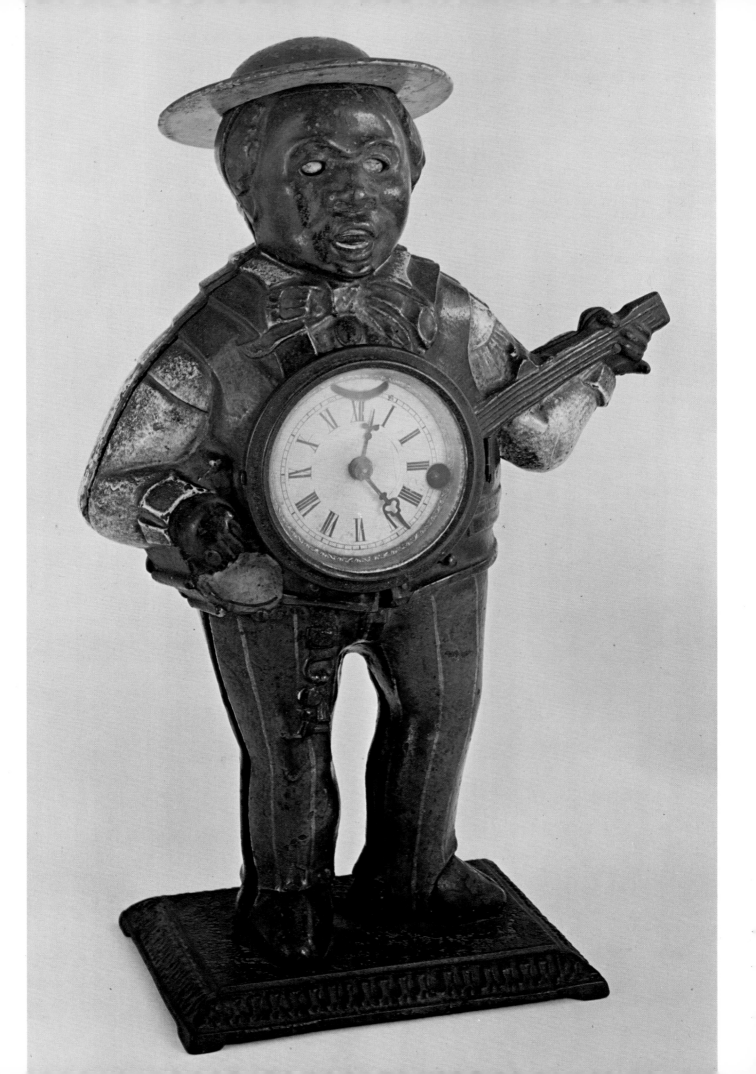

Watch Company, first in the field in 1875, made a watch to sell for about fifty cents, but this attempt failed. Then in 1880 the Waterbury Watch Company started to produce watches well-known by that name to every collector; by the time that that design was discontinued, in 1891, total production had exceeded one million. Finally, of course, R. H. Ingersoll and his brother initiated the famous 'dollar watch' in 1892. There were many other adventurous attempts to mass-manufacture watches during the last quarter of the nineteenth century, and most met with inevitable failure. One famous maker that survives to the present time but which started in 1892 is the Hamilton Watch Company.

The story of horology in America is one of development and exploitation of the mass market immediately that this became a profitable expedient. It may be significant, in this context, that America had no real craft tradition to withstand – had it so chosen – this course of events, as happened in England. Also, of course, it followed exactly the same pattern as occurred in other industries, even though clocks were the first peacetime product to be so affected; there is a marginally earlier American mass-production contract for war material. If the self-evident contrast with the course of events in Japan may seem to be extreme, it is no more than a clear demonstration of the proposition with which this chapter commenced – that is to say, that the bands of the horological spectrum, on a global view, take such an infinity of shapes and forms, and the concepts range over such a variety of ingenious inventions, as to make the mastery of the entire field, in all its minutest detail, both a physical and an intellectual impossibility. Within that one limitation, the interest generated by this subject can be enormous and exceptionally enjoyable.

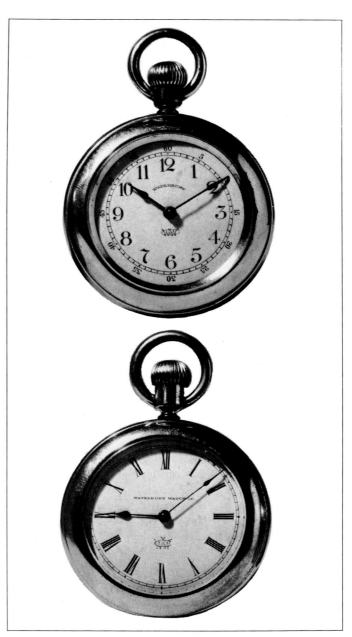

above
Early attempts to mass-produce cheap watches are represented by these examples of the series E and F produced by the Waterbury Watch Company in the last two decades of the nineteenth century. Series E (top) has the famous 'longwind' 9ft spring, requiring 140 half-turns of the button to wind the watch fully. Series F (below) was the first series using a spring of normal length.

right
The 'Yankee' was a very early model designed by R. H. Ingersoll, and it was made by the Waterbury Watch Company to be sold for $1. Museum of the Worshipful Company of Clockmakers, Guildhall, London.

left
Widely known as a 'Sambo' clock, this replica of an American 'nigger minstrel' is in a painted cast iron case with eyes that move in time with the escapement. It dates from about 1875. British Museum, London.

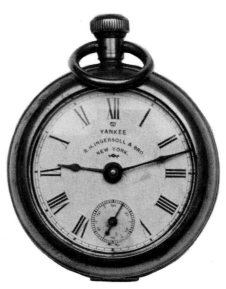

Collectors and Collecting

Now, in the mid 1970s, antiquarian horology as a hobby and pastime, and involving varying degrees of serious study on the part of its proponents, is big business. The world's great auction houses, but perhaps especially those in London, New York and Geneva, handle many thousands of pounds' worth of artefacts and related literature in this category each year, and membership of learned societies devoted to the subject continues to grow by leaps and bounds.

But it has not always been so. Until about twenty years ago, the number of serious collectors in England – to give one example – could almost be counted on the fingers of two hands. Many people believe that a significant side effect of the Second World War was a speeding-up in the steady decline of the hand-made article, and that one aspect of horology that gives it such a wide appeal today is that it can put back into appreciative hands objects that have been made individually, with great care and craftsmanship, and which consequently possess some indefinable but nonetheless recognisable characteristics not to be found in the wholly machine-made commodity. Such a phenomenon – a widespread hunger for the craftsman-made as opposed to the mass-produced article – manifests itself in many other directions at the present time and, when related to new goods, has of necessity become increasingly expensive to assuage.

In England, at different times, horology has been the fashionable recreation of kings. Charles II concentrated his attention upon Edward East's watches and the establishment of Greenwich Observatory, as we have seen, while George III built his own Royal Observatory at Kew, on the outskirts of London, in 1769, and there has survived to the present day notes written in his own hand on the correct method of disassembling a watch. Apparently he was given instruction in such things when a young man, as part of his education; and he retained the great interest he thus acquired into later life, for not only did he commission the first watch with a lever escapement from Thomas Mudge, but he was also intimately concerned with John Harrison's chronometer experiments and himself tested H.5 at his observatory at Kew.

There were in the eighteenth century, too, a number of wealthy collectors and patrons of the arts who included clocks and watches incidentally in the 'cabinets' of curiosities and bygones which they assembled with such loving care: prominent among these was, of course, Sir Hans Sloane whose library and collections formed the nucleus from which the British Museum was established. This kind of general collecting has carried on, among the wealthiest of families, right to the present century with such remarkable accumulations as that assembled by John Pierpoint Morgan, the American financier and merchant banker, whose tastes embraced not only pictures, but ceramics, books, watches and other items of artistic value and interest. He was in his time – he died in 1913 – the greatest art collector in the world, and, in the field of horology, one of the great rarities among the literature on the subject is the *Catalogue* of the Morgan watch collection, which was sumptuously printed in a tiny edition in 1912. A mere forty-five copies of this *Catalogue* were produced on hand-made paper, and a handful more upon vellum, and they were all privately distributed to friends and to a few of the most important libraries. His watches are now in the Metropolitan Museum in New York.

It was probably not until the years between the two World Wars that the specialist horological collector really came into his own. To the older generation of collectors today, the magic names of Wetherfield, Iden, Prestige and others still conjure

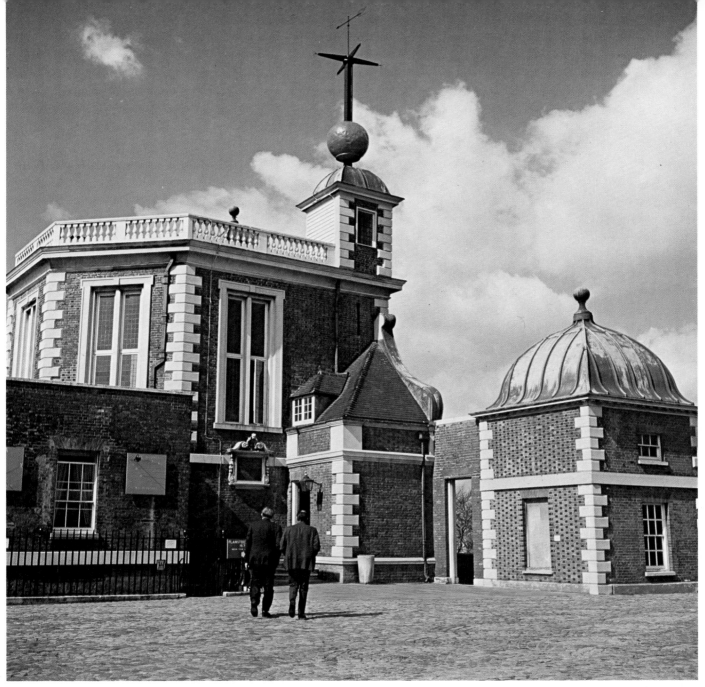

The heart of Old Greenwich Observatory is Flamsteed House, named after the first Astronomer Royal, appointed by Charles II in 1675. It contains the famous Octagon Room, on the roof of which is the Time Ball, a visual time signal installed in 1833. Royal Greenwich Observatory, as it is now called, moved to Herstmonceux Castle, in the heart of the Sussex countryside, in the early 1950s, since London's 'smog' made observational astronomy virtually impossible.

The Octagon Room, the focal point of the old Observatory, was fitted out with equipment by the best makers, including the pair of clocks with two-seconds pendulums by Thomas Tompion.

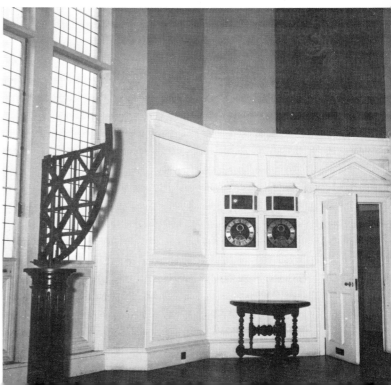

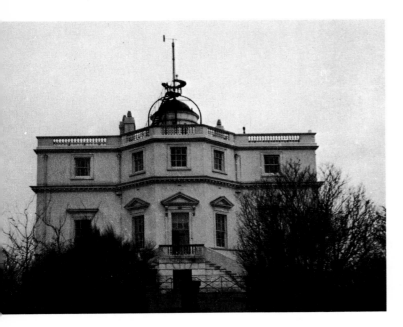

Founded by George III as his private observatory – for he was keenly interested in horology and allied sciences – Kew Observatory, in the Old Deer Park at Richmond, on the outskirts of London, has been used to rate timekeepers and issue performance certificates for them since 1885, a duty taken over by the National Physical Laboratory in 1912. More recently it has been a Meteorological Office.

up a stream of anecdotes and recollections of specific clocks and watches associated with their collections. These, too, are inevitably linked with the names of the great dealers of those days – Malcolm Gardner, the Websters father and son, James Oakes and others, not to mention the famous 'old school' of craftsmen restorers. Nowadays, however, the sheer weight of numbers of people fascinated by the subject, each striving to follow that particular one of its multitudinous threads which especially appeals to him, makes the emergence of any one personality as a subject for admiration, respect, envy, speculation or any of the other passions or emotions associated with ardent collecting, that much more unlikely. Many would feel some slight loss as a result; it is almost as if the craftsman-orientated collector had been converted into some kind of movement representing 'horology for the masses'.

Much is to be learnt, nevertheless, from any study of these single-minded student-collectors of the 1920s and the 1930s since, being so early in the field, they had a much wider spectrum of choice – especially if they had only limited means – than will ever be available again. Sometimes, too, their collections became so important as entities that it was obvious that they should be preserved in their entirety when their owners died. Such a collection was, of course, that formed by Courtenay Ilbert and now in the British Museum. Another that has been preserved complete and is located at his home town of Bury St Edmunds is that formed by the late Gershom Parkington, the famous cellist. Existing photographs of famous collectors of international status in their own surroundings are usually revealing, and it is important that they be preserved. Here we shall examine two such photographs, of a British and an American collector respectively.

Courtenay Adrian Ilbert has been mentioned sufficiently frequently to need little introduction. Born in 1888, he was educated at Eton and Cambridge, taking an honours degree in engineering, and then became professionally associated with a firm specialising in railways in India. During the Second World War he was engaged with the Ministry of Supply in that division dealing with the control of timber supplies. But principally, throughout his life from schooldays onwards, he was fascinated by horology and collected avidly. He was a man of retiring disposition, gentle and quiet but shrewd and, in his own way, both friendly and generous. His encyclopedic knowledge of horology became legendary in his own lifetime, as did his collection and supporting library, both without doubt the finest of their kind in the world of his day. He was generous in helping others of like interests with explanations illustrated by examples from among his own acquisitions, and frequently lent his greatest treasures for public exhibition, losing thereby on occasion when they came back from some overseas commitment deranged or damaged; yet he never grumbled. He lived in a large double-fronted Georgian house in Chelsea, in central London, which had been in his family for several hundred years. The clock room, which led off on the left of a large hallway, ran the full depth of the house, of which it had once clearly been the drawing-room. Although it was a large room by any standards, one had to pick one's way with the greatest care between the enormous number of 'exhibits' – of all shapes and sizes – which included a double line of clocks, placed back to back, and running the length of the room, all available wall-space being already occupied by others of the same species. The carillon clock by Nicholas Vallin of 1598, mentioned elsewhere in this book, was elevated upon a scaffolding in order to obtain a reasonable drop for the weights, and anyone wishing to inspect it closely had to do so by ladder. Yet another famous feature of Ilbert's clockroom was the huge chest of drawers – the type is generally described as a Wellington chest – in which he kept his working 'library' of watches. Its twenty-four drawers contained over one thousand specimens spanning three hundred years of watchmaking, and it was in constant use as a reference source when enquirers brought watches

right
One of the greatest collectors of this century, the American financier John Pierpoint Morgan published this catalogue of his watches which has become a great rarity on its own account.

234

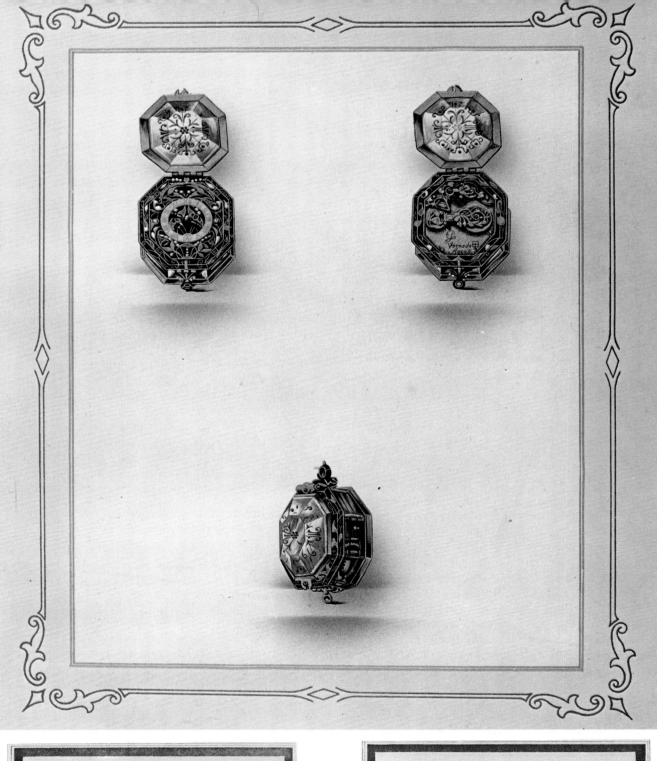

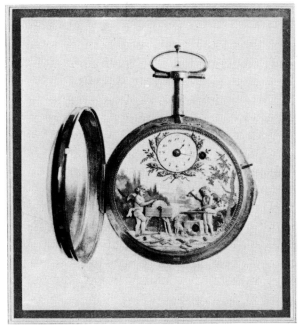

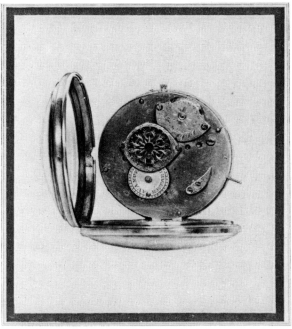

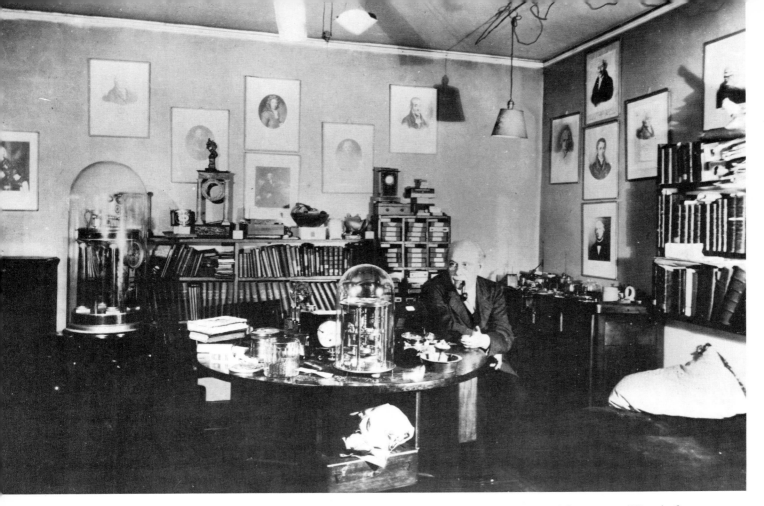

Major Paul Chamberlain, seen in his workroom. His bench has a brass plate upon its facing end bearing the name of Jules Jurgensen, a very celebrated Danish craftsman, and its original owner.

An outstanding feature of Courtenay Ilbert's famous collection of clocks and watches, now in the British Museum, was this giant chest of drawers, in which he kept his 'reference library' of over 1,000 watches and watch movements. As shown here, he used this constantly to identify timepieces brought to him.

to show him or dealers to sell to him. Ilbert enjoyed the friendliest relations with the trade at large, since he never tried to purchase behind their backs or outdo them at auctions. The result was that he was always given first refusal of anything of special interest that came on the market, and one dealer in particular – whom Ilbert had helped to establish himself – acted virtually as his agent. The two used to go on protracted purchasing expeditions abroad, especially in Europe where Ilbert made some remarkable discoveries.

Ilbert died in 1956 after a lengthy illness which, towards its climax, was both painful and excessively disabling. Yet his indomitable spirit enabled him to continue the work he loved right to the very end, even after he had to a substantial extent lost the power of speech. He had concerned himself with the production of a fresh edition of the clock and watch collector's 'bible' – Britten's *Old Clocks and Watches and their Makers* – as co-editor with two other eminent horologists, one of whom had already predeceased him. The finishing touches were put to the text only while he was confined to his bed in hospital, and it is a fitting memorial to such a man that at least some part of his enormous knowledge did find its way on to the printed page

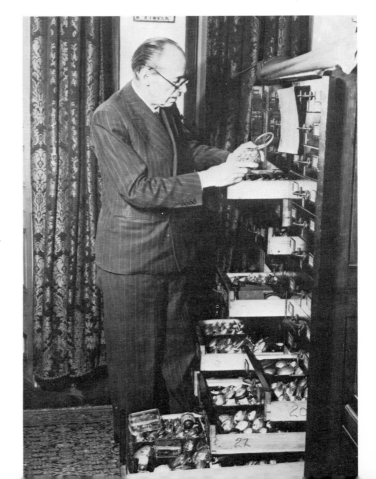

for the benefit of many who will always try, however unsuccessfully, to emulate him.

Major Paul Chamberlain, an American born in Three Oaks, a small town in the state of Michigan, in 1865 was, like Courtenay Ilbert, an engineer by profession. Educated at Michigan State College and Cornell University, he had established himself as a successful structural engineer by the advent of the First World War. He had also amassed a collection of some three hundred watches which, now that he had to turn his attention from his hobby to the exacting task of producing the much needed 75mm gun, he presented to the Chamberlain Memorial Museum in his home town. He subsequently prepared a detailed catalogue in which every item of this collection was described and classified.

When Chamberlain was finally demobilised from the army with distinction, his engineering practice had virtually disappeared, and his health was impaired sufficiently as to discourage him from attempting to rebuild it. He therefore turned the full force of his intellect and enthusiasm upon antiquarian horology, starting a second collection of watches which, when he died in 1940, numbered some twelve hundred specimens.

Thus, for a substantial number of years, Chamberlain lived in and for that special ambience of antiquarian horology which he constructed in his home in the Adirondacks and which became the staff of life not only to him but also to the many students in the field who visited him and came to regard his workroom almost as a shrine. There appeared in 1941 – sadly, he never lived to see it in print – what most horologists regard as a fitting epitaph, his book *It's About Time* which, without any shadow of doubt, is the most original and competent book on any aspect of antiquarian horology ever to emanate from the American continent. It reflects the travels far and wide of the author in search of material – in this respect, too, he resembled Ilbert – and also his interest in people, for he was able to cultivate the friendship and, inevitably, command the respect of leading craftsmen in many countries. He had a formidable memory which was well stocked with a bank of historical, technical and biographical detail, any minutest part of which he could instantly recall and from which, over some twenty-five years, he was able to formulate the many articles, certainly over one hundred, which he contributed to domestic and foreign trade and technical journals. In America, Chamberlain was regarded as just as great a horological guru as Ilbert was in Britain, yet both were modest, retiring men who would have been horrified at the thought of themselves as anything other than mere students and researchers, more experienced perhaps than the great majority of those who came to sit at their feet, but 'experts' never!

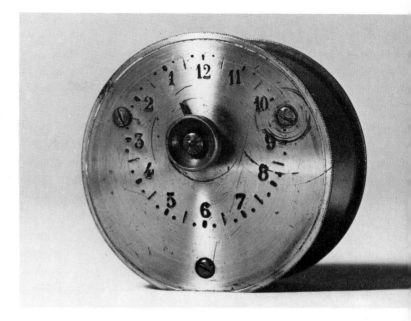

This small device – a mere 2½in in diameter and just over 1in thick – is an alarm mechanism of French origin, known as a 'reveille-matin' and made in enormous quantities by Antoine Redier in the mid nineteenth century. The pointer is turned to a figure corresponding with the difference in hours between the hour of setting and the alarm going off. A spring-driven train drives a tiny pendulum, gradually turning the hand back to zero – twelve o'clock – when the alarm sounds.

William Gossage, who died in 1877, became a famous industrial chemist, and his only horological patent, taken out in 1823, was for an alarm device which he is said to have needed to awake him at five o'clock in the morning to pursue his studies. His alarm is used in conjunction with a pocket watch, placed on top with its winding square fitted into a similarly squared pipe, connected to the mechanism. As the watch runs down, the pipe is turned and this, correspondingly, turns back the alarm dial to zero, when the bell sounds.

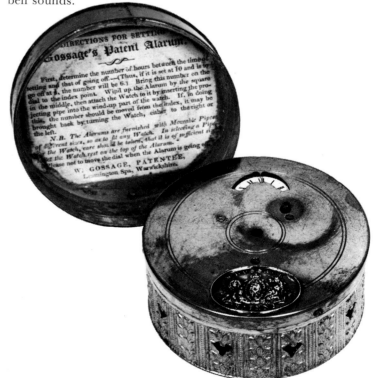

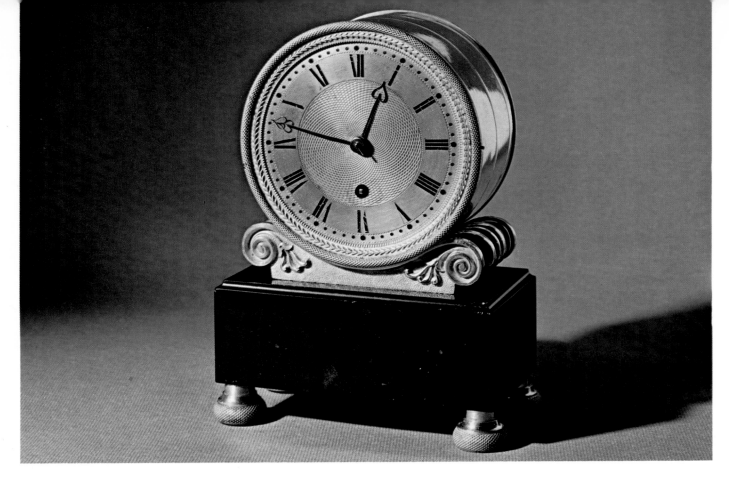

The environment with which such a man as Chamberlain surrounds himself and in which he can work best is well demonstrated by the photograph of him in his workroom – always, seemingly, called the Schoolroom, because it was constructed from the remains of a demolished schoolhouse and added, as an extension, on to his home. His workbench – he is facing away from it in the photograph – was originally the property of Jules Jurgensen, a nineteenth-century member of a very famous Danish family of craftsmen, who were based in Copenhagen and much respected by collectors everywhere. The brass nameplate on the side is just visible. At the left, clearly discernible under its glass shade, is his astronomical clock by an early nineteenth-century Paris maker who became famous for the handful of such clocks he made. His name was Raingo – nobody ever seems to have recorded any Christian name for him – and his surviving planetary clocks, a more appropriate description than just astronomical clocks, include specimens in the possession of the Queen and located at Windsor Castle, in the Sir John Soane Museum in London, and in the Musée des Arts et Métiers in Paris. The last-mentioned was incomplete when Raingo died, and it was finished by Paul Garnier, another famous French craftsman of the day.

Other elements which contribute to the sheer atmosphere of this photograph include the portraits of clockmakers on the walls, and even on this small scale, the faces of Ellicott, Graham, Tompion and Mudge can be clearly identified. Cham-

While hardly in the mass-produced range, this small clock by Payne, South Molton Street, London, is a delightful relic of Regency London which, because it is a timepiece only, will be somewhat less expensive than a clock with additional trains.

berlain possessed many books on horology in a variety of languages – some of which can be seen – and also collected old clock- and watchmaking tools, which, of course, he used. The lights, adjustable if in somewhat primitive manner, reflect precisely that air of disregard for everything but the mechanically important which so many of the old school of craftsmen adopted. Their workshops customarily dusty and, to the lay eye, untidy to the point of chaos, they yet knew where everything was and, in the tiny space upon their benches in which they actually worked – for the remainder of the work-top would be teeming with hand tools and other paraphernalia, in total disarray – they could turn out the most immaculate results, achieving fit and finish such as would never be believed possible simply by viewing their working conditions. Yet this is the way they liked it.

This photograph of Chamberlain's workroom acts as a good starting point for anybody surveying the horological scene today with, perhaps, a view to starting up a collection, even if only on modest lines. The Raingo clock is but one example of the many classes of antique clocks that have priced themselves out of the market so far as anyone but the wealthy is concerned – the figure fetched by one of his clocks when it was sold in Zürich in 1970,

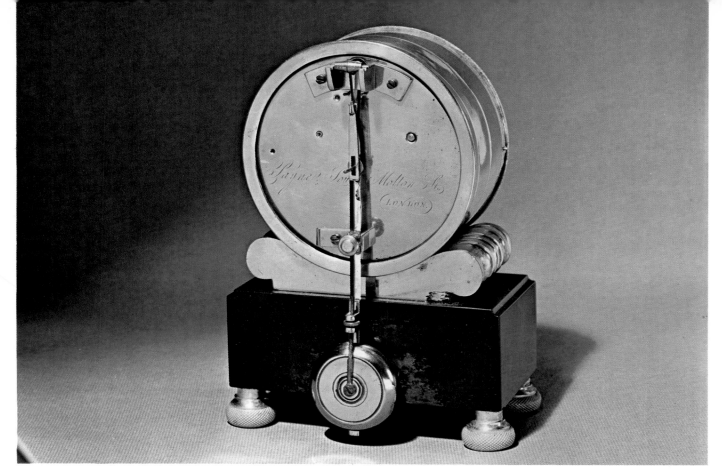

Seen from the back, the Payne clock shows obvious signs of quality, from the style of the pendulum to the provision of a capability to anchor it, when the clock is to be carried about. The movement is spring-driven, with a fusee and a duration of eight days.

when the peak of the market had by no means been reached, was 27,500 Swiss francs, and this was just for a *pendule de cheminée* – so that it can be disregarded for all practical purposes. Those who are sufficiently fortunate as to be able to muster the funds needed to acquire horological articles in the top flight of artistic and technical achievement for their collections have no need of advice from this book: they will without doubt be able to afford the professional advice of dealers and others who are active in the marketplace for such objects. Here it is the intention to deal with more moderately priced yet collectable items such as can still be found from time to time in the average antique shop or auction room. Some of the fringe items – that is to say, ephemera associated with clocks and watches rather than the timekeepers themselves – come up regularly in the bigger auction rooms, too, but as yet have not become popular enough to force up the price beyond the reach of the average small collector's purse.

So what clocks can such a novice collector of meagre means aspire to? It has to be recognised that, except for the magical exception that proves the rule, the seventeenth century is wholly out of court. So, too, is most of the eighteenth century except possibly for the odd and inevitably rather coarse provincial item.

The nineteenth century, however, offers some scope provided the collector does not aspire too high. English clocks of this period were, of course, still craft-made, and the Victorian over-elaboration of case that so many exhibit – although restraint in such details is by no means unknown – has taken on, in the appreciation of many connoisseurs, a kind of 'folksy' quaintness which makes them now far more widely accepted than ever before. Looking at Europe, the commonplace and, from the collector's point of view, once universally despised Vienna regulator nowadays fetches anything between one and two hundred pounds, but is an interesting and relatively unresearched subject for study, as is, too, the round French factory-made clock movement fitted into so many different kinds of case. Both are admirably functional as well as collectable. Black Forest clocks are not yet popular among collectors although they certainly merit attention, if only on account of the ingenuity of their wooden movements; but the early specimens are rather unlikely to be encountered and would probably make a good price if they were. The postman's alarm is a perfectly serviceable clock, simple though it is. Cuckoo clocks and similar extravagances – the other well-known style is the trumpeter clock – have a novelty value that perhaps serves to inflate their intrinsic worth for the average collector, especially if they can also be construed as 'antique'.

None of the clock styles mentioned so far has derived wholly from the true mass-production systems pioneered in the last century – even the

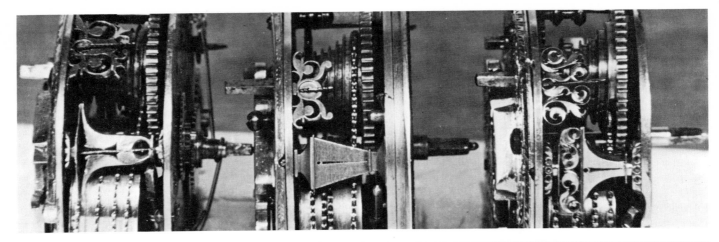

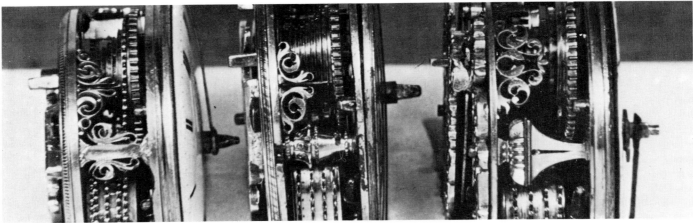

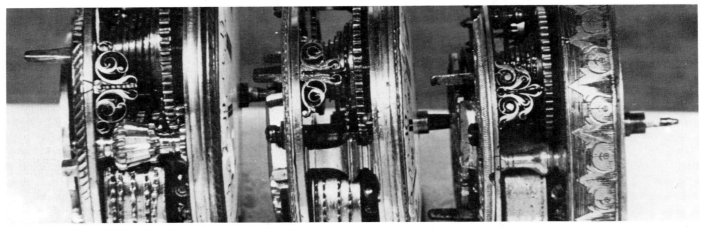

The plates of antique watch movements have customarily been separated by pillars which, at first comparatively plain, soon became the subject of embellishment. The potance, which is riveted to the underside of the plate and forms part of the fusee stop work, was also the subject of decoration, often elaborate, but not so varied in style as the pillars. Some of the many different designs of pillars are shown here (left to right, top to bottom): Tulip, Roman, Elaborated Roman; Ellicott, Decorated baluster (English provincial usage), Roman (Dutch version); Decorated baluster (Dutch version), Square baluster, Bombé baluster.

factory-made French round movement has its roots in the eighteenth century – so at some point a collector will start a fashion in this area. It could be profitable; mass-produced items are consumable and instantly replaced once they become even moderately unserviceable. Fashion, too, plays a large part. It is likely, therefore, that far fewer still survive than superficial consideration might suggest. The same thing applies as our survey of the field advances into the present century. The period before, during and for a few years after the First World War saw interesting things happening horologically: the folding travelling clock came into its own, often based on the so-called Goliath watch, and the wristwatch was in its initial stages of development. But it is very much an unexplored field up to now.

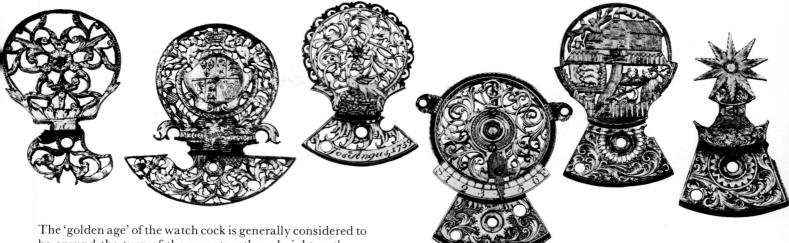

The 'golden age' of the watch cock is generally considered to be around the turn of the seventeenth and eighteenth centuries when the cock had reached both its largest size and the peak of its decorative style. As time passed, the cock tended to get smaller, and its decoration to degenerate, until eventually, following an experimental period in which various random shapes were employed for the table, it gradually settled into the plain wedge-shape which is common to the present time.

Clocks have hardly ever suffered that sad fate of so many thousands of watches, of being uncased for the sake of the melting value of the precious metal involved. However, their movements are sometimes found to have been rehoused in cases which the discriminating collector recognises as being so unrelated in period and anachronistic as to render them undesirable, and he may then impose an arbitrary divorce upon such an unhappy 'marriage'. If he cannot afford a reproduction case in the correct style, he may still run the movement on show, as an exhibition piece. The best practice does not accept the philosophy, therefore, that any case is better than none at all: if the case is blatantly inappropriate it will detract so very substantially from any merit the movement may possess. In this the pure layman might very well disagree, being possibly concerned more with the clock's function than with its original appearance.

So what about the multitude of watch movements, long since separated from their cases – the biggest melting-down of precious metal watch cases of all time took place in the great British Depression of the 1930s – which appear on the market with fair regularity? They make marvellously collectable objects, from all sorts of points of view. The mainly mechanically minded collector will want them, perhaps, to demonstrate the workings of various kinds of escapements, some common and not too expensive, others rare and rather costly, or to show the lay-out of different trains or the idiosyncrasies of particular makers. If a principal interest is in the decoration of the watch movement through the ages, then the watch cock and slide plate – the latter houses the balance

spring regulator – and also the pillars separating the plates of older movements will be the main focus of attention. Most such decorated movements might very well be relatively uninteresting mechanically: the verge escapement in watches went on for so many centuries that it is most unlikely to be collected on its own account, yet from the decorative viewpoint many such movements are highly desirable, displaying an enormous variety of styles and qualities of craftsmanship. National styles, too, can be well defined in this kind of collection.

Mention of the watch cock brings to mind the collector who specialises in this single component, on account of its intrinsic beauty or perhaps because of the huge variety of designs with which it has been decorated, or yet again because certain designs are very rare and therefore desirable. But how has it happened that so very many watch cocks have come to be separated from their movements – for they appear in large quantities from time to time in the sale rooms?

The answer is again to be found in the dreadful economic crisis of the 1930s. Watch cases were destroyed wholesale for their metal value, but antique watch movements had intrinsic value too. Although the basic structural materials were common metals like brass and steel, all visible brasswork, the plates, the wheels and decorative elements already mentioned like the pillars, cock and slide plate were gilded, and the gold thus deposited upon these surfaces could be recovered. The gilding process used, incidentally, bears no relationship to the electro-deposition commonplace today; it was variously called mercurial gilding, fire gilding or water gilding and consisted essentially of brushing on to the preheated brass surface a sponge-like amalgam of gold and mercury which had previously been prepared. When the amalgam had taken hold and a good surface obtained, the mercury was driven off as vapour by the application of more heat, leaving the gold

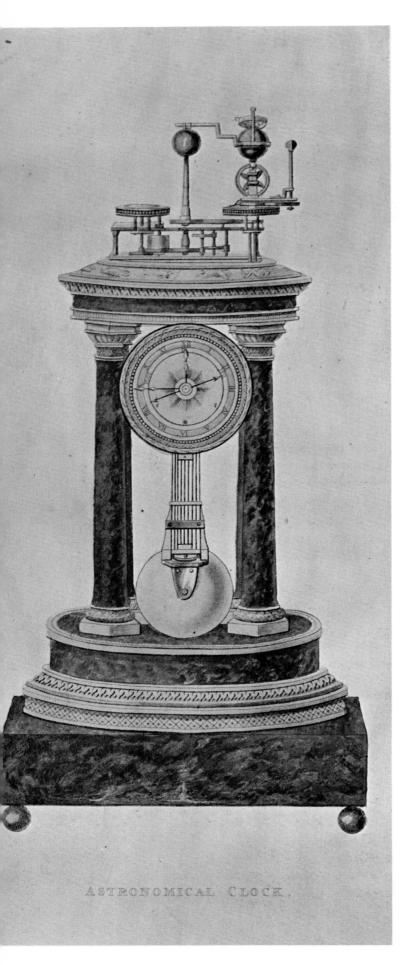

ASTRONOMICAL CLOCK.

'fired' on to the brass. The finish that can be obtained by this process cannot be duplicated by any other, according to enthusiasts; but it is a very hazardous one to carry out, since mercury vapour is an accumulative and highly toxic gas, and those who operated the process risked an abnormally high death rate.

So when bullion dealers melted watch cases nearly fifty years ago, they were also on the lookout for movements that would be worth scrapping for their gold content. The watch cock, however, being very highly decorated, was often separated from the rest of the movement and put aside, to be mounted up subsequently as a piece of jewellery. In consequence, many watch cocks reappeared as necklaces, brooches and the like, and collectors today will frequently go to some trouble to have such items reconstituted and all traces of mounting-up removed, so that the cocks can take their rightful places again as intricate and often beautiful examples of handiwork, upon which the

left
This hand-coloured print from the *Repository of the Arts*, published by R. Ackermann in 1824, illustrates one of Raingo's famous astronomical clocks. A similar one can be identified under its glass dome to the left of the picture of Chamberlain's workshop.

below
The keys forming the main feature of this illustration are mounted upon a gold 'Albert' chain, which is now intended for use as a bracelet, an example of the tendency to make items of jewellery out of such objects. Styles to be found in this circle include the plain crank key – said to be one of the earliest forms – the folding crank, the continental decorated crank key, and a variety of other later forms. In the centre are male and female versions of the Breguet or 'tipsy' key, while on the other side, and bordering the picture, are eight steel Victorian keys in virtually mint condition, all found together in the same old-established London jeweller's shop, where they may well have stayed since first being taken into stock.

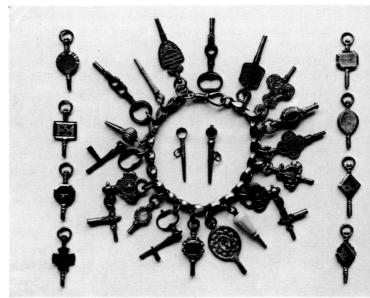

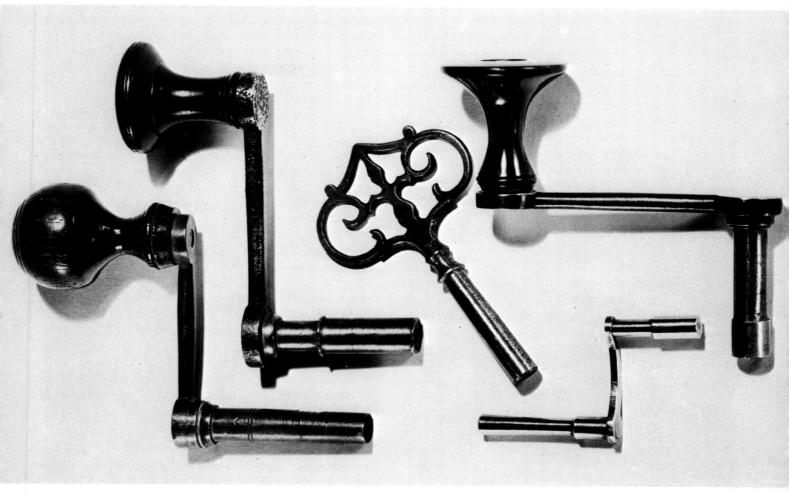

Cranked keys for clocks are customary for the conventional longcase and bracket designs, and these usually have a turned wooden handle. The wholly brass cranked key comes from a Vienna regulator, while the steel cast key with pierced plate is a mass-produced late nineteenth-century key.

greatest skill has been lavished. Much of this work, it is thought, was done by women; and, even in Tompion's day, the specialist watch cock maker charged substantial sums for the finest examples of his work.

Much speculation has focussed upon the source of the designs incorporated into watch cock decoration. No two cocks will ever be found to be identical, but the differences are often so slight that they can only be attributed to individual hand-working, and one celebrated collector in this field, a few years ago, reckoned to have amassed over forty cocks which were clearly based on the same original design. This suggests that watch cock makers may have had pattern books – in the same way as decorative engravers did – from which to work, but although a few such items have survived in other European countries, evidence of an equivalent English practice is so far rather limited.

A separate book could easily be based upon watch cock decoration: the motifs, ranging from geometric to pictorial, from 'inhabited foliage', as the auctioneers describe it, to all kinds of arabesques, from grotesque masks to mythical birds and beasts, reflects a vast gamut of invention. Then there is the matter of symmetry on either side of an imaginary line through the centre of the cock table; at certain periods this is popular, at others not. In the later stages of the development of the watch cock, all sorts of strange shapes of cock table were tried out. The conventional circular table gave place to squares, rectangles, stars, crowns and a host of others that defy easy description. By contrast, in the earlier stages, around the turn of the seventeenth century, strangely shaped features, generally described as 'wings', projected from the neck of the cock. Cocks can be found into which the balance spring regulator has been integrated, so that, to operate it, the whole centre of the cock table must be rotated. The index, or pointer, is fixed to this table and indicates the degree of regulation against a scale engraved upon the wide neck of the cock. Most watch cocks are made of brass that has been fire-gilt. The use of silver as a decorative metal for watch movements is found, but has never been common; silver cocks, as a result, are scarce and sought after. The decorative content of a watch cock is sometimes important. On either side of the year 1700, for instance, watch cocks

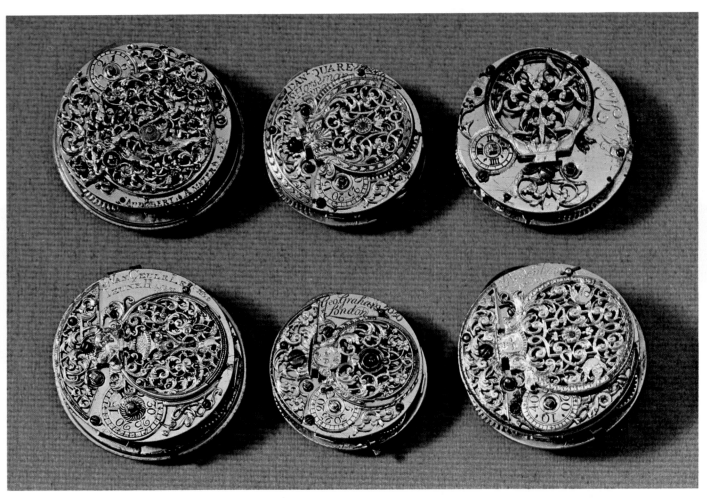

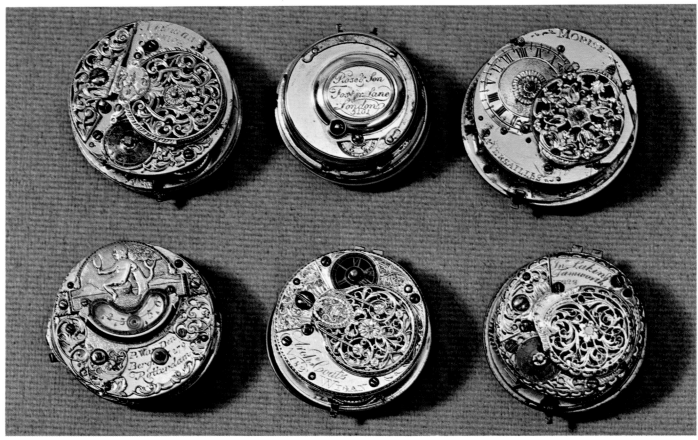

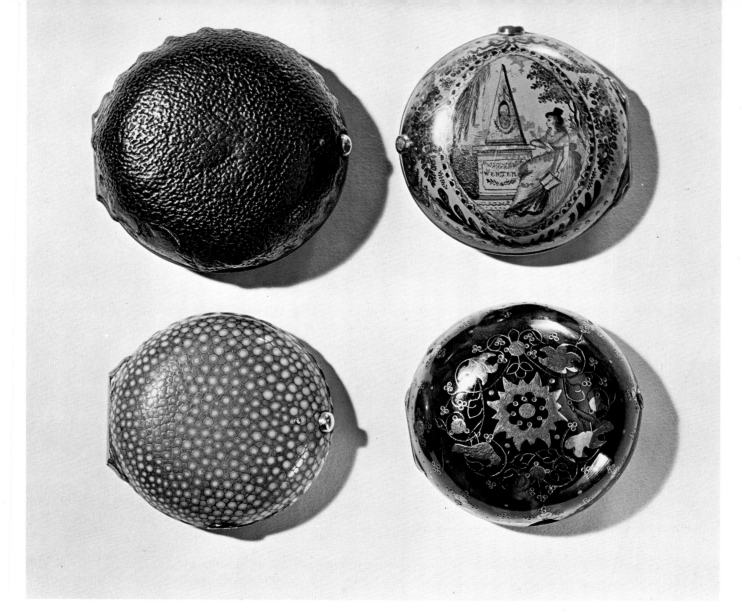

above

It is not uncommon for the outer case of a pair-cased watch to have become separated from the rest and, especially if it is decorative, for it to have survived as a separate entity. The four such outer cases shown here are clad in leather, reverse-painted horn (a cheaper alternative to enamelled work), tortoiseshell inlaid with silver, and shagreen. An interesting collection can be formed from items such as these.

above left

These verge watch movements display a variety of decoration ranging over the period from about 1680 to the end of the eighteenth century. Features of significance include regular or irregular borders to the cock feet, which also may be either pierced or solid according to the period, and the size and complexity of decoration of the slide plate housing the balance spring regulator.

left

Most watch movements are enriched with fire-gilding on the base metal, which is generally brass. Silver has been used only very sparingly in this context, but is found in the heritage of several European countries. This illustration includes British, French and Dutch movements of the eighteenth century.

decorated with the royal coat of arms seem, for some reason which is not at present understood, to have been confined to a particular type of watch, the so-called 'wandering-hour dial' watch, which has been described on page 128. It is inconceivable that all such watches, and there must have been plenty of them since a fair number have survived intact, can have had royal connections; yet there is almost always either a portrait of the monarch on dial or movement, or a coat of arms, or both. Other rare and desirable forms of decoration on watch cocks include the monogrammed cock, in which initials, generally those of the watchmaker, are woven into the decoration of the cock table; the masonic cock, which features the emblems and symbols of Freemasonry, such symbolism often being repeated upon the watch dial; cocks with signatures and dates, displayed on an otherwise blank area around the edge of the cock foot, a fashion which seems to have lasted a few years only around 1750 and which also seems confined to a type of cock generally described as having a 'lace edge' to the cock table; and finally the only wholly pictorial watch cock, which features a farmyard

245

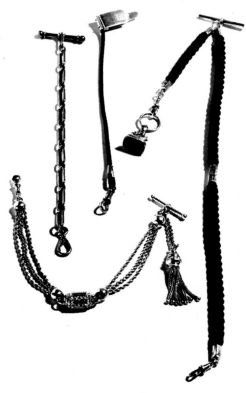

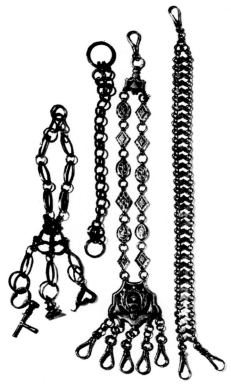

Short fob chains can be found in an enormous variety of styles and materials, from the elegance of enamelled and gem-set gold to the more simple cut steel versions shown here. The double fob chain is steel inlaid with multicoloured gold, and is most probably of Italian origin or made by immigrant craftsmen from that country. The folding bed-hook shown attached to the right-hand chain was used to suspend the watch from the drapes of the bed when retiring for the night. An alternative to this procedure was to use a watch stand (see page 247).

above right
Watch chains emerged in their final form during the second half of the nineteenth century, and many different linkages are to be found. Among those shown here are a Queen's chain, distinguished by its metal tassel, and an Albert made of plaited elephant's hair reminiscent of the Indian Empire.

scene, and of which several closely related but nonetheless different arrangements survive.

The watch, as such, has many more ancillaries associated with its operation than has the clock. There have been, and perhaps still are, collectors specialising in clock keys, but the range of these is very limited. The normal type of crank-shaped key will have a turned wood – or, very exceptionally, ivory – handle, and they come in sizes varying from the normal domestic bracket and longcase key to the very much larger type needed for a turret clock. Later types of keys for such as carriage clocks and the Vienna regulator are normally made entirely of brass, sometimes cranked and sometimes straight. Many of the mass-produced clocks had cheap cast steel keys, sometimes with flat pierced and shaped plates by which to turn them. That more or less covers the whole range.

Watch keys, on the other hand, come in as many varieties as do watch cocks, and a far wider range of materials was used in their construction. The

cranked key, usually in gilt metal, is considered to be the earliest style devised, but it is also believed to have had a very long life. Apart from this it is exceedingly difficult to be specific about dates or the currency of styles. Watch keys are often so elaborate and have been worked in such unfamiliar materials that they must have been the product of jewellers or perhaps specialists; watch key makers are almost unknown as a branch of any craft, however. There is hardly any literature on this subject, which never seems to have attracted the attention of researchers, perhaps because watch keys so often appeal to ladies as an item of adornment – they are frequently worn mounted as charms on bracelets – and have not yet come into their own as objects for serious study. Mechanically they comprise very few types: firstly the crank key with its near relation the folding crank which has its two joints hinged so that, when not in the functional Z-shape as used for winding, it lies completely flat, and secondly the resilient type are the only departures from the conventional straight one-piece key. The resilient key – sometimes called the Breguet or 'tipsy' key – has a ratchet arrangement built into it to prevent the key, and therefore the watch, being wound up the wrong way. Rotated in the right direction the key winds up normally; in the reverse direction the handle of the key simply freewheels, accompanied by the sound of the click riding over the tops of the ratchet wheel teeth. Both 'male' and 'female' keys are known – the latter is the conventional kind which fits over the winding square, while the former is the reverse, that is to say, the key itself terminates in a solid square which fits into a corresponding aperture on the watch, generally not for winding up but for such functions as altering the hands or setting an

246

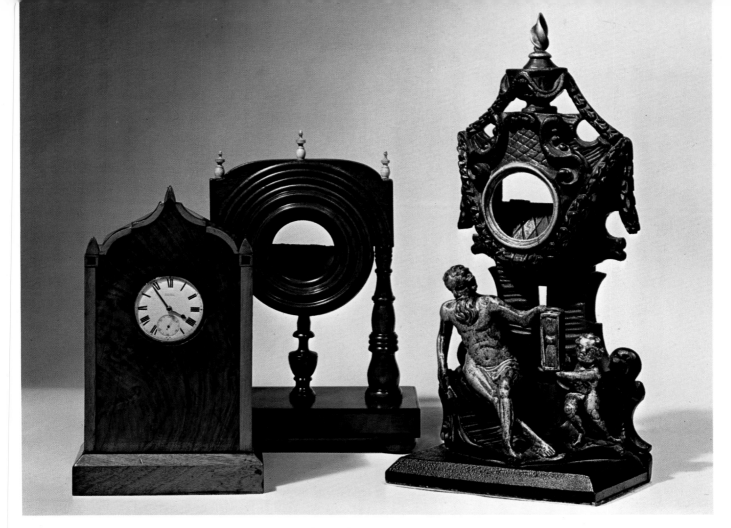

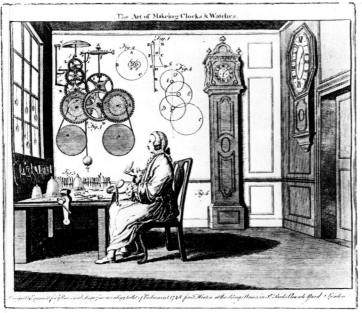

The alternative to using the folding bed-hook for securing the watch at night was to place it in a watch stand, and it may be that hooks were used only when travelling. Watch stands, like the other watch ancillaries, come in a profusion of designs and materials, the latter ranging from wood and metal to papier-mâché and pottery. The Rococo example showing Father Time with putto and hourglass is of eighteenth-century German origin, and the inside of the watch compartment has been carved in a quilted effect. The turned mahogany stand surmounted by ivory finials is a relic of Georgian England, while the third, made of fruitwood edged in box, is a nineteenth-century provincial piece.

The most famous workshop print is the Stradanus version of about 1578. This print, which appeared in the *Universal Magazine* in 1748, lacks perspective but is interesting on account of the octagonally dialled 'Act of Parliament' clock hanging on the wall, especially since it predates the Act itself by half a century.

alarm dial. Breguet, the famous French craftsman, not only favoured the resilient key, which is sometimes called after him, but also used male keys for various purposes. There are several large collections of watch keys in museums throughout the world. In London one of the best is that in possession of the Worshipful Company of Clockmakers and exhibited with the rest of its collection at Guildhall Library. In America a large privately owned collection was presented some years back to the Rollins College Art Museum in Winter Park, Florida, and must be one of the best collections in that country.

Keys are but one of several kinds of ancillary to the watch, and the others, being often decorative as well as functional and therefore popularly collected for themselves, will bear brief scrutiny. The watch key was generally carried with the watch,

247

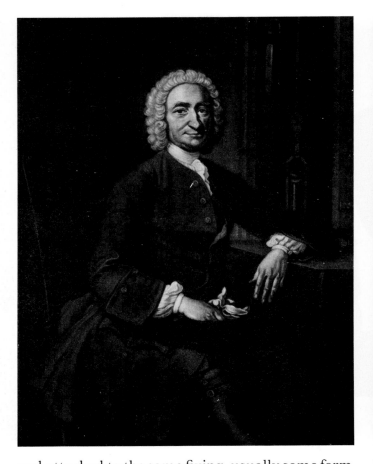

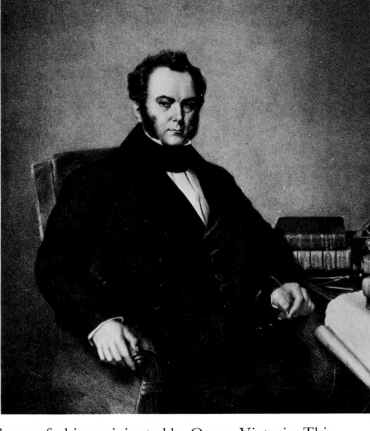

and attached to the same fixing, usually some form of watch-chain, that connected it to the wearer. When pockets were first introduced, about 1625, they were confined to the breeches and remained thus until the long waistcoat made its appearance about 1675. The fob, as it came to be known, was the pocket in the waistband of the trousers in which the valuables might well come to be carried, hence the highwayman's cry of 'Turn out your fobs!' The short chains called fob-chains, on one end of which would be attached the watch, had one or more swivel hooks at the other end which would be allowed to hang out of the top of the fob pocket and from which dangled watch key, seal and other small accessories. When waistcoats came into fashion, the short fob-chain continued in use but was allowed to hang out of the waistcoat pocket instead. The long chain, extending across the front of the wearer and terminating in opposite pockets of the waistcoat is a relatively modern development, certainly not earlier than mid nineteenth century. Indeed, various styles of long watch-chain are often referred to as 'Alberts', after the Prince Consort, while a particular style of chain which incorporates metal tassels is always known as a 'Queen's chain'. Such tassels were a commonplace decorative addition to certain ladies' accoutrements, such as muff and skirt guards – the latter used to hoist the hem of the skirt out of reach of mud and puddles in the streets, without any necessity for bending down – and might well have

been a fashion originated by Queen Victoria. This would explain the extension of the term 'Queen's' to a watch-chain, since it hardly seems likely that the monarch would have sported one herself.

The ladies' version of the fob-chain is called the chatelaine. An ornamental arrangement of chains and swivel hooks, the whole device hangs from the belt or waistband by a large hook located behind the main boss from which the rest is suspended. The chatelaine was originally used by the mistress of a medieval castle, as a means of carrying about the various keys she needed; in its later forms, it not only accommodated the watch, with its key and odd seals, but also such other small but useful accessories as scissors, thimbles and trinkets of various kinds. In some chatelaines – especially those very decorative and nowadays enormously expensive versions enriched with costly enamelling and pearls, and in which watch, chatelaine and all associated items are decorated *en suite* – the suspension hook has disappeared, and it would seem that such are really just highly elaborate fob-chains.

Fob seals, interesting study though they are, cannot be defined as part of the horological lineage and are therefore outside the scope of the present work. One accessory that will often be found both on fob-chain and on chatelaine, and which can be included, however, is the folding bed hook. Whether at home or *en voyage,* the owner of a watch did not necessarily leave it in his dressing-table

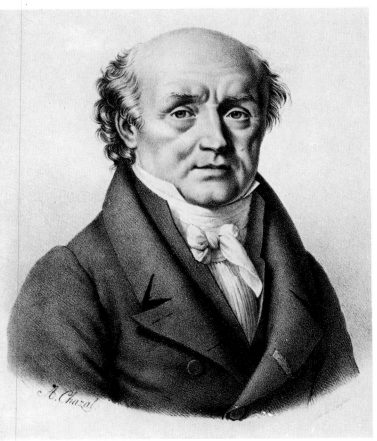

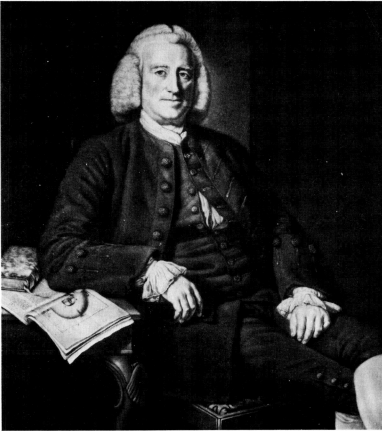

drawer when he retired at night; if it was a repeater, he could discover the time at will and without any need of a light by setting off the repeating action. He therefore hung it from the drapes of the bedstead by a bed hook, or placed it in a watch stand. Bed hooks were generally made retractable, like the blade of a pocket knife, because they were of necessity sharp and could not be carried about except with some kind of protection for the wearer. Sometimes the hook forms part of the watch key, and pivots into the body of it when not in use. Others were made as entities in their own right, and purely on stylistic grounds – for, like the watch key, the history of the bed hook remains largely a mystery to the present day – it would seem that they may have been used for several centuries, certainly well into Victorian times.

Mention of the watch stand brings to mind again the photograph of Chamberlain's workshop, for two of these can be seen on top of the bookcase at the back of the room. Left of centre is a very handsome type, in which the watch is framed in an arch supported by two pillars. From a black and white photograph it is difficult to be certain, but it looks as if this stand is surfaced in tortoiseshell. On the same level but right of centre, is a smaller rectangular watch stand of a well-established type, with the main panels in a finely figured wood and the edges banded with box. Such stands as this were essentially country-made pieces, but the graining and colour contrast between the woods

Portrait prints of clockmakers, usually copied from original paintings which, in many cases, no longer exist, cover a wide range of periods and personalities.

far left
This portrait of George Graham is of interest as being a nineteenth-century reproduction of an eighteenth-century mezzotint by J. Fabre, after a painting by T. Hudson.

centre left
William James Frodsham, F.R.S., one of the few clockmakers to have achieved this distinction, is here seen in a lithograph by Ada Cole from a painting by an unknown artist. Printed by Day & Son.

centre right
Abraham-Louis Breguet, probably the most famous horologist of all time, is known from several portraits as well as a sculptured bust. This lithograph by Langlumé is taken from a painting by A. Chazal.

above
One of the rarer portrait mezzotints of clockmakers of the later eighteenth century, this representation of John Ellicott, F.R.S., was executed by Robert Dunkarton after a painting by Nathaniel Dance. Like so many of these prints, it incorporates a wealth of period detail in the clothes and furniture, making it a fascinating social document.

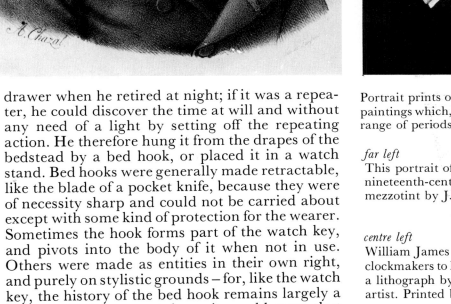

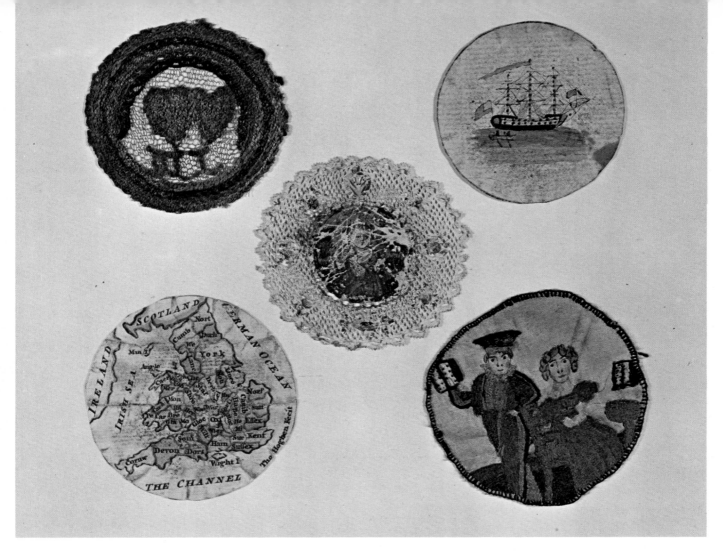

One kind of watch paper is the hand-worked type, employing one or more of quite a range of techniques, which serves a purely decorative and possibly sentimental function. Apart from colouring, these can include cut paper, drawn thread, embroidery and the like.

opposite page
The second kind of watch paper is the one placed within the watch case by the repairer to advertise his wares and services. Occasionally such repairers noted upon the back of the paper the work done on the watch, the amount charged, and other useful information.

left
The third category of horological print of which examples might be sought concerns the illustration of some complex clock, such as this astronomical clock by Jos. Naylor of Nantwich, Cheshire. Britten mentions two clocks by this maker, one in the Cluny Museum, Paris. The print is dated 1751, and Naylor died the following year. Museum of the Worshipful Company of Clockmakers, Guildhall, London.

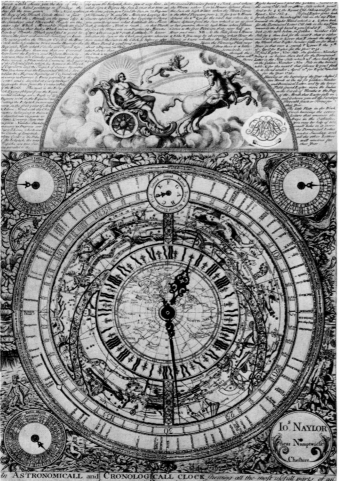

give them great appeal. They are unlikely to be earlier than of nineteenth-century provenance, but examples of eighteenth-century watch stands do survive, often in exuberant styles involving allegorical figures of Time with putti in Rococo settings, or with Atlas supporting the watch as though it were the world. There are innumerable varieties of this useful adjunct to the watch, mainly in wood but sometimes in metal, while there are versions in porcelain and pottery, as well as in less obvious materials like ivory, which was also used for turned finials surmounting wooden stands, especially those in more typically architectural styles. Museum collections do not seem to embrace this kind of artefact in any organised way, and one of the finest collections was formed privately at the beginning of the present century by Sir Gerald Ryan. This collection was extensively illustrated in the December 1919 issue of *The Connoisseur*, which even now forms almost the total corpus of literature on the subject. The styles and qualities of watch stands included in the Ryan collection seem almost entirely to have disappeared, and examples that do appear from time to time in the auction rooms are generally of much lesser merit. It would be interesting to know where some of the finer of these objects are now located.

There is just one more somewhat ephemeral ancillary to the pocket watch, and that is the watch paper. Essentially this takes the form of a liner placed between the inner and outer cases of a pair-cased watch to ensure a good tight fit, and since many such watches will still be found to have a rose silk liner rather than a paper one, and often obviously antique silk at that, it may be that this was the original form of the watch 'paper', placed between the cases by the maker of the watch himself.

In its generally understood and most frequently encountered form, however, the watch paper takes the shape of a printed advertisement for a watch-maker, who when traceable, usually turns out to be a craftsman who has repaired or overhauled the watch at some time in its career. Sometimes he will be found to have written on the back of the watch paper a note of the exact work he has carried out as well as the charge made for it, while his printed inscription will certainly contain useful information about his business address and the type of work or wares which he offers. It is not unusual to find several such papers compressed into the outer case of a watch – even occasionally to the extent of nine or ten – and where they have been annotated by the craftsmen concerned they provide an interesting chronological record of the performance of the watch often over quite a span of years. There is a fine collection amounting to some twelve hundred such papers, arranged in three volumes, in the Library of the Worshipful Company of Clockmakers of the City of London.

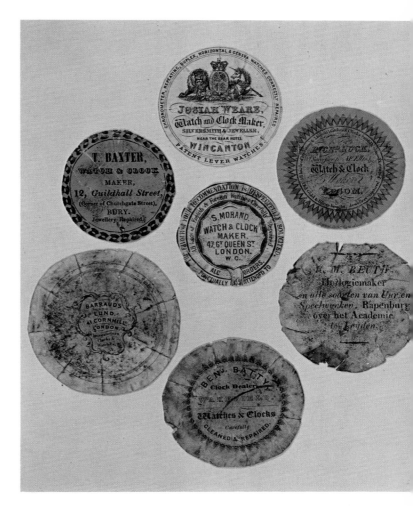

There are other varietes of watch papers, however, whose provenance is not quite so well understood. It was once believed, for instance, that the embroidered fabric 'papers', often with entwined initials or a heart motif, were worked by the love-lorn maiden for her betrothed, and indeed such is probably the case. But certain versions of these, notably the one portraying a sailor with his sweetheart which is usually both painted and stitched, recur frequently in nearly identical form and so must have been worked from some kind of pattern. Quite a range of techniques was used in making these decorative papers of the non-advertising sort, such as drawn thread, cut paper – often in the most intricate and minute patterns, so that one wonders not only at the patience needed but at the size of the scissors used – and painting upon paper or silk, not to mention the hand-colouring of printed decorative motifs such as maps and marine scenes. Another form used was the calendar, while equation tables are commonly found as watch papers, but usually with a watch-maker's name and address in the central space. Very occasionally a watch paper will be found to advertise some kind of business other than watch-making, but these are combined with a calendar and were obviously given away as a gimmick with the commodity concerned.

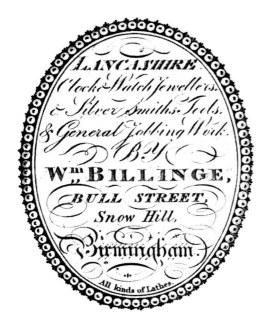

Although advertising had not reached the advanced state that prevails today, it was quite normal during the last century for craftsmen to solicit custom by taking space in street directories to display what they could offer. This typical page comes from Wrightson & Webb's *Directory* of Birmingham for 1835.

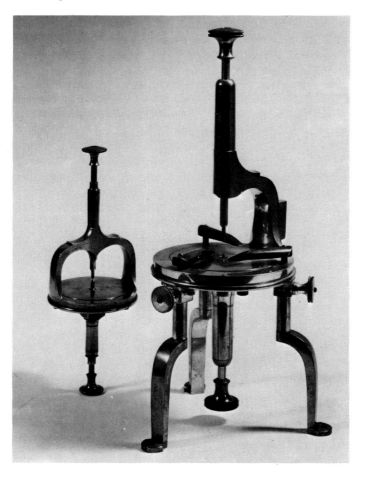

These are nineteenth-century chronometermakers' uprighting tools, which allow the craftsman to translate accurately the marking out of the pivot holes of his z movement from one plate to the other. The smaller tool bears the name of Charles Mill Frodsham.
right
A few of the commoner hand tools used by the craftsman at the bench, including pin tongs and vices, calipers of various designs, gauges, screw plates, and a Birch universal bench key, which will fit any size of a watch winding square. At the top is a fusee testing rod for watches, a stake for riveting verge balance wheels on to their arbors, and a special kind of small lathe for turning verge balance wheels.

Before leaving printing in its association with things horological, the field of prints connected with clock- and watchmaking is an enormous one and makes a very interesting study. It can, for convenience, be divided up into categories according to the subject matter, and such a classification might have one section devoted to clockmakers' workshop scenes, another to portraits of the craftsmen themselves, a third to specific clocks, usually of the monumental kind, and finally a miscellaneous category for the oddments that do not fit easily into any of the first three. In the first of these classes there is a wide range of prints to be collected, from the famous Stradanus version of 1578, the earliest record of such an establishment, through various English and European depictions in the eighteenth century, and finishing perhaps with nineteenth-century photographs illustrating factory working in its early stages. In the second category, probably the best-known are the mezzotints made in the eighteenth century, usually copied from painted portraits, the originals of which have only in very few cases survived. There are about a dozen or so of these, including all the most eminent English craftsmen from Tompion and Graham to Arnold and Mudge.

The prints of monumental clocks are of great importance since they can show any changes that have been made superficially to the appearance of a surviving example. Mention has been made previously of prints of Richard Greene's Lichfield clock and Jacob Lovelace's Exeter clock, both being important in this respect. There are innumerable representations of the Strasbourg cathedral clock, and these may still be found for a reasonable price; but most horological prints of any substance in all categories have become rare and expensive of recent years, and they are perhaps best sought in places off the beaten track where the existence of a horological plate as one illustration, say, in a book about crafts and trades, would not be recognised as significant.

Horological literature must play an ancillary role in any type of collecting in the field of clocks and watches; but the older works, long out of print, will be found only with difficulty, even from booksellers specialising in the subject, and they will be very expensive. There are plenty of modern works, however, which are useful to the student if not yet collectable for themselves, and some attempt has been made to outline these in the Further Reading lists (page 254). The bibliography on clocks and watches is vast, and now grows apace from year to year as a direct result of the growing enthusiasm for horological knowledge shown by ever-increasing numbers of people throughout the developed world. In the last year or two, there has been a movement by certain specialist publishers to produce facsimile reproductions of some of the rarest and most famous works on horology and, if it serves to bring such works to the hands of those who otherwise would never be able to aspire to the originals, then such action can only be applauded.

Finally, there remains one obvious field for the horological collector to consider, that of the tools of the trade. The first difficulty here is for the uninitiated collector to recognise a clock- or watchmaking tool if he meets one, unless he has first familiarised himself by spending time in a suitable workshop with the right kind of guidance at hand. Very many old tools, as they have been superseded, have been broken up for their brass content and, even to the present time, the occasional tool will turn up whose purpose puzzles the experts. The aspiring collector will keep a watchful eye open for any clockmaking or similar business that is being dispersed, in the hope of acquiring an old lathe, perhaps, or some useful hand tools; and he will clearly recognise that the best way to acclimatise himself to what such objects look like and are used for is to learn to handle them himself. Many tools were made, as part of their apprenticeship, by the craftsmen who subsequently used them. They will be found to have been beautifully worked, so that not only are they a joy to handle but also they are a pleasure simply to look at. Their shapes and intricacies often reflect the sheer excellence of the horological craft at its prime, and the student who formulates his approach to the subject only after a careful contemplation of the make-up and purpose of such objects as these is unlikely to go very far wrong in recognising the best in craft standards and thus eventually acquiring an intuitive appreciation for the quality of a piece which is so essential to the forming of any worthwhile collection.

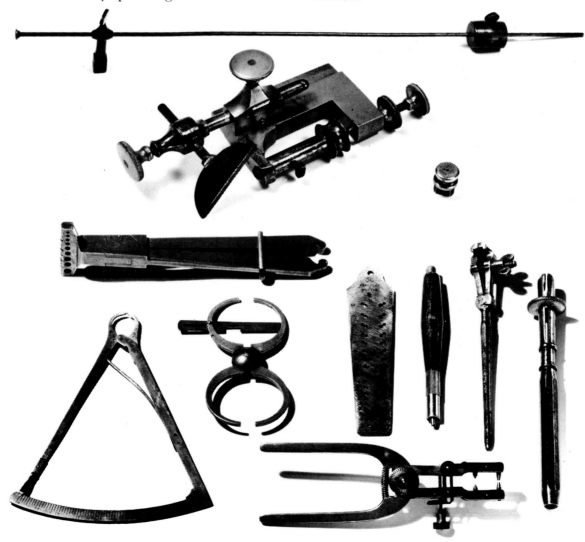

Bibliography

FURTHER READING

General Books
Baillie, G. H., *Watches, their history, decoration and mechanism*, London, 1929.
Baillie, G. H., Cecil Clutton and Courtney A. Ilbert, *Britten's Old Clocks and Watches and their Makers*, 7th edition, London, 1956 (8th edition revised and enlarged by Clutton, London, 1973).
Bassermann-Jordan and Hans V. Bertelet, *Uhren*, Braunschweig, 1961.
Beckett, Sir Edmund, *A Rudimentary Treatise on Clocks and Watches and Bells*, London, various editions to 1903.
Bruton, Eric, *Clocks and Watches*, London, 1968.
Camerer Cuss, T. P., and T. A. Camerer Cuss, *The Camerer Cuss Book of Antique Watches*, Woodbridge, 1976.
Chamberlain, Paul, *It's About Time*, New York, 1941.
Cipolla, Carlo M., *Clocks and Culture: 1300–1700*, London, 1967.
Clutton, C., and George Daniels, *Watches*, London, 1965.
Defossez, L., *Les Savants du XVIIe Siècle et la Mesure du Temps*, Lausanne, 1946.
Gelif, Edouard, *L'Horlogerie Ancienne*, Paris, 1949.
Jagger, Cedric, *Clocks*, London, 1973. Revised edition, 1975.
Joy, Edward T., *The Country Life Book of Clocks*, London, 1967.
Lloyd, H. Alan, *Some Outstanding Clocks over Seven Hundred Years*, London, 1958.
Milham, Willis, *Time and Timekeepers*, New York, various editions from 1923.
Moore, N. Hudson, *The Old Clock Book*, 2nd edition, New York, 1936.
Pioneers of Precision Time-Keeping, a symposium by the Antiquarian Horological Society, London, n.d. (about 1962).
Robertson, J. Drummond, *The Evolution of Clockwork*, London, 1931.
Tallquist, Prof. H., *Uhren och Urteknikens Historia*, Helsinki, 1939.
Tyler, E. J., *European Clocks*, London, 1968.

Dictionaries, General and Technical
Britten, F. J., *Watch and Clockmakers' Handbook, Dictionary and Guide*, London, various editions from 1881.
Carle, D. de, *Watch and Clock Encyclopaedia*, London, 1976.
Lloyd, H. Alan, *The Collector's Dictionary of Clocks*, London, 1964.

Technical Books
Carle, D. de, *Clock and Watch Repairing, including Complicated Watches*, London, 1974. This author has written a number of other technical books of value.
Gazeley, W. J., *Clock and Watch Escapements*, London, 1956.
Gazeley, W. J., *Clock and Watch Making and Repairing*, London, 1956.
Haswell, Eric, *Horology*, London, various editions from 1928.
Holtzapffel's Turning and Mechanical Manipulation, London, various editions to 1894.
Rawlings, A. L., *The Science of Clocks and Watches*, London, 1944.
Reid, Thomas, *Treatise on Clock and Watchmaking*, Edinburgh; 7 editions, 1826–1859.
Saunier, Claude, *Treatise on Modern Horology in Theory and Practice*, London, various editions from 1867.

Lists of Makers
In England there are already in print a number of lists by counties or large towns, and more appear every year. Neither Switzerland nor Germany has yet produced national lists of craftsmen, though there are some local studies in the former and on Augsburg in the latter. America is well served, with representative lists of makers in most of the authoritative works, as well as a number of specialist studies, in particular covering the early manufacturers.
Baillie, G. H., *Watchmakers and Clockmakers of the World*, London, various editions to 1972.
Campos, J. L. Basanta, *Relojeros de España: Diccionario Bio-Bibliográfico*, 1972.
Chenakal, V. L., *Watchmakers and Clockmakers in Russia: 1400–1850*, London, 1972.
Loomes, B. *Watchmakers and Clockmakers of the World*, vol. 2, London, 1976. (For vol. 1 see under G. H. Baillie above.)
Morpurgo, E., *Dizionario degli Orologiai Italiani 1300–1800*, 1950.
Morpurgo, E., *Nederlandse Klokken en Horlogemakers*, 1970.
Peate, I. C. *Clock and Watchmakers in Wales*, Cardiff, 1960.
Smith, J., *Old Scottish Clockmakers from 1453 to 1850*, Wakefield, 1975.
Sidenbladh, Elis, *Urmakare i Sverige*, Stockholm, 1947.
Tardy, *Dictionnaire des Horlogers Français*, Paris, 1972.

INDIVIDUAL MAKERS
Daniels, George, *The Art of Breguet*, London, 1975.
Ditisheim, Lallier, Reverchon and Vivielle, *Pierre Le Roy et la Chronométrie*, Paris, 1940.
Hawkins, J. B., *Thomas Cole and Victorian Clockmaking*, Sydney, 1975.
Jagger, Cedric, *Paul Philip Barraud*, London, 1968.
Lee, R. A., The Knibb Family – *Clockmakers*, London, 1964.
Mercer, Vaudrey, *John Arnold & Son*, London, 1972
Quill, Humphrey, *John Harrison – The Man Who Found Longitude*, London, 1966.
Salomons, David, *Breguet*, London, 1921 (French edition 1923).
Shenton, Rita, *Christopher Pinchbeck*, Ashford, 1976.
Symonds, R. W., *Thomas Tompion, His Life and Work*, London, 1951.

INDIVIDUAL COUNTRIES
England
Beeson, C. F. C., *English Church Clocks 1280–1850*, London, 1971.
Goamen, Muriel, *English Clocks*, London, 1967.
France
Tardy, *La Pendule Française des origines à nos jours*, Paris, various editions to the present time.
Edey, Winthrop. *French Clocks*, London, 1967.
Japan
Hyoe Takabayashi, *Tokei Hattatsu-shi* ('Development of Clocks'), 1927.
Mody, N. H. N., *Japanese Clocks*, original limited edition of 200 copies, London, 1932 (facsimile reprint, London, 1968).
Rambaut, A. A., *Notes on Some Japanese Clocks*, Dublin, 1889.
Switzerland
Jaquet, E., and Alfred Chapuis, *Histoire et Technique de la Montre Suisse*, Basle, 1945 (English edition, London, 1970).
United States of America
Daniels, G., *English and American Watches*, London, 1967.
Palmer, Brooks, *A Treasury of American Clocks*, New York, 1967.
Palmer, Brooks, *The Book of American Clocks*, New York, 1974.

Types of Clock and Watch
Allix, Charles, and Peter Bonnert, *Carriage Clocks – Their History and Development*, Woodbridge, 1974.
Bain, Alexander, *A Short History of the Electric Clock, With Explanations*, London, 1852
Bruton, Eric, *The Grandfather Clock*, London. 2nd Edit.
Chapuis, A., and Eugène Jaquet, *The History of the Self-Winding Watch 1770–1931*, Geneva, 1956.
Coole, P. G., and E. Neumann, *The Orpheus Clock*, London, 1972.
Edwardes, Ernest L., *The Grandfather Clock*, Altrincham, 1971.
Edwardes, Ernest L., *Weight-driven Chamber Clocks of the Middle Ages and Renaissance*, Altrincham, 1965.
Gould, Lt-Cdr R. T., *The Marine Chronometer*, London, 1923.
Hope-Jones, F., *Electrical Timekeeping*, London, 1940 (recently reproduced in facsimile).
Mortensen, Otto, *Jens Olsen's Clock*, Copenhagen, 1957.
Needham, Joseph, Derek Price and Wang Ling, *Heavenly Clockwork*, Cambridge, 1960.
Royer-Collard, F. B., *Skeleton Clocks*, London, 1969.

Exhibition and Collection Catalogues
This is only a tiny selection of English catalogues. Many museums round the world have published literature on their own collections.
Art-Journal Illustrated Catalogue to the Industry of All Nations, The, Great Exhibition catalogue, London, 1851.
Britten, F. J., *Old English Clocks – The Wetherfield Collection*, London, 1907.
Clutton, C., and George Daniels, *Clocks and Watches in the Collection of the Worshipful Company of Clockmakers*, London, 1975.
Ilbert Collection of Clocks, Catalogue of the, London, 1958: printed by Christie's as a sale catalogue, but not issued as the collection was bought privately for the British Museum.
Lee, Ronald, A., *The First Twelve Years of the English Pendulum Clock*, exhibition catalogue, London, 1969.
Tait, Hugh, *Clocks in the British Museum*, London, 1968.

Bibliographies
Baillie, G. H., *Clocks and Watches – An Historical Bibliography*, London, 1951.
Tardy, *Bibliographie Générale de la Mesure du Temps*, Paris, 1943.

Related Subjects
Chapuis, A., and Edmond Droz, *Automata – a Historical and Technological Study*, Neuchatel, 1958.
Cousins, Frank W., *Sundials*, London, 1969.
Goodison, N., *English Barometers 1680–1860*, London, 1969.
Gunther, R. T., *Early Science in Oxford*, Oxford, 1923.
Michel, Henri, *Scientific Instruments*, London, 1967.
Smith, G. H., and E. R. Smith, *Watch Keys as Jewelry*, New York, 1967.
Tardy, *Les Coqs de Montre*, Paris, n.d.

Horological Societies
Antiquarian Horological Society, New House, High Street, Ticehurst, Wadhurst, Sussex TN5 7AL, England.
Freunde Alter Uhren (President: Prof. Dr Richard Mühe), 7743 Furtwangen, Ilbenstrasse 54, Germany.
National Association of Clock and Watch Collectors, P.O. Box 33, Columbia (Pa) 17512, USA.

There are also comparable bodies in France and Switzerland. The American organisation is both the oldest and the largest: 30,000 members at the last count, and it has been in existence well over thirty years. The British society, next in order of seniority and with the more serious-minded approach to the subject, to judge by its literary output, was founded in 1953 and has something over 4000 members. It is also the most cosmopolitan, having a membership spread throughout the world, while the other organisations in the field tend to be more local. Each of the three bodies listed arrange foreign horological tours for their members from time to time, to take in museums and private collections outside their own countries. These and other events add a social dimension, to leaven what is fundamentally an academic and research-orientated interest.

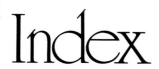

Index

Numbers in italics refer to illustrations